Emotion Explained

Emotion Explained

Edmund T. Rolls

University of Oxford
Department of Experimental Psychology
Oxford
England

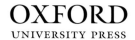
OXFORD
UNIVERSITY PRESS

OXFORD

UNIVERSITY PRESS

Great Clarendon Street, Oxford OX2 6DP

Oxford University Press is a department of the University of Oxford.
It furthers the University's objective of excellence in research, scholarship,
and education by publishing worldwide in

Oxford New York

Auckland Cape Town Dar es Salaam Hong Kong Karachi
Kuala Lumpur Madrid Melbourne Mexico City Nairobi
New Delhi Shanghai Taipei Toronto

With offices in

Argentina Austria Brazil Chile Czech Republic France Greece
Guatemala Hungary Italy Japan Poland Portugal Singapore
South Korea Switzerland Thailand Turkey Ukraine Vietnam

Oxford is a registered trade mark of Oxford University Press
in the UK and in certain other countries

Published in the United States
by Oxford University Press Inc., New York

British Library Cataloguing in Publication Data

Data available

Library of Congress Cataloging in Publication Data

Data available

Typeset by the author and Newgen Imaging Systems (P) Ltd., Chennai, India
Printed in Great Britain
on acid-free paper by
Ashford Colour Press Ltd., Gosport, Hants

ISBN 978–0–19–857004–2

1 3 5 7 9 10 8 6 4 2

Preface

What produces emotions? Why do we have emotions? How do we have emotions? Why do emotional states feel like something? This book seeks explanations of emotion by considering these questions.

One of the distinctive properties of this book is that it develops a conceptual and evolutionary approach (see for example Chapters 2 and 3) to emotion. This approach shows how cognitive states can produce and modulate emotion, and in turn how emotional states can influence cognition. Another distinctive property is that this book links these approaches to studies on the brain, at the level of neuronal neurophysiology, which provides much of the primary data about how the brain operates; but also to neuropsychological studies of patients with brain damage; to functional magnetic resonance imaging (fMRI) (and other neuroimaging) approaches; and to computational neuroscience approaches. The author performs research in all these areas, and this may help the approach to emotion described here to span many levels of investigation. The empirical evidence that is brought to bear is largely from non-human primates and from humans, because of the considerable similarity of their visual and emotional systems associated with the great development of the prefrontal cortex and temporal lobes in primates, and because the overall aim is to understand how emotion is implemented in the human brain, and the disorders that arise after brain damage.

To understand how the brain works, including how it functions in emotion, it is necessary to combine different approaches, including neural computation. Neurophysiology at the single neuron level is needed because this is the level at which information is exchanged between the computing elements of the brain. Evidence from the effects of brain damage, including that available from neuropsychology, is needed to help understand what different parts of the system do, and indeed what each part is necessary for. Neuroimaging is useful to indicate where in the human brain different processes take place, and to show which functions can be dissociated from each other. Knowledge of the biophysical and synaptic properties of neurons is essential to understand how the computing elements of the brain work, and therefore what the building blocks of biologically realistic computational models should be. Knowledge of the anatomical and functional architecture of the cortex is needed to show what types of neuronal network actually perform the computation. And finally the approach of neural computation is needed, as this is required to link together all the empirical evidence to produce an understanding of how the system actually works. This book utilizes evidence from all these disciplines to develop an understanding of how emotion is implemented by processing in the brain.

The overall plan of the book is as follows. Chapter 1 outlines the ways in which this book approaches different types of explanation of emotion, and introduces some of the concepts. Chapter 2 then considers the nature of emotion, producing a theory of emotion, and comparing it to some other theories. Chapter 3 considers the functions of emotion, and leads to a Darwinian theory of the adaptive value of emotion, which helps to illuminate many aspects of brain design and behaviour. Chapter 4 takes the explanation of emotion to the level of how emotion is implemented in the brain. Chapters 5 and 6 extend and complement this by extending the approach to motivated behaviour in which affect is an important component. In Chapter 5 the motivated behaviour considered is hunger, and in Chapter 6 thirst. Chapter 7 extends the approach to reward and affect produced by brain stimulation, and Chapter 8 to the pharmacology of emotion and addiction. Chapter 9 extends the approach further, to sexual behaviour. Chapter 10 then considers the issue of emotional feelings, which is part of the much larger issue of consciousness. Chapter 11 then synthesizes some of the points made, including how decisions are made and are influenced by emotions. Appendix 1 describes some of the computational framework for understanding how systems in the brain in the form of neural networks perform emotion-related learning. Appendix 2 describes an example of a more detailed neural network approach to emotion-related learning in which the analysis extends from the level of the spiking activity of single neurons up through many levels of investigation to global properties of the system such as the signals measured in functional neuroimaging investigations, and the resulting behaviour. Appendix 3 provides a Glossary of some of the terms. The book thus seeks to explain emotions in terms of the following: What produces emotions? Why do we have emotions? How do we have emotions? Why do emotional states feel like something?

This book evolved from my earlier book *The Brain and Emotion* (Rolls 1999a) in some of the following ways:

Emotion Explained goes beyond brain mechanisms of emotion, in that it seeks to explain emotions in terms of the following: What produces emotions? (The general answer I propose is reinforcing stimuli, that is rewards and punishers, but with other factors too.) Why do we have emotions? (The overall answer I propose is that emotions are evolutionarily adaptive as they provide an efficient way for genes to influence our behaviour to increase their success.) How do we have emotions? (I answer this by describing what is known about the brain mechanisms of emotion.) Why do emotional states feel like something? This is part of the large problem of consciousness, which I address in Chapter 10. It is in this sense that a broad-ranging explanation of emotion going beyond the brain mechanisms of emotion is the theme of this book.

Emotion Explained goes beyond the brain mechanisms of emotion by developing my approach and theory of the nature of emotion, and comparing my approach to a range of different approaches to the nature of emotion, including the approaches of A.Damasio, J.LeDoux, J.Panksepp, and appraisal theorists such as K.Scherer.

Another way in which this book goes beyond brain mechanisms of emotion is to propose in Chapter 3 a Darwinian account of why animals (including humans) have emotions. The theory will I believe stand the test of time, in the same way as Darwin's theory of evolution by natural selection, and argues that emotions have the important evolutionary role of enabling genes to specify the goals (i.e. the rewards etc that produce emotions) for actions, rather than the actions themselves. The advantage of this Darwinian design is that although the genes specify the goals, the actual actions are not prespecified by the genes, so that there is great flexibility of the actions themselves. This provides a new approach to the nature vs nurture debate in animal behaviour, for it shows how genes can influence behaviour without specifying a fixed, instinctive, behavioural response. I hope that this will make the book of interest to a wide audience, including many interested in evolution and evolutionary biology.

Although in evolution Darwinian processes lead to gene-defined goals, it is also the case that in humans goals may be influenced by other processes, including cultural processes. Indeed, some goals are defined within a culture, for example writing a novel like one by

Tolstoy vs one by Virginia Woolf. But it is argued that it is primary reinforcers specified by genes of the general type shown in Table 2.1 on page 18 that make us want to be recognised in society because of the advantages this can bring, to solve difficult problems, etc, and therefore to perform actions such as writing novels (see further Ridley (2003) Chapter 8, Ridley (1993a) pp. 310 ff, Laland and Brown (2002) pp. 271 ff, and Dawkins (1982)). Indeed, culture is influenced by human genetic propensities, and it follows that human cognitive, affective, and moral capacities are the product of a unique dynamic known as *gene-culture coevolution* (Gintis 2007, Bowles and Gintis 2005, Gintis 2003, Boyd, Gintis, Bowles and Richerson 2003).

We may also note that the theory that genes set many goals for action does not mean that our behaviour is determined by genes. Modern evolutionary theory has led to the understanding that many traits, particularly behavioural ones, may have some genetic basis but that does not mean that they will inevitably appear, because much depends on the environment (Dawkins 1995, Ridley 2003). Further, part of the power of the theory of emotion described here is that in evolution genes specify rewards and punishers that are goals for action, but do not specify the actions themselves, which are flexible and can be learned.

Emotion Explained goes beyond the brain mechanisms of emotion with a treatment (in Chapter 4) of the many different learning processes that become engaged in relation to emotion. The book also includes a formal treatment (in Appendix 1) of reinforcement learning and temporal difference (TD) learning, which are increasingly being used to understand emotion-related learning, as well as its brain mechanisms.

Emotion Explained goes beyond the brain mechanisms of emotion with a treatment of the functions of affective states in motivated behaviour (including hunger, thirst, and sexual behaviour), and indeed proposes a fundamental and simple relation between emotion and motivation. The role of sexual selection in the evolution of affective behaviour is included in Chapter 9.

The book has an integrated section on decision-making (in Chapter 11), and includes links to the developing new field of neuroeconomics.

At the same time, *Emotion Explained* does consider research on how emotion is implemented in the brain, including much new research in the areas of neurophysiology, and functional neuroimaging and clinical neuropsychology in humans. This treatment of the brain mechanisms of emotion is important not only for providing a basis for understanding disorders of emotion, but also turns out to be important in unravelling the many different ways in which emotions can influence our behaviour, because the different brain mechanisms themselves are being unravelled. The book includes a new theory of how the orbitofrontal cortex supports rapid reversals of emotional behaviour, by using a short term memory network for the current rule which acts in a biased competition mode to influence neurons known to be present in the orbitofrontal cortex. This helps to provide a contrast between the functions of the orbitofrontal cortex and amygdala in emotion. A description of the theory is given in Chapter 4, and a formal treatment of how the system operates is given in Appendix 2.

Appendix 2 also shows how it is possible to model the processing involved in emotional learning from the synaptic and neuronal level up through the neuronal network level to predict fMRI neuroimaging signals and behaviour, and thus illustrates a foundation for linking the many different levels of investigation of the brain mechanisms of emotion into a consistent account of precisely how findings at these different levels of exploration are related to each other. This cross-disciplinary approach is a feature of this book. Appendix 1 includes a treatment of autoassociation attractor networks that can maintain stable activity in a brain region, and shows how interacting attractor networks help to provide a foundation for understanding the interactions between mood, and cognition and memory.

The book links to research in psychiatry, with for example discussions of the impulsive behaviour that is a feature of borderline personality disorder, and to research in neurology, with for example assessment of the effects on emotion of damage produced by discrete lesions of the human brain.

Emotion Explained also goes beyond the brain mechanisms involved in emotion, by addressing (in Chapter 10) emotional feelings, part of the much larger problem of consciousness. One issue developed here is the concept that there is a credit assignment problem if a multiple step plan does not succeed, and that higher order thoughts provide a solution to this problem. The book also describes many recent functional neuroimaging investigations in which it has been possible to show that the activations of some brain regions are directly correlated with subjective feelings of affective state.

The material in this text is the copyright of Edmund T. Rolls. Part of the material described in the book reflects work done over many years in collaboration with many colleagues, whose tremendous contributions are warmly appreciated. The contributions of many will be evident from the references cited in the text. In addition, I have benefited enormously from the discussions I have had with a large number of colleagues and friends, many of whom I hope will see areas of the text that they have been able to illuminate. Much of the work described would not have been possible without financial support from a number of sources, particularly the Medical Research Council of the UK, the Human Frontier Science Program, the Wellcome Trust, the McDonnell-Pew Foundation, and the Commission of the European Communities.

The book was typeset in Latex using the WinEdt editor by the author.

The cover shows part of the picture 'Psyche Opening the Door into Cupid's Garden' painted in 1904 by John William Waterhouse.

Updates to the publications cited in this book are available at http://www.cns.ox.ac.uk.

Edmund T. Rolls dedicates this work to the overlapping group: his family, friends, and colleagues: *in salutem praesentium, in memoriam absentium.*

Contents

1 Introduction: the issues

1.1 Introduction

What are emotions? Why do we have emotions? What is their adaptive value? What are the brain mechanisms of emotion, and how can disorders of emotion be understood? Why does it feel like something to have an emotion? Why do emotions sometimes feel so intense? This book aims to provide answers to all these questions. When we know what emotions are, why we have them, how they are produced by our brains, and why it feels like something to have an emotion, we will have a broad-ranging explanation of emotion. It is in this sense that the title of this book is Emotion Explained.

We can similarly ask what motivates us: What is motivation? How is motivation controlled? How is motivation produced and regulated by the brain? What goes wrong in motivational disorders, for example in appetite disorders which produce overeating and obesity? How do these motivational control systems operate to ensure that we eat approximately the correct amount of food to maintain our body weight, or drink just enough to replenish our thirst? What are some of the underlying reasons for the different patterns of sexual behaviour found in different animals and humans? Why (and how) do we like some types of touch (e.g. a caress), and what is the relation of this to motivation? What brain processes underlie addiction? What is the relation between emotion, and motivational states such as hunger, appetite, and sexual behaviour? It turns out that the explanations for motivational behaviour are in many ways similar to those for emotional behaviour, and therefore I also treat motivation in this book.

The aims of the book are to explain emotions in terms of the following: What produces emotions? (The general answer I propose is reinforcing stimuli, that is rewards and punishers.) Why do we have emotions? (The overall answer I propose is that emotions are evolutionarily adaptive as they provide an efficient way for genes to influence our behaviour to increase their fitness.) How do we have emotions? (I answer this by describing what is known about the brain mechanisms of emotion.) Why do emotional states feel like something? This is part of the large problem of consciousness, which I address in Chapter 10.

Emotion and motivation are linked by the property that both involve rewards and punishers. Emotions can be thought of as states elicited by rewards or punishers. A full definition of emotion, and theory of emotion, with a starting point as the relation to rewards and punishers is described in Chapter 2. Motivation can be thought of as a state in which a reward is being sought, or a punisher is being avoided or escaped from. This is made clear in Chapters 2, 3, 5, 6 and 9. Because of the importance of reward and punishment for emotion and motivation, I define in Section 1.2 reward and punishment, and describe some of the types of learning that involve rewards and punishers. This is useful groundwork for what follows in the rest of this book. However, for those who wish in a first reading to skip the definitions in Section 1.2 (which are provided to ensure that there is a firm foundation for understanding emotion and motivation), it may be useful simply to think of a reward as something for which an animal (which includes humans) will work, and a punisher as something that an animal will work to escape from or avoid.

Some stimuli are innately rewarding or punishing and are called primary reinforcers (for example no learning is necessary to respond to pain as aversive), while other stimuli are learned or secondary reinforcers (for example the sight of a chocolate cake is not innately rewarding, but may become a learned reinforcer, for which we may work, by the process of association learning between the sight of the cake and its taste, where the taste is a primary reward or reinforcer). This type of learning, which is important in emotion and motivation, is called stimulus–reinforcement association learning. (A better term is stimulus–reinforcer association learning, where reinforcer is being used to mean a stimulus that might be a reward or a punisher.)

1.2 Rewards and punishers, and learning about rewards and punishers: instrumental learning and stimulus–reinforcer association learning

A reward is something for which an animal (including of course a human) will work. A punisher is something that an animal will work to escape or avoid (or that will decrease the probability of actions on which it is contingent). In order to exclude simple reflex-like behaviour, the concept invoked here by the term 'work' is to perform an arbitrary behaviour (called an operant response) in order to obtain the reward or avoid the punisher. An example of an operant response might be putting money in a vending machine to obtain food, or for a rat pressing a lever to obtain food. In these cases, the food is the reward. Another example of an operant response might be moving from one place to another in order to escape from or avoid an aversive (punishing) stimulus such as a cold draught. If the aversive stimulus starts and then the response is made, this is referred to as *escape* from the punisher. If a warning stimulus (such as a flashing light) indicates that the punisher will be delivered unless the operant response is made, then the animal may learn to perform the operant response when the warning stimulus is given in order to *avoid* the punisher.

Because the definitions of reward and punisher make it a requirement that it must be at least possible to demonstrate learning of an arbitrary operant response (made to obtain the reward or to escape from or avoid the punisher), we see that learning is implicit in the definition of reward and punisher. (Merely swimming up a chemical gradient towards a source of food as occurs in single cell organisms is called a taxis as described in Chapter 3; it does not require learning, and does not make the food qualify as a reward under the definition.) In that rewards and punishers do imply the ability to learn what to do to obtain the reward or escape from or avoid the punisher, we call rewards and punishers 'reinforcers'.

This introduction leads to the definition of **reinforcers** as stimuli that if their occurrence, termination, or omission is made contingent upon the making of a response, alter the probability of the future emission of that response (as a result of the contingency (i.e. dependency) on the response). The alteration of the probability of a response (or action) is the measure that learning has taken place. A positive reinforcer (such as food) increases the probability of emission of a response on which it is contingent; the process is termed **positive reinforcement**, and the outcome is a reward (such as food). A negative reinforcer (such as a painful stimulus) increases the probability of emission of a response which causes the negative reinforcer to be omitted (as in active avoidance) or terminated (as in escape), and the procedure is termed **negative reinforcement**. In contrast, **punishment** refers to procedures in which the probability of an action is decreased. Punishment thus describes procedures in which an action decreases in probability if it is followed by a painful stimulus, as in passive avoidance. Punishment can also be used to refer to a procedure involving the omission or termination of a reward ('extinction' and 'time out' respectively), both of which decrease the probability of responses (Gray 1975, Mackintosh 1983, Dickinson 1980, Lieberman 2000). My argument is that an affectively positive or 'appetitive' stimulus (which produces a state of pleasure) acts operationally as a **reward**, which when delivered acts instrumentally as a positive reinforcer, or when not delivered (omitted or terminated) acts to decrease the probability of responses on which it is contingent. Conversely I argue that an affectively negative or aversive stimulus (which produces an unpleasant state) acts operationally as a **punisher**, which when delivered acts instrumentally to decrease the probability of responses on which it is contingent, or when not delivered (escaped from or avoided) acts as a negative reinforcer in that it then increases the probability of the action on which its non-delivery is contingent[1].

Reinforcers, that is rewards or punishers, may be unlearned or **primary reinforcers**, or learned or secondary reinforcers. An example of a primary reinforcer is pain, which is innately a punisher. The first time a painful stimulus is ever delivered, it will be escaped from, and no learning that it is aversive is needed. Similarly, the first time a sweet taste is delivered, it can act as a positive reinforcer, so it is a primary positive reinforcer or reward. Other stimuli become reinforcing by learning, because of their association with primary reinforcers, thereby becoming '**secondary reinforcers**'. For example, a (previously neutral) sound that regularly precedes an electric shock can become a secondary reinforcer. Animals will learn operant responses reinforced by the secondary reinforcer, for example jumping to a place where the secondary reinforcer is not present or terminates. Secondary reinforcers are thus important in enabling animals to avoid primary punishers such as pain.

There is a close relation of all these processes to emotion, for as we will see in Chapter 2, fear is an emotional state that might be produced by a sound that has previously been associated with an electric shock. Shock in this example is the primary punisher, and fear is the emotional state that occurs to the tone stimulus as a result of the learning of the stimulus (i.e. tone)–reinforcer (i.e. shock) association. Another example of a secondary reinforcer is a visual stimulus associated with the taste of a food. For example, the first time we see a new type of food we do not treat the sight of the new visual stimulus as reinforcing, but if the stimulus has a good taste, the sight of the object becomes a positive secondary reinforcer, and we may choose the food when we see it in future by virtue of its association with a primary reinforcer. This type of learning is thus called stimulus–reinforcer association learning. (The operation is often referred to as stimulus–reinforcement association learning.) This type of learning is very important in many emotions, because it is as a result of this type of learning that many previously neutral stimuli come to elicit emotional responses, as in the example of fear above.

Unconditioned reinforcing stimuli often elicit autonomic responses. (Autonomic responses are those mediated through the autonomic nervous system, via the vagus and sympathetic nerves, which affect smooth muscle.) Examples include alterations of heart rate

---

[1] Note that my definition of a punisher, which is similar to that of an aversive stimulus, is of a stimulus or event that can either decrease the probability of actions on which it is contingent, or increase the probability of actions on which its non-delivery is contingent. The term punishment is restricted to situations where the probability of an action is being decreased.

and of blood pressure which might be produced by a painful stimulus; and salivation which might be produced by the taste of food. Many endocrine (hormonal) responses are also mediated through the autonomic nervous system and so are autonomic responses, for example the release of adrenaline (epinephrine) from the adrenal gland during emotional excitement. Previously neutral stimuli, such as the sound in our previous example, can by pairing with unconditioned stimuli, such as shock in the previous example, come by learning the association, to produce learned autonomic responses. In the example the tone might by pairing with shock come to elicit a change in heart rate, and sweating. This type of learning is called **classical conditioning**, and also **Pavlovian conditioning** after Ivan Pavlov who performed many of the original studies of this type of learning, including learned salivation to the sound of a bell that predicted the taste of food. It is a type of learning that is very similar to stimulus–reinforcer association learning, except that in the case of classical conditioning the responses involved are autonomic and endocrine responses.

In the case of stimulus–reinforcer association learning, the effects of the learning are mediated through the skeletal motor system, in that actions are performed that are instrumental in enabling animals to obtain rewards or avoid punishers, and are described as voluntary in humans. A key difference between **instrumental learning** and classical conditioning apart from the response systems involved lies in the contingencies that operate. In classical conditioning the animal has no control over whether the unconditioned stimulus is delivered (as in the experiments of Pavlov just described). In contrast, the whole notion of instrumental learning is that what the animal does is instrumental in determining whether the reinforcer (the goal) is obtained, or escaped from or avoided. Both types of learning are important in emotions because (as we will see in Chapter 2) instrumental reinforcers produce emotional responses, but also typically produce autonomic responses that therefore typically occur during emotional states, and indeed mediate important effects of emotions such as preparing the body for action by increasing heart rate etc.

A more detailed description of the nature of classical (Pavlovian) conditioning and instrumental learning, and how both are related to emotion, is provided in Section 4.6.1.

Motivation refers to the state an animal is in when it is willing to work for a reward or to escape from or avoid a punisher. So for example we say that an animal is motivated to work for the taste of food, and in this case the motivational state is called hunger. The definition of motivation thus implies the capacity to perform any, arbitrary, operant response in order to obtain the reward or escape from or avoid the punisher. By implying an operant response, we exclude simple behaviours such as reflexes and taxes (such as swimming up a chemical gradient), as described above and in Chapter 2. By implying learning of any response to obtain a reward (or avoid a punisher), motivation thus focuses on behaviours in which a goal is defined. Motivation is one of the states that are involved in the large area of brain design related to the fundamental issue of how goals for behaviour are defined, and an appropriate behaviour is selected, as described in this book and brought together into a theory in Chapter 2.

1.3   The approaches taken to emotion and motivation: their causes, functions, adaptive value, and brain mechanisms

To explain emotion, and motivation, a number of different approaches are taken, and some of these need some introduction. To examine the causes of emotion, the environmental stimuli and situations that elicit emotions are identified. This is part of the subject of Chapter 2. It is shown how the different environmental stimulus conditions that produce emotions provide the basis for a classification of different emotions. Understanding the functions of emotion also provides part of the explanation of why we have emotions, and many of the functions of emotion are described in Chapter 3. These functions of emotion explain in part the adaptive value of emotion, and give part of an explanation about why emotion has evolved. However, it turns out that emotions provide a fundamental solution to the issue of how genes design brains to produce behaviour that is advantageous to the genes, and this deep understanding of the adaptive value of emotion, and in a sense the cause of emotion, is elaborated in Chapter 3. When considering the adaptive value of emotion in the context of evolution, we must remember that animals are generally social, and that evolution may have led to the development of special reward and punishment systems to help to produce emotional behaviour that is adaptive in social situations. This area, of understanding and explaining aspects of social behaviour in terms of its evolutionary adaptive value, is the field of sociobiology, and this approach is introduced especially in the context of sexual behaviour in Chapter 9.

Another major approach taken to explain emotion and motivation, and their underlying reward and punishment systems, is in terms of the brain mechanisms that implement them. Understanding the brain processing and mechanisms of behaviour is one way to ensure that we have the correct explanation for how the behaviour is produced. Another important reason for investigating the actual brain mechanisms that underlie emotion and motivation, and reward and punishment, is not only to understand how our own brains work, but also to have the basis for understanding and treating medical disorders of these systems. Now it turns out that many of the brain systems that are involved in emotion and motivation have undergone considerable development in primates (e.g. monkeys and humans) compared to non-primates (for example rats and mice)[2]. It is because of the intended relevance to understanding human emotion and its disorders that emphasis is placed in this book on findings from research in non-human primates, including monkeys. Another reason for focusing interest on the primate brain is that there has been great development of the visual system in primates, and this itself has had important implications for the types of sensory stimuli that are processed by brain systems involved in emotion and motivation. One example is the importance of face identity and face expression decoding, which are both important in primate emotional behaviour, and indeed provide an important part of the foundation for much primate social behaviour. These are among the reasons why emphasis is placed on brain systems in primates, including humans,

---

[2] For example, the temporal lobe has undergone great development in primates, and several systems in the temporal lobe are either involved in emotion (e.g. the amygdala), or provide some of the main sensory inputs to brain systems involved in emotion and motivation. The prefrontal cortex has also undergone great development in primates, and one part of it, the orbitofrontal cortex, is very little developed in rodents, yet is one of the major brain areas involved in emotion and motivation in primates including humans. The development of some of these brain areas has been so great in primates that even evolutionarily old systems such as the taste system appear to have been rewired, compared with that of rodents, to place much more emphasis on cortical processing, taking place in areas such as the orbitofrontal cortex (see Rolls (1999a) and Rolls and Scott (2003)).

in the approach taken here. The overall medically relevant aim of the research described in this book is to provide a foundation for understanding the brain mechanisms of emotion and motivation, and thus their disorders, including depression, anxiety, addiction, sociopathy, and borderline personality disorder, in humans.

When considering brain mechanisms involved in emotion in primates, recent findings with the human brain imaging approaches are described. These approaches include functional magnetic resonance imaging (fMRI) to measure changes in brain oxygenation level locally (using a signal from deoxyhaemoglobin) to provide an index of local brain activity, as well as positron emission tomography (PET) studies to estimate local regional cerebral blood flow, again to provide an index of local brain activity. It is, however, important to note that these functional neuroimaging approaches provide rather coarse approaches to brain function, in that the spatial resolution is seldom better than 2 mm, so that the picture given is one of 'blobs on the brain', which give some indication of what is happening where in the brain, and what types of dissociation of functions are possible.

However, because there are millions of neurons in each of the areas that can be resolved with functional neuroimaging, such imaging techniques give rather little evidence on how the brain works. For this, one needs to know what information is represented in each brain area at the level at which information is exchanged between the computing elements of the brain, the neurons (brain cells). One also needs to know how the representation of information (for example about stimuli or events in the world) changes from stage to stage of the processing in the brain, to understand how the brain works as a system. It turns out that one can 'read' this information from the brain by recording the activity of single neurons, or groups of single neurons. The reason that this is an effective procedure for understanding what is represented is that each neuron has one information output channel, the firing of its action potentials, so that one can measure the full richness of the information being represented in a region by measuring the firing of its neurons. This can reveal fundamental evidence crucial for understanding how the brain operates. For example, neuronal recording can reveal all the information represented in an area even if parts of it are encoded by relatively small numbers, perhaps a few percent, of its neurons. (This is impossible with brain-imaging techniques, which also are susceptible to the interpretation problem that whatever causes the largest activation is interpreted as 'what' is being encoded in a region).

Neuronal recording also provides evidence for the level at which it is appropriate to build computational models of brain function, the neuronal network level. Such neuronal network computational models consider how populations of neurons with the connections found in a given brain area, and with biologically plausible properties such as learning rules for altering the strengths of synaptic connections between neurons, actually could perform useful computation to implement the functions being performed by that brain area. This approach should not really be considered as a metaphor for brain operation, but as a theory of how each part of the brain operates. The neuronal network computational theory, and any model or simulation based on it, may of course be simplified to some extent to make it tractable, but nevertheless the point is that the neuron-level approach, coupled with neuronal network models, together provide some of the fundamental elements for understanding how the brain actually works. For this reason, emphasis is also placed in this book on what is known about what is being processed in each brain area as shown by recordings from neurons. Such evidence, in terms of building theories and models of how the brain functions, can never be replaced by brain imaging evidence, although these approaches do complement each other very effectively. The approach to brain function in terms of computations performed by neuronal networks in different brain areas is the subject of the books *Neural Networks and Brain Function* by Rolls and Treves (1998) and *Computational Neuroscience of Vision* by Rolls and Deco (2002). The reader is referred to these books for more comprehensive accounts of this biologically plausible approach to brain function. In this book, some of the neurophysiological evidence and its computational implications for understanding how our brains work to produce emotion and motivation are described.

One of the main points made in this section is that rapid progress is being made now in understanding emotion and motivation, and part of this advance is related to the fact that we are just starting to be able to understand how the brain actually works, in terms of how its neuronal networks transform inputs into behaviour. Given that this basis for understanding how our own brains work does depend very much on understanding in detail how the brains of relatively close relatives, non-human primates such as monkeys, work, research on non-human primate brain information processing is quite crucial. We are really at the start of understanding in full detail how this works, but one aim of this book is to show how coming from that research new understanding into how our own brains work is being produced to the extent that even such complex processes as emotion and motivation are now seen to be at the heart of brain design. Moreover, that understanding is important for understanding the rich variety of human emotional behaviour, and also for understanding and treating disorders in emotion and motivation.

1.4   Reward, punishment, emotion, and motivation: the plan of the book

It may be useful to make it clear why the brain mechanisms of both emotion and motivation (with the examples of motivated behaviour considered being hunger, thirst, addiction, and sexual behaviour) are being considered together in this book. The reason is that for both emotion and motivation, rewards and punishers are assessed in order to provide the goals for behaviour. Operation of the brain to evaluate rewards and punishers is the fundamental solution of the brain to interfacing sensory systems to action selection and execution systems. Computing the reward and punisher value of sensory stimuli, and then using selection between different rewards and avoidance of punishers in a common reward-based currency appears to be the fundamental design that brains use in order to produce appropriate behaviour (see Chapter 2). The behaviour selected can be thought of as appropriate in the sense that it is based on the sensory systems and reward decoding that our genes specify (through the process of natural selection) in order to maximize their fitness (reproductive potential). Having reward and punishment systems is the solution that evolution has developed to produce appropriate behaviour. It happens that motivational and emotional behaviour are the types of behaviour in which rewards and punishers operate.

Considering both emotional and motivational behaviour in this book means that we can describe many of the principles that underlie the decoding of many types of rewarding and punishing stimuli, which have in common that they produce affective states. We can also see to some extent how the common currency of reward works to enable different rewards to be compared, and in particular how the reward value of all the different potential rewards that our genes specify is kept within a comparable range, so that we select different behaviours as appropriate. That is, we can examine many of the different ways in which the reward value of different sensory stimuli is modulated, both by internal signals as physiological needs are satisfied, and in addition to some extent by sensory-specific satiety (the mechanism by which repeating one reward causes it gradually to decrease its reward value somewhat, assisting the selection of other rewards in the environment).

However, perhaps the most important reason for treating reward and punishment systems, and the brain systems dealing with rewards and punishers, together is that we can develop an overall theory of how this set of issues, which might sometimes appear mysterious, is actually at the heart of brain design. Much of sensory processing, at least through the brain systems that are concerned with object identification (whether by sight, sound, smell, taste, or touch), can be seen to have the goal of enabling the correct reward value to be decoded and represented after the object has been identified. This means for example that in vision, representations of objects that can be accessed regardless of the view of the object shown, the size of the object on the retina, etc, must be formed. Moreover, these invariant representations of objects must be encoded in an appropriate way for the brain to associate in simple neuronal networks the object with primary (unlearned) reinforcers, such as the taste associated with the object, or the pain produced by the object. The actual motivational and emotional parts of the processing, the parts where the reward or punisher value is made explicit in the representation, should indeed no longer be seen as mysterious or perhaps superfluous aspects of brain processing. Instead, they are at the heart of which behavioural actions are selected, and how they are selected. Moreover, a large part of the brain's action and motor systems can be seen as having the goal in systems-level design of producing behaviour that will obtain the rewards decoded from sensory (and memory) inputs by the motivational and emotional systems of the brain. In particular, the implication is that the action systems for implicit (unconscious) behaviour have as part of their design principle the property that they will perform actions to optimize the output of the reward and punishment systems involved in motivation and emotion. Put another way, the brain systems involved in motivation and emotion must pass reward or punisher signals to the action systems, which must be built to attempt to obtain and maximize the reward signals being received; to switch behaviour from one reward to another as the reward values being received alter; and to switch behaviour also if signals indicating possible punishers are received (see Chapter 4).

This book is thus intended to uncover some of the most important and fundamental aspects and principles of brain function and design. The book is also intended to show that the way in which the brain works in motivation and emotion can be seen to be the result of natural selection operating to select genes that optimize our behaviour by building into us the appropriate reward and punisher systems, and the appropriate rules for the operation of these systems.

The plan of the book is that we consider in Chapters 2 and 3 the major issue of emotion, and its functions. These Chapters address the explanation of emotion by defining emotion, and elucidating its functions. Another part of the explanation of emotion is how it actually works, that is how it is implemented in the brain, which is described in Chapter 4. By understanding its mechanisms, we not only understand better the different processes that contribute to emotion, but also we provide a fundamental basis for starting to understand many disorders of emotion, including for example depression, and how they can be treated. Affective (emotional) states, and rewards, are involved in motivated behaviour such as eating, drinking, addiction, and sexual behaviour, and we consider these in Chapters 5, 6 and 9. These topics provide many clear examples of how the pleasantness or reward value of stimuli reflect a fundamental aspect of the design of both the brain and behaviour, and help to show the rewards, and punishers, that actually influence many aspects of our behaviour. In Chapter 10 the issue of emotional feelings, which is part of the big issue of consciousness, is considered, together with the brain processing involved in conscious feelings.

The aims of this book are thus to explain emotions in terms of:

1. What produces emotions? The answer developed in Chapter 2 is that emotions are produced by reinforcing stimuli.

2. Why do we have emotions? The most fundamental, and thoroughly Darwinian, explanation, developed in Chapter 3, is that the evolutionary adaptive value of emotions is that they provide an efficient way for genes to influence our behaviour to increase their (the genes') success.

3. How do we have emotions, that is, what are the brain and body processes that implement emotions, and motivational states such as hunger? These processes are described in Chapters 4–9.

4. Why do emotional states feel like something, which is part of the very large problem of consciousness. This is considered in Chapter 10.

2 The nature of emotion

2.1 Introduction

What are emotions? This is a question in which almost everyone is interested. There have been many answers, many of them surprisingly unclear and ill-defined. William James (1884) was at least clear about what he thought. He believed that emotional experiences were produced by sensing bodily changes, such as changes in heart rate or in skeletal muscles (the muscles involved in voluntary movements). His view was that "We feel frightened because we are running away". But he left unanswered the crucial question even for his theory, which is: Why do some events make us run away (and then feel emotional), whereas others do not?

A more modern theory is that of Frijda (1986), who argues that a change in action readiness is the central core of an emotion. Oatley and Jenkins (1996) (page 96) make this part of their definition too, stating that "the core of an emotion is readiness to act and the prompting of plans". But surely subjects in reaction time experiments in psychology who are continually for thousands of trials altering their action readiness are very far indeed from having normal or strong emotional experiences? Similarly, we can perform an action in response to a verbal request (e.g. open a door), yet may not experience great emotion when performing this action. Another example might be the actions that are performed in driving a car on a routine trip – we get ready, and many actions are performed, often quite automatically, yet little emotion occurs. So it appears that there is no necessary link between performing actions and emotion. This may not be a clear way to define emotion.

Because it is important to be able to specify what emotions are, in this Chapter we consider a systematic approach to this question. Part of the approach is to ask what causes emotions. Can clear conditions be specified for the circumstances in which emotions occur? This is considered in Section 2.2. Continuing with this theme, when we have come to understand the conditions under which emotions occur, does this help us to classify and describe different emotions systematically, in terms of differences between the different conditions that cause emotions to occur. A way in which a systematic account of different emotions can be provided is described in Section 2.3. A major help in understanding emotions would be provided by understanding what the functions of emotion are. It turns out that emotions have quite a number of different functions, each of which helps us to understand emotions a little more clearly. These different functions of emotion are described in Chapter 3. Understanding the different functions of emotion helps us to understand also the brain mechanisms of emotion, for it helps us to see that emotion can operate to affect several different output systems of the brain.

These analyses leave open though a major related question, which is why emotional states feel like something to us. This it transpires is part of the much larger, though more speculative, issue of consciousness, and why anything should feel like something to us. This aspect of emotional feelings, because it is part of the much larger issue of consciousness, is deferred until Chapter 10.

In Chapter 2, in considering the function of emotions, the idea is presented that emotions are part of a system that helps to map certain classes of stimuli, broadly identified as rewarding and punishing stimuli (i.e. aversive stimuli or 'punishers'), to action systems. Part of the idea is that this enables a simple interface between such stimuli and actions. This is an important area in its own right, which goes to the heart of why animals are built to respond to rewards and punishments, and have emotions.

The suggestion made in this book is that we now have a way of systematically approaching the nature of emotions, their functions, and their brain mechanisms. Doubtless in time there will be changes and additions to the overall picture. But the suggestion is that the ideas and theory presented here do provide a firm and systematic foundation for understanding emotions, their functions, and their brain mechanisms in a well-founded evolutionary context.

2.2 The outline of a theory of emotion

I will first introduce the essence of the definition of emotion that I propose. *The definition of emotions is that emotions are states elicited by rewards and punishers, that is, by instrumental reinforcers.* As described in Section 1.2, a reward is anything for which an animal will work. A punisher is anything that an animal will work to escape or avoid, or that will suppress actions on which it is contingent[3]. I note that any change in the regular delivery of a reward or a punisher acts as a reinforcer. The relevant states elicited by the reinforcers are those with the particular functions described in Chapter 3.

An example of an emotion might thus be happiness produced by being given a reward, such as a hug, a pleasant touch, praise, winning a large sum of money, or being with someone whom one loves. All these things are rewards, in that we will work to obtain them. Another example of an emotion might be fear produced by the sound of a rapidly approaching bus when we are cycling, or the sight of an angry expression on someone's face. We will work to avoid such stimuli, which are punishers. Another example might be frustration, anger, or sadness produced by the omission of an expected reward such as a prize, or the termination of a reward such as the death of a loved one. Another example might be relief, produced by the omission or termination of a punishing stimulus, for example the removal of a painful stimulus, or sailing out of danger. These examples indicate how emotions can be produced by the delivery, omission, or termination of rewarding or punishing stimuli, and go some way to indicate how different emotions could be produced and classified in terms of the rewards and punishers received, omitted, or terminated.

Before accepting this proposal, we should consider whether there are any exceptions to the proposed rule. Indeed, at first this may appear to be a rather reductionist hypothesis about what produces emotions. However, one way to test the suggested definition of the events that cause emotions is to ask whether there are any rewards or punishers that do not produce emotions. Conversely, we should ask whether there are any emotions that are produced by stimuli, events, or remembered events that are not rewarding or punishing. If we cannot find exceptions, then we should accept the suggestion as a useful identification, summary, and working definition of the conditions that produce emotions. Therefore in the next few pages we consider the questions: 'Are any emotions caused by stimuli, events, or remembered events that are not rewarding or punishing? Do any rewarding or punishing stimuli not cause

---

[3]A full definition in terms of reinforcement contingencies is given below.

emotions?' But first it is worth pointing out that in fact many approaches to or theories of emotion have in common that part of the process involves 'appraisal' (e.g. Frijda (1986); Oatley and Johnson-Laird (1987); Lazarus (1991); Izard (1993); Stein, Trabasso and Liwag (1994)). This is part, for example, of the suggestion made by Oatley and Jenkins (1996), who on page 96 write that "an emotion is usually caused by a person consciously or unconsciously evaluating an event as relevant to a concern (a goal) that is important; the emotion is felt as positive when a concern is advanced and negative when a concern is impeded". The concept of appraisal presumably involves in all these theories assessment of whether something is rewarding or punishing, that is whether it will be worked for or avoided. The description in terms of reward or punisher adopted here simply seems much more precisely and operationally specified.

The idea that rewards and punishers, that is instrumental reinforcers, are the stimuli that produce emotions has a considerable history, with origins that can be traced back to Watson (1929), Watson (1930), Harlow and Stagner (1933), Amsel (1958), and Amsel (1962). More recently, the approach was developed by Millenson (1967), Weiskrantz (1968), and Jeffrey Gray (1975, 1981). We can introduce some of the emotions that result from different reinforcement contingencies as follows. Consider the emotional effects of delivery of a 'reward': a state such as pleasure or happiness will be produced. An example might be receiving a prize for excellent work. Now consider the emotional effects of delivery of a 'punisher': pain or fear may be produced. For example, fear is an emotional state that might be produced by a sound that has previously been associated with a painful electrical shock. Shock in this example is the primary reinforcer, and fear is the emotional state that occurs to the tone stimulus as a result of the learning of the stimulus (i.e. tone)–reinforcer (i.e. shock) association. The tone in this example is a conditioned stimulus because of stimulus–reinforcer association learning, and has secondary reinforcing properties in that responses will be made to escape from it and thus avoid the primary reinforcer, shock.

The converse reinforcement contingencies produce the opposite effects on behaviour, and produce different emotions. The omission or termination of a reward ('extinction' and 'time out' respectively) reduce the probability of responses, and may produce the emotions of frustration, disappointment, or rage. (Imagine not receiving a prize that you deserved.) Behavioural responses followed by the omission or termination of a punisher increase in probability (this pair of reinforcement operations being termed 'active avoidance' and 'escape', respectively), and are associated with emotions such as relief.

The classification of emotions in terms of reinforcement contingencies is developed further in Section 2.3, and more formal definitions of rewards and punishers, and how they are related to learning theory concepts such as reinforcement and punishment are given in the footnote[4],

---

[4]Instrumental reinforcers are stimuli that, if their occurrence, termination, or omission is made contingent upon the making of an action, alter the probability of the future emission of that action (Gray 1975, Mackintosh 1983, Dickinson 1980, Lieberman 2000). Rewards and punishers are instrumental reinforcing stimuli. The notion of an action here is that an arbitrary action, e.g. turning right vs turning left, will be performed in order to obtain the reward or avoid the punisher, so that there is no pre-wired connection between the response and the reinforcer. Some stimuli are primary (unlearned) reinforcers (e.g., the taste of food if the animal is hungry, or pain); while others may become reinforcing by learning, because of their association with such primary reinforcers, thereby becoming 'secondary reinforcers'. This type of learning may thus be called 'stimulus–reinforcer association', and occurs via an associative learning process. A positive reinforcer (such as food) increases the probability of emission of a response on which it is contingent, the process is termed **positive reinforcement**, and the outcome is a reward (such as food). A negative reinforcer (such as a painful stimulus) increases the probability of emission of a response that causes the negative reinforcer to be omitted (as in active avoidance) or terminated (as in escape), and the procedure is termed **negative**

and in Sections 1.2 and 4.6.1. My argument is that an affectively positive or 'appetitive' stimulus (which produces a state of pleasure) acts operationally as a **reward**, which when delivered acts instrumentally as a positive reinforcer, or when not delivered (omitted or terminated) acts to decrease the probability of responses on which it is contingent. Conversely I argue that an affectively negative or aversive stimulus (which produces an unpleasant state) acts operationally as a **punisher**, which when delivered acts instrumentally to decrease the probability of responses on which it is contingent, or when not delivered (escaped from or avoided) acts as a negative reinforcer in that it then increases the probability of the action on which its non-delivery is contingent[5].

The link between emotion and instrumental reinforcers being made is partly an operational link. Most people find that it is not easy to think of exceptions to the statements that emotions occur after rewards or punishers are given (sometimes continuing for long after the eliciting stimulus has ended, as in a mood state); or that rewards and punishers, but not other stimuli, produce emotional states. But the link is deeper than this, as we will see, in that the theory has been developed that genes specify primary reinforcers in order to encourage the animal to perform arbitrary actions to seek particular goals, thus increasing the probability of their own (the genes') survival into the next generation (Rolls 1999a). The emotional states elicited by the reinforcers have a number of functions, described below, related to these processes.

Before considering how different emotions are related to different reinforcement contingencies in Section 2.3, I clarify a matter of terminology about moods vs emotions. A useful convention to distinguish between emotion and a mood state is as follows. An emotion consists of cognitive processing that results in a decoded signal that an environmental event (or remembered event) is reinforcing, together with the mood state produced as a result. If the mood state is produced in the absence of the external sensory input and the cognitive decoding (for example by direct electrical stimulation of the brain, see Chapter 7), then this is described only as a mood state, and is different from an emotion in that there is no object in the environment towards which the mood state is directed. (In that emotions are produced by stimuli or objects, and thus emotions 'take or have an object', emotional states are examples of what philosophers call intentional states.) It is useful to emphasize that there is great opportunity for cognitive processing (whether conscious or not) in emotions, for cognitive processes will very often be required to determine whether an environmental stimulus or event is reinforcing (see further Section 2.4).

2.3 Different emotions

As introduced in Section 2.2, the different emotions can in part be described and classified according to whether the reinforcer is positive or negative, and by the reinforcement contingency. An outline of such a classification scheme, elaborated by Rolls (1990d), Rolls (1999a)

reinforcement. In contrast, **punishment** refers to procedures in which the probability of an action is decreased. Punishment thus describes procedures in which an action decreases in probability if it is followed by a painful stimulus, as in passive avoidance. Punishment can also be used to refer to a procedure involving the omission or termination of a reward ('extinction' and 'time out' respectively), both of which decrease the probability of responses (Gray 1975, Mackintosh 1983, Dickinson 1980, Lieberman 2000).

[5]Note that my definition of a punisher, which is similar to that of an aversive stimulus, is of a stimulus or event that can either decrease the probability of actions on which it is contingent, or increase the probability of actions on which its non-delivery is contingent. The term punishment is restricted to situations where the probability of an action is being decreased.

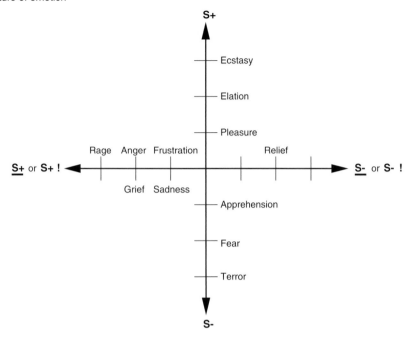

Fig. 2.1 Some of the emotions associated with different reinforcement contingencies are indicated. Intensity increases away from the centre of the diagram, on a continuous scale. The classification scheme created by the different reinforcement contingencies consists with respect to the action of (1) the delivery of a reward (S+), (2) the delivery of a punisher (S–), (3) the omission of a reward (S+) (extinction) or the termination of a reward (S+!) (time out), and (4) the omission of a punisher (S–) (avoidance) or the termination of a punisher (S–!) (escape). Note that the vertical axis describes emotions associated with the delivery of a reward (up) or punisher (down). The horizontal axis describes emotions associated with the non-delivery of an expected reward (left) or the non-delivery of an expected punisher (right).

and Rolls (2000f), is shown in Fig. 2.1. Movement away from the centre of the diagram represents increasing intensity of emotion, on a continuous scale. The diagram shows that emotions associated with the delivery of a reward (S+) include pleasure, elation and ecstasy. Of course, other emotional labels can be included along the same axis. Emotions associated with the delivery of a punisher (S–) include apprehension, fear, and terror (see Fig. 2.1). Emotions associated with the omission of a reward (S+) or the termination of a reward (S+!) include frustration, anger and rage. Emotions associated with the omission of a punisher (S–) or the termination of a punisher (S–!) include relief. Although the classification of emotions presented here (and by Rolls (1986c), Rolls (1986a), Rolls (1990d) and Rolls (1999a)) differs from earlier theories, the approach adopted here of defining and classifying emotions by reinforcing effects is one that has been developed in a number of earlier analyses (e.g. Millenson (1967), Gray (1975), Gray (1981); see Strongman (2003)).

I should make it clear that the scheme shown in Fig. 2.1 is not intended to be a dimensional scheme. [A dimensional scheme is one in which independent factors or dimensions have been identified that account for the major and independent sources of variation in a data set. Some investigators then work to show that these dimensions can be interpreted both biologically (for example as differing in autonomic, endocrine, or arousal-related ways) and psychologically (e.g. as representing anger vs fear), as described in Section 2.6.3.] However, the import of what is shown in Fig. 2.1 is to set out a set of logical possibilities of ways in which reinforcement contingencies can vary, and to show how they may be related to some different types of emotion.

It is actually a possibility that the four directions shown in Fig. 2.1 are at least partly independent from each other, and that a four-dimensional space is spanned by what is shown in Fig. 2.1. For example, sensitivity to (that is the ability to respond to) reward (S+) could be at least partly independent from sensitivity to punishers (S−), sensitivity to non-reward (S+ and S+!), and sensitivity to non-delivery of a punisher (S− and S−!). The dimensions or independent ways in which emotions may differ from each other could thus span 4 dimensions even with what is shown in Fig. 2.1, and these ways are expanded greatly as shown by the following further effects that make different emotions different to each other.

One important point about Fig. 2.1 is that there are a large number of different primary reinforcers, and that for example the reward label S+ shows states that might be elicited by just one type of reward, such as a pleasant touch. There will be a different reward axis (S+) and non-reward axis (S+ and S+!) for each type of reward (e.g. pleasant touch vs sweet taste); and, correspondingly, a different punisher axis (S−) and non-punisher axis (S− and S−!) for each type of punisher (e.g. pain vs bitter taste).

Different reinforcement contingencies can thus be used to classify a wide range of emotions. However, some of my tutorial pupils at Oxford sometimes expressed the view that reinforcement contingencies alone might not be able to account for the full range of human emotions. I therefore set out for them ways in which a system based on reinforcement contingencies could be developed in a number of different ways to give an account of most emotions. This extended set of ways of accounting for different emotions was published in 1986 (Rolls (1986c), Rolls (1986a)), and developed a little in later publications (e.g. Rolls (1995b), Rolls (1999a)). It is described, and elaborated further next. If the reader can think of any emotions that cannot be accounted for by a combination of the ways described next, then it would be interesting to consider what further extensions might be needed.

1. **Reinforcement contingency**

The first way in which different classes of emotion could arise is because of different reinforcement contingencies, as described above and indicated in Fig. 2.1.

2. **Intensity**

Second, different intensities within these classes can produce different degrees of emotion (see above and Millenson (1967)). For example, as the strength of a positive reinforcer being presented increases, emotions might be labelled as pleasure, elation, and ecstasy. Similarly, as the strength of a negative reinforcer being presented increases, emotions might be labelled as apprehension, fear, and terror (see Fig. 2.1). It may be noted here that anxiety can refer to the state produced by stimuli associated with the non-delivery of a reward or the delivery of a punisher (Gray 1987).

3. **Multiple reinforcement associations**

Third, any environmental stimulus might have a number of different reinforcement associations. For example, a stimulus might be associated both with the presentation of a reward and of a punisher, allowing states such as conflict and guilt to arise. The different possible combinations greatly increase the number of possible emotions.

4. **Different primary reinforcers**

Fourth, emotions elicited by stimuli associated with different primary reinforcers will be different even within a reinforcement category (i.e. with the same reinforcement contingency), because the original reinforcers are different. Thus, for example, the state elicited by a stimulus associated with a reward such as the taste of food will be different from that elicited by a reward such as being groomed. Indeed, it is an important feature of the association memory mechanisms described here that when a stimulus is applied, it acts as a key which 'looks up' or recalls the original primary reinforcer with which it was associated. Thus emotional stimuli will differ from each other in terms of the original primary reinforcers with which they were associated.

A summary of many different primary reinforcers is provided in Table 2.1, and inspection of this will help to show how some different emotions are produced by different primary reinforcers. For example, from Table 2.1 it might be surmised that one of the biological origins of the emotion of jealousy might be the state elicited in a male when his partner is courted by another male, because this threatens his parental investment in the offspring he raises with his partner, as described in Chapter 9. Jealousy in females would arise in a corresponding way. Examples of how further emotions including guilt, shame, anger, forgiveness, envy and love may arise in relation to particular primary reinforcers are provided later in this Section, throughout this Chapter, in Chapters 3 and 9, and in many other places in this book.

5. **Different secondary reinforcers**

A fifth way in which emotions can be different from each other is in terms of the particular (conditioned) stimulus that elicits the emotion, and the situation in which it occurs. Thus, even though the reinforcement contingency and even the unconditioned reinforcer may be identical, emotions will still be different cognitively, if the conditioned stimuli that give rise to the emotions are different (that is, if the objects of the emotion are different). For example, the emotional state elicited by the sight of one person may be different from that elicited by the sight of another person because the people, and thus the cognitive evaluations associated with the perception of the stimuli, are different. In another example, not obtaining a monetary reward in a gambling task might lead to frustration, but being blocked by another person from obtaining a reward might lead to anger directed at the person.

Thus evolution may have shaped different reinforcers to contribute in different ways and depending on the environmental circumstances to the exact emotion produced. For example, some emotions may be related to social reinforcers (e.g. love, anger, envy, and breaking rules of society so that shame is produced, see further Section 11.3), others to non-social reinforcers (such as fear of a painful stimulus), and others to solving difficult problems. By taking into account the nature of the primary reinforcer, the nature of the secondary reinforcer, and the environmental circumstances in which these apply, many different emotions can thus be accounted for, and cognitive factors taken into account. The common underlying basis of emotion remains however that it is related to goals/instrumental reinforcers, and the reinforcement contingencies that operate. The variety of different goals, and the contingencies and environmental situations in which they occur, combine to contribute to the richness in the variety of emotional states.

The gene-specified reinforcer approach to emotion advocated in this book is somewhat different to the domain-specific (vs domain general) approach of some evolutionary biologists (see Nesse (2000b)). In the domain-specific approach, a modular approach to different emotions may be taken, and the temptation is to end with a large number of specialized emotional systems, each promoting particular types of action. In contrast, in the approach described here, different genes build different reinforcement systems that define the goals for actions, and arbitrary actions appropriate for reaching the goal (i.e. instrumental actions) are then performed, with action–outcome learning guiding the actions produced. This can result in a rich variety of actions being selected in different emotion-provoking situations, without a tendency to suggest that particular perhaps instinctive actions are coupled to particular emotions. Instead, 'instinct' is involved in the process whereby the *goals* for actions, which are reinforcing stimuli, are specified by genes as a result of natural selection, and the behavioural response itself is not specified or 'determined' (see further Section 3.5).

Further, in the approach described here, modular neural systems useful for face identification, face expression recognition, and head gesture and movement may evolve because of the different specialized computational requirements for each and the importance of minimizing wiring length in the brain (see Section 4.4), and because the presence of these systems helps to provide representations that are useful in defining which stimulus or object-related events in the environment are associated with primary reinforcers.

6. **The behavioural responses that are available**

A sixth possible way in which emotions can vary arises when the environment constrains the types of behavioural response that can be made. For example, if an active behavioural response can occur to the omission of an expected reward, then anger might be produced and directed at the person who prevented the reward being obtained, but if only passive behaviour is possible, then sadness, depression or grief might occur.

By realizing that these six possibilities can occur in different combinations, it can be seen that it is possible to account for a very wide range of emotions, and this is believed to be one of the strengths of the approach described here. It is also the case that the extent to which a stimulus is reinforcing on a particular occasion (and thus an emotion is produced) depends on the prior history of reinforcements (both recently through processes that include sensory-specific satiety, and in the longer term), and that the current mood state can affect the degree to which a stimulus (a term that includes cognitively decoded events and remembered events) is reinforcing (see Section 4.10).

If we wish to consider the number of independent ways in which emotions may differ from each other (for comparison with the 'dimensional' theories described in Section 2.6.3) we see immediately that a vast subtlety of emotions can be systematically described using the approach described here. For example, based on the four different reinforcement contingencies shown in Fig. 2.1 we have four at least potentially independent 'dimensions', which are combined with perhaps another 100–500 independently varying (in that they are gene-specified) primary reinforcers, some of which are included in Table 2.1. These are combined with constraints to the actions that may be possible when a reinforcer is received (the 'coping potential' of appraisal theorists), which potentially at least doubles the number of emotions that can be described. We add further combinatorial possibilities by noting (point 3 above) that a given stimulus in the world may have many different reinforcement associations producing states such as conflict. The possible number of different emotions can be further multiplied by

Table 2.1 Some primary reinforcers, and the dimensions of the environment to which they are tuned

Taste

Salt taste	reward in salt deficiency
Sweet	reward in energy deficiency
Bitter	punisher, indicator of possible poison
Sour	punisher
Umami	reward, indicator of protein; produced by monosodium glutamate and inosine monophosphate
Tannic acid	punisher; it prevents absorption of protein; found in old leaves; probably somatosensory rather than strictly gustatory; see Critchley and Rolls 1996c

Odour

Putrefying odour	punisher; hazard to health
Pheromones	reward (depending on hormonal state)

Somatosensory

Pain	punisher
Touch	reward
Grooming	reward; to give grooming may also be a primary reinforcer
Washing	reward
Temperature	reward if tends to help maintain normal body temperature; otherwise punisher

Visual

Snakes, etc.	punisher for, e.g., primates
Youthfulness	reward, associated with mate choice
Beauty, e.g. symmetry	reward
Secondary sexual characteristics	rewards
Face expression	reward (e.g. smile) or punisher (e.g. threat)
Blue sky, cover, open space	reward, indicator of safety
Flowers	reward (indicator of fruit later in the season?)

Auditory

Warning call	punisher
Aggressive vocalization	punisher
Soothing vocalization	reward (part of the evolutionary history of music, which at least in its origins taps into the channels used for the communication of emotions)
courtship	reward
sexual behaviour	reward (a number of different reinforcers, including a low waist-to-hip ratio, and attractiveness influenced by symmetry and being found attractive by members of the other sex, are discussed in Chapter 9)

Table 2.1 continued **Some primary reinforcers, and the dimensions of the environment to which they are tuned**

Reproduction

mate guarding	reward for a male to protect his parental investment; jealousy results if his mate is courted by another male, because this may ruin his parental investment
nest building	reward (when expecting young)
parental attachment	reward
infant attachment to parents	reward
crying of infant	punisher to parents; produced to promote successful development

Other

Novel stimuli	rewards (encourage animals to investigate the full possibilities of the multidimensional space in which their genes are operating)
Sleep	reward; minimizes nutritional requirements and protects from
Altruism to genetically related individuals	danger reward (kin altruism)
Altruism to other individuals	reward while the altruism is reciprocated in a 'tit-for-tat' reciprocation (reciprocal altruism) Forgiveness, honesty, and altruistic punishment are some associated heuristics (May provide underpinning for some aspects of what is felt to be moral)
Altruism to other individuals	punisher when the altruism is not reciprocated
Group acceptance, reputation	reward (social greeting might indicate this) These goals can account for why some culturally specified goals are pursued
Control over actions	reward
Play	reward
Danger, stimulation, excitement	reward if not too extreme (adaptive because of practice?)
Exercise	reward (keeps the body fit for action)
Mind reading	reward; practice in reading others' minds, which might be
Solving an intellectual problem	adaptive reward (practice in which might be adaptive)
Storing, collecting	reward (e.g. food)
Habitat preference, home, territory	reward
Some responses	reward (e.g. pecking in chickens, pigeons; adaptive because it is a simple way in which eating grain can be programmed for a relatively fixed type of environmental stimulus)
Breathing	reward

the fact that each primary reinforcer may have associated with it almost any neutral stimulus to produce a secondary reinforcer.

The resulting number of emotional states that can be described and categorized is clearly enormous, even if we do not assume that each of the above factors operates strictly independently (factorially). For example, it is likely that if a gene were to specify a particular reward as being particularly intense in an individual, for example the pleasantness of touch, then omitting (S+) or terminating (S+!) this reward might also be expected to be particularly intense, so the contributions of reinforcement contingency and identity of the primary reinforcer might combine additively rather than multiplicatively. Even if there is only partial independence of the different processes 1–6 above, and of variation within each process, then nevertheless many different emotions can be systematically classified and described. It does of course remain an interesting issue of how the processes described above do combine, and of the extent to which a few factors actually do account for a great deal in the variation between different emotions. For example, if in an individual's sensitivity to non-reward is generally much more intense than the individual's sensitivity to reward, then this will shape the emotions in that individual, and account for quite a deal of the variance between that individual's emotional states. Such a factor might also account for quite an amount of the variation in emotions and personality between individuals (see Section 2.7).

Some examples of how different emotions might be classified using the above criteria now follow. Fear is a state that might be produced by a stimulus that has become a secondary reinforcer by virtue of its learned association with a primary negative reinforcer such as pain (see Fig. 2.1). Anger is a state that might be produced by the omission of an expected reward, frustrative non-reward, when an active behavioural response is possible (see Fig. 2.1). (In particular, anger may occur if another individual prevents an expected reward from being obtained.) Guilt may arise when there is a conflict between an available reward and a rule or law of society. Jealousy is an emotion that might be aroused in a male if the faithfulness of his partner seems to be threatened by her liaison (e.g. flirting) with another male. In this case the reinforcement contingency that is operating is produced by a punisher, and it may be that males are specified genetically to find this punishing because it indicates a potential threat to their paternity and paternal investment, as described in Chapters 9 and 3. Similarly, a female may become jealous if her partner has a liaison with another female, because the resources available to the 'wife' useful to bring up her children are threatened. Again, the punisher here may be gene-specified, as described in Chapter 3. Envy or disappointment might be produced if a prize is obtained by a competitor. In this case, part of the way in which the frustrative non-reward is produced is by the cognitive understanding that this is a competition in which there will be a winner, and that the person has set himself or herself the goal of obtaining it.

The partial list of primary reinforcers provided in Table 2.1 should provide readers with a foundation for starting to understand the rich classification scheme for different types of emotion that can be classified in this way.

Many other similar examples can be surmised from the area of evolutionary psychology (see e.g. Ridley (1993b), Buss (1999) and Barrett, Dunbar and Lycett (2002)). For example, there may be a set of reinforcers that are genetically specified to help promote social cooperation and even reciprocal altruism. Such genes might specify that emotion should be elicited, and behavioural changes should occur, if a cooperating partner defects or 'cheats' (Cosmides and Tooby 1999). Moreover, the genes may build brains with genetically specified rules that are useful heuristics for social cooperation, such as acting with a strategy of 'generous tit-for tat', which can be more adaptive than strict 'tit-for-tat', in that being generous occasionally is a good strategy to help promote further cooperation that has failed when both partners defect in a strict 'tit-for-tat' scenario (Ridley 1996). Genes that specify good heuristics to promote social cooperation may thus underlie such complex emotional states as feeling forgiving.

It is suggested that many apparently complex emotional states have their origins in designing animals to perform well in such sociobiological and socioeconomic situations (Ridley 1996, Glimcher 2003, Glimcher 2004). Indeed, many principles that humans accept as ethical may be closely related to strategies that are useful heuristics for promoting social cooperation, and emotional feelings associated with ethical behaviour may be at least partly related to the adaptive value of such gene-specified strategies. These ideas are developed in Section 11.3.

These examples indicate that an emotional state can be systematically specified and classified using the six principles described above in this Section. The similarity between particular emotions will depend on how close they are in the space defined by the above principles.

2.4 Refinements of the theory of emotion

The definition of emotions given above, that they are states produced by instrumental reinforcing stimuli, and have particular functions, is refined now.

First, when positively reinforcing (rewarding) stimuli (such as the taste of food or water) are relevant to a drive state produced by a change in the *internal milieu* (such as hunger and thirst), then we do not normally classify these stimuli as emotional, though they do produce pleasure, and indeed we describe the state they produce as affective (see Chapters 5 and 6). In contrast, emotional states are normally initiated by reinforcing stimuli that have their origin in the external environment, such as an (external) noise associated with pain (delivered by an external stimulus). We may then have identified a class of reinforcers (in our example, food) that we do not want to say cause emotions. This then is a refinement of the definition of emotions given above. Fortunately, we can encapsulate the set of reinforcing stimuli that we wish to exclude from our definition of stimuli that produce emotion. They are the set of external reinforcers (such as the sight of food) that are relevant to motivational states such as hunger and thirst, which are controlled by internal need-related (i.e. homeostatic) signals such as the concentration of glucose in the plasma (see Chapter 5). However, there is room for plenty of further discussion and refinement here. Perhaps some people (especially French people?) might say that they do experience emotion when they savour a wonderful food. There may well be cultural differences here in the semantics of whether such reinforcing stimuli should be included within the category that produce emotions.

Another area for discussion is how we wish to categorize the reinforcers associated with sexual behaviour. Such stimuli may be made to be rewarding, and to feel pleasurable, partly because of the internal hormonal state. Does this mean that we wish to exclude such stimuli from the class that we call emotion-provoking, in the same way that we might exclude food reward from the class of stimuli that are said to cause emotion, because the reward value of food depends on an internal controlling signal? I am not sure that there is a perfectly clear answer to this. But this may not matter, as long as we understand that there are some rewarding stimuli that some may wish to exclude from those that cause emotional states.

Second, emotional states can be produced by *remembered reinforcing stimuli*. (Indeed, when we remember stimuli or events, many of the cortical areas activated by the original sensory stimulus are also activated by the remembered stimuli or events. This is the case for most of the cortical areas in each sensory system, apart perhaps from the first (see Rolls (1989a), and Rolls and Treves (1998)). Thus if we recall a particular event, and this leads to reinstatement of activity in the higher parts of the visual system, this activity will provide inputs to the later parts of the brain involved in emotion, so that emotional states may then be produced.

Third, the stimulus that produces the emotional state does not have to be shown to be a reinforcer when producing the emotional state – it simply has to be *capable of being shown to have instrumental reinforcing properties*. An emotion-provoking stimulus can act as a reward or punisher, and is a goal for possible action.

Fourth, the definition given provides great opportunity for *cognitive processing* (whether conscious or not) in emotions, for cognitive processes will very often be required to determine whether an environmental stimulus or event is a reward or punisher. Normally an emotion consists of this cognitive processing that results in a decoded signal that the environmental event is reinforcing, together with the mood state produced as a result. If the mood state is produced in the absence of the external sensory input and the cognitive decoding (for example by direct electrical stimulation of the amygdala, see Rolls (1975) and Rolls (1999a)), then this is described only as a mood state, and is different from an emotion in that there is no object in the environment towards which the mood state is directed. The external reinforcing stimulus may alter the mood state very rapidly, and then the firing of the neurons that represent the mood state may gradually return back to their baseline firing rate, depending on the time course of the emotional state that is produced by the external reinforcing stimulus.

While discussing *mood*, it is worth pointing out that mood may be a particularly difficult state for the brain to maintain at a relatively constant level. In sensory systems the situation is different, for most sensory systems work by contrast, rather than absolute level. For example, early in the visual system it is the difference in brightness levels present at an edge, rather than the absolute brightness that is signaled. This is achieved by a process of lateral inhibition, which means that neighbouring neurons effectively inhibit each other. The result is that it is only at a dark–light boundary, where there is contrast, that neurons are firing. (In fact the firing will be fast on the bright side of the edge, and low, below a spontaneous level of firing, on the dark side of the edge. In the middle of a large bright area few neurons will be active, because the nearby neurons will be inhibiting each other.) However, for mood, the situation may be different. Here, the absolute firing rates of the neurons that represent mood state must be set to fire at the appropriate rate for long periods. Any drift in firing rates would represent a change of mood level. The situation for a brain system that represents mood may thus be different from that involved in most sensory and motor processing in the brain, both because in sensory systems it is the local contrast of firing rate that is important, not the absolute level, and because in sensory systems the inputs keep changing, so that it is not necessary to maintain an absolute value for long. The difficulty of maintaining a constant absolute level of firing in neurons may contribute to 'spontaneous' mood swings, depression that occurs without a clear external cause, and the multiplicity of hormonal and transmitter systems that seem to be involved in the control of mood (see Chapters 4 and 8).

Having said this, it also seems to be the case that there is some '*regression to a constant value*' for emotional states. What I mean by this is that we are sensitive to some extent not just to the absolute level of reinforcers being received, but also to the change in the rate, prob-

Positive and Negative Contrast

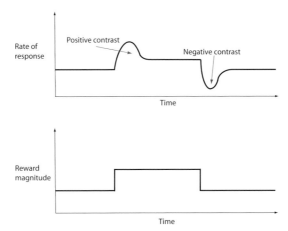

Fig. 2.2 Positive and negative contrast. If the magnitude of a moderate reward (positive reinforcer) is increased, then the rate of working increases markedly, but then drops back to a rate just greater than that to the moderate reinforcer. The positive overshoot is positive contrast. The converse happens if the magnitude of the reward is decreased.

ability, or magnitude of reinforcers being received. This is well shown by the phenomenon of *positive and negative contrast* effects with rewards. Imagine that an animal is working at a moderate rate for a moderate reward. If the reward is suddenly increased, the animal will work very much harder for a period (perhaps lasting for minutes or longer), but will then gradually revert back to work at a rate close to that at which the animal was working for the moderate reinforcement. This is called positive contrast (see Fig. 2.2). A comparable contrast effect is seen when the reward magnitude (or rate at which rewards are obtained, or the probability of obtaining rewards) is reduced – there is a negative overshoot in the rate of working for a time, but then the rate reverts back to a value close to that at which the animal worked for the moderate reward. This phenomenon is adaptive. It is evidence that animals are in part sensitive to a change in reinforcement, and this helps them to 'climb reward gradients' to obtain better rewards. In effect, regardless of the absolute level of reinforcement being received, it is adaptive to be sensitive to a change in reinforcement. If this were not true, an animal receiving very little reinforcement but then obtaining a small increase in positive reinforcement might still be working very little for the reward. But it is much more adaptive to work hard in this situation, as the extra little bit of reward might make the difference between survival or not, and might lead the animal in the direction of even better rewards if what has just been done leads to an improvement in rewards. A similar phenomenon may be evident in humans. People who have very little in the way of rewards, who may be poor, have a poor diet, and may suffer from disease, may nevertheless not have a baseline level of happiness that is necessarily very different from that of a person in an affluent society who in absolute terms apparently has many more rewards. This may be due in part to resetting of the baseline of expected rewards to a constant value, so that we are especially sensitive to changes in rewards (or punishers).

Fifth, in a case where the sight of a stimulus associated with pain produces fear, some philosophers categorize fear as an emotion, but not pain. The distinction they make may be that primary (unlearned) reinforcers do not produce emotions, whereas secondary reinforcers (stimuli associated by stimulus–reinforcement learning with primary reinforcers) do. They describe the pain as a sensation. But neutral stimuli (such as a table) can produce sensations when touched. It accordingly seems to be much more useful to categorize stimuli according to whether they are reinforcing (in which case they produce emotions), or are not reinforcing (in which case they do not produce emotions). Clearly there is a difference between primary reinforcers and learned reinforcers; but this is most precisely caught by noting that this is the difference, and that it is whether a stimulus is reinforcing that determines whether it is related to emotion. Primary and secondary reinforcers have in common that they produce affective states, whereas neutral, non-reinforcing, stimuli do not produce affective states. The major division thus seems to be between stimuli that produce affective states and those that do not; and it is reinforcing stimuli that produce affective states.

Sixth, as we are about to see, emotional states (i.e. those elicited by instrumental reinforcers) have many functions, and the implementations of only some of these functions by the brain are associated with emotional feelings (see Chapters 10 and 4, and Rolls (1999a)). Indeed there is evidence for interesting dissociations in some patients with brain damage between actions performed to reinforcing stimuli and what is subjectively reported. In this sense it is biologically and psychologically useful to consider emotional states to include more than those states associated with feelings of emotion.

Seventh, the role of learning in many emotions should be emphasized. The approach described above shows that the learning of stimulus–reinforcer (i.e. stimulus–reward and stimulus–punisher) associations is the learning involved when emotional responses are learned. In so far as the majority of stimuli that produce our emotional responses do so as a result of learning, this type of learning, and the brain mechanisms that underlie it, are crucial to the majority of our emotions. This, then, provides a theoretical basis for understanding the functions of some brain systems such as the amygdala in emotion, as described in Chapter 4.

It also follows from this approach towards a theory of emotion that brain systems involved in disconnecting stimulus–reinforcer associations when they are no longer appropriate will also be very important in emotion. Failure of this function would be expected to lead, for example, in frustrating situations to inappropriate perseveration of behaviour to stimuli no longer associated with rewards. The inability to correct behaviour when reinforcement contingencies change would be evident in a number of emotion-provoking situations, such as frustration (i.e. non-reward), and the punishment of previously rewarded behaviour. It will be shown in Chapter 4 that this approach, which emphasizes the necessity, in for example social situations, to update and correct the decoded reinforcement value of stimuli continually and rapidly, helps to provide a basis for understanding the functions of some other brain regions such as the orbitofrontal cortex in emotion.

Eighth, understanding the functions of emotion is also important for understanding the nature of emotions, and for understanding the brain systems involved in the different types of response that are produced by emotional states. Emotion appears to have many functions, which are not necessarily mutually exclusive. Some of these functions are described in Chapter

3.

However, a fundamentally important function of emotion that I will propose in Chapter 3 draws out a close link with the definition given here of emotions as states elicited by instrumental reinforcing stimuli, which are the goals for action. I show in Chapter 3 that genes define the goals for (instrumental) actions, and that this is an important Darwinian, adaptive, aspect of brain design. These goals for action are instrumental reinforcers, and this thus helps us to see that by understanding emotions as states elicited by reinforcers, we gain important insight into the nature of emotions. The treatment of the nature of emotion given in this Chapter is thus seen to be directly relevant to understanding this fundamentally important role of emotion in brain design which is related to the role that reinforcers have in guiding actions.

2.5 Summary of the classification of emotion

The theory of emotion outlined above provides systematic and principled ways to categorise different emotions.

One useful way to categorise emotions is to note that the main dimensions of the space of possible emotional responses can well be specified by the different primary reinforcers, examples of which are given in Table 2.1. Within each of these gene-specified dimensions, different reinforcement contingencies would lead to different emotional states, for example pleasure produced by a given taste, and disappointment (frustrative non-reward) if that taste is not available. Also within each of these reinforcer-defined dimensions the exact nature of the primary reinforcing stimulus, including its intensity and variations in its quality (for example in the nature of its texture if it is a somatosensory stimulus), would lead to differences in the emotion elicited. Also within each gene-specified dimension, many states could be cognitively different depending on which different stimulus (e.g. person) had become associated by learning with the primary reinforcer to become a secondary reinforcer. If we then remember that each secondary reinforcer may have many different reinforcement associations, then we see that very large numbers of possible emotions can be described and categorized in this way. Although the description leads to an enormously large numbers of different categories, nevertheless it is systematic, principled, and fairly complete.

Another possible way to categorize emotions might be by reinforcement contingency. For example we might group together into one category all emotions elicited by frustrative non-reward (S+ and S+! in Fig. 2.1). Gray (1987) went even further than this, grouping into one category not only the emotions elicited by frustrative non-reward (the non-delivery of rewards), but also those elicited by the delivery of punishers (S− in Fig. 2.1). Part of his reason for combining these two was that both can lead to decreases in behaviour, which led him to believe that there was a "behavioural inhibition system" (which he identified with the hippocampus) common to both. Clearly at some level the processing is inherently different, in that frustrative non-reward implies a neural system that predicts reward and produces an output if that outcome is not realised, whereas punishment may often involve activation of different sensory systems involved in for example pain. The whole operation and pharmacology of the different circuitry involved in frustrative non-reward and in the effects of punishers must at some level be different, and this is likely to be exploitable in treating emotional states that arise in these two different ways, so it may be very helpful not to combine them into a single category.

In general, categorising emotions by reinforcement contingency alone produces few emotional categories, which is a disadvantage given the many different emotions that can be distinguished, but does have an advantage in producing a rough grouping together of emotional states that do have something in common. However, it should be noted that the reinforcement contingency alone is not a good predictor of the appropriate emotion and emotional behaviour, as shown for example in Fig. 2.1 by the anger that might result from frustrative non-reward if action is possible, and the sadness that might arise if no action is possible to retrieve the lost reward. Further, I note that the axes in Fig. 2.1 refer to only one particular reinforcer (such as a food reward), and are effectively replicated for each different primary reinforcer.

2.6 Other theories of emotion

In the following subsections, I outline some other theories of emotion, and compare them with the above (Rolls') theory of emotion. Surveys of some of the approaches to emotion that have been taken in the past are provided by Strongman (2003) and Oatley and Jenkins (1996).

2.6.1 The James–Lange and other bodily theories of emotion including Damasio's theory

James (1884) believed that emotional experiences were produced by sensing bodily changes, such as changes in heart rate or in skeletal muscles. Lange (1885) had a similar view, although he emphasized the role of autonomic feedback (for example from the heart) in producing the experience of emotion. The theory, which became known as the James–Lange theory, suggested that there are three steps in producing emotional feelings (see Fig. 2.3). The first step is elicitation by the emotion-provoking stimulus of peripheral changes, such as skeleto-muscular activity to produce running away, and autonomic changes, such as alteration of heart rate. But, as pointed out above, the theory leaves unanswered perhaps the most important issue in any theory of emotion: Why do some events make us run away (and then feel emotional), whereas others do not? This is a major weakness of this type of theory. The second step is the sensing of the peripheral responses (e.g. running away, and altered heart rate). The third step is elicitation of the emotional feeling in response to the sensed feedback from the periphery.

The history of research into peripheral theories of emotion starts with the fatal flaw that step one (the question of which stimuli elicit emotion-related responses in the first place) leaves unanswered this most important question. The history continues with the accumulation of empirical evidence that has gradually weakened more and more the hypothesis that peripheral responses made during emotional behaviour have anything to do with producing the emotional behaviour (which has largely already been produced anyway according to the James–Lange theory), or the emotional feeling. Some of the landmarks in this history are as follows.

First, the peripheral changes produced during emotion are not sufficiently distinct to be able to carry the information that would enable one to have subtly different emotional feelings to the vast range of different stimuli that can produce different emotions. The evidence suggests that by measuring many peripheral changes in emotion, such as heart rate, skin conductance, breathing rate, and hormones such as adrenaline and noradrenaline (known in the United States by their Greek names epinephrine and norepinephrine), it may be possible to make coarse distinctions between, for example, anger and fear, but not much finer distinctions (Wagner 1989, Cacioppo, Klein, Berntson and Hatfield 1993, Oatley and Jenkins 1996).

James-Lange theory of emotion

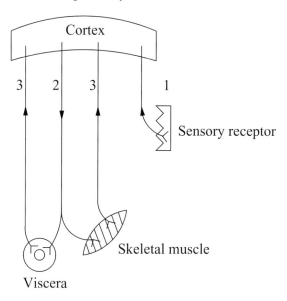

Fig. 2.3 The James–Lange theory of emotion proposes that there are three steps in producing emotional feelings. The first step is elicitation by the emotion-provoking stimulus (received by the cortex via pathway 1 in the Figure) of peripheral changes, such as skeleto-muscular activity to run away, and autonomic changes, such as alteration of heart rate (via pathways labelled 2 in the Figure). The second step is the sensing of the peripheral responses (e.g. altered heart rate, and somatosensory effects produced by running away) (via pathways labelled 3 in the Figure). The third step is elicitation of the emotional feeling in response to the sensed feedback from the periphery.

Second, when emotions are evoked by imagery, then the peripheral responses are much less marked and distinctive than during emotions produced by external stimuli (Ekman, Levenson and Friesen 1983, Stemmler 1989, Levenson, Ekman and Friesen 1990). This makes sense in that although an emotion evoked by imagery may be strong, there is no need to produce strong peripheral responses, because no behavioural responses are required.

Third, disruption of peripheral responses and feedback from them either surgically (for example in dogs, (Cannon 1927, Cannon 1929, Cannon 1931), or as a result of spinal cord injury in humans (Hohmann 1966, Bermond, Fasotti, Niewenhuyse and Schuerman 1991)), does not abolish emotional responses. What was found was that in some patients there was apparently some reduction in emotions in some situations (Hohmann 1966), but this could be related to the fact that some of the patients were severely disabled (which could have produced its own consequences for emotionality), and that in many cases the patients were considerably older than before the spinal cord damage, and this could have been a factor. What was common to both studies was that emotions could be felt by all the patients; and that in some cases, emotions resulting from mental events were even reported as being stronger (Hohmann 1966, Bermond, Fasotti, Niewenhuyse and Schuerman 1991).

Fourth, when autonomic changes are elicited by injections of, for example, adrenaline or noradrenaline, particular emotions are not produced. Instead, the emotion that is produced depends on the cognitive decoding of the reinforcers present in the situation, for example an actor who insults your parents to make you angry, or an actor who plays a game of hula hoop to make you feel happy (Schachter and Singer 1962). In this situation, the hormone adrenaline or noradrenaline can alter the magnitude of the emotion, but not which emotion is felt. This is further evidence that it is the decoded reinforcement value of the input stimulus or events that determines which emotion is felt. The fact that the hormone injections produced some change in the magnitude of an emotion is not very surprising. If you felt your heart pounding for no explicable reason, you might wonder what was happening, and therefore react more or abnormally.

Fifth, if the peripheral changes associated with emotion are blocked with drugs, then this does not block the perception of emotion (Reisenzein 1983).

Sixth, it is found that in normal life, behavioural expressions of emotion (for example smiling when at a bowling alley) do not usually occur when one might be expected to feel happy because of a success, but instead occur when one is looking at one's friends (Kraut and Johnson 1979). These body responses, which can be very brief, thus often serve the needs of communication, or of action, not of producing emotional feelings.

Despite this rather overwhelming evidence against an important role for body responses in producing emotions or emotional feelings, Damasio (1994) has effectively tried to resurrect a weakened version of the James–Lange theory of emotion from the 19th century, by arguing with his somatic marker hypothesis that after reinforcers have been evaluated, a bodily response ('somatic marker') normally occurs, then this leads to a bodily feeling, which in turn is appreciated by the organism to then make a contribution to the decision-making process[6]. The James–Lange theory has a number of major weaknesses just outlined that apply also to the somatic marker hypothesis.

The somatic marker hypothesis postulates that emotional decision-making is facilitated by peripheral feedback from for example the autonomic nervous system. In a direct test of this, Heims, Critchley, Dolan, Mathias and Cipolotti (2004) measured emotional decision making using the Iowa Gambling Task (Bechara, Damasio, Damasio and Anderson 1994, Bechara, Tranel, Damasio and Damasio 1996, Bechara, Damasio, Tranel and Damasio 1997, Damasio 1994) (described in Section 4.5.6) in patients with pure autonomic failure. In this condition, there is degeneration of the peripheral autonomic system, and thus autonomic responses are severely impaired, and there can be no resulting feedback to the brain. It was found that performance in the Iowa Gambling Task was not impaired, and nor were many other tests of emotion and emotional performance, including face expression identification, theory of mind tasks of social situations, and social cognition tasks. Thus emotional decision-making does not depend on the ongoing feedback from somatic markers related to autonomic function. Damasio might argue that feedback from the autonomic system is not actually important, and that it is feedback from skeletomotor responses such as arm movements or muscle tension that is important. He might also argue that the autonomic feedback is not usually necessary for emotional decision making, because it can be 'simulated' by the rest of the brain. However,

---

[6]In the James–Lange theory, it was emotional feelings that depend on peripheral feedback; for Damasio, it is the decision of which behavioural response to make that is normally influenced by the peripheral feedback. A quotation from Damasio (1994, p190) follows: "The squirrel did not really think about his various options and calculate the costs and benefits of each. He saw the cat, was jolted by the body state, and ran." Here it is clear that the pathway to action uses the body state as part of the route. Damasio would also like decisions to be implemented using the peripheral changes elicited by emotional stimuli. Given all the different reinforcers that may influence behaviour, Damasio (1994) even suggests that the net result of them all is reflected in the net peripheral outcome, and then the brain can sense this net peripheral result, and thus know what decision to take.

the study by Heims et al. (2004) does show that ongoing autonomic feedback is not necessary for normal emotional decision-making, and this leaves the somatic marker hypothesis more precarious.

Part of the evidence for the somatic marker hypothesis was that normal participants in the Iowa Gambling Task were described as deciding advantageously before knowing the advantageous strategy (Bechara, Damasio, Tranel and Damasio 1997). The interpretation was that they had implicit (unconscious) knowledge implemented via a somatic marker process that was used in the task, which was not being solved by explicit (conscious) knowledge. Maia and McClelland (2004) (see also Maia and McClelland (2005)) however showed that with more sensitive questioning, normal participants at least had available to them explicit knowledge about the outcomes of the different decks that was as good as or better than the choices made, weakening the arguments of Bechara et al. (1997) and Bechara, Damasio, Tranel and Damasio (2005) that the task was being solved implicitly and using somatic markers. Further evidence on factors that contribute to the effects found in the Iowa Gambling Task are described in Section 4.5.6.

Another argument against the somatic marker hypothesis is that there can be dissociations between autonomic and other indices of emotion, thus providing evidence that behaviour may not follow from autonomic and other effects. For example, lesions of different parts of the amygdala influence autonomic responses and instrumental behaviour differently, as shown in Section 4.6.3 and Fig. 4.52.

Another major weakness, which applies to both the James–Lange and to Damasio's somatic marker hypothesis, is that they do not take account of the fact that once an information processor has determined that a response should be made or inhibited based on reinforcement association, a function attributed in the theory proposed in this Chapter and by Rolls (Rolls 1986c, Rolls 1986a, Rolls 1990d, Rolls 1999a) to the orbitofrontal cortex, it would be very inefficient and noisy to place in the execution route a peripheral response, and transducers to attempt to measure that peripheral response, itself a notoriously difficult procedure (see, e.g., Grossman (1967)). Even for the cases when Damasio (1994) might argue that the peripheral somatic marker and its feedback can be by-passed using conditioning of a representation in, e.g., the somatosensory cortex to a command signal (which might originate in the orbitofrontal cortex), he apparently would still wish to argue that the activity in the somatosensory cortex is important for the emotion to be appreciated or to influence behaviour. (Without this, the somatic marker hypothesis would vanish.) The prediction would apparently be that if an emotional response were produced to a visual stimulus, then this would necessarily involve activity in the somatosensory cortex or other brain region in which the 'somatic marker' would be represented. This prediction could be tested (for example in patients with somatosensory cortex damage), but it seems most unlikely that an emotion produced by a visual reinforcer would require activity in the somatosensory cortex to feel emotional or to elicit emotional decisions. However, Adolphs, Tranel and Denburg (2000) have pursued this general line of enquiry, and report that the more damage there is to somatosensory cortex, the greater the impairment in the emotional state reported by patients. However, the parts of the somatosensory system that appear to be damaged most frequently in the patients with emotional change are often in the anterior and ventral extensions of the somatosensory cortex in insular and nearby areas, and it would be useful to know whether this damage interrupted some of the connections or functions of the orbitofrontal cortex areas just anterior.

More recently, Damasio has stated the somatic marker hypothesis in a weak form, suggesting that somatic markers do not even reflect the valence of the reinforcer, but just provide a signal that depends on the intensity of the emotion, independently of the type of emotion. On this view, the role of somatic markers in decision making would be very general, providing, as Damasio says, just a jolt to spur the system on (A.R.Damasio, paper delivered at the 6th Annual Wisconsin Symposium on Emotion, April 2000).

The alternative view proposed here (and by Rolls (1986c), Rolls (1986a), Rolls (1990d), Rolls (1999a), and Rolls (2000f)) is that where the reinforcement value of the visual stimulus is decoded, namely in the orbitofrontal cortex and the amygdala, is the appropriate part of the brain for outputs to influence behaviour (via, e.g., the orbitofrontal-to-striatal connections), and that the orbitofrontal cortex and amygdala, and brain structures that receive connections from them, are the likely places where neuronal activity is directly related to emotional states and to felt emotions (see further Chapter 10 and Rolls (1999a)).

2.6.2 Appraisal theory

Appraisal theory, developed and described by Frijda (1986), Oatley and Johnson-Laird (1987), Lazarus (1991), Izard (1993), Stein, Trabasso and Liwag (1994), Oatley and Jenkins (1996), and Scherer (1999) (see also Scherer (2001) and Scherer, Schorr and Johnstone (2001)) generally holds that two types of appraisal are involved in emotion. Primary appraisal holds that "an emotion is usually caused by a person consciously or unconsciously evaluating an event as relevant to a concern (a goal) that is important; the emotion is felt as positive when a concern is advanced and negative when a concern is impeded" (from Oatley and Jenkins (1996), p. 96). As noted above, the concept of appraisal presumably involves assessment of whether something is a reward or punisher, that is whether it will be worked for or avoided. The description in terms of rewards and punishers adopted here simply seems much more precisely and operationally specified. If primary appraisal is defined with respect to goals, it might be helpful to note that goals may just be the reinforcers specified in Rolls' theory, and if so the reinforcer/punisher approach provides clear definitions of goals (as reinforcers, see Appendix 3), which is helpful, precise, and makes a link to what may be specified by genes.

Secondary appraisal is concerned with coping potential, that is with whether for example a plan can be constructed, and how successful it is likely to be.

I note that appraisal theory is in many ways quite close to the theory that I outline here and in *The Brain and Emotion* (Rolls 1999a), and I do not see them as rivals. Instead, I hope that those who have an appraisal theory of emotion will consider whether much of what is encompassed by primary appraisal is not actually rather close to assessing whether stimuli or events are reinforcers; and whether much of what is encompassed by secondary appraisal is rather close to taking into account the actions that are possible in particular circumstances, as described above in Section 2.2.

An aspect of some flavours of appraisal theory with which I do not agree is that emotions have as one of their functions releasing particular actions, which seems to make a link with species-specific action tendencies or responses (Tomkins 1995, Panksepp 1998) or more 'open motor programs' (Ekman 2003). I argue in Chapter 3 that rarely are behavioural responses programmed by genes (see Table 2.1), but instead genes optimise their effects on behaviour if they specify the goals for (flexible) actions, that is if they specify rewards and punishers. The difference is quite considerable, in that specifying goals is much more economical in terms of the information that must be encoded in the genome; and in that specifying goals for actions allows much more flexibility to the actual actions that are produced. Of course I acknowledge that there is some preparedness to learn associations between particular types of secondary and primary reinforcers, and see this just as an economy of sensory–sensory convergence in the brain, whereby for example it does not convey much advantage to be able to learn that flashing lights (as contrasted with the taste of a food just eaten) are followed by sickness.

2.6.3 Dimensional and categorical theories of emotion

These theories suggest that there are a number of fundamental or basic emotions. Charles Darwin for example in his book *The Expression of the Emotions in Man and Animals* (1872) showed that some basic expressions of emotion are similar in animals and humans. Some of the examples he gave are shown in Table 2.1. His focus was on the continuity between animals and humans of how emotion is expressed.

In a development of this approach, Ekman and colleagues (Ekman 1982, Ekman 1992, Ekman 1993, Ekman, Friesen and Ellsworth 1972, Ekman, Levenson and Friesen 1983) have suggested that humans categorize face expressions into a number of basic categories that are similar across cultures. These face expression categories include happy, fear, anger, surprise, grief and sadness.

A related approach is to identify a few clusters of variables or factors that result from multidimensional analysis of questionnaires, and to identify these factors as basic emotions. (Multidimensional analyses such as factor analysis seek to identify a few underlying sources of variance to which a large number of data values such as answers to questions are related.) The categories of emotions identified in these ways may be supported by correlating them with autonomic measures (e.g. Ekman et al. (1983)).

One potential problem with some of these approaches is that they risk finding seven plus or minus two categories, which is the normal maximal number of categories with which humans normally operate, as described in a famous paper by George Miller (1956). A second problem is that there is no special reason why the first few factors (which account for most of the variance) in a factor analysis should provide a complete or principled classification of different emotions, or of their functions. In contrast, the theory described here does produce a principled classification of different emotions based on reinforcement contingencies, the nature of the primary and secondary reinforcers, etc, as set out in Sections 2.2 and 2.3. Moreover, the present theory links the functions of emotions to the classification produced, by showing how the functions of emotion can be understood in terms of the gene-specified reinforcers that produce different emotions (see Chapter 3).

An opposite approach to the dimensional or categorical approach is to attempt to describe the richness of every emotion (e.g. Ben-Ze'ev (2000)). Although it is important to understand the richness of every emotion, I believe that this is better performed with a set of underlying principles of the type set out above (in Section 2.2), rather than without any obvious principles to approach the subtlety of emotions.

2.6.4 Other approaches to emotion

LeDoux (LeDoux 1992, LeDoux 1995, LeDoux 1996) has described a theory of the neural basis of emotion that is probably conceptually similar to that of Rolls (Rolls 1975, Rolls 1986c, Rolls 1986a, Rolls 1990d, Rolls 1995b, Rolls 1999a, Rolls 2000f) (and this book), except that he focuses mostly on the role of the amygdala in emotion (and not on other brain regions such as the orbitofrontal cortex, which are poorly developed in the rat); except that he focuses mainly on fear (based on his studies of the role of the amygdala and related structures in fear conditioning in the rat); and except that he suggests from his neurophysiological findings that an important route for conditioned emotional stimuli to influence behaviour is via the subcortical inputs (especially auditory from the medial part of the medial geniculate nucleus of the thalamus) to the amygdala. This theory is discussed further on pages 169–170.

Panksepp's (1998) approach to emotion has its origins in neuroethological investigations of brainstem systems that when activated lead to behaviours like fixed action patterns, including escape, flight and fear behaviour. His views about consciousness include the postulate that "feelings may emerge when endogenous sensory and emotional systems within the brain that receive direct inputs from the outside world as well as the neurodynamics of the SELF (a Simple Ego-type Life Form) begin to reverberate with each other's changing neuronal firing rhythms" (Panksepp 1998) (p. 309).

Other approaches to emotion are summarized by Strongman (2003).

2.7 Individual differences in emotion, personality, and emotional intelligence

Hans J. Eysenck developed the theory that personality might be related to different aspects of conditioning. He analysed the factors that accounted for the variance in the differences between the personality of different humans (using, for example, questionnaires), and suggested that the first two factors in personality (those which accounted for most of the variance) were introversion vs extraversion, and neuroticism (related to a tendency to be anxious). He performed studies of classical conditioning on groups of subjects, and also obtained measures of what he termed arousal. Based on the correlations of these measures with the dimensions identified in the factor analysis, he suggested that introverts showed greater conditionability (to weak stimuli) and are more readily aroused by external stimulation than extraverts; and that neuroticism raises the general intensity of emotional reactions (see Eysenck and Eysenck (1968) and Eysenck and Eysenck (1985)).

Jeffrey A. Gray (1970) reinterpreted the findings, suggesting that introverts are more sensitive to punishment and frustrative non-reward than are extraverts; and that neuroticism reflects the extent of sensitivity to both reward and punishment (see Matthews and Gilliland (1999)). A related hypothesis is that extraverts may show enhanced learning in reward conditions, and may show enhanced processing of positively valent stimuli (Rusting and Larsen 1998). Matthews and Gilliland (1999), reviewing the evidence, show that there is some support for both hypotheses about introversion vs extraversion, namely that introverts may in general condition readily, and that extraverts may be relatively more responsive to reward stimuli (and correspondingly, introverts to punishers). However, Matthews and Gilliland (1999) go on to show that extraverts may perform less well at vigilance tasks (in which the subject must detect stimuli that occur with low probability); may tend to be more impulsive; and perform better when arousal is high (e.g. later in the day), and when rapid responses rather than reflective thought is needed (see also Matthews, Zeidner and Roberts (2002)). With respect to neuroticism and trait anxiety, anxious individuals tend to focus attention on potentially threatening information (punishers) at the cost of neglecting neutral or positive information sources; and may make more negative judgements, especially in evaluating self-worth and personal competence (Matthews, Zeidner and Roberts 2002).

More recent evidence comes from recent functional neuroimaging studies. For example, Canli, Sivers, Whitfield, Gotlib and Gabrieli (2002) have found that happy face expressions are more likely to activate the human amygdala in extraverts than in introverts. In addition, positively affective pictures interact with extraversion, and negatively affective pictures with neuroticism to produce activation of the amygdala (Canli, Zhao, Desmond, Kang, Gross and Gabrieli 2001, Hamann and Canli 2004). This supports the conceptually important point made above that part of the basis of personality may be differential sensitivity to different rewards and punishers, and omission and termination of different rewards and punishers.

The observations just described are consistent with the hypothesis that part of the basis of extraversion is increased reactivity to positively affective (as compared to negatively affective) face expressions and other positively affective stimuli including pictures. The exact mechanisms involved may be revealed in the future by genetic studies, and these might potentially address for example whether genes control responses to positively affective stimuli, or whether some more general personality trait by altering perhaps mood produces differential top-down biasing of face expression decoding systems in the way outlined in Section 4.10.

Another example is the impulsive behaviour that is a part of Borderline Personality Disorder (BPD), which could reflect factors such as less sensitivity to the punishers associated with waiting for rational processing to lead to a satisfactory solution, or changes in internal timing processes that lead to a faster perception of time (Berlin, Rolls and Kischka 2004, Berlin and Rolls 2004) (see Section 4.5.6). It was of considerable interest that the BPD group (mainly self-harming patients), as well as a group of patients with damage to the orbitofrontal cortex, scored highly on a Frontal Behaviour Questionnaire that assessed inappropriate behaviours typical of orbitofrontal cortex patients including disinhibition, social inappropriateness, perseveration, and uncooperativeness. In terms of measures of personality, using the Big Five personality measure, both groups were also less open to experience (i.e. less open-minded). In terms of other personality measures and characteristics, the orbitofrontal and BPD patients performed differently: BPD patients were less extraverted and conscientious and more neurotic and emotional than the orbitofrontal group (Berlin, Rolls and Kischka 2004, Berlin and Rolls 2004, Berlin, Rolls and Iversen 2005). Thus some aspects of personality, such as impulsiveness and being less open to experience, but not other aspects, such as extraversion, neuroticism and conscientiousness, were differentially related to orbitofrontal cortex function.

Daniel Goleman (1995) has popularized the concept of *emotional intelligence*. The rather sweeping definition given was "Emotional intelligence [includes] abilities such as being able to motivate oneself and persist in the face of frustrations, to control impulse and delay gratification; to regulate one's moods and keep distress from swamping the ability to think; to empathize and to hope" (Goleman (1995), p. 34).

One potential problem with this definition of emotional intelligence as an ability is that different aspects within this definition (such as impulse control and hope) may be unrelated, so a unitary ability described in this way seems unlikely. An excellent critical evaluation of the concept has been produced by Matthews, Zeidner and Roberts (2002). They note (p. 368) that in a rough and ready way, one might identify personality traits of emotional stability (low neuroticism), extraversion, agreeableness, and conscientiousness/self-control as dispositions that tend to facilitate everyday social interaction and to promote more positive emotion. (Indeed, one measure of emotional intelligence, the EQ-i (Bar-On 1997), has high correlations with some of the Big Five personality traits, especially, negatively, with neuroticism, and the EQ-i may reflect three constructs, self-esteem, empathy, and impulse control (Matthews et al. 2002).) But these personality traits are supposed to be independent, so linking them to a single ability of emotional intelligence is inconsistent. Moreover, this combination of personality traits might well not be adaptive in many circumstances, so the concept of this combination as an 'ability' is inappropriate (pp. 368–370).

However, the concept of emotional intelligence does appear to be related in a general way to the usage of the (mainly clinical) term 'alexithymia', in a sense the opposite, which includes the following components: (a) difficulty in identifying and describing emotions and distinguishing between feelings and the bodily sensations of arousal, (b) difficulty in describing feelings to other people, (c) constricted imaginal processes, as evidenced by a paucity of fantasies, and (d) a stimulus-bound externally oriented cognitive style, as evidenced by preoccupation with the details of external events rather than inner emotional experiences (Matthews et al. 2002). In terms of personality, alexithymia converges with the first three dimensions of the Five Factor Model of personality (FFM, the Big Five model), with high N (vulnerability to emotional distress), low E (low positive emotionality), and a limited range of imagination (low O) (Matthews et al. 2002). Indeed, alexithymia is strongly inversely correlated with measures of emotional intelligence, suggesting that emotional intelligence may be a new term that encompasses much of the opposite of what has been the important concept of alexithymia in the clinical literature for more than 20 years (Matthews et al. 2002). Alexithymics have difficulties in identifying face expressions (Lane, Sechrest, Reidel, Weldon, Kaszniak and Schwartz 1996), suggesting some impairments in the fundamental processing of emotion-related information, in particular capacities known to require the orbitofrontal and anterior cingulate cortices (Hornak, Bramham, Rolls, Morris, O'Doherty, Bullock and Polkey 2003). Consistently, it has been found that anterior cingulate cortex activation is correlated across individuals with their ability to recognize and describe emotions induced either by films or by the recall of personal experiences (Lane, Reiman, Axelrod, Yun, Holmes and Schwartz 1998). In summary, emotional intelligence, and what is largely its opposite, alexithymia, is probably not a particular ability, is not independent of existing personality measures, but does encompass a number of probably different ways in which individuals may differ in their emotion-related processing (Rolls 2007d).

I do not consider this research area in much more detail. However, I do point out that insofar as sensitivity to rewards and punishers, and the ability to learn and be influenced by rewards and punishers, may be important in personality, and are closely involved in emotion according to the theory developed here, there may be close links between the neural bases of emotion, to be described in Chapter 4, and personality. An extreme example might be that if humans were insensitive to social punishers following orbitofrontal cortex damage, we might expect social problems, and indeed Tranel, Bechara and Denburg (2002) have used the term 'acquired sociopathy' to describe some of these patients.

More generally, we might expect sensitivity to different types of reinforcer (including social reinforcers) to vary between individuals both as a result of gene variation and as a result of learning, and this, operating over a large number of different social reinforcers, might produce many different variations of personality based on the sensitivity to a large number of different reinforcers. Further, insofar as the functions of particular brain regions may be related to particular processes involved in emotion [with evidence for example that the human orbitofrontal cortex is involved in face expression decoding, and in impulsiveness, but not in some other aspects of personality (see Section 4.5.6)], then it may be possible in future to understand different particular modules for inter-relations between reward/punishment and personality systems.

The concept of the relation between differential sensitivity to different types of reward and punisher might produce individuals showing many types of conditional evolutionarily stable strategies (see footnote 19 on page 358), where the conditionality of the strategy might be influenced in different individuals by differential sensitivity to different rewards and punishers. Examples of behaviours that might be produced in this way are included in Chapter 9.

2.8   Cognition and Emotion

It may be noted that while the definition of emotions as states elicited by reinforcers (with particular functions) is operational, it should not be criticized as behaviourist (Katz 2000). For example, the definition has nothing to do with stimulus–response (habit) associations, but instead with a two-stage type of learning, in which a first stage is learning which environmental stimuli or events are associated with reinforcers, which potentially is a very rapid and flexible process; and a second stage produces appropriate instrumental and arbitrary actions performed in order to achieve the goal (which might be to obtain a reward or avoid a punisher). In the instrumental stage, animals learn about the outcomes of their actions (see Dickinson (1994), Pearce (1997)).

To determine what is a goal for an action, every type of cognitive operation may be involved. The proposal is that whatever cognitive operations are involved, then if the outcome is that a certain event, stimulus, thought (or any one of these remembered) leads to the evaluation that the event is a reward or punisher, then an emotion will be produced. So cognition is far from excluded.

Indeed, cognitive operations may produce emotions when operating at three levels of the architecture, as described more fully in Chapter 3. The first is the implicit level (see Fig. 10.4), where a primary reinforcer, or a stimulus or event associated with a primary reinforcer, may lead to emotions. The second level is where a (first order) syntactic symbol processing system performing "what ... if" computations to implement planning results in identification of a rewarding or punishing outcome. The third level is the higher order linguistic thought level described in Chapter 10, where thinking about and evaluating the operations of a first order linguistic processor may result in a reinforcing outcome such as "I should not spend further time thinking about that set of plans, as it would be better now to devote my linguistic resources (which are limited and serial) to this other set of plans".

Another way in which cognition influences emotion is that cognitive states, even at the level of language, can modulate subjective and brain responses to affective stimuli, as analysed in Section 4.5.5.7. There an experiment is described in which a word label ('cheese' vs 'body odour') influences the pleasantness ratings, and the activations in olfactory stages at least as early as the secondary olfactory cortex in the orbitofrontal cortex, to a standard test odour (De Araujo, Rolls, Velazco, Margot and Cayeux 2005). An implication of these findings is that language-based cognitive states can influence even relatively early cortical representations of rewards and punishers, and thus potentially modulate how much emotion is felt subjectively to an emotion-provoking stimulus.

I suggest that this top-down modulation occurs in a way that is exactly analogous to top-down attentional effects, which are believed to be implemented by a top-down biased competition mechanism (Rolls and Deco 2002, Deco and Rolls 2003, Deco and Rolls 2005b, Rolls and Stringer 2001b). In this case, the semantic, language-based, representation is the source of the biased competition, and the effect could be not only to bias the early cortical representation of a reward or punisher in one direction or another, but also by providing much or little top-down modulation, to influence how much emotion is felt (see Chapter 10), by modulating the processing of emotion-related stimuli (including remembered stimuli or events) at relatively early processing stages. This could be a mechanism by which cognition can influence how much emotion is felt under conditions in which emotions such as empathy and pity may occur, and when for example reading a novel, attending a play, listening to music, etc (see Section 11.4). Analysis of the mechanisms by which the top-down biased competition operates are becoming detailed (Desimone and Duncan 1995, Rolls and Deco 2002, Deco and Rolls 2003, Deco and Rolls 2004, Deco and Rolls 2005b), and are included in the model described in Appendix 2 in which a rule module exerts a top-down influence on neurons that represent stimulus–reward and stimulus–punisher combinations to influence which stimulus should currently be interpreted as reward-related (see also Deco and Rolls (2005d)).

Another way in which cognitive factors are related to emotion is that mood can affect cognitive processing, and one of the effects of this is to promote continuity of behaviour (see Chapter 3). One of the mechanisms described (in Section 4.10) utilizes backprojections to cortical areas from the amygdala and orbitofrontal cortex, so that reciprocal interactions between cognition and emotion are made possible.

2.9   Emotion, motivation, reward, and mood

It is useful to be clear about the difference between motivation, emotion, reward, and mood (cf. Rolls (2000f)). **Motivation** makes one work to obtain a reward, or work to escape from or avoid a punisher. One example of motivation is hunger, and another thirst, which in these cases are states set largely by internal homeostatically-related variables such as plasma glucose concentration and plasma osmolality. A reward is a stimulus or event that one works to obtain, such as food, and a punisher is what one works to escape from or avoid (or which suppresses an action on which its delivery is contingent), such as a painful stimulus or the sight of an object associated with a painful stimulus. Obtaining the reward or avoiding the punisher is the goal for the action. A motivational state is one in which a goal is *desired*. An **emotion** is a state elicited when a goal is obtained, that is by an instrumental reinforcer (i.e. a reward or punisher, or omission or termination of a reward or punisher), for example fear produced by the sight of the object associated with pain. This makes it clear that emotions are states elicited by rewards or punishers that have particular functions.

Of course, one of the functions of emotions is that they are motivating, as exemplified by the case of the fear produced by the sight of the object that can produce pain, which motivates one to avoid receiving the painful stimulus, which is the goal for the action. In that emotion-provoking stimuli or events produce motivation, then arousal is likely to occur, especially for reinforcers that lead to the active initiation of actions. However, arousal alone is not sufficient to define motivation or emotion, in that the motivational state must specify the particular type of goal that is the object of the motivational state, such as water if we are thirsty, food if we are hungry, and avoidance of the painful unconditioned stimulus signalled by a fear-inducing conditioned stimulus.

A **mood** is a continuing state normally elicited by a reinforcer, and is thus part of what is an emotion. The other part of an emotion is the decoding of the stimulus in terms of whether it is a reward or punisher, that is, of what causes the emotion, or in philosophical terminology of what the emotion is about or the object of the emotion. Mood states help to implement some of the persistence-related functions of emotion, can continue when the originating stimulus may be forgotten (by the explicit system described in Chapter 10), and may occur spontaneously not because such spontaneous mood swings may have been selected for, but because of the difficulty of maintaining stability of the neuronal firing that implements mood (or affective) state (see *The Brain and Emotion*, Rolls (1999a), pp. 62, 66). Mood states are thus not necessarily about an object.

Thus, motivation may be seen as a state in which one is working for a goal, and emotion as a state that occurs when the goal, a reinforcer, is obtained, and that may persist afterwards. The concept of gene-defined reinforcers providing the goals for action helps to understand the relation between motivational states (or desires) and emotion, as the organism must be built to be motivated to obtain the goals, and to be placed in a different state (emotion) when the goal is or is not achieved by the action. Emotional states may be motivating, as in frustrative non-reward. The close but clear relation between motivation and emotion is that both involve what humans describe as affective states (e.g. feeling hungry, liking the taste of a food, feeling happy because of a social reinforcer), and both are about goals. The Darwinian theory of the functions of emotion developed in Chapter 3 which shows how emotion is adaptive because it reflects the operation of a process by which genes define goals for action applies just as much to motivation (see further Section 3.6), in that emotion can be thought of as states elicited by goals (rewards and punishers), and motivation can be thought of as states elicited when goals are being sought. By specifying goals the genes must specify both that we must be motivated to obtain those goals, and that when the goals are obtained, further states, emotional states with further functions, are produced.

2.10   Is the concept of emotion still useful when we understand its mechanisms?

Kralik and Hauser (2000) ask whether it is helpful to maintain the concept of an emotional state when one starts to understand the mechanisms of reward and punisher decoding, the selection of actions, etc. My view is that emotion is a helpful concept, for a number of reasons.

First, the state is produced by clearly defined stimuli (see above).

Second, the state has many different functions, summarized in Chapter 3, so that a model in which a stimulus is connected to a single output is inappropriate. In these circumstances, an intervening state that implements many functions is useful.

Third, one of the functions of emotion is to support the selection of any appropriate action to a reward or punisher, or its omission or termination, as in two-process learning. In the first stage, an emotional state is produced, and in the second stage, any action is selected that is appropriate given the emotional state. For example, if fear is the emotional state produced by a pain-associated stimulus, an action will be selected to escape from or avoid the emotion-provoking stimulus. In that emotion is a state that guides the elicitation of an action to a stimulus, the emotional state is not itself a behavioural response.

Fourth, other functions of emotional states include the biasing of cognitive function to influence the interpretation of future events, which is clearly not a response.

Fifth, emotional states have the important properties that they persist for times in the order of minutes or hours, thus maintaining persistence of behaviour and consistency of action even after the emotion-provoking stimulus has disappeared.

Sixth, the concept of emotional states just described maps neatly onto folk-psychological concepts of emotions, and provides a convenient conceptual level that bridges to the low-level description of exactly how the stimuli are decoded to elicit the state, how the state is maintained, and how it performs its many functions.

The concept of an emotional state is thus clearly defined in terms of how stimuli elicit the state, and of the many functions of the state including the selection of action. Emotional states are not the stimuli themselves, nor the stimulus decoding, nor the responses finally selected, but consist of on-going states elicited by stimuli in the way described, and performing the functions described. We are indeed starting to understand how the different types of processing involved are implemented in the brain, and these are some of the types of advance described in *The Brain and Emotion* (Rolls 1999a) and in this book. But understanding the implementation of the processes involved in emotion does not mean that emotion itself as a useful concept at its own level will disappear.

In addition, understanding 'how' emotion works will not address a number of important questions about emotion, including the 'why' questions about for example the evolutionary adaptive value of emotions (see Section 3.1).

2.11 Advantages of the approach to emotion described here (Rolls' theory of emotion)

I now evaluate the advantages of and justifications for starting with the concept that emotions are states elicited by instrumental reinforcers, even though one proposes that a full definition requires the principles summarized in section 2.2, and incorporating a statement of the functions elicited by those states.

One advantage is that this definition in terms of rewards and punishers may provide a concise operational definition of the environmental stimuli or events that actually lead to emotions. If we can agree that the environmental conditions that lead to emotions are those that can be described as rewarding or punishing, and that those that are not rewards or punishers do not lead to states that are described as emotional, then we are a long way forward in producing a conceptualization of what emotions may be. No commentators on the *Précis of The Brain and Emotion* (Rolls 2000f) actually produced clear exceptions to this correspondence. If we accept this operational definition, it provides us with a powerful way forward to start to examine emotions (because we accept that they are states elicited by rewards or punishers, and have a useful delimitation of what events produce emotion). This leads directly to an analysis of the brain mechanisms that implement emotions as those brain mechanisms that decode environmental stimuli as primary reinforcers, those brain mechanisms that implement stimulus–reinforcer association learning, and the brain mechanisms that link the resulting emotional states to actions.

A second advantage of this definition is that it enables us to see emotions in the context of what I propose is their most important function, namely as a way to provide a mechanism for the genes to influence behaviour in a brain that evolves by gene selection. It is argued in Chapter 3 that the genes do this by specifying the stimuli or events that the animal is built to find rewarding or punishing, i.e. to find reinforcing, so that the genes specify the goals for action, not the actions themselves. The definition of emotions as states elicited by reinforcers thus links directly to the Darwinian theory I propose for why we have emotions, which is that some genes specify reinforcers, that is goals for action, that will increase the fitness of these genes. It is these particular genes that specify reinforcers that provide the foundation I propose for emotional states. The definition of emotion in terms of states elicited by reinforcers should not be seen thus as behaviourist, but instead as part of a much broader theory that takes an adaptive, Darwinian, approach to the functions of emotion, and how they are important in brain design (see Section 3.5).

A third advantage is that the definition offers a principled way to approach emotion. Different emotions can be classified and understood in terms of different reinforcement contingencies and different reinforcers, and hence directly in terms of their functions. This is recommended as being more advantageous than categorizing emotions based on clusters of variables or factors that result from multidimensional analysis of questionnaires etc, or by correlation with autonomic or face expression measures, which do not lead directly to an understanding of the different functions of different emotions (and run the risk of producing seven plus or minus two categories, cf. Miller (1956)), as described in section 2.6.3. This definition of emotion also leads to an operational, and thus clearly specified, approach to emotions, whereas approaches such as appraisal theory may suffer from the disadvantage that they quickly become somewhat under-specified and intractable, as described in section 2.6.2. Moreover, this principled way of understanding emotions provides a systematic and fundamental way to approach the brain mechanisms involved in emotion, in that brain regions involved in decoding primary reinforcers, and brain regions involved in learning associations of events to primary reinforcers, can be seen to have a clear information-processing role in emotion. Analysing the information processing performed by each connected stage in the brain provides a fruitful approach to understanding neural computation (Rolls and Treves 1998, Rolls and Deco 2002).

In the context of emotion, this approach is also more principled and systematic than identifying categories of (sometimes ethologically described) behaviour such as playfulness and aggression, and looking for brain centres specialized for each category of behaviour (cf. Panksepp (1998)). The specification of actions such as fixed action patterns (in contrast to goals) by genes is not only genetically expensive, but having brain regions specialized for actions (such as playfulness and rage, cf Panksepp (1998)) would lead to a multitude of specialized brain action/emotion systems, with potentially one for every possible type of emotional response. In contrast, specifying emotions as states elicited by reinforcers leaves open and flexible the particular action that may be taken in particular circumstances, and has the great advantage of economy of genetic specification (the genes need only specify what is rewarding and punishing). (Of course, as described above, the type of coping by actions that is possible may influence the emotional state, as in the case of sadness vs anger.)

Specifying emotions in terms of the types of rewards and punishers that elicit the emotion may of course also lead to spatially separated brain systems especially involved in different types of emotion, for the primary reinforcers (such as taste, touch, pain, the failure to receive an expected reward, or a face expression, and learning about these reinforcers) may be decoded and represented in different brain regions. This is because of their different input pathways to the brain, and the utility of forming representations to the object level within each sensory modality before reward value is made explicit in the representation, leading to some specialization of different brain regions and systems in different types of emotion (see Chapter 4).

A fourth advantage of conceptualizing emotions as states elicited by reinforcers is that this provides an immediate way into understanding the relation between emotion and personality (see section 2.7).

A complex issue related to one's definition of emotion is where the boundaries for emotional states should be set. Should our definition result in emotions being states that occur in invertebrates such as Aplysia, as suggested by Kupferman (2000)? My own answer to this is to set off from emotions those behaviours that are performed with fixed responses, that is without the possibility for selecting arbitrary types of behaviour as the goals for actions (see Chapter 3). Such fixed-response behaviours include taxes, such as might be performed by a single cell organism swimming up a chemical gradient towards a source of nutrient. One reason why these types of behaviour with fixed responses are excluded from emotion (though they may be forerunners to it) is that the behaviour does not occur by elicitation of a persistent or continuing state to a reinforcing stimulus that provides the motivation for (arbitrary) instrumental responses to obtain the goal. (That an instrumental (or operant) response is being made is demonstrated most precisely by the bidirectional criterion that either a response, or its opposite, may be performed as an action to obtain a goal.) It is the intervening persistent state elicited by reinforcing stimuli and the ability to allow stimuli to be interfaced to arbitrary instrumental responses or actions that is one of the prime functions of emotion described here (see Chapter 3), and is therefore incorporated into the definition of emotion. The definition thus provides a clear way of dividing states into emotional or not, as it includes only those states that allow instrumental learning, that is arbitrary actions to be performed to obtain reinforcing outcomes (such as obtaining rewards and avoiding punishers). Although animals that do not perform instrumental learning may not qualify according to this criterion as having emotions, they may of course have states that are precursors to emotions. This discussion thus leads to one possible way to separate animals that have emotions from those that do not, a way that is related to one of the fundamental functions of emotion, but it is realised that the separation made at this point should be seen as a useful separating point with a clear principle underlying it, but not a separating point that need be thought of as more than a useful convention in this context.

3 The functions of emotion: reward, punishment, and emotion in brain design

3.1 Introduction

We now confront the fundamental issue of why we, and other animals, are built to have emotions, as well as motivational states. I will propose that it is because we (and many other animals) use rewards and punishers to guide or determine our behaviour, and that this is a good design for a system that is built by genes where some of the genes are increasing their survival by specifying the goals for behaviour. The emotions arise and are an inherent part of such a system because they are the states, typically persisting, that are elicited by the rewards and punishers. I will show that this is a very adaptive way for evolution to design complex animals without having to specify the details of the behavioural responses.

What results from this analysis is thus a thoroughly Darwinian theory (though not anticipated by Darwin, and operating at the level of individual genes) that places emotion at the heart of brain design because it reflects the way in which genes build our brains in such a way that our genes can specify the goals of our actions, and thus what we do. There is thus a close conceptual link between instrumental learning and emotion, for primary reinforcers (primary rewards and punishers) are the gene-specified goals for our actions, and we use instrumental learning to learn any actions during our life-times that will lead to the gene-specified goals.

In Section 3.2, I outline several types of brain design, with differing degrees of complexity, and suggest that evolution can operate much better with only some of these types of design.

Understanding the functions of emotion is important not only for understanding the nature of emotions, but also for understanding the different brain systems involved in the different types of response that are produced by emotional states. Indeed, answers to 'why' questions in nature (for example, 'Why do we have emotions? What are the functions of emotion?') are important, as are answers to 'how' questions (for example, 'How is emotion implemented in the brain? How do disorders of emotion arise, and how can they be understood and treated?').

In this book, the question of why we have emotions is a fundamental issue that I answer in terms of a Darwinian, functional, approach, producing the answer that emotions are states elicited by goals (rewards and punishers), and that this is part of an adaptive process by which genes can specify the behaviour of the animal by specifying goals for behaviour rather than fixed responses. I believe that this is approach leads to a fundamental understanding of why we have emotions which is likely to stand the test of time, in the same way that Darwinian thinking itself provides a fundamental way of understanding biology and many 'why' questions about life.

While considering 'why' (or 'ultimate') questions (which are important in their own right, and will not be answered by answers to 'how' or 'proximate' questions), it may be helpful to place into perspective the approaches taken to understanding the adaptive value of behaviour (Tinbergen 1963) that have led to sociobiology (Wilson 1975) and evolutionary psychology (see Buss (1999)). These approaches are relevant to understanding why we have emotions, including many of the issues discussed in Chapter 9 on sexual behaviour. 'Adaptation' refers to characteristics of living organisms – such as their colour, shape, physiology, and behaviour – that enable them to survive and reproduce successfully in the environments in which they live (Dawkins 1995).

Sociobiology and evolutionary psychology have sometimes been criticized as producing 'just-so' stories in which the purported adaptive explanation for a behaviour seems too facile and untestable (Gould and Lewontin 1979), but we should note that there are rigorous approaches to testing evolutionary hypotheses for the adaptive value of a behaviour or other characteristic (see Dawkins (1995), Chapter 1). The tests include the following:

1. *Making use of existing genetic variation.* A famous example is that of the peppered moth, *Biston betularia*. In its dark form it is found to survive better than the light form when both are released into industrial areas in which the genetically specified black form is better camouflaged (Kettlewell 1955).

2. *Using artificially produced variation.* The variation could be genetically produced, or variation produced in the testing conditions in an experiment. Using the latter approach, Tinbergen, Broekhuysen, Feekes, Houghton, Kruuk and Szule (1967) showed that black-headed gulls' newly born chicks survive better if the parents remove broken egg shells to a good distance from the nest. This supports the hypothesis that the behaviour is adaptive because removing the shells, which are white inside, makes the nest less conspicuous to predators.

3. *The comparative method.* Comparing species in which a trait has evolved genetically and independently can provide good evidence at the correlative level. For example, kittiwakes do not remove hatched egg shells from their nest, and in contrast with black-headed gulls, this is related to the fact that kittiwakes nest in places on cliffs that are inaccessible even to other birds (Cullen 1957).

4. *Adaptation through design features.* If it can be shown that design features such as the bat sonar echolocation system are very well suited to detecting small animals of prey such as moths, then that provides some evidence that the features are genetically selected because of their adaptive value. Even more telling are examples where the behaviour is not as adaptive as it might be – for example, in some schooling fish, the spacing during swimming is not hydrodynamically optimal, and this implies that the details of the behaviour are under selective pressure other than only swimming efficiency (Dawkins 1995).

Thus adaptive accounts of behaviour can be tested, and need not be 'just-so' stories.

We should also note that by no means all behaviour reflects optimal adaptation (see Dawkins (1982) Chapter 3, 'Constraints on Perfection'), for six reasons:

1. There is a *time lag*, and present animals may have evolved under somewhat different selection pressures.

2. *Historical constraints*, which can be important in that natural selection always operates in an 'adaptive landscape' with local optima, not global optima (i.e. natural selection can improve an existing animal, but cannot start from nothing and build towards a particular overall design).

3. *Available genetic variation*, an example of which is that it has not proved possible to breed cattle with more female (cows) than male (bulls) offspring.

4. *Constraints of costs and materials.*

5. Imperfections at one level due to *selection at another level.* An important point here is that evolution through natural selection can be best understood not at the level of what is adaptive for the group or species, but at the level of what increases the fitness of the genes.

6. Mistakes due to *environmental unpredictability* or 'malevolence'. Genes must specify behaviour that is on average good for them, and there are limited numbers of genes that influence behaviour. These constraints mean that genes cannot take into account all possible combinations of environmental contingencies that may arise.

3.2   Brain design and the functions of emotion

3.2.1   Taxes, rewards, and punishers: gene-specified goals for actions, and the flexibility of actions

3.2.1.1   Taxes

A simple design principle is to incorporate mechanisms for taxes into the design of organisms. Taxes consist at their simplest of orientation towards stimuli in the environment, for example the bending of a plant towards light that results in maximum light collection by its photosynthetic surfaces. (When just turning rather than locomotion is possible, such responses are called tropisms.) With locomotion possible, as in animals, taxes include movements towards sources of nutrient, and movements away from hazards such as very high temperatures. The design principle here is that animals have, through a process of natural selection, built receptors for certain dimensions of the wide range of stimuli in the environment, and have linked these receptors to response mechanisms in such a way that the stimuli are approached or escaped from.

3.2.1.2   Rewards and punishers

As soon as we have approach to stimuli at one end of a dimension (e.g. a source of nutrient) and away from stimuli at the other end of the dimension (in this case lack of nutrient), we can start to wonder when it is appropriate to introduce the terms 'rewards' and 'punishers' for the stimuli at the different ends of the dimension. By convention, if the response consists of a fixed response to obtain the stimulus (e.g. locomotion up a chemical gradient), we shall call this a taxis not a reward. On the other hand, if an arbitrary operant response can be performed by the animal in order to approach the stimulus, then we will call this rewarded behaviour, and the stimulus that the animal works to obtain a reward. (The arbitrary operant response can be thought of as any arbitrary response the animal will perform to obtain the stimulus. It can be thought of as an action.) This criterion, of an arbitrary operant response, is often tested by bidirectionality. For example, if a rat can be trained to either raise its tail, or lower its tail, in order to obtain a piece of food, then we can be sure that there is no fixed relationship between the stimulus (e.g. the sight of food) and the response, as there is in a taxis. Some authors reserve the term 'motivated behaviour' for that in which an arbitrary operant response will be performed to obtain a reward or to escape from or avoid a punisher. If this criterion is not met, and only a fixed response can be performed, then the term 'drive' can be used to describe the state of the animal when it will work to obtain or escape from the stimulus.

We can thus distinguish a first level of approach/avoidance mechanism complexity in a taxis, with a fixed response available for the stimulus, from a second level of complexity in which any arbitrary response (or action) can be performed, in which case we use the term reward when a stimulus is being approached, and punisher when the action is to escape from or avoid the stimulus.

The role of natural selection in this process is to guide animals to build sensory systems that will respond to dimensions of stimuli in the natural environment along which actions of the animals can lead to better survival to enable genes to be passed on to the next generation, which is what we mean by fitness[7]. The animals must be built by such natural selection to perform actions that will enable them to obtain more rewards, that is to work to obtain stimuli that will increase their fitness. Correspondingly, animals must be built to perform actions that will enable them to escape from, or avoid when learning mechanisms are introduced, stimuli that will reduce their fitness. There are likely to be many dimensions of environmental stimuli along which actions of the animal can alter fitness. Each of these dimensions may be a separate reward–punisher dimension. An example of one of these dimensions might be food reward. It increases fitness to be able to sense nutrient need, to have sensors that respond to the taste of food, and to perform behavioural responses to obtain such reward stimuli when in that need or motivational state. Similarly, another dimension is water reward, in which the taste of water becomes rewarding when there is body-fluid depletion (see Rolls and Rolls (1982a), Rolls (1999a), and Chapter 6).

One aspect of the operation of these reward–punisher systems that these examples illustrate is that with very many reward–punisher dimensions for which actions may be performed, there is a need for a selection mechanism for actions performed to these different dimensions. In this sense, rewards and punishers provide a common currency that provides one set of inputs to action selection mechanisms. Evolution must set the magnitudes of each of the different reward systems so that each will be chosen for action in such a way as to maximize overall fitness. Food reward must be chosen as the aim for action if some nutrient depletion is present, but water reward as a target for action must be selected if current water depletion poses a greater threat to fitness than does the current degree of food depletion. This indicates that for a competitive selection process for rewards, each reward must be carefully calibrated in evolution to have the right value in the common currency in the selection process. Other types of behaviour, such as sexual behaviour, must be performed sometimes, but probably less frequently, in order to maximize fitness (as measured by gene transmission into the next generation).

There are many processes that contribute to increasing the chances that a wide set of different environmental rewards will be chosen over a period of time, including not only need-related satiety mechanisms that reduce the rewards within a dimension, but also sensory-specific satiety mechanisms, which facilitate switching to another reward stimulus (sometimes within and sometimes outside the same main dimension), and attraction to novel stimuli. (As noted in Sections 3.4.6 and 4.6.5, attraction to novel stimuli, i.e. finding them rewarding, is one way that organisms are encouraged to explore the multidimensional space within which their genes are operating. The suggestion is that animals should be built to find somewhat novel stimuli rewarding, for this encourages them to explore new parts of the environment in which their genes might do better than others' genes. Unless animals are built to find novelty somewhat rewarding, the multidimensional genetic space being explored by genes in

---

[7] Fitness refers to the fitness of genes, but this must be measured by the effects that the genes have on the organism.

the course of evolution might not find the appropriate environment in which they might do better than others' genes.)

3.2.1.3 Stimulus–response learning reinforced by rewards and punishers

In this second level of complexity, involving reward or punishment, learning may occur. If an organism performs trial-and-error responses, and as the result of performing one particular response is more likely to obtain a reward, then the response may become linked by a learning process to that stimulus as a result of the reward received. The reward is said to reinforce the response to that stimulus, and we have what is described as stimulus–response or habit learning. The reward acts as a positive reinforcer in that it increases the probability of a response on which it is made contingent. A punisher reduces the probability of a response on which it is made contingent. (It should be noted that this is an operational definition, and that there is no implication that the punisher feels like anything – the punisher just has in the learning mechanism to reduce the probability of responses followed by the punisher.) Stimulus–response or habit learning is typically evident after over-training, and once habits are being executed, the behaviour becomes somewhat independent of the reward value of the goal, as shown in experiments in which the reward is devalued. This is described in more detail in Section 4.6.1 on page 149.

3.2.1.4 Stimulus–reinforcer association learning, and two-factor learning theory

Two-process learning introduces a third level of complexity and capability into the ways in which behaviour can be guided. Rewards and punishers still provide the basis for guiding behaviour within a dimension, and for selecting the dimension towards which action should be directed.

The first stage of the learning is stimulus–reinforcer association learning, in which the reinforcing value of a previously neutral, e.g. visual or auditory, stimulus is learned because of its association with a primary reinforcer, such as a sweet taste or a painful touch. This learning is of an association between one stimulus, the conditioned or secondary reinforcer, and the primary reinforcer, and is thus stimulus–stimulus association learning. This stimulus–reinforcer learning can be very fast, in as little as one trial. For example, if a new visual stimulus is placed in the mouth and a sweet taste is obtained, a simple approach response such as reaching for the object will be made on the next trial. Moreover, this stimulus–reinforcer association learning can be reversed very rapidly. For example, if subsequently the object is made to taste of salt, then approach no longer occurs to the stimulus, and the stimulus is even likely to be actively pushed away.

The second process or stage in this type of learning is instrumental learning of an operant response made in order to obtain the stimulus now associated with reward (or avoid a stimulus associated by learning with the punisher). This is action–outcome learning. The outcome could be a primary reinforcer, but often involves a secondary reinforcer learned by stimulus–reinforcer association learning. The action–outcome learning may be much slower, for it may involve trial-and-error learning of which action is successful in enabling the animal to obtain the stimulus now associated with reward or avoid the stimulus now associated with a punisher. However, this second stage may be greatly speeded if an operant response or strategy that has been learned previously to obtain a different type of reward (or avoid a different punisher) can be used to obtain (or avoid) the new stimulus now known to be associated with reinforcement. It is in this flexibility of the response that two-factor learning has a great advantage over stimulus–response learning. The advantage is that any response (even, at its simplest, approach or withdrawal) can be performed once an association has been learned between a stimulus and a primary reinforcer. This flexibility in the response is much more adaptive (and could provide the difference between survival or not) than no learning, as in taxes, or stimulus–response learning. The different processes that are involved in instrumental learning are described in more detail in Section 4.6.1.

Another key advantage of this type of two-stage learning is that after the first stage the different rewards and punishers available in an environment can be compared in a selection mechanism, using the common currency of rewards and punishers for the comparison and selection process. In this type of system, the many dimensions of rewards and punishers are again the basis on which the selection of a behaviour to perform is made.

Part of the process of evolution can be seen as identifying the factors or dimensions that affect the fitness of an animal, and providing the animal with sensors that lead to rewards and punishers that are tuned to the environmental dimensions that influence fitness. The example of sweet taste receptors being set up by evolution to provide reward when physiological nutrient need is present has been given above.

We can ask whether there would need to be a separate sensing mechanism tuned to provide primary (unlearned) reinforcers for every dimension of the environment to which it may be important to direct behaviour. (The behaviour has to be directed to climb up the reward gradient to obtain the best reward, or to climb a gradient up and away from punishers.) It appears that there may not be. For example, in the case of the so-called specific appetites, for perhaps a particular vitamin lacking in the diet, it appears that a type of stimulus–reinforcer association learning may actually be involved, rather than having every possible flavour set up to be a primary reward or punisher. The way that this happens is by a form of association learning. If an animal deficient in one nutrient is fed a food with that nutrient, it turns out that the animal 'feels better' some time after ingesting the new food, and associates this 'feeling better' with the taste of that particular food. Later, that food will be chosen. The point here is that the first time the animal is in the deficient state and tastes the new food, that food may not be chosen instead of other foods. It is only after the post-ingestive conditioning that, later, that particular food will be selected (Rozin and Kalat 1971). Thus in addition to a number of specific primary (unlearned) reward systems (e.g. sweet taste for nutrient need, salt taste for salt deficiency, pain for potentially damaging somatosensory stimulation), there may be great opportunity for other arbitrary sensory stimuli to become conditioned rewards or punishers by association with some quite general change in physiological state. Another example to clarify this might be the way in which a build-up of carbon dioxide is aversive. If we are swimming deep, we may need to come to the surface in order to expel carbon dioxide (and obtain oxygen), and we may indeed find it very rewarding to obtain the fresh air. Does this mean that we have a specific reward/punisher system for carbon dioxide that can directly guide our actions towards a goal? It may be that too much carbon dioxide has been conditioned to be a negative reinforcer or punisher, because we feel so much better after we have breathed out the carbon dioxide. The implication here is that a number of bodily signals can influence a general bodily state, and we learn to improve the general state, rather than to treat the signal as a specific reinforcer that directs us to a particular goal. Another example might be social reinforcers. It would be difficult to build-in a primary reinforcer system for every possible type of social reinforcer. Instead, there may be a number of rather general primary social reinforcers, such as acceptance within a group, approbation, greeting, face expression, and pleasant touch which are among the primary rewards by association with which other stimuli become secondary social reinforcers.

To help specify the way in which stimulus–reinforcer association learning operates, a list of what may be in at least some species primary reinforcers is provided in Table 2.1 on page 18. The reader will doubtless be able to add to this list, and it may be that some of the reinforcers in the list are actually secondary reinforcers. The reinforcers are categorized where possible by modality, to help the list to be systematic. Possible dimensions to which each reinforcer is tuned are suggested.

3.2.2   Explicit systems, language, and reinforcement

A fourth level of complexity to the way in which behaviour is guided is by processing that includes syntactic operations on semantically grounded symbols (see Section 10.2). This allows multistep one-off plans to be formulated. Such a plan might be: if I do this, then B is likely to do this, C will probably do this, and then X will be the outcome. Such a process cannot be performed by an animal that works just to obtain a reward, or secondary reinforcers. The process may enable an available reward to be deferred for another reward that a particular multistep strategy could lead to. What are the roles of rewards and punishers in such a system?

The language system can still be considered to operate to obtain rewards and avoid punishers. This is not merely a matter of definition, for many of the rewards and punishers will be the same as those described above, those which have been tuned by evolution to the dimensions of the environment that can enable an animal to increase fitness. The processing afforded by language can be seen as providing a new type of strategy to obtain such gene-specified rewards or avoid such punishers. If this were not generally the case, then the use of the language system would not be adaptive: it would not increase fitness.

However, once a language system has evolved, a consequence may be that certain new types of reward become possible. These may be related to primary reinforcers already present, but may develop beyond them. For example, music may have evolved from the system of non-verbal communication that enables emotional states to be communicated to others. An example might be that lullabies could be related to emotional messages that can be sent from parents to offspring to soothe them. Music with a more military character might be related to the sounds given as social signals to each other in situations in which fighting (or co-operation in fighting) might occur. The prosodic quality of voice expression may be part of the same emotion communication system, and brain systems that are activated by prosody may be strongly engaged in women even in tasks that do not require prosody to be analysed (Schirmer, Zysset, Kotz and von Cramon 2004). Then on top of this, the intellectualization afforded by linguistic (syntactic) processing would contribute further aspects to music. Another example here is that solving problems by intellectual means should itself be a primary reinforcer as a result of evolution, for this would encourage the use of intellectual abilities that have potential advantage if used. A further set of examples of how, when a language system is present, there is the possibility for further types of reinforcer, comes from the possibility that the evolution of some mental abilities may have been influenced by sexual selection (see Section 9.6.2).

3.2.3 Special-purpose design by an external agent vs evolution by natural selection

The above mechanisms, which operate in an evolutionary context to enable animals' behaviour to be tuned to increase fitness by evolving reward–punisher systems tuned to dimensions in the environment that increase fitness, may be contrasted with typical engineering design. In the latter, we may want to design a robot to work on an assembly line. Here there is an external designer, the engineer, who defines the function to be performed by the robot (e.g. picking a nut from a box, and attaching it to a particular bolt in the object being assembled). The engineer then produces special-purpose design features that enable the robot to perform this task, by for example providing it with sensors and an arm to enable it to select a nut, and to place the nut in the correct position in the 3D space of the object to enable the nut to be placed on the bolt and tightened. This contrast with a real animal allows us to see important differences between these types of control for the behaviour of the system.

In the case of the animal, there is a multidimensional space within which many optimizations to increase fitness must be performed. The solution to this is to evolve multiple reward–punisher systems tuned to each dimension in the environment that can lead to an increased fitness if the animal performs the appropriate actions. Natural selection guides evolution to find these dimensions. In contrast, in the robot arm, there is an externally defined behaviour to be performed, of placing the nut on the bolt, and the robot does not need to tune itself to find the goal to be performed. The contrast is between design by evolution that is 'blind' to the purpose of the animal, and design by a designer who specifies the job to be performed (cf. Dawkins (1986b)).

Another contrast is that for the animal the space will be high-dimensional, so that selection of the most appropriate reward for current behaviour (taking into account the costs of obtaining each reward) is needed, whereas for the robot arm, the function to perform at any one time is specified by the designer. Another contrast is that the behaviour, that is the instrumental action, that is most appropriate to obtain the reward must be selected by the animal, whereas the movement to be made by the robot arm is specified by the design engineer.

The implication of this comparison is that operation by animals using reward and punisher systems tuned to dimensions of the environment that increase fitness provides a mode of operation that can work in organisms that evolve by natural selection. It is clearly a natural outcome of Darwinian evolution to operate using reward and punisher systems tuned to fitness-related dimensions of the environment, if arbitrary responses are to be made by the animals rather than just preprogrammed movements such as are involved in tropisms and taxes. Is there any alternative to such a reward–punisher-based system in this evolution by natural selection situation? I am not clear that there is. This may be the reason why we are built to work for rewards, avoid punishers, have emotions, and feel needs (motivational states). These concepts start to bear on developments in the field of artificial life (see, e.g. Boden (1996)).

The sort of question that some philosophers might ponder is whether if life evolved on Mars it would have emotions. My answer to this is 'Yes', if the organisms have evolved genetically by natural selection, and the genes have elaborated behavioural mechanisms to maximize their fitness in a flexible way, which as I have just argued would imply that they have evolved reward and punisher systems that guide behaviour. They would have emotions in the sense introduced in Chapter 2, in that they would have states that would be produced by rewards or punishers, or by stimuli associated with rewards and punishers (Rolls 2002, Rolls 2005). It is of course a rather larger question to ask whether our extraterrestrial organisms would have emotional feelings. My answer to this arises out of the theory of consciousness introduced in Chapter 10, and would be 'Only if the organisms have a linguistic system that can think about and correct their first order linguistic thoughts'. However, even if such higher-order thought processes are present, it is worth considering whether emotional feelings might despite these higher-order thoughts not be present. After all, we know that much behaviour can be guided unconsciously, implicitly, by rewards and punishers. My answer to this issue is that the organisms would have emotional feelings; for as suggested above, the explicit system has to work in general for rewards of the type that are rewarding to the implicit system, and for the explicit system to be guided towards solutions that increase fitness, it should feel good when the explicit system works to a correct solution. Otherwise, it is difficult to explain how the explicit system is guided towards solutions that are not only solutions to problems, but that are also solutions that tend to have adaptive value. If the system has evolved so that it feels like something when it is performing higher-order thought processing, then it seems likely that it would feel like something when it obtained a reward or punisher, for this is the way that the explicit, conscious, thoughts would be guided (see Chapter 10 for further explanation).

3.3   Selection of behaviour: cost–benefit 'analysis'

One advantage of a design based on rewards and punishers is that the decoding of stimuli to a reward or punisher value provides a common currency for the mechanism that selects which behavioural action should be performed. Thus, for example, a moderately sweet taste when little hunger is present would have a smaller reward value than the taste of water when thirst is present. An action-selection mechanism could thus include in its specification competition between the different rewards, all represented in a common currency, with the most rewarding stimulus being that most likely to be selected for action. As described above, to make sure that different types of reward are selected when appropriate, natural selection would need to ensure that different types of reward would operate on similar scales (from minimum to maximum), so that each type of reward would be selected if it reaches a high value on its scale. Mechanisms such as sensory-specific satiety can be seen as contributing usefully to this mechanism which ensures that different types of reward will be selected for action.

However, the action selection mechanisms must take into account not only the relative value of each type of reward, but also the cost of obtaining each type of reward. If there is a very high cost of obtaining a particular reward, it may be better, at least temporarily, until the situation changes, to select an action that leads to a smaller reward, but is less costly. It appears that animals do operate according to such a cost–benefit analysis, in that if there is a high cost for an action, that action is less likely to be performed. One example of this comes from the fighting of deer. A male deer is less likely to fight another if he is clearly inferior in size or signalled prowess (Dawkins 1995).

There may also be a cost to switching behaviour. If the sources of food and water are very distant, it would be costly to switch behaviour (and perhaps walk a mile) every time a mouthful of food or a mouthful of water was swallowed. This may be part of the adaptive value of incentive motivation or the 'salted nut' phenomenon — that after one reward is given early on in working for that reward the incentive value of that reward may increase. This may be expressed in the gradually increasing rate of working for food early on in a meal. By increasing the reward value of a stimulus for the first minute or two of working for it, hysteresis may be built into the behaviour selection mechanism, to make behaviour 'stick' to one reward for at least a short time once it is started.

When one refers to a 'cost–benefit analysis', one does not necessarily mean at all that the animal thinks about it and plans with 'if ... then' multistep linguistic processing the benefits and costs of each possible course of action. Instead, in many cases 'cost–benefit analysis' is likely to be built into animals to be performed with simple implicit processing or rules. One example would be the incentive motivation just described, which provides a mechanism for an animal to persist for at least a short time in one behaviour without having to explicitly plan to do this by performing as an individual a cost–benefit analysis of the relative advantages and costs of continuing or switching. Another example might be the way in which the decision to fight is made by male deer: the decision may be based on simple processes such as reducing the probability of fighting if the other individual is larger, rather than thinking through the consequences of fighting or not on this occasion. Thus, many of the costs and benefits or rewards that are taken into account in the action selection process may in many animals operate according to simply evaluated rewards and costs built in by natural selection during evolution (Krebs and Kacelnik 1991, Dawkins 1995). Animals may take into account, for example, quite complex information, such as the mean and variance of the rewards available from different sources, in making their selection of behaviour, yet the actual selection may then be based on quite simple rules of thumb, such as, 'if resources are very low, choose a reliable source of reward'. It may only be in some animals, for example humans, that explicit, linguistically based multistep cost–benefit analysis can be performed. It is important when interpreting animal behaviour to bear these arguments in mind, and to be aware that quite complex behaviour can result from very simple mechanisms. It is important not to over-interpret the factors that underlie any particular example of behaviour.

Reward and punisher signals provide a common currency for different sensory inputs, and can be seen as important in the selection of which actions are performed. Evolution ensures that the different reward and punisher signals are made potent to the extent that each will be chosen when appropriate. For example, food will be rewarding when hungry, but as hunger falls, the current level of thirst may soon become sufficient to make the reward produced by the taste of water greater than that produced by food, so that water is ingested. If however a painful input occurs or is signalled at any time during the feeding or drinking, this may be a stronger signal in the common currency, so that behaviour switches to that appropriate to reduce or avoid the pain. After the painful stimulus or threat is removed, the next most rewarding stimulus in the common currency might be the taste of water, and drinking would therefore be selected. The way in which a part of the brain such as the striatum and rest of the basal ganglia may contribute to the selection of behaviour by implementing competition between the different rewards and punishers available, all expressed in a common currency, is described by Rolls and Treves (1998), Chapter 9, by Rolls (1999a), and in Chapter 8. The functions of the orbitofrontal cortex and cingulate cortex in behavioural switching are considered in Chapter 4.

Many of the rewards for behaviour consist of stimuli, or remembered stimuli. Examples of some primary reinforcers are included in Table 2.1. However, for some animals, evolution has built-in a reward value for certain types of response. For example, it may be reinforcing to a pigeon or chicken to peck. The adaptive value of this is that for these animals, simply pecking at their environment may lead to the discovery of rewards. Another example might be exercise, which may have been selected to be rewarding in evolution because it keeps the body physically fit, which could be adaptive. While for some animals making certain responses may thus act as primary reinforcers (see Glickman and Schiff (1967)), this is likely to be adaptive only if animals operate in limited environmental niches. If one is built to find pecking very rewarding, this may imply that other types of response are less able to be made, and this tends to restrict the animal to an environmental niche. In general, animals with a wide range of behavioural responses and strategies available, such as primates, are able to operate in a wider range of environments, are in this sense more general-purpose, are less likely to find that particular responses are rewarding per se, and are more likely to be able to select behaviour based on which of a wide range of stimuli is most rewarding, rather than based on which response-type they are pre-adapted to select.

The overall aim of the cost–benefit analysis in animals is to maximize fitness. By fitness we mean the probability that an animal's genes will be passed on into the next generation. To maximize this, there may be many ways in which different stimuli have been selected during evolution to be rewards and punishers (and among punishers we could include costs). All these rewards and punishers should operate together to ensure that over the lifetime of the animal there is a high probability of passing on genes to the next generation; but in doing this, and maximizing fitness in a complex and changing environment, all these rewards and punishers may be expected to lead to a wide variety of behaviour.

Once language enables rewards and punishers to be intellectualized, so that, for example, solving complex problems in language, mathematics, or music becomes rewarding, behaviour might be less obviously seen as adapted for fitness. However, it was suggested above that the ability to solve complex problems may be one way in which fitness, especially in a changing environment, can be maximized. Thus we should not be surprised that working at the level of ideas, to increase understanding, should in itself be rewarding. These circumstances, that humans have developed language and other complex intellectual abilities, and that natural selection in evolution has led problem-solving to be rewarding, may lead to the very rapid evolution of ideas (see also Section 9.6.2).

3.4   Further functions of emotion

The fundamental function of emotion, to enable an efficient way for the goals for actions to be defined by genes during evolution and to be implemented in the brain, has been described in Sections 3.2 and 3.3. The simple brain implementation provided as a result of evolution allows the different goals to be selected and compared by using reward and punisher evaluation or appraisal of stimuli, and of the stimuli that may be obtained by different courses of action. This function allows flexibility of the behavioural responses that will be performed to obtain gene-specified goals. Next we consider some further functions and properties of emotion, and also highlight some particularly interesting examples of the types of emotional behaviour that result from the fundamental operation of emotional systems described above.

3.4.1   Autonomic and endocrine responses

An additional function of emotion is the elicitation of autonomic responses (e.g. a change in heart rate) and endocrine responses (e.g. the release of adrenaline). It is of clear survival value to prepare the body, for example by increasing the heart rate, so that actions such as running which may be performed as a consequence of the reinforcing stimulus can be performed more efficiently. The neural connections from the amygdala and orbitofrontal cortex via the hypothalamus as well as directly towards the brainstem autonomic motor nuclei may be particularly involved in this function (see Chapter 4). The James–Lange theory (see Chapter 2, and Schachter and Singer (1962); Grossman (1967); and Reisenzein (1983)), and theories that are closely related to it in supposing that feedback from parts of the periphery, such as the face (Adelmann and Zajonc 1989) or body (Damasio 1994), leads to emotional feelings, have the major weakness that they do not give an adequate account of how the peripheral change is produced only by stimuli that happen to be emotion-provoking. Perhaps the most important issue in emotion is why only some stimuli give rise to emotions. We have prepared the way for answering this by identifying the stimuli that produce emotions as reinforcers. This prepares the way for answering the question of how emotions are produced, by investigating which parts of the brain decode whether stimuli are reinforcing, and produce responses that include autonomic responses (see Chapter 4).

Mechanisms that lead animals to perform taxes such as swimming up chemical gradients are clearly required extremely early in animal evolution, and indeed are present in single cell animals such as *Amoeba*. At some later time in evolution, when specialized systems are present in the body, the autonomic and endocrine responses just described can be adaptive in enabling the animal to cope effectively with changes in the environment, and it is frequently appropriate for these states of autonomic and or endocrine activation to persist for considerable periods. At this stage in evolution there are thus likely to be brain systems that ensure that autonomic, and probably endocrine, states can be maintained for considerable periods. By this stage in evolution we have two key aspects of processing in place that later become important in emotion, namely guidance of behaviour towards stimuli that are useful (as determined by gene-specification), and guidance of responses away from noxious stimuli; and the persistence of such states after the evoking stimulus has disappeared. Later in evolution, when arbitrary (or operant) instrumental behaviour becomes possible in order to obtain what can now be called reinforcers, is one convenient stage at which to say that emotions are present. In this sense, the autonomic and endocrine aspects of emotional states may be precursors in evolution to the full emotional states that it is convenient to define as present when arbitrary actions can be performed.

3.4.2   Flexibility of behavioural responses, because emotions are related to the rewards and punishers that specify the goals for action

A function of emotion inherent in the gene-based theory described above is providing flexibility of behavioural responses, and this function of emotion is elaborated now. The thesis here is that when a rewarding or punishing stimulus in the environment elicits an emotional state, we can perform any appropriate and arbitrary response to obtain the reward, or avoid the punisher. That is, the reward or punisher defines the goal for the action, but does not specify the action itself. The action itself can be selected by the animal as appropriate in the current circumstances as that most appropriate for obtaining the reward or avoiding or escaping from the punisher. This is more flexible than simply learning a fixed behavioural response to a stimulus, which is what was implied by the stimulus–response (S–R) or habit learning theories of the 1930s.

This flexibility of behavioural responses is made very clear when we consider the learning processes that typically occur when emotion-provoking stimuli occur. Let us consider as an example avoidance learning. An example of this might be learning an action to perform when a tone sounds in order to avoid an electrical shock. The learning would take place in two stages, with different processes involved in each stage. In the first stage, stimulus–reinforcer association learning would produce an emotional state such as fear to a tone associated with the shock. This learning stage may be very rapid, and may occur in one trial. (We will see in Chapter 4 that the amygdala and orbitofrontal cortex are especially involved in this type of learning.) The second stage of the avoidance learning would be instrumental learning of an operant response, motivated by and performed in order to terminate the fear-inducing stimulus. Finding an appropriate behavioural response to remove the fear-inducing stimulus may occur by trial-and-error, and may take many trials. This two-stage learning process was suggested as being important for avoidance learning by N. E. Miller and O. H. Mowrer (see Gray (1975) and Section 4.6.1.2).

The suggestion made here is that this general type of two-stage learning process is closely related to the design of animals for many types of behaviour, including emotional behaviour. It simplifies the interface of sensory systems to motor systems. Instead of having to learn a particular response or habit to a particular stimulus by slow, trial-and-error, learning, two-stage learning allows very fast (often one trial) learning of an emotional state to a rewarding or punishing stimulus. Then the motor system can operate in a quite general way, sometimes using new trial-and-error learning, but often using many previously learned strategies, to approach the reward or avoid the punisher, which act as goals. This not only gives great flexibility to the interface between the sensory stimulus and an action, but also makes it relatively simple. It means that the reward value of a number of different stimuli can be decoded at roughly the same time. A behavioural decision system can then compare the different rewards available, in that they have a form of 'common currency'. (The value of each type of reward in this 'common currency' will be affected by many different factors, such as need state, e.g. hunger; how recently that reward has been obtained; the necessity in evolution to set each type of reward so that it sometimes is chosen if it is important for survival; etc.) The decision system can then choose between the rewards, based on their value, but also on the cost of obtaining each reward (see earlier in this Chapter). After the choice has been made, the action or motor system can then switch on any behavioural responses possible, whether learned or not, in order to maximize the reward signal being obtained. The magnitude of the reward signal being obtained would be indicated just by the firing of the neurons that reflect the value of the reward being obtained (e.g. the taste of a food if hungry, the pleasantness of touch, etc.), as described in Chapters 4–9. The actual way in which the appropriate response or action is learned may depend on response-reinforcer (i.e. action–outcome) association learning, or on some more general type of purposive behaviour that can be learned to obtain goals. It may be emphasized that emotions are thus an important part of brain design by enabling actions to be selected on the basis of goals, in allowing flexibility of the action performed, but also, and extremely importantly, by enabling a very simple type of one-trial learning, stimulus–reinforcer association learning, which is also very fast, to enable animals to respond to new attractive or dangerous stimuli with learning that may take as little as one trial.

3.4.3 Emotional states are motivating

Another function of emotion is that it is motivating. For example, fear learned by stimulus–reinforcer association formation provides the motivation for actions performed to avoid noxious stimuli. Similarly, positive reinforcers elicit motivation, so that we will work to obtain the rewards. Another example where emotion affects motivation is when a reward becomes no longer available, that is frustrative non-reward (see Fig. 2.1). If an action is possible, then increased motivation facilitates behaviour to produce harder working to obtain that reinforcer again or another reinforcer. If no action is possible to obtain again that reward (e.g. after a death in the family), then as described in Chapter 2, grief or sadness may result. This may be adaptive, by preventing continuing motivated attempts to regain the positive reinforcer that is no longer available, and helping the animal in due course to therefore be sensitive to other potential reinforcers to which it might be adaptive to switch. As described in Chapter 2, if such frustrative non-reward occurs in humans when no action is possible, depression may occur.

A depressed state that lasts for a short time may be seen as being adaptive for the reason just given. However, the depression may last for a very long time perhaps because long-term explicit (conscious) knowledge in humans enables the long-term consequences of loss of the positive reinforcer to be evaluated and repeatedly brought to mind as described in Chapter 10, and this may make long-term (psychological) depression maladaptive. Thus a discrepancy between the evolutionary and current environment caused by the rapid development of an explicit system may contribute to some emotional states that are no longer adaptive.

In an interesting evolutionary approach to depression, Nesse (2000a) has argued that humans may set long-term goals for themselves that are difficult to attain, and may spend years trying to attain these goals. An example of such a goal might be obtaining a particular position in one's career, or professional qualification, which may take years of a person's life. If the goal is not attained, then the lack of the reinforcer may lead to prolonged depression. Humans may find it difficult to reorganize their long-term aims to identify other, replacement and more attainable, goals, and without facility at this reorganization of long-term goals, the depression may be prolonged. The evolutionary aspect of this is that with our long-term explicit planning system (described in Chapter 10) and the value that society places on long-term goals and the status that attaining these may confer, humans find themselves in an environmental situation in which their explicit long-term planning system did not evolve, so that it is not well adapted to identifying goals that are realistic. The explicit system then provides a long-lasting non-reward signal to the emotion system (which in addition did not evolve to deal with such long-lasting non-reward inputs), and this contributes to long-lasting depression. A therapeutic solution would be to help depressed people identify possible precipitating factors such as unachieved long-term goals, and readjust their life aims so that positive reinforcers start to be obtained again, helping to lift the person out of the depression.

As described in Chapter 2, motivation is an important aspect of an emotional state, but does not require an inherently different mechanism, in that if genes are specifying the reward value of some stimuli ('primary reinforcers'), then the behavioural system must be built to seek to obtain these stimuli (i.e. be motivated to treat them as goals), for otherwise the stimuli would be operationally describable as rewards.

3.4.4 Communication

Because of its survival value, the ability to decode signals from other animals as being rewarding or punishing is important. The reward or punisher value may in some cases be innate, and in other cases learned. It may also be adaptive to send such signals, and in some cases the sending of such signals may be 'honest' and in other cases 'deceptive'. These communicated signals may indicate for example the extent to which animals are willing to compete for resources, and they may influence the behaviour of other animals (Hauser 1996). Communicating emotional states may have survival value, for example by reducing fighting.

Darwin (1872), in his book entitled 'The Expression of the Emotions in Man and Animals' had as a goal emphasizing the similarity, and therefore the possible phylogenetic closeness, of the expressions of man and his closest living relatives, but nevertheless noted the communicative value of such expressions.

The observation that expressions can evoke a response in the receiver underlies the idea that expressions can also be communicative rather than simply outward signs of affect (Chevalier-Skolnikoff 1973). Expression can be seen as a way of inviting/inducing certain responses in the receiver, much as a smile can appease, a laugh can invite participation, and fear could enlist assistance. In non-human primates, expression is used as a tool with which to regulate and maintain social relations. For example, in the macaque if a subordinate grimaces in an aggressive encounter with a dominant, this signals submission. However, the use of expression is not necessarily so straightforward, for if the same expression were to be given by a dominant individual approaching a subordinate, it no longer signals submission but the positive intention of the dominant. In this way, the communicative effect of expression can be said to be context-dependent, and it depends on the age, sex, dominance and kinship of the senders and receivers (Chevalier-Skolnikoff 1973).

Zeller (1987) also describes what may be said to be the manipulation of social relations through facial expression in non-human primates, that is threat faces are given to coerce another into a desired activity, and friendly expressions are given to enlist co-operation from another.

To argue that the expression of emotion is utilized in social communication, then the ability to decode these signals must be demonstrated. That is, are others able to perceive the content of an individual's expression? Humans have been shown to be remarkable in this ability, even cross-culturally (Ekman 1998), and many would say the happiness in a smile and the anger in furrowed brows are intuitively easy signals to understand.

If the facial expression cannot be transmitted, then this might also on this hypothesis be expected to influence the social and emotional behaviour of others. Izard (1971) showed that a rhesus macaque with impaired facial motor nerve (VIII) function received an increased number of aggressive assaults, and that its position in the social dominance hierarchy fell. Further, humans who have difficulties in producing facial expressions (e.g. patients with Bell's palsy or Parkinson's disease) say that their social interactions are made difficult (Sutherland 1997).

A powerful method of looking at adaptation is to compare different groups of related species in order to uncover the evolutionary history (phylogeny) of particular adaptations, and to uncover what particular selection pressures were at work on such adaptations. Such evidence, described in the following, can be used to underscore the communicative value of the expression of emotion. Expression cannot be produced without the relevant facial muscles contracting or relaxing, and therefore expression is dependent on the musculature of the face. The primate order has undergone some dramatic shifts in the evolution of the facial musculature that can be witnessed in the detectable difference in the use of facial expression between the strepsirhines (prosimians) and haplorhines (simians), and the hominoids (apes) and hominids, as follows.

The facial musculature of the strepsirhines is not very differentiated and relatively primitive. Facial innervation is also significantly less (Zeller 1987). Accordingly, the strepsirhines have a meagre set of expressions and a mask-like face (Chevalier-Skolnikoff 1973). In the haplorhines, the muscles of the mid-facial region become more differentiated and afford the face greater expressiveness when compared to the strepsirhines. This can be related to the reduction in the reliance on auditory and olfactory communication, corresponding to the shift from nocturnal to diurnal living. With the great apes, there is a still greater differentiation of the mid-facial muscles, and also the development of new muscles around the mouth. The new muscles offer a mobility that can produce a facial expression which a macaque, for instance, could not perform (Chevalier-Skolnikoff 1973). This trend continues in man, and the even greater differentiation and the complex interlacing of muscles provide the potential for new movements. For example, the *zygomaticus major* muscle can pull the mouth corners into the human smile (Chevalier-Skolnikoff 1973). Thus, we can see how there have been successive shifts in the muscular differentiation of the face, which has had a concomitant effect on the use of facial expression.

Interestingly, the evolution of the facial anatomy and the expressions that depend on it also correspond to the evolution of sociality through the primate order (Andrew 1963). While the first proliferation of facial expression occurred after the switch to a diurnal way of life, the continuation of this trend accords with the gregariousness of the species. Communication by expression would be more or less pointless in solitary and/or nocturnal species such as the Galago, but would become much more useful in group living, diurnal and terrestrial, species. Consistent with this, highly gregarious and 'socially complex' species of Old World monkeys and apes (e.g. baboons, chimpanzees) have the most exaggerated facial expression repertoire, culminating with that of man. This evidence corroborates the idea that one of the functions of emotion lies in the communicative value of its expression.

Chapter 4 describes the brain systems in the temporal lobe visual cortex, the amygdala, and the orbitofrontal cortex that are specialized for the decoding of face-related information such as expression and identity. Here we note some interesting comparative evidence. Barton and Aggleton (2000) measured the relative volume of the amygdala (by plotting the volume of the amygdala nuclei against medulla volume) across the primate order. They revealed a successive relative enlargement of the cortico-basolateral (CBL) nuclei of the amygdala between the insectivores and the strepsirhines, and strepsirhines and haplorhines. The insectivores were used as a representative of the ancestor of the primate lineage. Further, the size of the CBL group of amygdala nuclei correlated with social group size. Part of the relevance of this is that we know that neurons selectively responsive to faces are found in the basolateral/basal accessory group of amygdala nuclei (Leonard, Rolls, Wilson and Baylis 1985). Thus a part of the amygdala especially concerned with processing face stimuli shows particular evolutionary development through the primates, and correlates with the size of the social group. This evidence is thus also consistent with the importance of communication in social behaviour and emotion, in this case involving probably both face identity and expression.

As social groups are at once both competitive and cooperative, one of the adaptive functions of emotion, and its display, could be to signal, whether honestly or dishonestly, the shifting intentions and dispositions of an individual to another in the social group. Overall, it would be expected that the emphasis on the communicative value of emotion would be greater in species with a socially complex organization, and the evidence above seems to bear this out.

3.4.5   Social attachment

Another area in which emotion is important is in social bonding. Examples of this are the emotions associated with the attachment of the parents to their young, with the attachment of the young to their parents, and with the attachment of the parents to each other (see Section 9.2). In the theory of the ways in which the genes affect behaviour ('selfish gene' theory, see Dawkins (1989), Ridley (2003)), it is held that (because, e.g., of the advantages of parental care) all these forms of emotional attachment have the effect that genes for such attachment are more likely to survive into the next generation. Kin-altruism can also be considered in these terms (see e.g. Dawkins (1989) and Section 9.6.2). In these examples, social bonding is related to primary (gene-specified) reinforcers. In other cases, the emotions involved in social interactions may arise from reinforcers involved in reciprocal altruism, utilizing for example 'tit-for-tat' strategies. In these cases it is crucial to remember which reinforcers are exchanged with particular individuals, so that cheating does not lead to disadvantages for some of those involved. This type of social bonding can be stable when there is a net advantage to both parties in cooperating (see Section 11.3).

Some investigators have argued that the main functions of emotion are in social situations (see Strongman (2003)). While it is certainly the case that many emotions are related to social situations (as can be inferred from Table 2.1), many are not, including for example the fear of snakes by primates, or the fear that is produced by the sight of an object that has produced pain previously.

3.4.6   Separate functions for each different primary reinforcer

It is useful to highlight that each primary (gene-specified) reinforcer (of which a large number are suggested in Table 2.1) not only leads to a different set of emotions, but also implements a different function. A few examples of these functions are elaborated here. This should make it possible for the reader to complete the elaboration for the other primary reinforcers in Table 2.1. Before considering these examples, let us remember that each function is related to the survival or sexually selected value being provided by the specifying gene; and that in so far as emotional states are associated with feelings (see Chapter 10), anything that feels pleasant or unpleasant to the organism, and is reinforcing, is likely to have survival value, and to implement another function of emotion. (The argument given in Chapter 10 is that stimuli that act as implicit or unconscious rewards may also act to produce pleasant feelings in the explicit or conscious processing system, so that both the implicit and explicit routes to action operate largely consistently.)

One example of a primary reinforcer taken from Table 2.1 is slight novelty, which may feel good and be positively reinforcing because it may lead to the discovery of better opportunities for survival in the environment (e.g. a new food). It is crucial that animals that succeed in the genetic competition that drives evolution have genes that encourage them to explore new environments, for then it is possible for the genes that happen to be present in an individual to explore the large multidimensional space (or more colloquially, range of ways to vary) of the environment in which they might succeed.

Another example from Table 2.1 is gregariousness, which may assist the identification of new social partners, which could provide advantage.

Probably related to the effects of novelty is sensory-specific satiety, the phenomenon whereby pleasant tastes during a meal gradually become less pleasant as satiety approaches (see Chapter 5). This may be an aspect of a more general adaptation to ensure that behaviour does eventually switch from one reinforcer to another. Although these examples are of positive reinforcers, it is comparably the case that natural selection acting on genes will lead to the elaboration of other stimuli as punishers when avoiding these stimuli has survival value. Of course the genes may be misled sometimes and lead to behaviour that does not have survival value, as when for example the non-nutritive sweetener saccharin is eaten by animals. This does not disprove the theory, but only points out that the genes cannot specify correctly for every possible stimulus or event in the environment, but must only on average lead to behaviour feeling pleasant that increases fitness, i.e. is appropriate for gene survival.

3.4.7 The mood state can influence the cognitive evaluation of moods or memories

Another property of emotion is that the current mood state can affect the cognitive evaluation of events or memories (see Blaney (1986)), and this may have the function of facilitating continuity in the interpretation of the reinforcing value of events in the environment. A theory of how this occurs is presented in Section 4.10 'Effects of emotions on cognitive processing'.

3.4.8 Facilitation of memory storage

An eighth function of emotion is that it may facilitate the storage of memories. One way in which this occurs is that episodic memory (i.e. one's memory of particular episodes) is facilitated by emotional states. This may be advantageous in that storage of as many details as possible of the prevailing situation when a strong reinforcer is delivered may be useful in generating appropriate behaviour in situations with some similarities in the future. This function may be implemented in the brain by the relatively non-specific projecting systems to the cerebral cortex and hippocampus, including the cholinergic pathways in the basal forebrain and medial septum (see Section 4.9.5) (Rolls and Treves 1998, Rolls 1999a, Wilson and Rolls 1990c, Wilson and Rolls 1990b, Wilson and Rolls 1990a), and the ascending noradrenergic pathways (see Section 4.9.6).

A second way in which emotion may affect the storage of memories is that the current emotional state may be stored with episodic memories, providing a mechanism for the current emotional state to affect which memories are recalled. In this sense, emotion acts as a contextual retrieval cue, that as with other contextual effects influences the retrieval of episodic memories (see Rolls and Treves (1998)).

A third way in which emotion may affect the storage of memories is by guiding the cerebral cortex in the representations of the world that are set up. For example, in the visual system, it may be useful to build perceptual representations or analysers that are different from each other if they are associated with different reinforcers, and to be less likely to build them if they have no association with reinforcers. Ways in which backprojections from parts of the brain important in emotion (such as the amygdala) to parts of the cerebral cortex could perform this function are discussed in Section 4.10, 'Effects of emotions on cognitive processing'; by Rolls (1999a); and by Rolls and Treves (1998).

3.4.9 Emotional and mood states are persistent, and help to produce persistent motivation

A ninth function of emotion is that by enduring for minutes or longer after a reinforcing stimulus has occurred, it may help to produce persistent motivation and direction of behaviour. For example, if an expected reward is not obtained, the persisting state of frustrative non-reward may usefully keep behaviour directed for some time at trying to obtain the reward again.

3.4.10 Emotions may trigger memory recall and influence cognitive processing

A tenth function of emotion is that it may trigger recall of memories stored in neocortical representations. Amygdala and orbitofrontal cortex backprojections to cortical areas could perform this for emotion in a way analogous to that in which the hippocampus could implement the retrieval in the neocortex of recent memories of particular events or episodes (see Rolls and Treves (1998) and Rolls and Kesner (2006)). This is thought to operate as follows. When a memory is stored in a neocortical area or hippocampus, any mood state that is present and reflected in the firing of neurons in the orbitofrontal cortex or amygdala will become associated with that memory by virtue of the associatively modifiable synaptic connections from the backprojecting neurons onto the neocortical or hippocampal system neurons. Then later, a particular mood state represented by the firing of neurons in the amygdala or orbitofrontal cortex will by the associatively modified backprojection connections enhance or produce the recall of memories stored when that mood state was present. These effects have been formally modelled by Rolls and Stringer (2001b), and are described further in Section 4.10. One consequence of these effects is that once in a particular mood state, memories associated with that mood state will tend to be recalled and incoming stimuli will be interpreted in the light of the current mood state. The result may be some continuity of emotional state and thus of behaviour. This continuity may sometimes be advantageous, by keeping behaviour directed towards a goal, and making behaviour interpretable by others, but it may become useful in human psychiatric conditions to break this self-perpetuating tendency.

It is useful to have these functions of emotion in mind when considering the neural basis of emotion, for each function is likely to activate particular output pathways from emotional systems associated with it.

3.5 The functions of emotion in an evolutionary, Darwinian, context

In this book (see for example Section 3.2), the question of why we have emotions is a fundamental issue that I answer in terms of a Darwinian, functional, approach, producing the answer that emotions are states elicited by goals (rewards and punishers), and that this is part of an adaptive process by which genes can specify the behaviour of the animal by specifying goals for behaviour rather than fixed responses. The emotional states elicited with respect to the goals depend on the reinforcement contingencies, as illustrated in Fig. 2.1. The states themselves may be the goals for action, such as reducing fear, and additionally maintain behaviour by being persistent, and act in other ways as described in Section 3.4.

This theory of emotion provides I believe a powerful approach to understanding how genes influence behaviour. In much thinking in zoology, an approach has been to understand how genes may determine particular behaviours. For example, Tinbergen (1963) and Tinbergen (1951) considered that innate releasing stimuli might elicit fixed action patterns. An example is the herring gull chick's pecking response elicited as a fixed action pattern by the innate releasing stimulus of a red spot on its parent's bill. A successor in this approach in the context of emotion is Panksepp (1998). The instinctive pecking response may be improved by learning (Hailman 1967), but is not an arbitrary, flexible, response as in instrumental, action–outcome, learning (see Section 4.6.1.2). The details of the stimulus, or the context in which it occurs, may be taken into account, to influence the instinctive response (Dawkins 1995), but there is still no arbitrary relation between the stimulus and the action, as in instrumental learning.

In contrast, the most important function of emotion that I propose is for genes to specify the stimuli that are the goals for behaviour. This means that the genetic specification can be kept relatively simple, in that it is stimuli that are specified by the genes, such as a taste or touch, and this is generally simpler than specifying the details of a response (such as climbing a tree, running along a branch, picking an apple, and placing it into the mouth). It also means that relatively few genetic specifications are needed, for instead of having to encode many relations between particular stimuli and particular behavioural responses, the genes need to span the dimensionality of the stimulus space of primary reinforcers. Examples of some of these primary, gene-encoded, reinforcers are shown in Table 2.1.

Another way in which the genetic specification required can be kept low is that stimulus–reinforcer association learning can then be used to enable quite arbitrary stimuli occurring in the lifetime of an animal to become associated with primary reinforcers by stimulus–reinforcer association learning, and thus to lead to actions.

But the most important advantage conferred by emotion is that the behaviour required need not be genetically specified, for arbitrary actions can be learned in the lifetime of the animal by instrumental, action–outcome, learning to obtain or avoid the goals specified by the genes. The actions are arbitrary operants, in that any action may be made to obtain the goal (see Section 4.6.1.2). Thus the genetic specification of the behaviour that emotion allows is one in which the behaviour is not pre-programmed with respect to the stimulus (as in instinctive behaviour such as fixed action patterns), but instead the action is not specified by the genes, and the goals to which actions are directed are specified by the genes. Of course this does not deny that some behavioural responses are genetically specified as responses, and examples might include pecking to particular stimuli in birds, orientation to and suckling of the nipple in mammals, and some examples of preparedness to learn (see Section 4.6.1.2).

Darwinian natural selection of genes that encode the goals for action (i.e. encode reinforcers) rather than the actions themselves, and thus allows great flexibility of the resulting behaviour, can be thought of as liberating 'The Selfish Gene' (Dawkins 1976, Dawkins 1989). When Richard Dawkins wrote *The Selfish Gene* (Dawkins 1976), he was careful to make it clear that the concept that selection and competition operate at the level of genes (Hamilton 1964, Hamilton 1996) does not lead inevitably to genetic determinism of behaviour. Nevertheless the concept was criticised on these grounds, and Dawkins devoted a whole chapter of *The Extended Phenotype* to addressing this further (Dawkins 1982). The concepts developed in *Emotion Explained* help to resolve this further, for I argue that an important way in which genes influence hehaviour (and in doing so produce emotion), is by specifying the reinforcers, the goals for actions, rather than particular behaviours. This helps to avoid the charge that selfish genes 'determine' the behaviour. Instead, many of the genes that influence behaviour operate by competing with each other in a world of reinforcing stimuli or goals for actions, and thus there is great flexibility in the behaviour that results. We are led to think not of behaviours being inherited or 'determined by selfish genes', but instead of genes exploring by natural selection reinforcers that may guide behaviour successfully so that the fitness of the genes is increased. In this sense, the selfish gene (in particular, those involved in specifying reinforcers) is liberated from directly 'determining' behaviour, to providing goals for (instrumental) actions that can involve completely flexible behaviour made to obtain the goal. In these cases, the heritability of behaviour is best understood as the heritability of reinforcers in a stimulus space not in a behavioural or response space.

An interesting consequence of this fundamental adaptive value of emotion that I propose is that the genetic specification does need to include specification for several synapses through the nervous system from the sensory input to the brain region where the reward or punishment value of the goal stimulus is made explicit in the representation (see footnote 8 on page 66). It is thus a prediction that genes specify the connectivity to the stage of processing in the brain where goals are specified, so that appropriate actions can be learned to the goals. Evidence is described in Chapters 4 and 5 that the goals may not be made explicit, that is related to neuronal firing, until stages of information processing such as the orbitofrontal cortex and amygdala. An example of this specification is that sweet taste receptors on the tongue must be connected to neurons that specify food reward, and whose responses are modulated by hunger signals (see Chapter 5).

The definition I provide of emotions, that they are states (with particular functions) elicited by reinforcers (see Chapter 2), thus is consistent with what I see as the most important function of emotion, that of being part of a design by which genes can specify (some) goals or reinforcers of our actions. This means that the theory of emotion that I propose should not be seen as behaviourist, but instead as part of a much broader theory that takes an adaptive, Darwinian, approach to the functions of emotion, and how they are important in brain design. Further, the theory shows how cognitive states can produce and modulate emotion (see Sections 2.8 and 4.5.5.7), and in turn how emotional states can influence cognition (see Section 4.10).

I believe that this approach leads to a fundamental understanding of why we have emotions that is likely to stand the test of time, in the same way that Darwinian thinking itself provides a fundamental way of understanding biology and many 'why' questions about life. This is thus intended to be a thoroughly Darwinian theory of the adaptive value of emotion in the design of organisms.

3.6 The functions of motivation in an evolutionary, Darwinian, context

Motivation may be seen as a state in which one is working for a goal, and emotion as a state that occurs when the goal, a reinforcer, is obtained, and that may persist afterwards. The concept of gene-specified reinforcers providing the goals for action helps to understand the relation between motivational states and emotion, as the organism must be built to be motivated to obtain the goals, and to be placed in a different state (emotion) when the goal is or is not achieved by the action. The close but clear relation between motivation and emotion is that both involve what humans describe as affective states (e.g. feeling hungry, liking the taste of a food, feeling happy because of a social reinforcer), and both are about goals. The

Darwinian theory of the functions of emotion developed in this Chapter, which shows how emotion is adaptive because it reflects the operation of a process by which genes define goals for action, applies just as much to motivation. By specifying goals, the genes must specify both that we must be motivated to obtain those goals, and that when the goals are obtained, further states, emotional states with further functions, are produced. In motivated behaviour, many factors influence how rewarding or punishing the goal is. In terms of motivated states relevant to internal homeostatic needs, the reward or goal value of a sensory stimulus such as the taste of food or water is set up genetically to be influenced by the relevant internal signals, such as plasma glucose concentration or plasma osmolality in the cases of hunger and thirst, as described in Chapters 5 and 6. If a gene-specified goal such as the taste of expected food is not obtained, then we are left in a state of frustrative non-reward in which the original goal remains rewarding, which will leave us motivated to still obtain it if it may still be available, or will lead to a learned change in its reward value, and to extinction of that behaviour, if we learn that no action will obtain the goal (see Section 3.4.3).

3.7   Are all goals for action gene-specified?

Finally in this Chapter, we can ask whether all goals are gene-specified. An important concept of this Chapter has been that part of the adaptive value of emotion is that it is part of the process that results from the way in which genes specify reinforcers, that is the goals for action. Emotions may thus be elicited by primary reinforcers, or by stimuli that become associated by learning with primary reinforcers, i.e. secondary reinforcers. But are there goals related to emotional and motivational states that are not related to goals defined in this way by gene-specified reinforcers?

I think it is likely that most reinforcers can be traced back to a gene-specified goal, even if they are in some cases rather general goals. Some examples of these types of reinforcer (and there are likely to be many others) are included in Table 2.1, such as goals for social cooperation and group acceptance, mind reading, and solving an intellectual problem. However, when an explicit, rational, reasoning system capable of syntactic operations on symbols (as described in Chapter 10) evolves, it is possible that goals that are not very directly related to gene specifications become accepted. This may be seen in some of the effects of culture. Indeed, some goals are defined within a culture, for example writing a novel. But it is argued that it is primary reinforcers specified by genes of the general type shown in Table 2.1 that make us want to be recognised in society because of the advantages this can bring, to solve difficult problems, etc, and therefore to perform actions such as writing novels (see further Chapters 9 and 10, Ridley (2003) Chapter 8, Ridley (1993a) pp. 310 ff, Laland and Brown (2002) pp. 271 ff, and Dawkins (1982)). Indeed, culture is influenced by human genetic propensities, and it follows that human cognitive, affective, and moral capacities are the product of a unique dynamic known as *gene-culture coevolution* (Gintis 2007, Bowles and Gintis 2005, Gintis 2003, Boyd et al. 2003). Nevertheless, there may be cases where the explicit, reasoning, system might specify a goal, and thus lead to emotions, that could not be related to any genetic adaptive value, whether current or specified in evolutionary history. In these cases I would argue that although emotion has evolved and is generally adaptive in relation to gene-specified reinforcers, when the explicit, reasoning, system evolves, this can set up alternative goals that tap into and utilize the existing emotional system for facilitating actions, but with respect to which the goals might be genetically unspecified and even non-adaptive.

4 The brain mechanisms underlying emotion

4.1 Introduction

Part of the explanation provided in this book of emotions is the way in which emotions are implemented in our brains. What happens in our brains during emotions? What processes taking place in our brains make us have emotions, and behave the way we do? We start with diagrams to show some of the brain regions we will be discussing. Then there is a short summary of the general principles involved in the brain mechanisms underlying emotion. Given that emotions can be considered as states elicited by reinforcers (Chapter 2), a principled approach is to consider where primary reinforcers are represented (Section 4.3), where and how potential secondary (learned) reinforcers are represented (Section 4.4), and then the brain regions that implement stimulus–reinforcer, i.e. emotional, learning, considering in turn the orbitofrontal cortex (Section 4.5), amygdala (Section 4.6), and cingulate cortex (Section 4.7). Then we consider output systems for emotion (Section 4.9).

Some of the main brain regions implicated in emotion will now be considered in the light of the introduction given in Chapters 2 and 3 on the nature and functions of emotion. These brain regions include the amygdala, orbitofrontal cortex, cingulate cortex, and basal forebrain areas including the hypothalamus, which are shown in Figs. 4.1 and 4.2. Particular emphasis is placed on investigations of the functions of these regions in non-human primates (usually monkeys), for in primates many areas of the neocortex undergo great development and provide major inputs to these regions, in some cases to parts of these structures thought not to be present in non-primates. An example of this is the projection from the primate neocortex in the anterior part of the temporal lobe to the basal accessory nucleus of the amygdala (see below). Studies in primates are thus particularly relevant to understanding the neural basis of emotion in humans.

4.2 Overview

The way in which recent studies in primates indicate that the neural processing of emotion is organized is as follows (see Fig. 4.3).

1. There are brain mechanisms that are involved in computing the reward value of primary (unlearned) reinforcers. The primary reinforcers include taste, touch (both pleasant touch and pain), and to some extent smell, and perhaps certain visual stimuli, such as face expression. There is evidence that there is a representation of the primary reinforcers taste and positive touch in the orbitofrontal cortex.

2. Then some brain regions are concerned with learning associations between previously

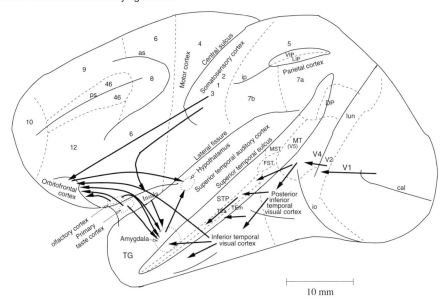

Fig. 4.1 Some of the pathways involved in emotion described in the text are shown on this lateral view of the brain of the macaque monkey. Connections from the primary taste and olfactory cortices to the orbitofrontal cortex and amygdala are shown. Connections are also shown in the 'ventral visual system' from V1 to V2, V4, the inferior temporal visual cortex, etc., with some connections reaching the amygdala and orbitofrontal cortex. In addition, connections from the somatosensory cortical areas 1, 2, and 3 that reach the orbitofrontal cortex directly and via the insular cortex, and that reach the amygdala via the insular cortex, are shown. as, arcuate sulcus; cal, calcarine sulcus; cs, central sulcus; lf, lateral (or Sylvian) fissure; lun, lunate sulcus; ps, principal sulcus; io, inferior occipital sulcus; ip, intraparietal sulcus (which has been opened to reveal some of the areas it contains); sts, superior temporal sulcus (which has been opened to reveal some of the areas it contains). AIT, anterior inferior temporal cortex; FST, visual motion processing area; LIP, lateral intraparietal area; MST, visual motion processing area; MT, visual motion processing area (also called V5); PIT, posterior inferior temporal cortex; STP, superior temporal plane; TA, architectonic area including auditory association cortex; TE, architectonic area including high order visual association cortex, and some of its subareas TEa and TEm; TG, architectonic area in the temporal pole; V1–V4, visual areas V1–V4; VIP, ventral intraparietal area; TEO, architectonic area including posterior visual association cortex. The numerals refer to architectonic areas, and have the following approximate functional equivalence: 1,2,3, somatosensory cortex (posterior to the central sulcus); 4, motor cortex; 5, superior parietal lobule; 7a, inferior parietal lobule, visual part; 7b, inferior parietal lobule, somatosensory part; 6, lateral premotor cortex; 8, frontal eye field; 12, part of orbitofrontal cortex; 46, dorsolateral prefrontal cortex.

neutral stimuli, such as the sight of objects or of individuals' faces, with primary reinforcers. These brain regions include the amygdala and orbitofrontal cortex. For the processing of primary reinforcers, and especially for secondary reinforcers, the brain is organized to process the stimulus first to the object level (so that if the input is visual, the object can be recognized independently of its position on the retina, or size, or view), and then to determine whether the stimulus is rewarding or punishing. Once the relevant brain regions have determined whether the input is reinforcing, whether primary or secondary, the signal is passed directly to output regions of the brain, with no need to produce peripheral body or autonomic responses.

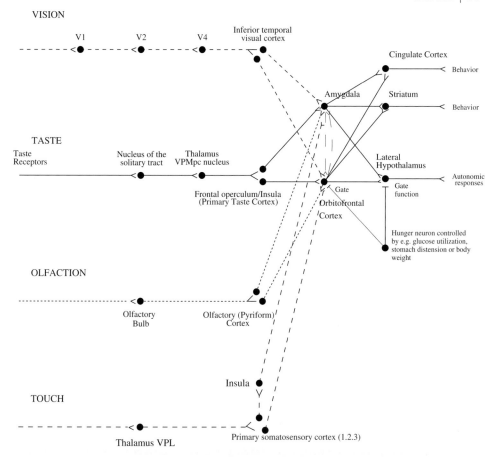

Fig. 4.2 Schematic diagram showing some of the connections of the taste, olfactory, somatosensory, and visual pathways in the brain. V1, primary visual (striate) cortex; V2 and V4, further cortical visual areas. VPL, ventro-postero-lateral nucleus of the thalamus, which conveys somatosensory information to the primary somatosensory cortex (areas 1, 2 and 3).

3. The brain regions in which the reinforcing, and hence emotional, value of stimuli are represented interface to three main types of output system:

The first is the autonomic and endocrine system, for producing such changes as increased heart rate and release of adrenaline, which prepare the body for action.

The second type of output is to brain systems concerned with performing actions unconsciously or implicitly, in order to obtain rewards or avoid punishers. These brain systems include the basal ganglia.

The third type of output is to a system capable of planning many steps ahead, and for example deferring short-term rewards in order to execute a long-term plan. This system may use syntactic processing to perform the planning, and is therefore part of a linguistic system which performs explicit (conscious) processing, as described more fully in Chapter 10.

Brain Mechanisms of Emotion

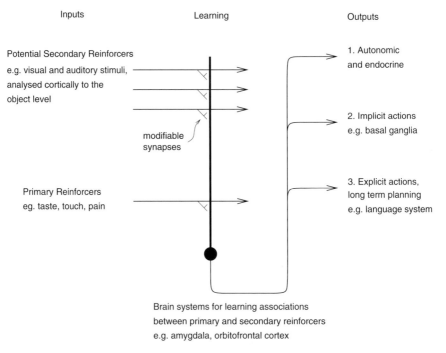

Fig. 4.3 Schematic diagram showing the organization of some of the brain mechanisms underlying emotion, including those involved in learning the reinforcement associations of visual stimuli.

4.3 Representations of primary reinforcers

Emotions can be produced by primary reinforcers. (Primary reinforcers are unlearned reinforcers, that is they are innately reinforcing.) Other, previously neutral, stimuli, such as the sight of an object, can by association learning with a primary reinforcer come to be a secondary (or learned) reinforcer, which can also produce an emotional response. For these reasons, in order to understand the neural basis of emotion it is necessary to know where in the processing systems in the brain a sensory input comes to be decoded[8] and treated by the rest of the brain (which may try to maximize or minimize its activity) as a primary reinforcer.

---

[8] By decoding, I mean what is made explicit in the representation. If the firing of neurons (in for example the inferior temporal visual cortex) reflects which object has been seen invariantly with respect to size, position, reward association, etc., then it can be said that representations of objects have been decoded from the sensory information reaching the retina. Although information about which object has been seen is of course present in the retinal neuronal firing, it is not made explicit at this stage of processing. Instead, local contrast over small regions of the retina is made explicit at the retinal level, in that retinal neurons have small concentric receptive fields responsive to small spots of light. If the firing of neurons in, for example, the orbitofrontal cortex reflects whether an object is currently associated with reward, then we can say that the reward value of objects has been decoded by this stage of processing. The most common way for information to be made explicit in the firing is by altering the firing rate of neurons, though it has been hypothesized that some additional information might be available in the relative time of firing of different neurons. This issue of the representation of information by populations of neurons is considered more comprehensively by Rolls and Treves (1998), Rolls and Deco (2002), Franco, Rolls, Aggelopoulos and Treves (2004) and Aggelopoulos, Franco and Rolls (2005).

4.3.1 Taste

In primates, the evidence that the representation of taste is independent of its rewarding properties as far as the primary taste cortex is described in Chapter 5. In the secondary taste cortex, which is part of the orbitofrontal cortex, the representation is of the food reward value of the taste, in that the taste responses of neurons are modulated by hunger, and decrease to zero when the animal is satiated, and the taste is no longer rewarding (see Section 4.5 and Chapter 5). There may be some though a less complete modulation by hunger of neuronal taste responses in the amygdala (see Section 4.6), and in this sense taste reward may be less well represented in the amygdala than the orbitofrontal cortex.

4.3.2 Smell

For olfaction, it is known that some orbitofrontal cortex olfactory neurons respond to the smell of food only when a monkey has an appetite for that food (Critchley and Rolls 1996a), and consistent results have been found in humans with functional neuroimaging (O'Doherty, Rolls, Francis, Bowtell, McGlone, Kobal, Renner and Ahne 2000). The responses of these neurons thus reflect the reward value of these food-related olfactory stimuli.

It is not yet known in primates whether this modulation of olfactory neuronal responses occurs at earlier processing stages. However, there is evidence in humans that the primary olfactory cortical areas (including the pyriform cortex and cortico-medial amygdala region) represent the identity and intensity of olfactory stimuli, in that in a functional magnetic resonance imaging (fMRI) investigation, activation of these regions was correlated with the subjective intensity ratings but not the subjective pleasantness ratings of six odours (Rolls, Kringelbach and De Araujo 2003c). In contrast, the reward value of odours is represented in the human medial orbitofrontal cortex, in that activation here was correlated with the pleasantness but not intensity ratings of six odours (Rolls et al. 2003c) (cf. Anderson, Christoff, Stappen, Panitz, Ghahremani, Glover, Gabrieli and Sobel (2003)). (In rats, there is some evidence that signals about hunger can influence olfactory processing as far peripherally as the olfactory bulb (Pager, Giachetti, Holley and LeMagnen 1972, Pager 1974).)

Although some of these primate orbitofrontal cortex olfactory neurons may respond because odours are secondary reinforcers as a result of olfactory-to-taste association learning (Rolls, Critchley, Mason and Wakeman 1996b), it is known that some olfactory neurons in the orbitofrontal cortex do not alter their responses during olfactory-to-taste association learning (Critchley and Rolls 1996b). The responses of these olfactory neurons could thus reflect information about whether the odour is a primary reinforcer. However, the neurons could also simply be representing the identity of the odour. This issue has not yet been settled.

In humans there is some evidence that pheromone-like odours can influence behaviour, though probably not through the vomero-nasal olfactory system, which appears to be vestigial in humans (see Section 9.8). In rodents and many mammals (but not humans and Old World monkeys), signals in an accessory olfactory system which includes the vomeronasal organ and the accessory olfactory bulb could act as primary reinforcers which affect attractiveness and aggression, and act as primary reinforcers (see Section 9.8).

4.3.3 Pleasant and painful touch

Experiments have recently been performed to investigate where in the human touch-processing system (see Figs. 4.1 and 4.2) tactile stimuli are decoded and represented in terms of their rewarding value or the pleasure they produce. In order to investigate this, Rolls, O'Doherty, Kringelbach, Francis, Bowtell and McGlone (2003d) performed functional magnetic resonance imaging (fMRI) of humans who were receiving pleasant, neutral, and painful tactile stimuli. They found that a weak but very pleasant touch of the hand with velvet produced much stronger activation of the orbitofrontal cortex than a more intense but affectively neutral touch of the hand with wood. In contrast, the pleasant stimuli produced much less activation of the primary somatosensory cortex S1 than the neutral stimuli (see Fig. 4.4). It was concluded that part of the orbitofrontal cortex is concerned with representing the positively affective aspects of somatosensory stimuli. Nearby, but separate, parts of the human orbitofrontal cortex were shown in the same series of experiments to be activated by taste and olfactory stimuli. Thus the pleasantness of tactile stimuli, which can be powerful primary reinforcers (Taira and Rolls 1996), is correlated with the activity of a part of the orbitofrontal cortex. This part of the orbitofrontal cortex probably receives its somatosensory inputs via the somatosensory cortex both via direct projections and via the insula (Mesulam and Mufson 1982a, Mesulam and Mufson 1982b, Rolls and Treves 1998). In contrast, the pleasantness of a tactile stimulus does not appear to be represented explicitly in the somatosensory cortex. The indication thus is that only certain parts of the somatosensory input, which reflect its pleasantness, are passed on (perhaps after appropriate processing) to the orbitofrontal cortex by the somatosensory cortical areas. It was also notable that the pleasant touch activated the most anterior (pregenual) part of the anterior cingulate cortex (see Fig. 4.4).

The issue of where the reinforcing properties of activation of the pain pathways is decoded is complex (Melzack and Wall 1996, Perl and Kruger 1996). There are clearly specialized peripheral nerves (including C fibres, with some activated via VR1 or capsaicin receptors) that convey painful stimulation to the central nervous system, and perhaps two main brain systems (Hunt and Mantyh 2001, Julius and Basbaum 2001). One is a spino-parabrachial pathway which originates from the superficial dorsal horn in the spinal cord and may have preferential access to brain areas involved in affect such as the amygdala, and the second is the spinothalamic pathway which distributes nociceptive information to parts of the brain involved in both discrimination and affect (Hunt and Mantyh 2001). At the spinal cord level, there are reflexes that enable a limb to be withdrawn from painful stimulation. But the essence of a reinforcer is that it should enable the probability of an arbitrary (that is any) instrumental response or action to be altered. For this learning to occur, it is probably necessary that the activity should proceed past the central gray in the brainstem, which is an important region for pain processing, to at least the diencephalic (hypothalamus/thalamus) level. This level may be sufficient for at least simple operant responses, such as lifting the tail, to be learned to avoid footshock (Huston and Borbely 1973). For more complex operant responses, it is likely that the basal ganglia must be intact (see Sections 4.9.2 and 8.4).

There appears to be a focus for pain inputs in part of area 3 of the primary somatosensory cortex, as shown by loss of pain sensation after a lesion to this region (Marshall 1951), and by activation measured in PET studies of regions in the primary and the secondary somatosensory cortex (Coghill, Talbot, Evans, Meyer, Gjedde, Bushnell and Duncan 1994), although a more recent PET study from the same Centre implicates the cingulate cortex rather than the somatosensory cortex in the affective aspects of pain (Rainville, Duncan, Price, Carrier and Bushnell 1997). However, there is evidence that structures as recently developed as the orbitofrontal cortex of primates are important in the subjective aspects of pain, for patients with lesions or disconnection of the orbitofrontal cortex may say that they

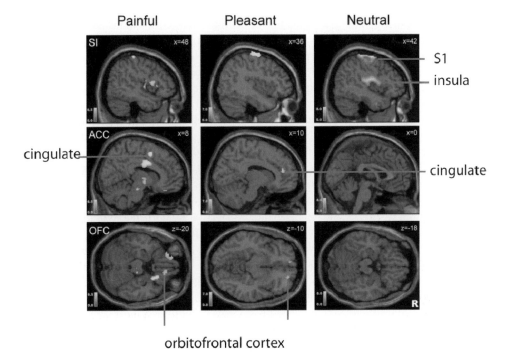

Painful   **Pleasant**   **Neutral**

orbitofrontal cortex

Fig. 4.4 Brain activation to painful, pleasant and neutral touch of the human brain. The top row shows strongest activation of the somatosensory cortex S1/insula by the neutral touch, on sagittal sections (parallel to the midline). The middle row shows activation of the most anterior part of the anterior cingulate cortex by the pleasant touch, and of a more posterior part by the painful touch, on sagittal sections. The bottom row shows activation of the orbitofrontal cortex by the pleasant and by the painful touch, on axial sections (in the horizontal plane). The activations were thresholded at p<0.0001 to show the extent of the activations. (After Rolls, O'Doherty et al., 2003d.) (See colour plates section.)

can identify the input as painful, but that it does not produce the same affective feeling as previously (Freeman and Watts 1950, Melzack and Wall 1996). In the fMRI study of Rolls, O'Doherty, Kringelbach, Francis, Bowtell and McGlone (2003d) painful inputs (produced by a stylus) were also applied to the hand, and we found that the orbitofrontal cortex was more strongly activated by the painful touch than by the neutral touch, whereas the somatosensory cortex was relatively more activated by the physically heavier neutral touch (see Fig. 4.4). This provides evidence that negative (see also Petrovich, Petersson, Ghatan, Ston-Elander and Ingvar (2000)) as well as positive aspects of affective touch are especially represented in the orbitofrontal cortex. In this study, as in many studies (Vogt and Sikes 2000), a part of the anterior cingulate cortex in or near to the cingulate motor area was also activated by pain (see example in Fig. 4.4 and Section 4.7).

4.3.4 Visual stimuli

Although most visual stimuli are not primary reinforcers, but may become secondary reinforcers as a result of stimulus–reinforcer association learning, it is possible that some visual stimuli, such as the sight of a smiling face or of an angry face, could be primary reinforcers.

It has been shown that there is a population of neurons in the cortex in the anterior part of the macaque superior temporal sulcus that categorize face stimuli based on the expression on the face, not based on the identity of the face (Hasselmo, Rolls and Baylis 1989a) (see Section 4.4.6). Thus it is possible that the reinforcing value of face expression could be being decoded by this stage of cortical processing (which is at the same stage approximately as the inferior temporal visual cortex; see Rolls and Deco (2002), and Baylis, Rolls and Leonard (1987)). This cortical region projects into the amygdala, in which face-selective neurons are also found (Leonard, Rolls, Wilson and Baylis 1985). Although it is not yet known whether amygdala face-selective neurons can code for expression or reward as well as identity (Leonard, Rolls, Wilson and Baylis 1985), this does seem likely given that these amygdala neurons receive some of their inputs from the neurons in the cortex in the superior temporal sulcus.

Another population of face-selective neurons is also found in the orbitofrontal cortex (Rolls, Critchley, Browning and Inoue 2006a) (see Section 4.5.5.6), and some of these neurons by being tuned to face expression could represent the primary reinforcing value of a face. Consistent with this, orbitofrontal and cingulate cortex lesions can impair humans' ability to identify the emotional expression in a face (Hornak, Rolls and Wade 1996, Rolls 1999b, Hornak, Bramham, Rolls, Morris, O'Doherty, Bullock and Polkey 2003) (see Section 4.5.6). However, it seems likely that, in addition, at least some of the face-selective neurons in the amygdala and orbitofrontal cortex reflect the secondary reinforcing value of a face, given the role these brain regions play in stimulus–reinforcer association learning (see Sections 4.5 and 4.6).

In humans, it has been found that activation of the orbitofrontal cortex is correlated with the attractiveness of the face being viewed (O'Doherty, Winston, Critchley, Perrett, Burt and Dolan 2003b). This may be an example of a visual primary reinforcer being represented in the orbitofrontal cortex.

It is possible that some auditory stimuli can be primary reinforcers. Where the reinforcement value may be decoded is not yet known, though auditory neurons that respond to vocalization have been found in the orbitofrontal cortex (Rolls, Critchley, Browning and Inoue 2006a) and amygdala (personal observations), and may also be present in the cingulate cortex (Jurgens 2002, West and Larson 1995); and orbitofrontal and cingulate cortex lesions can impair humans' ability to identify the emotional expression in a voice (Hornak, Rolls and Wade 1996, Hornak, Bramham, Rolls, Morris, O'Doherty, Bullock and Polkey 2003) (see Section 4.5.6).

As discussed in Chapter 3 and Section 4.6.5, novel stimuli are somewhat rewarding and in this sense act as primary reinforcers. The value of this type of reinforcer is that it encourages animals to explore new environments in which their genes might produce a fitness advantage. Neurons that respond to visual stimuli that are associated with rewards, and to novel stimuli, have been discovered in the primate amygdala, and this evidence suggests that these neurons are involved in the primary reinforcing properties of novel stimuli (Wilson and Rolls 1993, Wilson and Rolls 2005).

Further examples of visual primary reinforcers are given in Section 3.2.1.4 and Table 2.1.

4.4   Representing potential secondary reinforcers

Many stimuli, such as the sight of an object, have no intrinsic emotional effect. They are not primary reinforcers. Yet they can come as a result of learning to have emotional significance. This type of learning is called stimulus–reinforcer association, and the association is between the sight of the neutral visual stimulus (the potential secondary reinforcer) and the primary reward or punisher (the taste of food, or a painful stimulus). In that both the potential secondary reinforcer and the primary reinforcer are stimuli, stimulus–reinforcer association learning is a type of stimulus–stimulus association learning.

How are the representations of objects built in the brain, and what is the form of the representation appropriate for it to provide the input stimulus in stimulus–reinforcer association learning? These issues are addressed in detail by Rolls and Deco (2002), but some of the relevant issues in the present context of how stimuli should be represented if they are to be appropriate for subsequent evaluation by stimulus–reinforcer association learning brain mechanisms are described in this Section (4.4). The description of the functions of brain mechanisms that play a fundamental role in utilizing these representations for emotional learning and processing starts in Section 4.5.

4.4.1   The requirements of the representation

From an abstract, formal point of view we would want the representation of the to-be-associated stimulus, neutral before stimulus–reinforcer association learning, to have some of the following properties:

4.4.1.1   Invariance

The representation of the object should be invariant with respect to physical transforms of the object such as size (which varies with distance), position on the retina (translation invariance), and view. The reason that invariance is such an important property is that if we learned, for example, an association between one view of an object and a reward or punisher, it would be extremely unadaptive if when we saw the object again from a different view we did not have the same emotional response to it, or recognize it as a food with a good taste. We need to learn about the reward and punisher associations of objects, not of particular images with a fixed size and position on the retina. This is the fundamental reason why perceptual processing in sensory systems should proceed to the level at which objects are represented invariantly before the representation is used for emotional and motivation-related learning by stimulus–reinforcer association.

There are only exceptional circumstances in which we wish to learn, or it would be adaptive to learn, associations to stimuli represented early on in sensory processing streams, before invariant representations are computed. There are exceptional cases though, such as it being appropriate to learn an emotional response to a loud sound represented only as tones, as has been studied by LeDoux (1994) in his model system. We should realise that such cases are exceptions, and that the fundamental design principle is very different, with representations normally being at the object level before there is an interface to emotion learning systems, as described in the work considered below and elsewhere (e.g. Rolls (1986c), Rolls (1986a), Rolls (1990d), Rolls (1999a)).

While the example taken has been from vision, the same is true for other modalities. For example, in audition, we would want to make the same emotional decoding to the word 'Fire' independently of whether we hear it spoken (with extremely different pitches) by a child, by a woman, or by a man. This could not be decoded without high-level cortical processing, emphasizing the point that normally we need to have emotional responses to stimuli decoded correctly to the level where an object has been made explicit in the representation.

The capacity for view-invariant representation of objects may be especially well developed in primates, as implied for example by the great development in primates of the parts of the temporal lobe concerned with vision (inferior temporal visual cortex, cortex in the superior temporal sulcus, etc., see Sections 4.4.3 and 4.4.5).

The issue then arises of the organization of vision in non-primates, and whether view-invariant representations are formed when there is a much less well-developed temporal lobe. It may be that for many objects, a sufficiently good representation of objects which is effectively view-invariant can be formed without explicitly computing a view-invariant representation. Take for example the representation of a small fruit such as a raspberry. The nature of this object is that it can be recognized from almost any viewing angle based on the presence of three simple features, (two-dimensional) shape, surface texture, and colour. [Moreover, once one has been identified by, for example, taste, there are likely to be others present locally, and serial feeding (concentrating on one type of food, then switching to another) may take advantage of this.] Thus much behaviour towards objects may take place based on the presence of a simple list of identifying features, rather than by computing true view-invariant representations of objects that look different from different angles (see also Rolls and Deco (2002), Section 8.2.1). The sophisticated mechanism present in the primate temporal lobe for computing invariant representations of objects may be associated with the evolution of hands, tool use, and stereoscopic vision, and the necessity to recognize and manipulate objects from different angles to make artefacts. At a slightly simpler level, primates often eat more than 100 different types of food in a day, and the ability to perform view-invariant representations of large numbers of small objects is clearly adaptive in this situation too.

It is certainly of interest that apparently quite complex behaviour, including food selection in birds and insects, may be based on quite simple computational processes, such as in this case object identification based on a list of simple features. We should always be cautious about inferring more complex substrates for behaviour than is really necessary given the capacities. Part of the value of neurophysiological investigation of the primate temporal cortex is that it shows that view-invariant representations are actually computed, even for objects that look very different from different viewing angles (see Section 4.4.3 and Rolls and Deco (2002)).

4.4.1.2 Generalization

If we learn an emotional response to an object, we usually want to generalize the emotional response to other similar objects. An example might be the sight of a pin, which, after stimulus–reinforcer association learning, would generalize to the shape of other similar sharp-pointed objects such as a pencil, a pen, etc. Generalization occurs most easily if each object is represented by a population of neurons firing, each perhaps reflecting different properties of the object. Then if the object alters a little, in that some of its features change, there will still be sufficient similarity of the representation for it to be reasonably correlated with the original representation.

The way in which generalization occurs in the types of neuronal network found in the brain, and the nature of the representation needed, have been described by Rolls and Treves (1998) and Rolls and Deco (2002). A synopsis of some of the key ideas as they apply most directly to pattern associators, which are types of network involved in learning about which environmental stimuli are associated with reward or with punishment, is provided in Appendix 1. The approach is introduced in Fig. 4.5. The unconditioned or primary reinforcer activates the neuron shown (one of many) by unmodifiable synaptic connections (only one of which is drawn in Fig. 4.5). The to-be-conditioned stimulus activates the neuron through a population of modifiable synapses. The association is learned by strengthening those synapses from active conditioned stimulus input axons when the postsynaptic neuron is activated by the primary reinforcer. This is known as the Hebb learning rule (after D. O. Hebb, who in 1949 envisaged a synaptic learning rule of this general form). Later, when only the conditioned stimulus is presented, it activates the postsynaptic neuron through the modified synapses, producing the same firing as that originally produced by the unconditioned stimulus. If the conditioned stimulus is represented by the firing of a set of axons, then we can think of this as a vector. In the same way, we can think of the synaptic weights as another vector. If the input vector matches the weight vector, then the maximal activation of the neuron is produced. If the input vector uses distributed encoding (with perhaps each axon reflecting the presence of one or several features of the object), then a similar vector of firing will represent a similar object. Because many of the strengthened synapses activated by the original stimulus will also be activated by the similar stimulus, the similar stimulus will produce activation of the neuron that is similar to that produced by the original conditioned stimulus. The neuron can thus be thought of as computing the similarity of input patterns of firing, and it is this which results in good generalization (see Appendix 1).

This consideration leads to the suggestion that in order to enable good generalization to occur, the to-be-conditioned stimulus, i.e. the potential secondary reinforcer, should be represented with a distributed representation. If, in contrast to a distributed representation, there was a local representation (in which a single neuron would be so specifically tuned that it carried all the information about which stimulus was present), then generalization would be much more difficult. If one learned an association to a single neuron firing that represented the object, then any small alteration of the stimulus would lead to another neuron firing (so that small perceptual differences between stimuli could be represented), and there would be no generalization.

4.4.1.3 Graceful degradation

If there is minor damage to the nervous system, for example if some neurons die or some synapses are lost, there is no catastrophic change in performance. Instead, as the damage becomes more and more major, there is generally a gradual decline in the performance of the function affected. This is known as graceful degradation (and is a form of fault tolerance). Graceful degradation is a simple property of neural networks that use distributed representations. It arises in a very similar way to generalization. Because each object is represented by an ensemble (or vector) of neuronal activity, if a few of the input axons or the synapses are damaged, then the remainder of the input axons and synapses can still produce activation of the neuron that approximates the correct activation. [As explained in Appendix 1 and by Rolls and Treves (1998) and Rolls and Deco (2002), the operation performed by a neuron may be thought of as computing the inner or dot product of the input firing rate vector of neuronal activity and the synaptic weight vector. The result is a scalar value, the activation of the neuron. The dot product effectively measures the similarity of the input firing-rate vector and the stored synaptic-weight vector. Provided that the two vectors use distributed representations, then graceful degradation will occur.] Given that the output of the network is produced in practice not by a single neuron but by a population of neurons, loss of

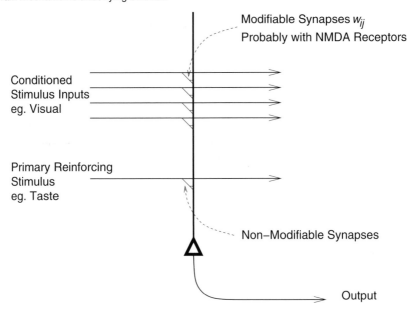

Fig. 4.5 Pattern association between a primary reinforcer, such as the taste of food, which activates neurons through non-modifiable synapses, and a potential secondary reinforcer, such as the sight of food, which has modifiable synapses on to the same neurons. Such a mechanism appears to be implemented in the amygdala and orbitofrontal cortex. (Homosynaptic) long-term depression (see Appendix 1) in a pattern associator in the amygdala could account for the habituating responses to novel visual stimuli which are not associated with primary reinforcers.

a few output neurons (which of course provide the input to the next stage) does not produce catastrophic degradation either (see further Rolls and Treves (1998), Rolls and Deco (2002), and Appendix 1).

4.4.2 High capacity

We would like the object representation to convey much information, that is to be capable of representing separately (discriminating between) many different objects. At the same time, we would like this high capacity representation to be readable by a pattern associator of the type just described, which reads out the information from the representation using a dot product operation. It turns out that this can be achieved by a distributed representation of the type found in the brain (Rolls and Deco 2002, Franco, Rolls, Aggelopoulos and Treves 2004, Franco, Rolls, Aggelopoulos and Jerez 2007).

One property of the representation is that each neuron should convey essentially independent information. The implication of this is that the number of stimuli that can be represented increases exponentially with the number of neurons in the population (because information is a log measure). Another property of the representation is that it should be readable by a simple operation such as a dot product, with each input neuron conveying an approximately similar amount of information. (This is described further in Appendix 1. The point is that a binary code would be too compact for the properties required.) It turns out that exactly the type of representation required is built for objects in the visual system, and is found elsewhere in the brain too (see Rolls and Treves (1998); Rolls and Deco (2002); Franco, Rolls, Aggelopoulos and Treves (2004); and Aggelopoulos, Franco and Rolls (2005); and Appendix 1). Another advantage of this type of representation is that a great deal of information about which object was shown can be read by taking the activity of any reasonably large subset of the population. This means that neurons in the brain do not need to have an input connection from every neuron in the sending population; and this makes the whole issue of brain wiring during development tractable (see Rolls and Treves (1998); Rolls and Deco (2002); and Rolls and Stringer (2000)).

It turns out that not only does the inferior temporal visual cortex have a representation of both faces and non-face objects with the properties described above (see Section 4.4.5), but also it transpires that the inferior temporal visual cortex does not contaminate its representation of objects (which must be used for many different functions in the brain) by having reward representations associated on to the neurons there (see Section 4.4.3). Instead, because its outputs are used for many functions, the reward value of objects is not what determines the response of inferior temporal cortex neurons. (If it did, then we might go blind to objects if they changed from being rewarding to being neutral. Exactly this change of reward value does occur if we eat a food to satiety, yet we can still see the food.) This issue, that the inferior temporal visual cortex is the stage in the object processing stream at which objects become represented, and from which there are major inputs to other parts of the brain which do learn reward and punishment associations of objects, the orbitofrontal cortex and amygdala, is considered next. The reasons for this architectural design are also considered.

4.4.3 Objects, and not their reward and punishment associations, are represented in the inferior temporal visual cortex

We now consider whether associations between visual stimuli and reinforcement are learned, and stored, in the visual cortical areas that proceed from the primary visual cortex, V1, through V2, V4, and the inferior temporal visual cortex (see Figs. 4.1 and 4.2). Is the emotional or motivational valence of visual stimuli represented in these regions? A schematic diagram summarizing some of the conclusions that will be reached is shown in Fig. 4.3.

One way to answer the issue just raised is to test monkeys in a learning paradigm in which one visual stimulus is associated with reward (for example glucose taste, or fruit juice taste), and another visual stimulus is associated with an aversive taste, such as strong saline. Rolls, Judge and Sanghera (1977) performed just such an experiment and found that single neurons in the inferior temporal visual cortex did not respond differently to objects based on their reward association. To test whether a neuron might be influenced by the reward association, the monkey performed a visual discrimination task in which the reinforcement contingency could be reversed during the experiment. (That is, the visual stimulus, for example a triangle, to which the monkey had to lick to obtain a taste of fruit juice, was after the reversal associated with saline – if the monkey licked to the triangle after the reversal, he obtained mildly aversive salt solution.) An example of such an experiment is shown in Fig. 4.6. The neuron responded more to the triangle, both before reversal when it was associated with fruit juice, and after reversal, when the triangle was associated with saline. Thus the reinforcement association of the visual stimuli did not alter the response to the visual stimuli, which was based on the physical properties of the stimuli (for example their shape, colour, or texture). The same was true for the other neurons recorded in this study.

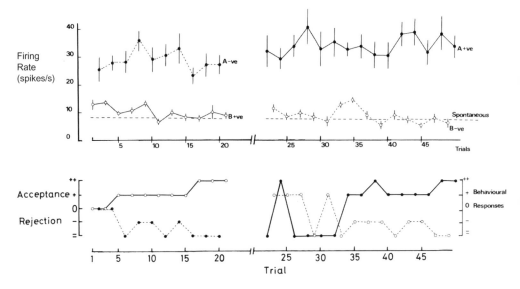

Fig. 4.6 Examples of the responses of a neuron in the inferior temporal visual cortex, showing that its responses (firing rate in spikes/s, upper panel) do not reverse when the reward association of the visual stimuli reverses. For the first 21 trials of the visual discrimination task, visual stimulus A was aversive (–ve, because if the monkey licked he obtained saline), and visual stimulus B was associated with reward (+ve, because if the monkey licked when he saw this stimulus, he obtained fruit juice). The neuron responded more to stimulus A than to stimulus B. After trial 21, the contingencies reversed (so that A was now +ve, and B –ve). The monkey learned the reversal correctly by about trial 35 (lower panel). However, the inferior temporal cortex neuron did not reverse when the reinforcement contingency reversed – it continued to respond to stimulus A after the reversal, even though the stimulus was now +ve. Thus this, and other inferior temporal cortex neurons, respond to the physical aspects of visual stimuli, and not to the stimuli based on their reinforcement association or the reinforcement contingency. (From Rolls, Judge and Sanghera 1977.)

This conclusion, that the responses of inferior temporal neurons during visual discriminations do not code for whether a visual stimulus is associated with reward or punishment, is also consistent with further findings (Ridley, Hester and Ettlinger 1977, Jarvis and Mishkin 1977, Gross, Bender and Gerstein 1979, Sato, Kawamura and Iwai 1980), including an investigation in which macaques search for food-related stimuli in complex visual scenes (Rolls, Aggelopoulos and Zheng 2003a). In the visual food reward search task the monkeys searched a complex natural visual scene to find and touch one of two objects in order to obtain fruit juice reward. If the wrong object was touched, the monkeys obtained mildly aversive hypertonic saline. The neurons responded to one of the selected stimuli in this experiment, and when the reward/punisher was reversed between the stimuli, the neuron continued to respond independently of whether the stimulus was associated with reward or with the punisher (Rolls, Aggelopoulos and Zheng 2003a). This independence from reward association seems to be characteristic of neurons right through the temporal visual cortical areas, and must be true in earlier cortical areas too, in that they provide the inputs to the inferior temporal visual cortex (Rolls and Deco 2002).

4.4.4   Why reward and punishment associations of stimuli are not represented early in information processing in the primate brain

The processing stream that has just been considered is that concerned with objects, that is with what is being looked at. Two fundamental points about pattern association networks for stimulus–reinforcer association learning can be made from what we have considered. The first point is that sensory processing in the primate brain proceeds as far as the invariant representation of objects (invariant with respect to, for example, size, position on the retina, and even view), independently of reward vs punisher association. Why should this be, in terms of systems-level brain organization? The suggestion that is made is that the visual properties of the world about which reward associations must be learned are generally objects (for example the sight of a banana, or of an orange), and are not just raw pixels or edges, with no invariant properties, which is what is represented in the retina and the primary visual cortex (V1). The implication is that the sensory processing must proceed to the stage of the invariant representation of objects before it is appropriate to learn reinforcer associations. The invariance aspect is important too, for if we had different representations for an object at different places in our visual field, then if we learned when an object was at one point on the retina that it was rewarding, we would not generalize correctly to it when presented at another position on the retina. If it had previously been punishing at that retinal position, we might find the same object rewarding when at one point on the retina, and punishing when at another. This is inappropriate given the world in which we live, and in which our brain evolved, in that the most appropriate assumption is that objects have the same reinforcer association wherever they are on the retina.

The same systems-level principle of brain organization is also likely to be true in other sensory systems, such as those for touch and hearing. For example, we do not generally want to learn that a particular pure tone is associated with a reward or punisher. Instead, it might be a particular complex pattern of sounds such as a vocalization that carries a reinforcement signal, and this may be independent of the exact pitch at which it is uttered. Thus, cases in which some modulation of neuronal responses to pure tones in parts of the brain such as the medial geniculate (the thalamic relay for hearing) (LeDoux 1994) where tonotopic tuning is found, may be rather special model systems (that is simplified systems on which to perform experiments), and not reflect the way in which auditory-to-reinforcer pattern associations are normally learned. The same may be true for touch in so far as one considers associations between objects identified by somatosensory input, and primary reinforcers. An example might be selecting a food object from a whole collection of objects in the dark.

The second point, which complements the first, is that the visual system is not provided with the appropriate primary reinforcers for such pattern-association learning, in that visual processing in the primate brain is mainly unimodal to and through the inferior temporal visual cortex (see Fig. 4.2). It is only after the inferior temporal visual cortex, when it projects to structures such as the amygdala and orbitofrontal cortex, that the appropriate convergence between visual processing pathways and pathways conveying information about primary reinforcers such as taste and touch/pain occurs (Fig. 4.2). We will later, therefore, turn our attention to the amygdala and orbitofrontal cortex, to consider whether they might be the brain regions that contain the neuronal networks for pattern associations involving primary reinforcers. We note at this stage that in order to make the results as relevant as possible to brain function and its disorders in humans, the system being described is that present in primates such as monkeys. In rats, although the organization of the amygdala may be similar, the areas that may correspond to the primate inferior temporal visual cortex and orbitofrontal cortex are less developed.

4.4.5 Invariant representations of faces and objects in the inferior temporal visual cortex

4.4.5.1 Processing to the inferior temporal cortex in the primate visual system

A schematic diagram to indicate some aspects of the processing involved in object identification from the primary visual cortex, V1, through V2 and V4 to the posterior inferior temporal cortex (TEO) and the anterior inferior temporal cortex (TE) is shown in Fig. 4.7. Their approximate location on the brain of a macaque monkey is shown in Fig. 4.8, which also shows that TE has a number of different subdivisions. The different TE areas all contain visually responsive neurons, as do many of the areas within the cortex in the superior temporal sulcus (Baylis, Rolls and Leonard 1987). For the purposes of this summary, these areas will be grouped together as the anterior inferior temporal cortex (IT), except where otherwise stated. Some of the information processing that takes place through these pathways that must be addressed by computational models is as follows. A fuller account is provided by Rolls (2000a), Rolls and Deco (2002) and Rolls (2007e). Many of the studies on neurons in the inferior temporal cortex and cortex in the superior temporal sulcus have been performed with neurons that respond particularly to faces, because such neurons can be found regularly in recordings in this region, and therefore provide a good population for systematic studies (Rolls 2000a, Rolls and Deco 2002, Rolls 2004d, Rolls 2007e).

4.4.5.2 Receptive field size and translation invariance

There is convergence from each small part of a region to the succeeding region (or layer in the hierarchy) in such a way that the receptive field sizes of neurons (for example 1 degree near the fovea in V1) become larger by a factor of approximately 2.5 with each succeeding stage. [The typical parafoveal receptive field sizes found would not be inconsistent with the calculated approximations of, for example, 8 deg in V4, 20 deg in TEO, and 50 deg in inferior temporal cortex (Boussaoud, Desimone and Ungerleider 1991) (see Fig. 4.7)]. Such zones of convergence would overlap continuously with each other (see Fig. 4.7). This connectivity provides part of the basis for the fact that many neurons in the temporal cortical visual areas respond to a stimulus relatively independently of where it is in their receptive field, and moreover maintain their stimulus selectivity when the stimulus appears in different parts of the visual field (Gross, Desimone, Albright and Schwartz 1985, Tovee, Rolls and Azzopardi 1994, Rolls, Aggelopoulos and Zheng 2003a). This is called translation or shift invariance. In addition to having topologically appropriate connections, it is necessary for the connections to have the appropriate synaptic weights to perform the mapping of each set of features, or object, to the same set of neurons in IT. How this could be achieved is addressed in the computational neuroscience models described by Wallis and Rolls (1997), Rolls and Deco (2002), Stringer, Perry, Rolls and Proske (2006), Rolls and Stringer (2006) and Rolls (2007c).

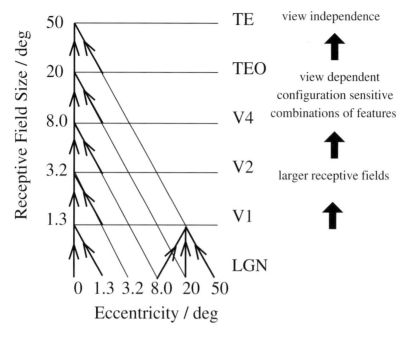

Fig. 4.7 Schematic diagram showing convergence achieved by the forward projections in the visual system, and the types of representation that may be built by competitive networks operating at each stage of the system from the primary visual cortex (V1) to the inferior temporal visual cortex (area TE) (see text). LGN, lateral geniculate nucleus. Area TEO forms the posterior inferior temporal cortex. The receptive fields in the inferior temporal visual cortex (for example in the TE areas) cross the vertical midline (not shown).

4.4.5.3 Reduced translation invariance in natural scenes, and the selection of a rewarded object

Until recently, research on translation invariance considered the case in which there is only one object in the visual field. What happens in a cluttered, natural, environment? Do all objects that can activate an inferior temporal neuron do so whenever they are anywhere within the large receptive fields of inferior temporal neurons (cf. Sato (1989))? If so, the output of the visual system might be confusing for structures that receive inputs from the temporal cortical visual areas. If one of the objects in the visual field was associated with reward, and another with punishment, would the output of the inferior temporal visual cortex to emotion-related brain systems be an amalgam of both stimuli? If so, how would we be able to choose between the stimuli, and have an emotional response to one but not perhaps the other, and select one for action and not the other?

In an investigation of this, it was found that the mean firing rate across all cells to a fixated effective face with a non-effective face in the parafovea (centred 8.5 degrees from the fovea) was 34 spikes/s. On the other hand, the average response to a fixated non-effective face with an effective face in the periphery was 22 spikes/s (Rolls and Tovee 1995a). Thus these cells gave a reliable output about which stimulus is actually present at the fovea, in that their response was larger to a fixated effective face than to a fixated non-effective face, even when there

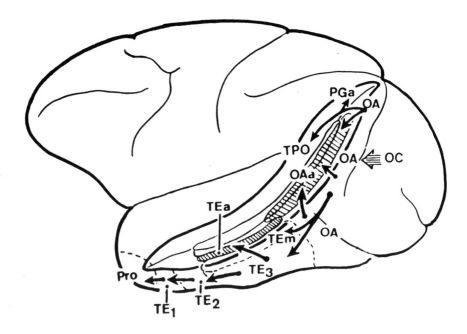

Fig. 4.8 Lateral view of the macaque brain (left hemisphere) showing the different architectonic areas (e.g. TEm, TPO) in and bordering the anterior part of the superior temporal sulcus (STS) of the macaque (see text).

were other parafoveal stimuli effective for the neuron. Thus the neurons provide information biased towards what is present at the fovea, and not equally about what is present anywhere in the visual field. This makes the interface to action simpler, in that what is at the fovea can be interpreted (e.g. by an associative memory) partly independently of the surroundings, and choices and actions can be directed if appropriate to what is at the fovea (cf. Ballard (1993)). These findings are a step towards understanding how the visual system functions in a normal environment (see also Gallant, Connor and Van-Essen (1998), and Stringer and Rolls (2000)).

To investigate further how information is passed from the inferior temporal cortex (IT) to other brain regions to enable stimuli to be selected from natural scenes for action, Rolls, Aggelopoulos and Zheng (2003a) analysed the responses of single and simultaneously recorded IT neurons to stimuli presented in complex natural backgrounds. In one situation, a visual fixation task was performed in which the monkey fixated at different distances from the effective stimulus. In another situation the monkey had to search for two objects on a screen, and a touch of one object was rewarded with juice, and of another object was punished with saline (see Fig. 4.9). In both situations neuronal responses to the effective stimuli for the neurons were compared when the objects were presented in the natural scene or on a plain background. It was found that the overall response of the neuron to objects was sometimes somewhat reduced when they were presented in natural scenes, though the selectivity of the neurons remained. However, the main finding was that the magnitudes of the responses of the neurons typically became much less in the real scene the further the monkey fixated in

Receptive Field Size
in Natural Scenes

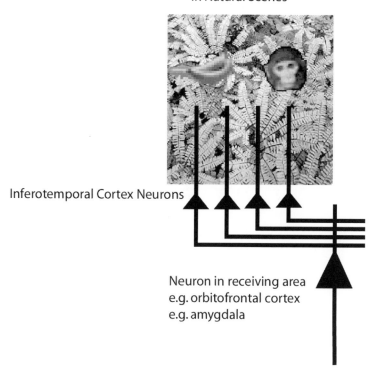

Inferotemporal Cortex Neurons

Neuron in receiving area
e.g. orbitofrontal cortex
e.g. amygdala

Fig. 4.9 Objects shown in a natural scene, in which the task was to search for and touch one of the stimuli. The objects in the task as run were smaller. The diagram shows that if the receptive fields of inferior temporal cortex neurons are large in natural scenes with multiple objects (in this scene, bananas and a face), then any receiving neuron in structures such as the orbitofrontal cortex and amygdala would receive information from many stimuli in the field of view, and would not be able to provide evidence about each of the stimuli separately.

the scene away from the object (see Fig. 4.10). It is proposed that this reduced translation invariance in natural scenes helps an unambiguous representation of an object which may be the target for action to be passed to the brain regions that receive from the primate inferior temporal visual cortex. It helps with the binding problem, by reducing in natural scenes the effective receptive field of inferior temporal cortex neurons to approximately the size of an object in the scene. The computational utility and basis for this is considered by Rolls and Deco (2002), Trappenberg, Rolls and Stringer (2002), Deco and Rolls (2004), Aggelopoulos and Rolls (2005) and Rolls and Deco (2006), and includes an advantage for what is at the fovea because of the large cortical magnification of the fovea, and shunting interactions between representations weighted by how far they are from the fovea.

These findings suggest that the principle of providing strong weight to whatever is close to the fovea is an important principle governing the operation of the inferior temporal visual cortex, and in general of the output of the visual system in natural environments. This principle of operation is very important in interfacing the visual system to action systems, because the

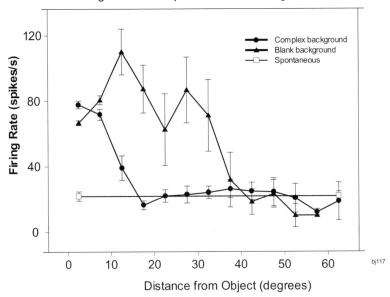

Fig. 4.10 Firing of a temporal cortex cell to an effective stimulus presented either in a blank background or in a natural scene, as a function of the angle in degrees at which the monkey was fixating away from the effective stimulus. The task was to search for and touch the stimulus. (After Rolls, Aggelopoulos and Zheng, 2003.)

effective stimulus in making inferior temporal cortex neurons fire is in natural scenes usually on or close to the fovea. This means that the spatial coordinates of where the object is in the scene do not have to be represented in the inferior temporal visual cortex, nor passed from it to the action selection system, as the latter can assume that the object making IT neurons fire is close to the fovea in natural scenes. Thus the position in visual space being fixated provides part of the interface between sensory representations of objects and their coordinates as targets for actions in the world. The small receptive fields of IT neurons in natural scenes make this possible. After this, local, egocentric, processing implemented in the dorsal visual processing stream using e.g. stereodisparity may be used to guide action towards reward-associated objects (Rolls and Deco 2002).

The reduced receptive field size in complex natural scenes also enables emotions to be selective to just what is being fixated, because this is the information that is transmitted by the firing of IT neurons to structures such as the orbitofrontal cortex and amygdala.

4.4.5.4　Size and spatial frequency invariance

Some neurons in the inferior temporal visual cortex and cortex in the anterior part of the superior temporal sulcus (IT/STS) respond relatively independently of the size of an effective face stimulus, with a mean size invariance (to a half maximal response) of 12 times (3.5 octaves) (Rolls and Baylis 1986). This is not a property of a simple single-layer network (see Fig. 8.1 of Rolls and Deco (2002)), nor of neurons in V1, which respond best to small stimuli, with a typical size-invariance of 1.5 octaves. (Some neurons in IT/STS also respond to face stimuli that are blurred, or that are line drawn, showing that they can also map the different spatial frequencies with which objects can be represented to the same representation in IT/STS, see Rolls, Baylis and Leonard (1985).)

Some neurons in the temporal cortical visual areas actually represent the absolute size of objects such as faces independently of viewing distance (Rolls and Baylis 1986). This could be called neurophysiological size constancy. The utility of this representation by a small population of neurons is that the absolute size of an object is a useful feature to use as an input to neurons that perform object recognition. Faces only come in certain sizes.

4.4.5.5 Combinations of features in the correct spatial configuration

Many cells in this processing stream respond to combinations of features (including objects), but not to single features presented alone, and the features must have the correct spatial arrangement. This has been shown, for example, with faces, for which it has been shown by masking out or presenting parts of the face (for example eyes, mouth, or hair) in isolation, or by jumbling the features in faces, that some cells in the cortex in IT/STS respond only if two or more features are present, and are in the correct spatial arrangement (Perrett, Rolls and Caan 1982, Rolls, Tovee, Purcell, Stewart and Azzopardi 1994b). Corresponding evidence has been found for non-face cells. For example, Tanaka, Saito, Fukada and Moriya (1990) showed that some posterior inferior temporal cortex neurons might only respond to the combination of an edge and a small circle if they were in the correct spatial relation to each other. Evidence consistent with the suggestion that neurons are responding to combinations of a few variables represented at the preceding stage of cortical processing is that some neurons in V2 and V4 respond to end-stopped lines, to tongues flanked by inhibitory subregions, or to combinations of colours (see Rolls and Deco (2002)). Neurons that respond to combinations of features but not to single features indicate that the system is non-linear (Elliffe, Rolls and Stringer 2002).

4.4.5.6 A view-independent representation

For recognizing and learning about objects (including faces), it is important that an output of the visual system should be not only translation- and size-invariant, but also relatively view-invariant. In an investigation of whether there are such neurons, we found that some temporal cortical neurons reliably responded differently to the faces of two different individuals independently of viewing angle (Hasselmo, Rolls, Baylis and Nalwa 1989b), although in most cases (16/18 neurons) the response was not perfectly view-independent. Mixed together in the same cortical regions there are neurons with view-dependent responses (for example Hasselmo, Rolls, Baylis and Nalwa (1989b) and Rolls and Tovee (1995b)). Such neurons might respond, for example, to a view of a profile of a monkey but not to a full-face view of the same monkey (Perrett, Smith, Potter, Mistlin, Head, Milner and Jeeves 1985, Hasselmo et al. 1989b).

These findings, of view-dependent, partially view-independent, and view-independent representations in the same cortical regions are consistent with the hypothesis discussed below that view-independent representations are being built in these regions by associating together the outputs of neurons that respond to different views of the same individual. These findings also provide evidence that one output of the visual system includes representations of what is being seen, in a view-independent way that would be useful for object recognition and for learning associations about objects; and that another output is a view-based representation that would be useful in social interactions to determine whether another individual is looking at one, and for selecting details of motor responses, for which the orientation of the object with respect to the viewer is required (Rolls and Deco 2002).

Further evidence that some neurons in the temporal cortical visual areas have object-based responses comes from a population of neurons that responds to moving faces, for example to a head undergoing ventral flexion, irrespective of whether the view of the head was full face, of either profile, or even of the back of the head (Hasselmo, Rolls, Baylis and Nalwa 1989b).

4.4.5.7 Distributed encoding

An important question for understanding brain function is whether a particular object (or face) is represented in the brain by the firing of one or a few gnostic (or 'grandmother') cells (Barlow 1972), or whether instead the firing of a group or ensemble of cells each with somewhat different responsiveness provides the representation. Advantages of distributed codes (see Appendix 1, Rolls and Treves (1998) and Rolls and Deco (2002)) include generalization and graceful degradation (fault tolerance), and a potentially very high capacity in the number of stimuli that can be represented (that is exponential growth of capacity with the number of neurons in the representation). If the ensemble encoding is sparse, this provides a good input to an associative memory, for then large numbers of stimuli can be stored (see Appendix 1 of this book, Chapters 2 and 3 of Rolls and Treves (1998), and Chapter 7 of Rolls and Deco (2002)). We have shown that in the inferior temporal visual cortex and cortex in the anterior part of the superior temporal sulcus (IT/STS), responses of a group of neurons, but not of a single neuron, provide evidence on which face was shown. We showed, for example, that these neurons typically respond with a graded set of firing to different faces, with firing rates from 120 spikes/s to the most effective face, to no response at all to a number of the least effective faces (Baylis, Rolls and Leonard 1985, Rolls and Tovee 1995b, Rolls and Deco 2002). In fact, the firing rate probability distribution of a single neuron to a set of stimuli is approximately exponential (Rolls and Tovee 1995b, Treves, Panzeri, Rolls, Booth and Wakeman 1999, Rolls and Deco 2002, Baddeley, Abbott, Booth, Sengpiel, Freeman, Wakeman and Rolls 1997, Franco, Rolls, Aggelopoulos and Jerez 2007). To provide examples, Fig. 4.11 shows typical firing rate changes of a single neuron on different trials to each of several different faces. This makes it clear that from the firing rate on any one trial, information is available about which stimulus was shown, and that the firing rate is graded, with a different firing rate response of the neuron to each stimulus.

The distributed nature of the encoding typical for neurons in the inferior temporal visual cortex is illustrated in Fig. 4.12, which shows that temporal cortical neurons typically responded to several members of a set of five faces, with each neuron having a different profile of responses to each face (Baylis, Rolls and Leonard 1985). It would be difficult for most of these single cells to tell which of even five faces, let alone which of hundreds of faces, had been seen. Yet across a population of such neurons, much information about the particular face that has been seen is provided, as shown below.

The single neuron selectivity or sparseness a^S of the activity of inferior temporal cortex neurons was 0.65 over a set of 68 stimuli including 23 faces and 45 non-face natural scenes, and a measure called the response sparseness a_r^S of the representation, in which the spontaneous rate was subtracted from the firing rate to each stimulus so that the responses of the neuron were being assessed, was 0.38 across the same set of stimuli (Rolls and Tovee 1995b). [For the definition of population sparseness see Section A.1.6. For binary neurons (firing for example either at a high rate or not at all), the single neuron sparseness is the proportion of stimuli that a single neuron responds to. These definitions are described further by Rolls and Deco (2002), by Franco et al. (2007), and by Franco et al. (2007).]

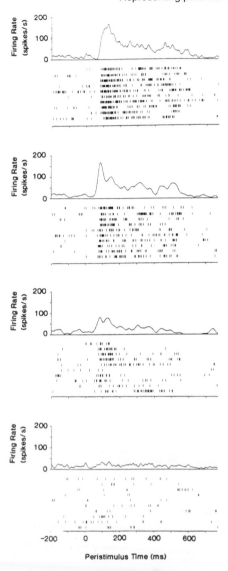

Fig. 4.11 Peristimulus time histograms and rastergrams showing the responses on different trials (originally in random order) of a face-selective neuron in the inferior temporal visual cortex to four different faces. (In the rastergrams each vertical line represents one spike from the neuron, and each row is a separate trial. Each block of the Figure is for a different face.) (From Tovee, Rolls, Treves and Bellis 1993.)

It has been possible to apply information theory to show that each neuron conveys on average approximately 0.4 bits of information about which face in a set of 20 faces has been seen (Tovee and Rolls 1995, Tovee, Rolls, Treves and Bellis 1993, Rolls, Treves, Tovee and Panzeri 1997d). If a neuron responded to only one of the faces in the set of 20, then it could convey (if noiseless) 4.6 bits of information about one of the faces (when that face was shown). If, at the other extreme, it responded to half the faces in the set, it would convey

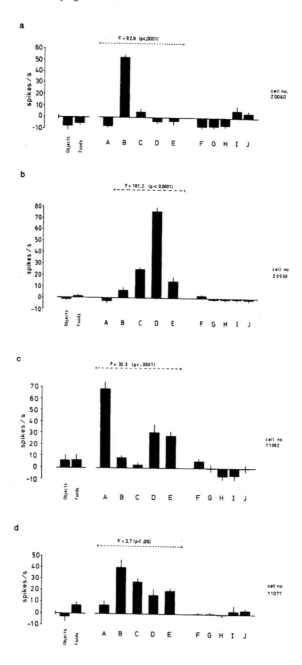

Fig. 4.12 Responses of four different temporal cortex visual neurons to a set of five faces (A–E), and, for comparison, to a wide range of non-face objects and foods. F–J are non-face stimuli. The means and standard errors of the responses computed over 8–10 trials are shown. (From Baylis, Rolls and Leonard, 1985.)

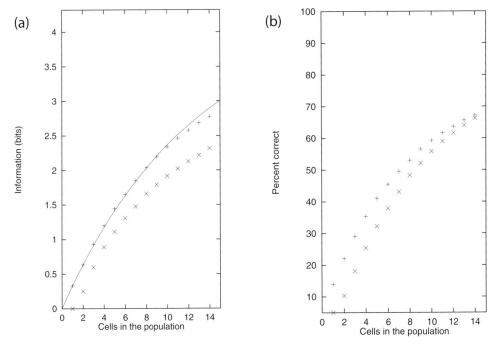

Fig. 4.13 (a) The values for the average information available in the responses of different numbers of these neurons on each trial, about which of a set of 20 face stimuli has been shown. The decoding method was Dot Product (DP, ×) or Probability Estimation (PE, +). The full line indicates the amount of information expected from populations of increasing size, when assuming random correlations within the constraint given by the ceiling (the information in the stimulus set, I = 4.32 bits). (b) The percent correct for the corresponding data to those shown in (a). (After Rolls, Treves and Tovee, 1997.)

1 bit of information about which face had been seen on any one trial. In fact, the average maximum information about the best stimulus was 1.8 bits of information. This provides good evidence not only that the representation is distributed, but also that it is a sufficiently reliable representation that useful information can be obtained from it.

The most impressive result obtained so far is that when the information available from a population of neurons about which of 20 faces has been seen is considered, the information increases approximately linearly as the number of cells in the population increases from 1 to 14 (Rolls, Treves and Tovee 1997b, Abbott, Rolls and Tovee 1996a) (see Fig. 4.13). Remembering that the information in bits is a logarithmic measure, this shows that the representational capacity of this population of cells increases exponentially (see Fig. 4.14). This is the case both when an optimal, probability estimation, form of decoding of the activity of the neuronal population is used, and also when the neurally plausible dot product type of decoding is used (Fig. 4.13). (The dot product decoding assumes that what reads out the information from the population activity vector is a neuron or a set of neurons that operates just by forming the dot product of the input population vector and its synaptic weight vector – see Rolls, Treves and Tovee (1997b), and Appendix 1.) By simulation of further neurons and further stimuli, we have shown that the capacity grows very impressively, approximately as shown in Fig. 4.14 (Abbott, Rolls and Tovee 1996a). The result has been replicated with

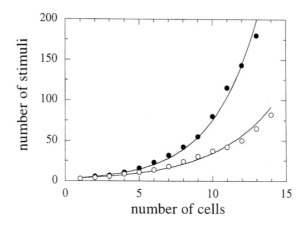

Fig. 4.14 The number of stimuli (in this case from a set of 20 faces) that are encoded in the responses of different numbers of neurons in the temporal lobe visual cortex, based on the results shown in Fig. 4.13. (After Rolls, Treves and Tovee, 1997; Abbott, Rolls and Tovee, 1996.)

simultaneously recorded neurons (Rolls, Franco, Aggelopoulos and Reece 2003b, Rolls, Aggelopoulos, Franco and Treves 2004). This result is exactly what would be hoped for from a distributed representation. This result is not what would be expected for local encoding, for which the number of stimuli that could be encoded would increase linearly with the number of cells. (Even if the grandmother cells were noisy, adding more replicates to increase reliability would not lead to more than a linear increase in the number of stimuli that can be encoded as a function of the number of cells.) Moreover, the encoding in the inferior temporal visual cortex about objects remains based on the spike count from each neuron, and not on the relative time of firing of each neuron or stimulus-dependent synchronization, when analysed with simultaneous single neuron recording (Franco, Rolls, Aggelopoulos and Treves 2004, Rolls, Franco, Aggelopoulos and Jerez 2006b) even in natural scenes while an attentional task is being performed (Aggelopoulos, Franco and Rolls 2005). Further, much of the information is available in short times of e.g. 20 or 50 ms (Tovee and Rolls 1995, Rolls, Franco, Aggelopoulos and Jerez 2006b), so that the receiving neuron does not need to integrate over a long time period to estimate a firing rate.

These findings provide very firm evidence that the encoding built at the end of the visual system is distributed, and that part of the power of this representation is that by receiving inputs from relatively small numbers of such neurons, neurons at the next stage of processing (for example in memory structures such as the hippocampus, amygdala, and orbitofrontal cortex) would obtain information about which of a very great number of stimuli had been shown.

This representational capacity of neuronal populations has fundamental implications for the connectivity of the brain, for it shows that neurons need not have hundreds of thousands or millions of inputs to have available to them information about what is represented in another population of cells, but that instead the real numbers of perhaps 8,000–10,000 synapses per neuron would be adequate for them to receive considerable information from the several different sources between which this set of synapses is allocated.

It may be noted that it is unlikely that there are further processing areas beyond those described where ensemble coding changes into grandmother cell encoding. Anatomically, there does not appear to be a whole further set of visual processing areas present in the brain; and outputs from the temporal lobe visual areas such as those described are taken to limbic and related regions such as the amygdala and via the entorhinal cortex to the hippocampus (see Rolls (1994b), Rolls (2000a), Rolls and Treves (1998), Rolls and Deco (2002) and Rolls and Stringer (2005)). Indeed, tracing this pathway onwards, we have found a population of neurons with face-selective responses in the amygdala, and in the majority of these neurons, different responses occur to different faces, with ensemble (not local) coding still being present (Leonard, Rolls, Wilson and Baylis 1985). The amygdala, in turn, projects to another structure that may be important in other behavioural responses to faces, the ventral striatum, and comparable neurons have also been found in the ventral striatum (Williams, Rolls, Leonard and Stern 1993). We have also recorded from face-responding neurons in the part of the orbitofrontal cortex that receives from the IT/STS cortex, and have found that the encoding there is also not local (Rolls, Critchley, Browning and Inoue 2006a).

4.4.6 Face expression, gesture and view represented in a population of neurons in the cortex in the superior temporal sulcus

In addition to the population of neurons that code for face identity, which tend to have object-based representations and are in areas TEa and TEm on the ventral bank of the superior temporal sulcus, there is a separate population in the cortex in the superior temporal sulcus (e.g. area TPO) that conveys information about facial expression (Hasselmo, Rolls and Baylis 1989a) (see e.g. Fig. 4.15). Some of the neurons in this region tend to have view-based representations (so that information is conveyed for example about whether the face is looking at one, or is looking away), and might respond to moving faces, and to facial gesture (Hasselmo, Rolls, Baylis and Nalwa 1989b).

Thus information in cortical areas that project to the amygdala and orbitofrontal cortex is about face identity, and about face expression and gesture. Both types of information are important in social and emotional responses to other primates (including humans), which must be based on who the individual is as well as on the face expression or gesture being made. One output from the amygdala for this information is probably via the ventral striatum, for a small population of neurons has been found in the ventral striatum with responses selective for faces (Rolls and Williams 1987a, Williams et al. 1993).

4.4.7 The brain mechanisms that build the appropriate view-invariant representations of objects required for learning emotional responses to objects, including faces

This book has the main goals of advancing understanding of the nature of emotion, of its functions and adaptive value in a Darwinian framework, and of how it is implemented in the brain taking mainly a systems-level approach. The main goal of the books by Rolls and Treves (1998) and Rolls and Deco (2002) was to provide some of the foundations for understanding at the computational and neuronal network level how the brain performs its functions. Some of the ways in which the visual system may produce the distributed invariant representations of objects needed for inputs to the emotion-learning systems described in this book have been described by Rolls and Deco (2002) and Rolls and Treves (1998), and include a hierarchical feed-forward series of competitive networks using convergence from

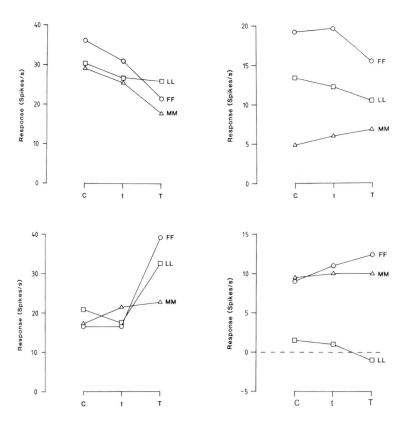

Fig. 4.15 There is a population of neurons in the cortex in the superior temporal sulcus with responses tuned to respond differently to different face expressions. The cells in the two left panels did not discriminate between individuals (faces MM, FF, and MM), but did discriminate between different expressions on the faces of those individuals (C, calm expression; t, mild threat; T, strong threat). In contrast, the cells in the right two panels responded differently to different individuals, and did not discriminate between different expressions. The neurons that discriminated between expressions were found mainly in the cortex in the fundus of the superior temporal sulcus; the neurons that discriminated between identity were in contrast found mainly in the cortex in lateral part of the ventral lip of the superior temporal sulcus (areas TEa and TEm). (From Hasselmo, Rolls and Baylis 1989.)

stage to stage; and the use of a modified Hebb synaptic learning rule that incorporates a short-term memory trace of previous neuronal activity to help learn the invariant properties of objects from the temporo-spatial statistics produced by the normal viewing of objects (Rolls and Deco 2002, Rolls 2004d, Wallis and Rolls 1997, Rolls and Milward 2000, Stringer and Rolls 2000, Rolls and Stringer 2001a, Elliffe, Rolls and Stringer 2002, Stringer and Rolls 2002, Deco and Rolls 2004, Rolls and Stringer 2006).

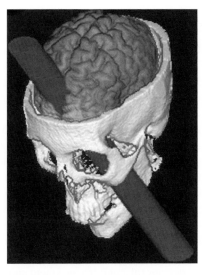

Fig. 4.16 Reconstruction of the possible entry and exit points of the tamping iron that went through Phineas Gage's frontal lobes by Damasio, Grabowski, Frank, Galaburda and Damasio (1994).

4.5 The orbitofrontal cortex

4.5.1 Historical background

The prefrontal cortex has for long been implicated in emotion, though it is only relatively recently that there has been a firm scientific foundation for understanding how it functions. Let us look first at some of the background.

4.5.1.1 Phineas Gage

One of the first indications that the prefrontal cortex is involved in emotion came from the remarkable case of Phineas Gage, who was working as a foreman for a railway development in Vermont in the USA (Harlow 1848). In 1848, he was tamping down explosives with a tamping iron when unexpectedly the tamping detonated the explosive. The tamping iron, a long bar like a crow bar approximately 3 ft 7 inches long, shot into the air and passed upwards through the front of Phineas Gage's brain (see Fig. 4.16) (Damasio, Grabowski, Frank, Galaburda and Damasio 1994). Gage survived but from that time on became a changed person. Formerly he had held responsibility as a foreman, but after the operation he became less reliable, and did not appear to be so concerned about the consequences of his actions. Moreover, in his personal life, he was described as being a changed person ("No longer Gage", short-tempered, capricious and profane). However, these personality and emotional changes took place without other general changes in Phineas Gage's intellectual abilities and intelligence. Hannah and Antonio Damasio and colleagues have reconstructed the site of the brain damage from the fractures found in the skull, and have shown that there would have been considerable damage to the lower (or ventral) part of the frontal cortex, which is where the orbitofrontal cortex is located (Damasio et al. 1994, Damasio 1994)). (It is so-called because it is just above the orbit of the eye.) The case of Phineas Gage suggested that the prefrontal cortex is involved in some way in emotion and personality, and that these functions are dissociable in the brain from many other types of brain function.

4.5.1.2 Prefrontal leucotomy

Another historical line of evidence implicates the frontal lobes in emotion. During an investigation of the effects of frontal lobe lesions in non-human primates on a short-term spatial memory task, Jacobsen (1936) noted that after the operation one of his animals became calmer and showed less frustration when reward was not given. Hearing of this emotional change, Moniz, a Portugeuse neurosurgeon, argued that anxiety, irrational fears, and emotional hyperexcitability in humans might be treated by damage to the frontal lobes. He operated on twenty patients and published an enthusiastic report of his findings (Moniz 1936) (see Fulton (1951)). This rapidly led to the widespread use of this surgical procedure, and more than 20,000 patients were subjected to prefrontal 'lobotomies' (in which a part of the frontal lobe was removed) or 'leucotomies' (in which some of the white matter connections of the frontal lobe were cut) of varying extent during the next 15 years. Although irrational anxiety or emotional outbursts were sometimes controlled, it was not clear that the surgery treated effectively the symptoms for which it was intended, side-effects were often apparent, and the effects were irreversible (Rylander 1948, Valenstein 1974). For these reasons these operations have been essentially discontinued. A lesson is that very careful and full assessment and follow-up of patients should be performed when a new neurosurgical (or any medical) procedure is being developed, before it is ever considered for widespread use. In relation to pain, patients who underwent a frontal lobotomy sometimes reported that after the operation they still had pain but that it no longer bothered them affectively (Freeman and Watts 1950, Melzack and Wall 1996).

4.5.2 Topology

Given this historical background, we now turn to a more systematic and fundamental consideration of how some parts of the frontal lobes are involved in emotion. The prefrontal cortex is the region of cortex that receives projections from the mediodorsal nucleus of the thalamus and is situated in front of the motor and premotor cortices (Areas 4 and 6) in the frontal lobe (see Fig. 4.1). Based on the divisions of the mediodorsal nucleus, the prefrontal cortex may be divided into three main regions (Fuster 1996). First, the magnocellular, medial (meaning towards the midline), part of the mediodorsal nucleus projects to the orbital (ventral) surface of the prefrontal cortex (which includes Areas 13 and 12) (see Fig. 4.17). It is called the orbitofrontal cortex, and is the part of the primate prefrontal cortex that appears to be primarily involved in emotion. The orbitofrontal cortex receives information from the part of the visual system concerned with forming representations of objects (the inferior temporal visual cortex), and taste, olfactory, and touch (somatosensory, body sensory) inputs (see Figs. 4.1 and 4.2). Second, the parvocellular, lateral, part of the mediodorsal nucleus projects to the dorsolateral prefrontal cortex. This part of the prefrontal cortex receives inputs from the parietal cortex, and is involved in tasks such as spatial short-term memory tasks, attention, and, in humans, functions such as planning (see Fuster (1996); Shallice and Burgess (1996); Rolls and Deco (2002); Deco and Rolls (2003)). Third, the pars paralamellaris (most lateral) part of the mediodorsal nucleus projects to the frontal eye fields (Area 8) in the anterior bank of the arcuate sulcus.

The orbitofrontal cortex is considered in the rest of this Section. The cortex on the orbital surface of the frontal lobe includes Area 13 caudally, Area 11 anteriorly, and Area 14 medially, and the cortex on the inferior convexity includes Area 12 (see Figs. 4.17, and 5.19 on page

ANTERIOR

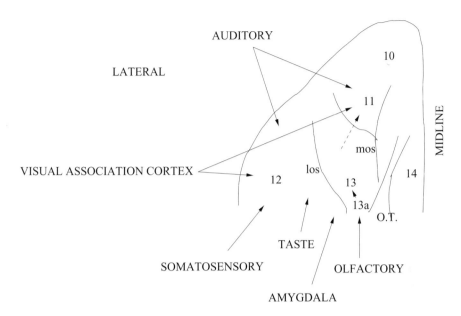

Fig. 4.17 Ventral view of the macaque orbitofrontal cortex. The midline is on the right of the diagram, and the inferior convexity is laterally, on the left. Subdivisions (after Barbas and Pandya 1989), and some afferents to the orbitofrontal cortex, are shown. mos, medial orbital sulcus; los, lateral orbital sulcus.

264, and Carmichael and Price (1994); Petrides and Pandya (1994); Ongur and Price (2000); Ongur, Ferry and Price (2003); and Kringelbach and Rolls (2004)). This brain region is poorly developed in rodents, but well developed in primates including humans. To understand the function of this brain region in humans, the majority of the studies described have therefore been performed with macaque monkeys or with humans. There is some variability in the sulcal patterns in the human orbitofrontal cortex (Chiavaras and Petrides 2001), and it is useful to take this into account in imaging studies (Kringelbach and Rolls 2004).

4.5.3 Connections

Some of the connections of the orbitofrontal cortex are shown schematically in Figs. 4.18, 4.1, 4.2 and 4.17.

Rolls, Yaxley and Sienkiewicz (1990) discovered a taste area in the lateral part of the primate orbitofrontal cortex by showing that neurons in it respond to taste placed into the mouth, and showed that this was the secondary taste cortex in that it receives a major projection from the primary taste cortex (Baylis, Rolls and Baylis 1994). More medially, there is an olfactory area (Rolls and Baylis 1994). Anatomically, there are direct connections from the primary olfactory cortex, pyriform cortex, to area 13a of the posterior orbitofrontal cortex, which in turn has onward projections to a middle part of the orbitofrontal cortex (area 11) (Price, Carmichael, Carnes, Clugnet and Kuroda 1991, Morecraft, Geula and Mesulam 1992, Barbas 1993, Carmichael, Clugnet and Price 1994) (see Figs. 4.17 and 4.18). Visceral inputs

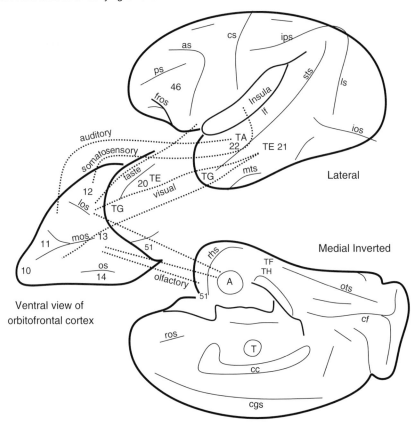

Fig. 4.18 Schematic diagram showing some of the gustatory, olfactory, and visual pathways to the orbito-frontal cortex, and some of the outputs of the orbitofrontal cortex. The secondary taste cortex and the secondary olfactory cortex are within the orbitofrontal cortex. V1, primary visual cortex. V4, visual corti-cal area V4. Abbreviations: as, arcuate sulcus; cc, corpus callosum; cf., calcarine fissure; cgs, cingulate sulcus; cs, central sulcus; ls, lunate sulcus; ios, inferior occipital sulcus; mos, medial orbital sulcus; os, orbital sulcus; ots, occipito-temporal sulcus; ps, principal sulcus; rhs, rhinal sulcus; sts, superior temporal sulcus; lf, lateral (or Sylvian) fissure (which has been opened to reveal the insula); A, amygdala; INS, in-sula; T, thalamus; TE (21), inferior temporal visual cortex; TA (22), superior temporal auditory association cortex; TF and TH, parahippocampal cortex; TG, temporal pole cortex; 12, 13, 11, orbitofrontal cortex; 35, perirhinal cortex; 51, olfactory (prepyriform and periamygdaloid) cortex.

may reach the posteromedial and lateral areas from the ventral part of the parvicellular division of the ventroposteromedial nucleus of the thalamus (VPMpc) (Carmichael and Price 1995b). Visual inputs reach the orbitofrontal cortex directly from the inferior temporal visual cortex, the cortex in the superior temporal sulcus, and the temporal pole (Jones and Powell 1970, Barbas 1988, Barbas 1993, Barbas 1995, Petrides and Pandya 1988, Barbas and Pandya 1989, Seltzer and Pandya 1989, Morecraft et al. 1992, Carmichael and Price 1995b). There are corresponding auditory inputs (Barbas 1988, Barbas 1993), and somatosensory inputs from somatosensory cortical areas 1, 2 and SII in the frontal and pericentral operculum, and from the insula (Barbas 1988, Preuss and Goldman-Rakic 1989, Carmichael and Price 1995b). The caudal orbitofrontal cortex has strong reciprocal connections with the amygdala (Price et al. 1991, Carmichael and Price 1995a). The orbitofrontal cortex also receives inputs via the mediodorsal nucleus of the thalamus, pars magnocellularis, which itself receives afferents from temporal lobe structures such as the prepyriform (olfactory) cortex, amygdala, and inferior temporal cortex (Nauta 1972, Krettek and Price 1974, Krettek and Price 1977). The medial orbital areas, and parts of lateral orbital area 12, receive connections from and project to the anterior cingulate cortex (Carmichael and Price 1995a). The medial orbitofrontal cortex receives connections from the subiculum (Carmichael and Price 1995a), which itself receives connections from the hippocampus (see Rolls and Treves (1998)).

The orbitofrontal cortex projects back to temporal lobe areas such as the inferior temporal visual cortex, and, in addition, to the entorhinal cortex (or 'gateway to the hippocampus') and cingulate cortex (Nauta 1964, Insausti, Amaral and Cowan 1987). The orbitofrontal cortex also projects to the preoptic region, lateral hypothalamus and brainstem autonomic areas such as the dorsal motor nucleus of the vagus and the nucleus of the solitary tract, to the ventral tegmental area (Nauta 1964, Johnson, Rosvold and Mishkin 1968, Van der Kooy, Koda, McGinty, Gerfen and Bloom 1984), and to the head of the caudate nucleus (Kemp and Powell 1970). Reviews of the cytoarchitecture and connections of the orbitofrontal cortex are provided by Petrides and Pandya (1994), Pandya (1996), Carmichael and Price (1994), Carmichael and Price (1995a), Carmichael and Price (1995b), Barbas (1995), Ongur and Price (2000), Ongur, Ferry and Price (2003), and Kringelbach and Rolls (2004).

4.5.4 Effects of damage to the orbitofrontal cortex

Damage to the caudal orbitofrontal cortex in the monkey produces emotional changes. These include reduced aggression to humans and to stimuli such as a snake and a doll, a reduced tendency to reject foods such as meat (Butter, Snyder and McDonald 1970, Butter and Snyder 1972, Butter, McDonald and Snyder 1969), and a failure to display the normal preference ranking for different foods (Baylis and Gaffan 1991). In the human, euphoria, irresponsibility, lack of affect, and impulsiveness can follow frontal lobe damage (Kolb and Whishaw 2003, Damasio 1994, Eslinger and Damasio 1985), particularly orbitofrontal cortex damage (Rolls, Hornak, Wade and McGrath 1994a, Hornak, Bramham, Rolls, Morris, O'Doherty, Bullock and Polkey 2003, Berlin, Rolls and Kischka 2004, Berlin, Rolls and Iversen 2005).

These changes that follow frontal lobe damage may be related to a failure to react normally to and learn from non-reward in a number of different situations. This failure is evident as a tendency to respond when responses are inappropriate, e.g. no longer rewarded. In particular, macaques with lesions of the orbitofrontal cortex are impaired at tasks that involve learning about which stimuli are rewarding and which are not, and especially in altering behaviour when reinforcement contingencies change. The monkeys may respond when responses are inappropriate, e.g. no longer rewarded, or may respond to a non-rewarded stimulus. For example, monkeys with orbitofrontal cortex damage are impaired on Go/NoGo task performance, in that they Go on the NoGo trials (Iversen and Mishkin 1970)[9], and in

---

[9] In a Go/NoGo task, on a Go trial one visual stimulus is shown, and a response such as licking a tube can be made to obtain a food reward; and on a NoGo trial, a different visual stimulus is shown, and no response must be made otherwise a punishment, of for example a taste of aversive saline, is obtained (Thorpe, Rolls and Maddison 1983, Rolls, Critchley, Mason and Wakeman 1996b). The task tests for stimulus–reward associations, in that one visual stimulus is associated with food reward, and the other with saline punishment if a response is made. There is a different version of a Go/NoGo task on which on NoGo trials no response must be made in order to obtain reward, and this version of the task with symmetrical reinforcement tests for whether one visual stimulus can be

an object-reversal task in that they respond to the object that was formerly rewarded with food, and in extinction in that they continue to respond to an object that is no longer rewarded (Butter 1969, Jones and Mishkin 1972, Meunier, Bachevalier and Mishkin 1997)[10]. There is some evidence for dissociation of function within the orbitofrontal cortex, in that lesions to the inferior convexity produce Go/NoGo and object reversal deficits, whereas damage to the caudal orbitofrontal cortex, area 13, produces the extinction deficit (Rosenkilde 1979). The visual discrimination learning deficit shown by monkeys with orbitofrontal cortex damage (Jones and Mishkin 1972, Baylis and Gaffan 1991) may be due to the tendency of these monkeys not to withhold responses to non-rewarded stimuli (Jones and Mishkin 1972), including foods that are not normally accepted (Butter et al. 1969, Baylis and Gaffan 1991).

Lesions more laterally, in for example the inferior convexity which receives from the inferior temporal visual cortex, can influence tasks in which objects must be remembered for short periods, e.g. delayed matching to sample and delayed matching to non-sample tasks (Passingham 1975, Mishkin and Manning 1978, Kowalska, Bachevalier and Mishkin 1991), and neurons in this region may help to implement this visual object short-term memory by holding the representation active during the delay period (Rosenkilde, Bauer and Fuster 1981, Wilson, O'Sclaidhe and Goldman-Rakic 1993). Whether this inferior convexity area is specifically involved in a short-term object memory is not yet clear, and a medial part of the frontal cortex may also contribute to this function (Kowalska et al. 1991). It should be noted that this short-term memory system for objects (which receives inputs from the temporal lobe visual cortical areas in which objects are represented) is different from the short-term memory system in the dorsolateral part of the prefrontal cortex, which is concerned with spatial short-term memories, consistent with its inputs from the parietal cortex (see, e.g., Williams, Rolls, Leonard and Stern (1993) but see also Deco and Rolls (2003) and Deco, Rolls and Horwitz (2004)). In any case, it is worth noting that this part of the prefrontal cortex could be involved in a function related to short-term memory for objects. This does not exclude this part of the prefrontal cortex from, in addition, being part of the more orbitofrontal system involved in visual to reinforcer association learning and reversal.

The effects of damage to the orbitofrontal cortex in humans are described in Section 4.5.6.

---

mapped to one behaviour, a response, and another visual stimulus to another behaviour, not responding, in order to obtain reward. Unless otherwise specified, it is the first version of the task that uses asymmetrical reinforcement and that tests for stimulus–reinforcer associations that is referred to in this book.

[10]In a visual discrimination reversal task as run in neurophysiological experiments (Thorpe, Rolls and Maddison 1983, Rolls, Critchley, Mason and Wakeman 1996b), on a trial on which one visual stimulus is shown, the S+ or positive discriminative stimulus S^D, a response such as licking a tube can be made to obtain a food reward; and on a trial on which the other visual stimulus is shown, the S– or negative discriminative stimulus S^Δ, no response must be made otherwise a punisher, of for example a taste of aversive saline, is obtained (Thorpe, Rolls and Maddison 1983, Rolls, Critchley, Mason and Wakeman 1996b). After good performance is obtained, the reward association is reversed, so that the visual stimulus that was formerly an S+ becomes an S–, and vice versa. Behaviour typically reverses over a number of trials, so that the new S+ become the stimulus that is worked for. The task tests for the ability to reverse stimulus–reward associations, and if reversal occurs, shows for example that the neuron being recorded encodes the reinforcement association of the visual stimuli, and not the physical identity of visual stimuli. The improvement in reversal learning performance so that after a number of reversal a reversal can take place in as little as one trial (Thorpe, Rolls and Maddison 1983) is referred to as reversal learning set (Deco and Rolls 2005d).

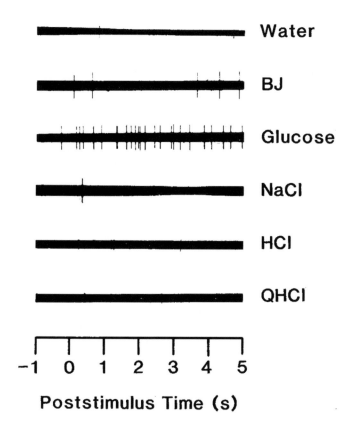

Fig. 4.19 Examples of the responses recorded from one caudolateral orbitofrontal taste cortex neuron to the six taste stimuli, water, 20% blackcurrant juice (BJ), 1 M glucose, 1 M NaCl, 0.01 M HCl, and 0.001 M quinine HCl (QHCl). The stimuli were placed in the mouth at time 0. (From Rolls, Yaxley and Sienkiewicz 1990.)

4.5.5 Neurophysiology and functional neuroimaging of the orbitofrontal cortex

The hypothesis that the orbitofrontal cortex is involved in correcting behavioural responses made to stimuli previously associated with reinforcement has been investigated by making recordings from single neurons in the orbitofrontal cortex while monkeys performed these tasks known to be impaired by damage to the orbitofrontal cortex. It has been shown that some neurons respond to primary reinforcers such as taste and touch; that others respond to learned secondary reinforcers, such as the sight of a rewarded visual stimulus, and thus predict or estimate a reward value; and that the rapid learning of associations between previously neutral visual stimuli and primary reinforcers is reflected in the responses of orbitofrontal cortex neurons in primates (Rolls 2004b, Rolls 2004a, Rolls 2004h, Rolls 2006d). These types of neuron are described next.

OFC

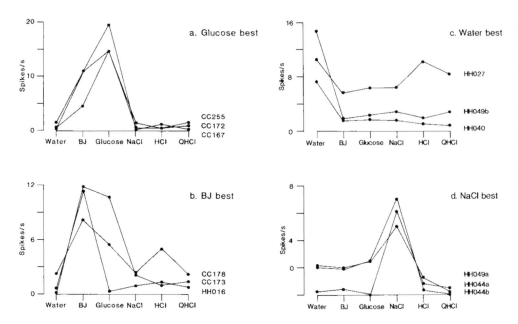

Fig. 4.20 Typical response profiles to different tastes of different orbitofrontal cortex taste neurons. Some responded best to the taste of 1 M glucose (a), to blackcurrant fruit juice (BJ) (b), to water (c), and to 0.1 M sodium chloride (NaCl) (d). HCl, 0.01 M HCl, sour; QHCl, 0.001 M quinine hydrochloride (bitter). (From Rolls, Yaxley and Sienkiewicz 1990.)

4.5.5.1 Taste

One of the discoveries that has helped us to understand the functions of the orbitofrontal cortex in behaviour is that it contains a major cortical representation of taste (Rolls 1989a, Rolls 1995b, Rolls 1997c, Rolls 1999a, Rolls and Scott 2003, Kadohisa, Rolls and Verhagen 2005a, Rolls 2007b) (cf. Fig. 4.2 and Chapter 5). Given that taste can act as a primary reinforcer, that is without learning as a reward or punisher, we now have the start for a fundamental understanding of the functions of the orbitofrontal cortex in stimulus–reinforcer association learning. We now know how one class of primary reinforcer reaches and is represented in the orbitofrontal cortex. A representation of primary reinforcers is essential for a system that is involved in learning associations between previously neutral stimuli and primary reinforcers, e.g. between the sight of an object, and its taste.

The most direct and precise evidence that taste is represented in the primate orbitofrontal cortex comes from recording the activity of single neurons in the macaque monkey orbitofrontal cortex. It has been shown that different single neurons respond differently to the prototypical tastes sweet, salt, bitter, and sour (Rolls, Yaxley and Sienkiewicz 1990), to the 'taste' of water (Rolls, Yaxley and Sienkiewicz 1990), and to the taste of protein or umami (Rolls 2001a) as exemplified by monosodium glutamate (Baylis and Rolls 1991) and inosine monophosphate (Rolls, Critchley, Wakeman and Mason 1996c). Each neuron typically responds to more than one taste, as shown in Figs. 4.19 and 4.20, but each taste can be clearly identified by considering the activity of a population of taste cells (Rolls, Critchley, Verhagen and Kadohisa 2007a). This is called population encoding, and it has many very useful properties that are described in Appendix 1 and Section 4.4.5.7, and by Rolls and Treves (1998) and Rolls and Deco (2002). In addition, other neurons are tuned to respond best to astringency (which is a flavour characteristic of tea) as exemplified by tannic acid (Critchley and Rolls 1996c). The input in this case comes through the somatosensory (touch) rather than taste pathways, so astringency is a tactile contribution to flavour. The mouth feel of fat (which contributes to the pleasantness of many foods including chocolate and ice cream) also activates a different population of primate orbitofrontal cortex neurons (see Chapter 5, Rolls, Critchley, Browning, Hernadi and Lenard (1999a), and Verhagen, Rolls and Kadohisa (2003)).

The caudolateral part of the orbitofrontal cortex has been shown anatomically to be the secondary taste cortex, in that it receives connections from the primary taste cortex just behind it in the insular/frontal opercular cortex (see Fig. 4.1) (Baylis, Rolls and Baylis 1994). This caudolateral orbitofrontal cortex region then projects on to other regions in the orbitofrontal cortex (Baylis et al. 1994), and neurons with taste responses (in what can be considered as a tertiary gustatory cortical area) can be found in many regions of the orbitofrontal cortex (see Rolls, Yaxley and Sienkiewicz (1990); Rolls and Baylis (1994); Rolls, Critchley, Wakeman and Mason (1996c); Critchley and Rolls (1996c); Rolls, Verhagen and Kadohisa (2003e); and Rolls and Scott (2003)).

There is also evidence from functional neuroimaging that taste can activate the human orbitofrontal cortex. For example, Francis, Rolls, Bowtell, McGlone, O'Doherty, Browning, Clare and Smith (1999) showed that the taste of glucose can activate the human orbitofrontal cortex, and O'Doherty, Rolls, Francis, Bowtell and McGlone (2001b) showed that the taste of glucose and salt activate nearby but separate parts of the human orbitofrontal cortex. De Araujo, Kringelbach, Rolls and Hobden (2003a) showed that umami taste (the taste of protein) as exemplified by monosodium glutamate is represented in the human orbitofrontal cortex as well as in the primary taste cortex as shown by functional magnetic resonance imaging (fMRI) (Fig. 5.15). The taste effect of monosodium glutamate (present in e.g. tomato, green vegetables, fish, and human breast milk) was enhanced in an anterior part of the orbitofrontal cortex in particular by combining it with the nucleotide inosine monophosphate (present in e.g. meat and some fish including tuna), and this provides evidence that the activations found in the orbitofrontal cortex are closely related to subjective taste effects. Small, Zald, Jones-Gotman, Zatorre, Petrides and Evans (1999) also found activation of the orbitofrontal cortex by taste.

The nature of the representation of taste in the orbitofrontal cortex is that the reward value of the taste is represented. The evidence for this is that the responses of orbitofrontal taste neurons are modulated by hunger in just the same way as is the reward value or palatability of a taste. In particular, it has been shown that orbitofrontal cortex taste neurons stop responding to the taste of a food with which the monkey is fed to satiety, and that this parallels the decline in the acceptability of the food (see Fig. 4.21) (Rolls, Sienkiewicz and Yaxley 1989b). In contrast, the representation of taste in the primary taste cortex (Scott, Yaxley, Sienkiewicz and Rolls 1986a, Yaxley, Rolls and Sienkiewicz 1990) is not modulated by hunger (Rolls, Scott, Sienkiewicz and Yaxley 1988, Yaxley, Rolls and Sienkiewicz 1988). Thus in the primary taste cortex of primates (and at earlier stages of taste processing), the reward value of taste is not represented, and instead the identity of the taste is represented (see further Scott, Yan and

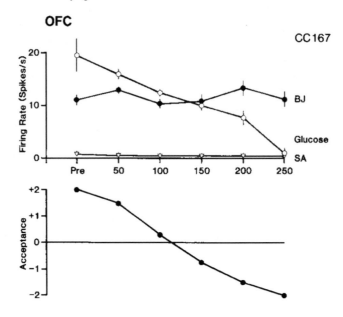

Fig. 4.21 The effect of feeding to satiety with glucose solution on the responses (rate ± s.e.m.) of a neuron in the secondary taste cortex to the taste of glucose and of blackcurrant juice (BJ). The spontaneous firing rate is also indicated (SA). Below the neuronal response data, the behavioural measure of the acceptance or rejection of the solution on a scale from +2 (strong acceptance) to –2 (strong rejection) is shown. The solution used to feed to satiety was 20% glucose. The monkey was fed 50 ml of the solution at each stage of the experiment as indicated along the abscissa, until he was satiated as shown by whether he accepted or rejected the solution. Pre is the firing rate of the neuron before the satiety experiment started. (From Rolls, Sienkiewicz and Yaxley 1989b.)

Rolls (1995) and Rolls and Scott (2003)).

Additional evidence that the reward value of food is represented in the orbitofrontal cortex is that monkeys work for electrical stimulation of the orbitofrontal cortex if they are hungry, but not if they are satiated (Mora, Avrith, Phillips and Rolls 1979). Thus the electrical stimulation of this brain region produces reward that is equivalent to food for a hungry animal. Further evidence implicating the firing of neurons in the orbitofrontal cortex in reward is that neurons in the orbitofrontal cortex are activated from many brain-stimulation reward sites (Rolls, Burton and Mora 1980c, Mora, Avrith and Rolls 1980). Thus there is clear evidence that it is the reward value of taste that is represented in the orbitofrontal cortex.

In humans, there is evidence that the reward value, and, what can be directly reported in humans, the subjective pleasantness, of food is represented in the orbitofrontal cortex. The evidence comes from an fMRI study in which humans rated the pleasantness of the flavour of chocolate milk and tomato juice, and then ate one of these foods to satiety. It was found that the pleasantness of the flavour of the food eaten to satiety decreased, and that this decrease in pleasantness was reflected in decreased activation in the orbitofrontal cortex (Kringelbach, O'Doherty, Rolls and Andrews 2003) (see Fig. 4.22). Further evidence that the pleasantness of flavour is represented here is that the flavour of the food not eaten to satiety showed very little

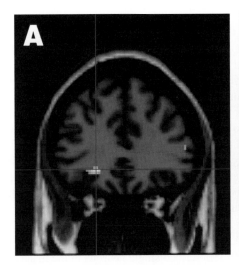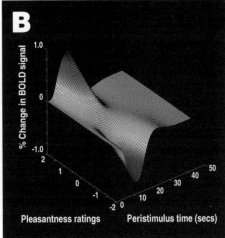

Fig. 4.22 Areas of the human orbitofrontal cortex with activations correlating with pleasantness ratings for food in the mouth. (A) Coronal section through the region of the orbitofrontal cortex from the random effects group analysis showing the peak in the left orbitofrontal cortex (Talairach co-ordinates X,Y,Z=−22,34,−8, z-score=4.06), in which the BOLD signal in the voxels shown in yellow was significantly correlated with the subjects' subjective pleasantness ratings of the foods throughout an experiment in which the subjects were hungry and found the food pleasant, and were then fed to satiety with the food, after which the pleasantness of the food decreased to neutral or slightly unpleasant. The design was a sensory-specific satiety design, and the pleasantness of the food not eaten in the meal, and the BOLD activation in the orbitofrontal cortex, were not altered by eating the other food to satiety. The two foods were tomato juice and chocolate milk. (B) Plot of the magnitude of the fitted haemodynamic response from a representative single subject against the subjective pleasantness ratings (on a scale from −2 to +2) and peristimulus time in seconds. (After Kringelbach, O'Doherty, Rolls and Andrews, 2003.) (See colour plates section.)

decrease, and correspondingly the activation of the orbitofrontal cortex to this food not eaten in the meal showed little decrease. The phenomenon itself is called sensory-specific satiety, is an important property of reward systems, and is described in more detail in Chapter 5. The experiment of Kringelbach, O'Doherty, Rolls and Andrews (2003) was with a whole food, but further evidence that the pleasantness of taste, or at least a stimulus very closely related to a taste, is represented in the human orbitofrontal cortex is that the orbitofrontal cortex is activated by water in the mouth when thirsty but not when satiated (De Araujo, Kringelbach, Rolls and McGlone 2003b) (see Fig. 6.7). Thus, the neuroimaging findings with a whole food, and with water when thirsty, provide evidence that the activation to taste *per se* in the human orbitofrontal cortex is related to the subjective pleasantness or affective value of the taste.

Consistent with these anatomical and neurophysiological findings, damage to the caudal orbitofrontal cortex in the monkey produces altered preferences for foods, including a reduced tendency to reject foods such as meat (Butter et al. 1970, Butter and Snyder 1972, Butter et al. 1969), and a failure to display the normal preference ranking for different foods (Baylis and Gaffan 1991). In humans there are few published descriptions of changes of affective reactions to foods after damage to the orbitofrontal cortex (when damage to the olfactory tract which runs just under the orbitofrontal cortex is excluded). However, of the patients in the groups with damage in the orbitofrontal cortex that we have studied (Rolls, Hornak, Wade and McGrath 1994a, Hornak, Rolls and Wade 1996, Hornak, Bramham, Rolls, Morris,

O'Doherty, Bullock and Polkey 2003, Hornak, O'Doherty, Bramham, Rolls, Morris, Bullock and Polkey 2004) and in similar patients, the most common complaint they make to the physician is about the quality of their taste and smell sensations. There are large changes in their emotional behaviour which will be described below (Section 4.5.6), but these patients do not usually actually complain about the emotional changes that others observe.

In conclusion, the evidence indicates that the reward value of taste is represented in the primate orbitofrontal cortex. There is also evidence that the corresponding subjective evaluation of taste, how pleasant it is, is related to activation of the orbitofrontal cortex. Thus evidence from studies of taste provide evidence that an aspect of affect is represented in the orbitofrontal cortex, and that this is not just general affect, but conveys a rich sensory representation of taste and its reward value, and is able to implement even the variation in the pleasantness of individual tastes as they vary during a meal.

4.5.5.2 An olfactory representation in the orbitofrontal cortex

Takagi, Tanabe and colleagues (see Takagi (1991)) described single neurons in the macaque orbitofrontal cortex that were activated by odours. A ventral frontal region has been implicated in olfactory processing in humans in PET[11] and fMRI studies (Jones-Gotman and Zatorre 1988, Zatorre and Jones-Gotman 1991, Zatorre, Jones-Gotman, Evans and Meyer 1992, Rolls, Kringelbach and De Araujo 2003c).

Rolls and colleagues have analysed the rules by which orbitofrontal olfactory representations are formed and operate in primates (Rolls 2001b). For 65% of neurons in the orbitofrontal olfactory areas, Critchley and Rolls (1996b) showed that the representation of the olfactory stimulus was independent of its association with taste reward (analysed in an olfactory discrimination task with taste reward, as some orbitofrontal cortex olfactory neurons are bimodal, with responses also to taste stimuli (Rolls and Baylis 1994)). For the remaining 35% of the neurons, the odours to which a neuron responded were influenced by the taste (glucose or saline) with which the odour was associated (Critchley and Rolls 1996b). Thus the odour representation for 35% of orbitofrontal neurons appeared to be built by olfactory-to-taste association learning.

This possibility that the odour representation of some primate orbitofrontal cortex olfactory neurons is built by olfactory-to-taste association learning was confirmed by reversing the taste with which an odour was associated in the reversal of an olfactory discrimination task. It was found that 73% of the sample of neurons analysed altered the way in which they responded to odour when the taste reinforcer association of the odour was reversed (Rolls, Critchley, Mason and Wakeman 1996b). Reversal was shown by 25% of the neurons (see, for example, Fig. 4.23), and 48% altered their activity in that they no longer discriminated after the reversal. These latter neurons thus respond to a particular odour only if it is associated with a taste reward, and not when it is associated with the taste of salt, a punisher. They do not respond to the other odour in the task when it is associated with reward. Thus they respond to a particular combination of an odour, and its being associated with taste reward and not a taste punisher. They may be described as *conditional olfactory-reward neurons*, and may be important in the mechanism by which stimulus–reinforcer (in this case olfactory-to-taste) reversal learning occurs (Deco and Rolls 2005d), as described in Section 4.5.7 and Appendix B.

---

[11] Positron emission tomography is a method of functional neuroimaging that uses radioactively labelled compounds to measure for example altered blood flow in an area to provide a measure of changing activity.

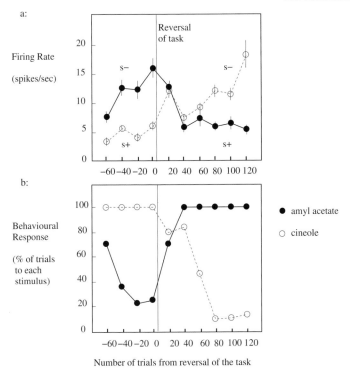

Fig. 4.23 Orbitofrontal cortex: olfactory to taste association reversal. (a) The activity of a single orbitofrontal olfactory neuron during the performance of a two-odour olfactory discrimination task and its reversal is shown. Each point represents the mean poststimulus activity of the neuron in a 500-ms period on approximately 10 trials of the different odourants. The standard errors of these responses are shown. The odourants were amyl acetate (closed circle) (initially S−) and cineole (o) (initially S+). After 80 trials of the task the reward associations of the stimuli were reversed. This neuron reversed its responses to the odourants following the task reversal. (b) The behavioural responses of the monkey during the performance of the olfactory discrimination task. The number of lick responses to each odourant is plotted as a percentage of the number of trials to that odourant in a block of 20 trials of the task. (After Rolls, Critchley, Mason and Wakeman 1996.)

The olfactory to taste reversal was quite slow, both neurophysiologically and behaviourally, often requiring 20–80 trials, consistent with the need for some stability of flavour (i.e. olfactory and taste combination) representations. The relatively high proportion of olfactory neurons with modification of responsiveness by taste association in the set of neurons in this experiment was probably related to the fact that the neurons were preselected to show differential responses to the odours associated with different tastes in the olfactory discrimination task. Thus the rule according to which the orbitofrontal olfactory representation was formed was for some neurons by association learning with taste.

We do not yet know whether this is the first stage of processing at which olfactory neuronal responses are determined in some cases by the (taste) reward with which the odour is associated, though this is a real possibility in that in an fMRI study in humans described below the pleasantness vs unpleasantness of odours did not affect activations in primary olfactory cortical areas (Rolls, Kringelbach and De Araujo 2003c). (In rodents the encoding may be

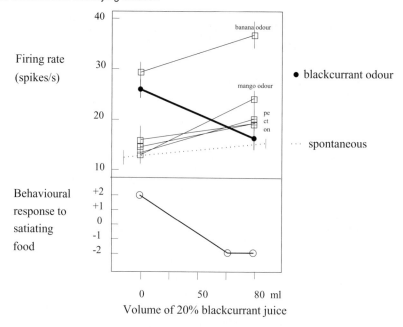

Firing rate (spikes/s)

Behavioural response to satiating food

Volume of 20% blackcurrent juice

banana odour

• blackcurrant odour

mango odour

pe ct on

··· spontaneous

Fig. 4.24 The effect of feeding to satiety on the responses of an olfactory neuron in the orbitofrontal cortex. The monkey was fed to satiety with blackcurrant juice, and the neuronal response to the odour of blackcurrant juice, but not to other odours, decreased as the monkey was being fed to satiety. The neuronal responses reflected the monkey's preference for the blackcurrant juice, as shown in the lower graph. (From Critchley and Rolls, 1996a.)

different, in that an influence of reward-association learning on olfactory neuronal responses in the pyriform cortex (a primary olfactory cortical area) has been reported (Schoenbaum and Eichenbaum 1995)).

The olfactory neurons that do not reverse in the reversal of the olfactory–taste reversal task may be carrying information that is in some cases independent of the reinforcer association (i.e. is about olfactory identity). In other cases, the olfactory representation in the orbitofrontal cortex may reflect associations of odours with other primary reinforcers (for example whether sickness has occurred in association with some smells), or may reflect primary reinforcer value provided by some olfactory stimuli. (For example, the smell of flowers may be innately pleasant and attractive and some other odours may be innately unpleasant – see Chapter 3.) In this situation, the olfactory input to some orbitofrontal cortex neurons may represent an unconditioned stimulus input with which other (for example visual) inputs may become associated.

To analyse the nature of the olfactory representation in the orbitofrontal cortex, Critchley and Rolls (1996a) measured the responses of olfactory neurons that responded to food while they fed the monkey to satiety. They found that the majority of orbitofrontal olfactory neurons reduced their responses to the odour of the food with which the monkey was fed to satiety (see Fig. 4.24). Thus for these neurons, the reward value of the odour is what is represented in the orbitofrontal cortex. We do not yet know whether this is the first stage of processing at

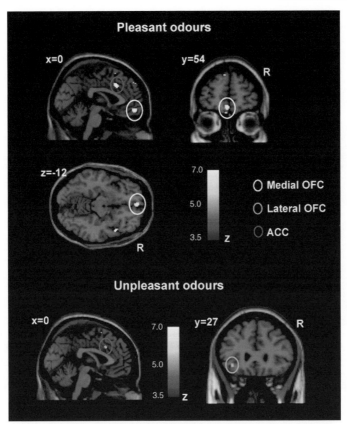

Fig. 4.25 The representation of pleasant and unpleasant odours in the human brain. Above : Group conjunction results for the 3 pleasant odours. Sagittal, horizontal and coronal views are shown at the levels indicated, all including the same activation in the medial orbitofrontal cortex, OFC (X,Y,Z = 0,54,−12; z=5.23). Also shown is activation for the 3 pleasant odours in the anterior cingulate cortex, ACC (X,Y,Z= 2,20,32; z=5.44). These activations were significant at p<0.05 fully corrected for multiple comparisons. Below : Group conjunction results for the 3 unpleasant odours. The sagittal view (left) shows an activated region of the anterior cingulate cortex (X,Y,Z= 0,18,36; z=4.42, p<0.05, S.V.C.). The coronal view (right) shows an activated region of the lateral orbitofrontal cortex (−36,27,−8; z=4.23, p<0.05 S.V.C.). All the activations were thresholded at p<0.00001 to show the extent of the activations. After Rolls, Kringelbach and De Araujo, 2003c. (See colour plates section.)

which the reward value as influenced by an internal homeostatic need state such as hunger[12] is represented in the primate olfactory system. (In rodents, there is some evidence that hunger can influence olfactory responses even in the olfactory bulb, but the fact that humans can still report accurately the intensity of an odour even when its reward value and pleasantness as influenced by feeding to satiety is decreased to zero suggests that this is not a general property of olfactory processing implemented at early stages in primates including humans, as described in Chapter 5 (Section 5.4.4.1).

---

[12]Homeostasis is the regulation of the internal milieu, and the controls of food and water intake described in Chapters 5 and 6 are examples of behaviours that maintain homeostasis.

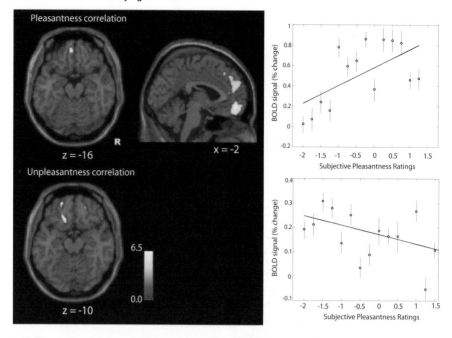

Fig. 4.26 The representation of pleasant and unpleasant odours in the human brain. Random effects group analysis correlation analysis of the BOLD signal with the subjective pleasantness ratings. On the top left is shown the region of the medio-rostral orbitofrontal (peak at [−2, 52, −10]; z=4.28) correlating positively with pleasantness ratings, as well as the region of the anterior cingulate cortex in the top middle. On the far top-right of the figure is shown the relation between the subjective pleasantness ratings and the BOLD signal from this cluster (in the medial orbitofrontal cortex at Y = 52), together with the regression line. The means and s.e.m. across subjects are shown. At the bottom of the figure are shown the regions of left more lateral orbitofrontal cortex (peaks at [−20, 54, −14]; z=4.26 and [−16, 28, −18]; z=4.08) correlating negatively with pleasantness ratings. On the far bottom-right of the figure is shown the relation between the subjective pleasantness ratings and the BOLD signal from the first cluster (in the lateral orbitofrontal cortex at Y = 54), together with the regression line. The means and s.e.m. across subjects are shown. The activations were thresholded at p<0.0001 for extent. After Rolls, Kringelbach and De Araujo, 2003c. (See colour plates section.)

Consistent with this finding at the neuronal level in non-human primates, activation of a part of the human orbitofrontal cortex is related to the pleasantness of food odour, in that the activation measured with fMRI produced by one food odour, banana, decreased after banana was eaten for lunch to satiety, but remained strong to another food odour, vanilla, not eaten in the meal (O'Doherty, Rolls, Francis, Bowtell, McGlone, Kobal, Renner and Ahne 2000).

Further evidence that pleasant odours are represented in the orbitofrontal cortex is that 3 pleasant odours (linalyl acetate [floral, sweet], geranyl acetate [floral], and alpha-ionone [woody, slightly food-related]) had overlapping activations in the medial orbitofrontal cortex in a region not activated by three unpleasant odours (hexanoic acid, octanol, and isovaleric acid) (Rolls, Kringelbach and De Araujo 2003c) (see Fig. 4.25). Moreover, activation of the medial orbitofrontal cortex was correlated with the subjective pleasantness ratings of the odours, and activation of the lateral orbitofrontal cortex with the subjective unpleasantness ratings of the odours (see Fig. 4.26). Other studies have also shown activation of the human orbitofrontal

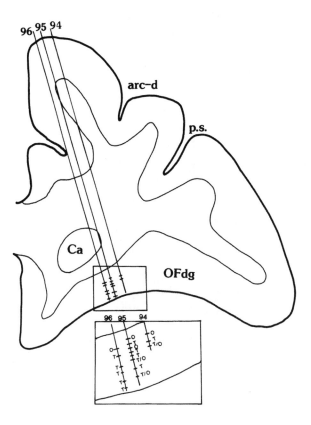

Fig. 4.27 Examples of tracks made into the orbitofrontal cortex in which taste (T) and olfactory (O) neurons were recorded close to each other in the same tracks. Some of the neurons were bimodal (T/O). arc-d, arcuate sulcus; Ca, head of Caudate nucleus; Ofdg, dysgranular part of the Orbitofrontal Cortex; p.s., principal sulcus. (After Rolls and Baylis 1994.)

cortex by odour (Zatorre et al. 1992, Zatorre, Jones-Gotman and Rouby 2000, Royet, Zald, Versace, Costes, Lavenne, Koenig, Gervais, Routtenberg, Gardner and Huang 2000, Anderson et al. 2003).

Although individual neurons do not encode large amounts of information about which of 7–9 odours has been presented, we have shown that the information does increase linearly with the number of neurons in the sample (Rolls, Critchley and Treves 1996a, Rolls and Critchley 2007). This ensemble encoding does result in useful amounts of information about which odour has been presented being provided by orbitofrontal olfactory neurons.

4.5.5.3 Convergence of taste and olfactory inputs in the orbitofrontal cortex: the representation of flavour

In the more medial and anterior parts of the orbitofrontal cortex, not only unimodal taste neurons, but also unimodal olfactory neurons are found (see Fig. 4.27). In addition some single neurons respond to both gustatory and olfactory stimuli, often with correspondence

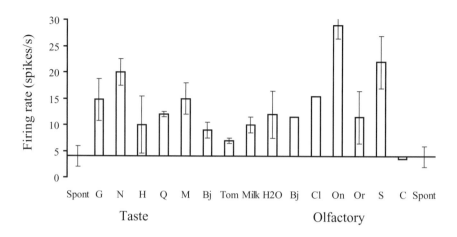

Fig. 4.28 The responses of a bimodal neuron with taste and olfactory responses recorded in the caudolateral orbitofrontal cortex. G, 1 M glucose; N, 0.1 M NaCl; H, 0.01 M HCl; Q, 0.001 M Quinine HCl; M, 0.1 M monosodium glutamate; Bj, 20% blackcurrant juice; Tom, tomato juice; B, banana odour; Cl, clove oil odour; On, onion odour; Or, orange odour; S, salmon odour; C, control no-odour presentation. The mean responses ± s.e.m. are shown. The neuron responded best to the savoury tastes of NaCl and monosodium glutamate and to the consonant odours of onion and salmon. (After Rolls and Baylis 1994.)

between the two modalities (Rolls and Baylis 1994) (see Fig. 4.28; cf. Fig. 4.2). It is probably here in the orbitofrontal cortex of primates that these two modalities converge to produce the representation of flavour (Rolls and Baylis 1994), and, consistent with this, neurons in the macaque primary taste cortex do not have olfactory responses (Verhagen, Kadohisa and Rolls 2004). Consistently, in a human fMRI investigation of olfactory and taste convergence in the brain, it was shown that there is a part of the human taste insula that is not activated by odour (De Araujo, Rolls, Kringelbach, McGlone and Phillips 2003c). The evidence described above (Section 4.5.5.2) indicates that these representations are built by olfactory–gustatory association learning, an example of stimulus–reinforcer association learning.

The human orbitofrontal cortex also reflects the convergence of taste and olfactory inputs, as shown for example by the fact that activations in the human medial orbitofrontal cortex are correlated with both the cross-modal consonance of combined taste and olfactory stimuli (high for example for sweet taste and strawberry odour), as well as for the pleasantness of the combinations, as shown in Fig. 4.29 (De Araujo et al. 2003c).

4.5.5.4 Visual inputs to the orbitofrontal cortex, and visual stimulus–reinforcer association learning and reversal

We have been able to show that there is a major visual input to many neurons in the orbitofrontal cortex, and that what is represented by these neurons is in many cases the reinforcer (reward or punisher) association of visual stimuli. Many of these neurons reflect the relative preference or reward value of different visual stimuli, in that their responses decrease to zero to the sight of one food on which the monkey is being fed to satiety, but remain unchanged to the sight of other food stimuli. In this sense the visual reinforcement-related neurons predict

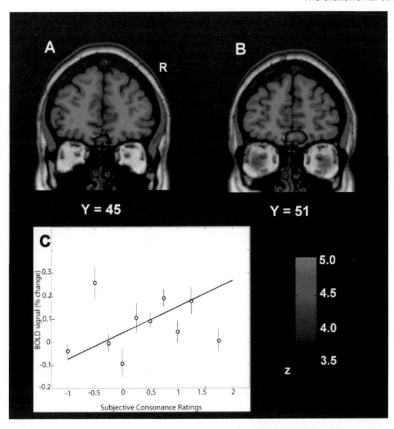

Fig. 4.29 Flavour formation in the human brain, shown by cross-modal olfactory–taste convergence. Brain areas where activations were correlated with the subjective ratings for stimulus (taste–odour) consonance and pleasantness. (A) A second-level, random effects analysis based on individual contrasts (the consonance ratings being the only effect of interest) revealed a significant activation in a medial part of the anterior orbitofrontal cortex. (B) Random effects analysis based on the pleasantness ratings showed a significant cluster of activation located in a (nearby) medial part of the anterior orbitofrontal cortex. The images were thresholded at p<0.0001 for illustration. (C) The relation between the BOLD signal from the cluster of voxels in the medial orbitofrontal cortex shown in (A) and the subjective consonance ratings. The analyses shown included all the stimuli included in this investigation. The means and standard errors of the mean across subjects are shown, together with the regression line, for which r=0.52. (After DeAraujo, Rolls, Kringelbach, McGlone and Phillips, 2003c.) (See colour plates section.)

the reward value that is available from the primary reinforcer, the taste. The visual input is from the ventral, temporal lobe, visual stream concerned with 'what' object is being seen, in that orbitofrontal visual neurons frequently respond differentially to objects or images (but depending on their reward association) (Thorpe, Rolls and Maddison 1983, Rolls, Critchley, Mason and Wakeman 1996b). The primary reinforcer that has been used is taste.

The fact that these neurons represent the reinforcer associations of visual stimuli has been shown to be the case in formal investigations of the activity of orbitofrontal cortex visual neurons, which in many cases reverse their responses to visual stimuli when the taste with which the visual stimulus is associated is reversed by the experimenter (Thorpe, Rolls and

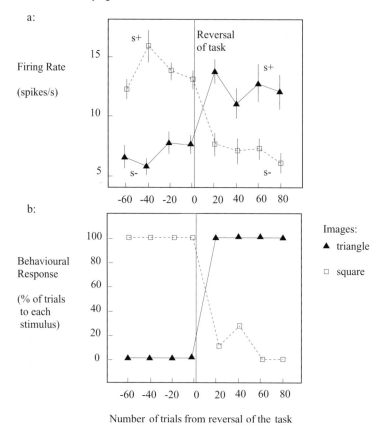

Fig. 4.30 Orbitofrontal cortex: visual discrimination reversal. The activity of an orbitofrontal visual neuron during performance of a visual discrimination task and its reversal. The stimuli were a triangle and a square presented on a video monitor. (a) Each point represents the mean poststimulus activity in a 500 ms period of the neuron based on approximately 10 trials of the different visual stimuli. The standard errors of these responses are shown. After 60 trials of the task the reward associations of the visual stimuli were reversed. (+ indicates that a lick response to that visual stimulus produces fruit juice reward; − indicates that a lick response to that visual stimulus results in a small drop of aversive tasting saline. This neuron reversed its responses to the visual stimuli following the task reversal. (b) The behavioural response of the monkey to the task. It is shown that the monkey performs well, in that he rapidly learns to lick only to the visual stimulus associated with fruit juice reward. (After Rolls, Critchley, Mason and Wakeman 1996.)

Maddison 1983, Rolls, Critchley, Mason and Wakeman 1996b). An example of the responses of an orbitofrontal cortex neuron that reversed the visual stimulus to which it responded during reward-reversal is shown in Fig. 4.30.

This reversal by orbitofrontal visual neurons can be very fast, in as little as one trial, that is a few seconds (see for example Fig. 4.31). The significance of the visual stimulus, a syringe from which the monkey was fed, was altered during the trials. On trials 1–5, no response of the neuron occurred to the sight of the syringe from which the monkey had been given glucose solution to drink from the syringe on the preceding trials. On trials 6–9, the neuron responded to the sight of the same syringe from which he had been given aversive hypertonic saline drink on the preceding trial. Two more reversals (trials 10–15, and 16–17) were performed. The

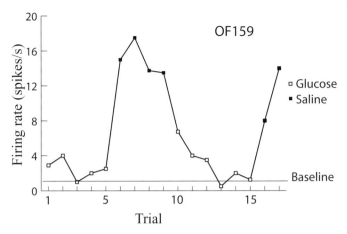

Fig. 4.31 Orbitofrontal cortex: one-trial visual discrimination reversal by a neuron. On trials 1–5, no response of the neuron occurred to the sight of a 2 ml syringe from which the monkey had been given orally glucose solution to drink on the previous trial. On trials 6–9, the neuron responded to the sight of the same syringe from which he had been given aversive hypertonic saline to drink on the previous trial. Two more reversals (trials 10–15, and 16–17) were performed. The reversal of the neuron's response when the significance of the same visual stimulus was reversed shows that the responses of the neuron only occurred to the sight of the visual stimulus when it was associated with a positively reinforcing and not with a negatively reinforcing taste. Moreover, it is shown that the neuronal reversal took only one trial. (After Thorpe, Rolls and Maddison 1983.)

reversal of the neuron's response when the significance of the visual stimulus was reversed shows that the responses of the neuron only occurred to the stimulus when it was associated with aversive saline and not when it was associated with glucose reward.

These neurons thus reflect the information about which stimulus is currently associated with reward during reversals of visual discrimination tasks – they are reward predicting neurons. If a reversal occurs, then the taste cells provide the information that an unexpected taste reinforcer has been obtained, another group of cells shows a vigorous discharge that reflects the error between the expected reward and the reward actually obtained (see below), and the visual cells with reinforcer association-related responses reverse the stimulus to which they are responsive. These neurophysiological changes take place rapidly, in as little as 5 s, and are presumed to be part of the neuronal learning mechanism that enables primates to alter their knowledge of the reinforcer association of visual stimuli so rapidly. This capacity is important whenever behaviour must be corrected when expected reinforcers are not obtained, in, for example, feeding, emotional, and social situations (see Chapters 3 and 5, Rolls (1999a), and Kringelbach and Rolls (2003)). In that these neurons reflect whether a visual stimulus is associated with reward or a punisher, they reflect the relative preference for different stimuli (Thorpe, Rolls and Maddison 1983, Rolls, Critchley, Mason and Wakeman 1996b) (as found also by Tremblay and Schultz (1999)). Consistent with this evidence that the responses of some orbitofrontal cortex neurons reflect the learned predictive reward value of visual stimuli, Thorpe, Rolls and Maddison (1983) and Tremblay and Schultz (2000) found that orbitofrontal cortex neurons learned to respond differently to new stimuli that did or did not predict reward.

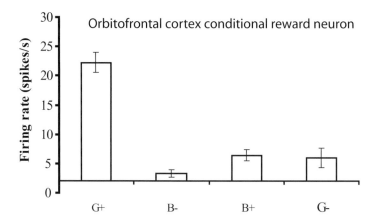

Fig. 4.32 A conditional reward neuron recorded in the orbitofrontal cortex by Thorpe, Rolls and Maddison (1983) which responded only to the Green stimulus when it was associated with reward (G+), and not to the Blue stimulus when it was associated with Reward (B+), or to either stimuli when they were associated with a punisher, the taste of salt (G– and B–). The mean firing rate ± the s.e.m. is shown.

Different neurons in the orbitofrontal cortex are tuned to different learned or conditioned reinforcers, with for example approximately 5% responding to visual stimuli associated with taste reward, and 3% to visual stimuli associated with taste punishment (see Table 4.3 on page 118) (Thorpe, Rolls and Maddison 1983, Rolls, Critchley, Mason and Wakeman 1996b).

In the visual discrimination reversal task, a second class of neuron was found that codes for particular stimuli only if they are associated with reward, and not if they are associated with punishment. Such a neuron might respond to a green stimulus associated with reward; after reversal not respond to the green stimulus when it was associated with punishment; and not respond to a blue stimulus irrespective of whether it was associated with reward or punishment (Thorpe, Rolls and Maddison 1983) (see example in Fig. 4.32). They may be described as *conditional visual stimulus-to-taste reward neurons*, and are analogous to their olfactory counterparts described above in Section 4.5.5.2.

The proportions of neurons showing reversal, or conditional visual stimulus–reinforcer related responses, are shown in Table 4.1. Most visual neurons showed full or conditional reversal, while the proportion of olfactory neurons (see Section 4.5.5.2) was lower (Rolls, Critchley, Mason and Wakeman 1996b).

Table 4.1 Proportion of neurons in the primate orbitofrontal cortex showing reversal, or conditional reversal (ceasing to discriminate or ceasing to respond after the reversal), or no change of responses, during visual or olfactory discrimination reversal (from Rolls, Critchley, Mason and Wakeman 1996).

	Olfactory	cells	Visual	cells
	Number	%	Number	%
Reversal	7	25.0	12	70.6
Conditional reversal	12	42.9	4	23.5
No change	9	32.1	1	5.9
Total	28	100.0	17	100.0

This reversal learning found in orbitofrontal cortex neurons probably is implemented in the orbitofrontal cortex, for it does not occur one synapse earlier in the visual inferior temporal cortex (Rolls, Judge and Sanghera 1977), and it is in the orbitofrontal cortex that there is convergence of visual and taste pathways on to the same neurons (Thorpe, Rolls and Maddison 1983, Rolls, Critchley, Mason and Wakeman 1996b).

A possible mechanism for this learning is Hebbian modification of synapses conveying visual input on to taste-responsive neurons, implementing a pattern-association network (Rolls and Treves 1998) (see Appendix 1). In this model the unconditioned stimulus forcing the output neurons to respond is the (taste) primary reinforcer, and the (visual or olfactory) conditioned stimulus becomes associated with this by associatively modifiable synapses) (Rolls and Treves 1998, Rolls 1999a, Rolls and Deco 2002). Such a pattern association network could in principle unlearn the association by using associative synapses that incorporate long term depression (Rolls and Treves 1998, Rolls and Deco 2002). Although reversal might be implemented by having long-term synaptic depression (LTD) for synapses that represented the reward-associated stimulus before the reversal, and long-term potentiation (LTP) of the synapses activated by the new stimulus that after reversal is associated with reward, this would require one-trial LTP and one-trial heterosynaptic LTD to account for one-trial stimulus–reward reversal (Thorpe et al. 1983, Rolls et al. 1996b, Rolls 2000e) (see Appendix 1 and Appendix 2). To implement the reversal learning very rapidly, in as little as one trial after a number of reversals when reversal learning set has been acquired, a special switching network in the orbitofrontal cortex may be required, and a model of this is described in Section 4.5.7 and Appendix 2.

These studies in macaques provide evidence on the details of the neuronal representations in the primate orbitofrontal cortex which are essential for building a computational under-standing for exactly what information is represented in it, how it is represented, how these differ from preceding and succeeding stages, and thus how the orbitofrontal cortex operates computationally (see Appendix 1 and Appendix 2). However, the types of visual-reward asso-ciation that have been studied in primates (and confirmed as applying in humans (O'Doherty, Deichmann, Critchley and Dolan 2002)) include objects associated with taste rewards or pun-ishers. It has therefore been useful not only to confirm that these concepts do indeed apply to humans, but also to extend the types of visual conditioned reinforcers to quite abstract rein-forcers such as monetary reward. In an fMRI study, O'Doherty, Kringelbach, Rolls, Hornak and Andrews (2001a) used a visual discrimination task in which one stimulus was associated with monetary reward, and a different visual stimulus with monetary loss (punishment). The actual amounts of money won on reward trials and lost on punishment trials were probabilistic. This part of the design, and the fact that unexpected visual discrimination reversals occurred so that there were trials on which money was lost, enabled us to show that the magnitude of the activation of the medial orbitofrontal cortex was correlated with the amount of money won on each trial, and the magnitude of the activation of the lateral orbitofrontal cortex was correlated with the amount of money lost on each trial, as shown in Figs. 4.33 and 4.34.

Another way in which it has been shown that the visual neurons in the orbitofrontal cortex reflect the expected reward value predicted by visual stimuli is by reducing the reward value by feeding to satiety. With this sensory-specific satiety (or reward devaluation) paradigm, it has been shown that the visual (as well as the olfactory and taste) responses of orbitofrontal cortex neurons in the macaque decrease to zero as the monkey is fed to satiety with one food, but remain unchanged to another food not eaten in the meal (Critchley and Rolls 1996a)

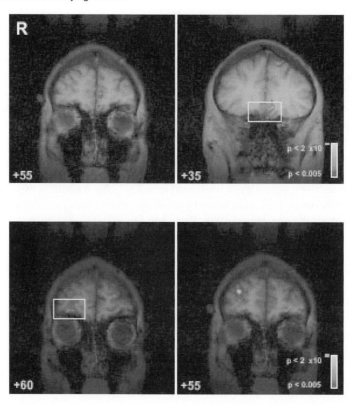

Fig. 4.33 Correlation of brain activations with the amount of money won or lost in a visual discrimination reversal task with probabilistic monetary reward and loss. Voxels in the OFC and other regions whose activity increases relative to the increasing magnitude of Reward or of Punishment obtained. Voxels in an area of left medial OFC (Talairach coordinates [X,Y,Z] : [–6,34,–28]) correlated positively with Reward, and voxels in an area of right lateral OFC (Talairach co-ordinates [X,Y,Z] : [28,60,–6]) correlated positively with Punishment. (After O'Doherty, Kringelbach, Rolls, Hornak and Andrews, 2001a.) (See colour plates section.)

(see example in Fig. 4.35). In that these neurons parallel the changing preference of the monkey for the food being eaten to satiety vs the food not being eaten to satiety, they reflect the relative preference for different visual stimuli (Thorpe, Rolls and Maddison 1983, Rolls, Critchley, Mason and Wakeman 1996b) (as found also by Tremblay and Schultz (1999) and Wallis and Miller (2003)). Wallis and Miller (2003) also showed that although some neurons in the dorsolateral prefrontal cortex also reflect the preferences of macaques for visual stimuli, the neurons in the orbitofrontal cortex responded earlier, and, as we found (Thorpe, Rolls and Maddison 1983, Rolls, Critchley, Mason and Wakeman 1996b, Critchley and Rolls 1996a, Rolls and Baylis 1994), did not reflect the motor responses being made by the macaques. These findings are consistent with the hypothesis that expected reward value is represented in the orbitofrontal cortex, reflects stimulus–reinforcer (sensory–sensory) association learning, and that this information is projected to the dorsolateral prefrontal cortex, where it can be used in tasks requiring planning, for example where rewarding stimuli must

b

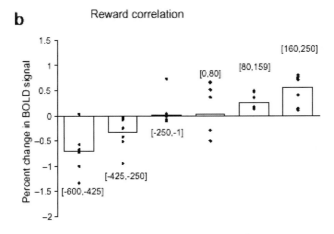

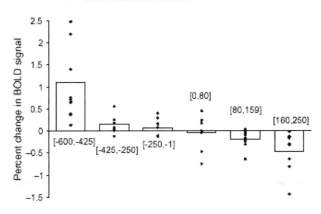

Fig. 4.34 Correlation of brain activations with the amount of money won or lost in a visual discrimination reversal task with probabilistic monetary reward and loss. The mean percent change in BOLD signal from baseline across subjects for 6 different category ranges of reward and punishment. The signal was averaged across a category range within each subject and then the average signal change from each category was averaged across subjects. This is plotted for voxels in the medial OFC that significantly correlated with reward and for voxels in the lateral OFC that significantly correlated with punishment. The ranges of monetary reward and punishment in each category are shown on the chart and were determined by their relative frequencies, which follow from the experimental design. (After O'Doherty, Kringelbach, Rolls, Hornak and Andrews, 2001a.)

to linked to particular responses, and where delays may be involved, in ways that have been modelled by Deco and Rolls (2003) and Deco and Rolls (2005d).

4.5.5.5 Error neurons in the orbitofrontal cortex, and visual stimulus–reinforcer association learning and reversal

In addition to the neurons that encode the reward association of visual stimuli, other neurons (3.5%) in the orbitofrontal cortex detect different types of non-reward (Thorpe, Rolls and

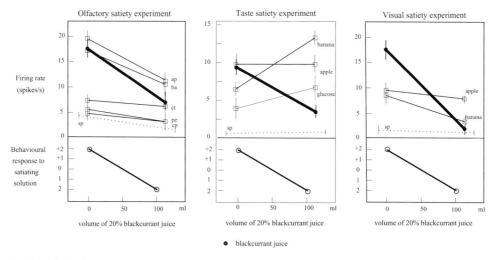

Fig. 4.35 Orbitofrontal cortex neuron with visual, olfactory and taste responses, showing the responses before and after feeding to satiety with blackcurrant juice. The solid circles show the responses to black-currant juice. The olfactory stimuli included apple (ap), banana (ba), citral (ct), phenylethanol (pe), and caprylic acid (cp). The spontaneous firing rate of the neuron is shown (sp). (After Critchley and Rolls 1996a).

Maddison 1983). For example, some neurons responded in extinction, immediately after a lick had been made to a visual stimulus that had previously been associated with fruit juice reward, and other neurons responded in a reversal task, immediately after the monkey had responded to the previously rewarded visual stimulus, but had obtained the punisher of salt taste rather than reward (see example in Fig. 4.36).

Different populations of such neurons respond to other types of non-reward, including the removal of a formerly approaching taste reward, and the termination of a taste reward (Thorpe, Rolls and Maddison 1983) (see Table 4.2). The fact that different non-reward neurons respond to different types of non-reward (e.g. some to the noise of a switch that indicated that extinction of free licking for fruit juice had occurred, and others to the first presentation of a visual stimulus that was not followed by reward in a visual discrimination task) potentially enables context-specific extinction or reversal to occur. (For example, the fact that fruit juice is no longer available from a lick tube does not necessarily mean that a visual discrimination task will be operating without reward.) Thus the error neurons can be specific to different tasks, and this could provide a mechanism for reversal in one task to be implemented, while at the same time not reversing behaviour in another task. Also, it provides additional evidence to that in Table 4.2 that these neurons did not respond simply as a function of arousal, or just in relation to a general frustrative non-reward/error signal.

The presence of these neurons is fully consistent with the hypothesis that they are part of the mechanism by which the orbitofrontal cortex enables very rapid reversal of behaviour by stimulus–reinforcer association relearning when the association of stimuli with reinforcers is altered or reversed (Rolls 1986c, Rolls 1986a, Rolls 1990d, Rolls 1999a). This information appears to be necessary for primates to rapidly alter behavioural responses when reinforcement contingencies are changed, as shown by the effects of damage to the orbitofrontal cortex described above. To the extent that the firing of some dopamine neurons may reflect error

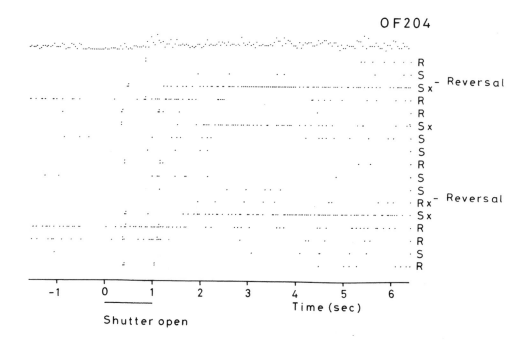

Fig. 4.36 Error neuron: Responses of an orbitofrontal cortex neuron that responded only when the monkey licked to a visual stimulus during reversal, expecting to obtain fruit juice reward, but actually obtaining the taste of aversive saline because it was the first trial of reversal. Each single dot represents an action potential; each vertically arranged double dot represents a lick response. The visual stimulus was shown at time 0 for 1 s. The neuron did not respond on most reward (R) or saline (S) trials, but did respond on the trials marked x, which were the first trials after a reversal of the visual discrimination on which the monkey licked to obtain reward, but actually obtained saline because the task had been reversed. It is notable that after an expected reward was not obtained due to a reversal contingency being applied, on the very next trial the macaque selected the previously non-rewarded stimulus. This shows that rapid reversal can be performed by a non-associative process, and must be rule-based. A model for this is the subject of Section 4.5.7 and Appendix 2. (After Thorpe, Rolls and Maddison 1983.)

Table 4.2 Numbers of orbitofrontal cortex neurons responding in different types of extinction or reversal (after Thorpe, Rolls and Maddison, 1983). The Table shows the tasks (rows) in which individual orbitofrontal neurons responded (1), did not respond (0), or were not tested (blank).

Neuron number	1	2	3	4	5	6	7	8	9	10	11	12	13	14	15	16	17	18
Visual discrim: Reversal	1	0	1	0	0	1	1	0						0				
Visual discrim: Extinction	1																	
Ad lib licking: Reversal	1	1		0	0	0		0	1									
Ad lib licking: Extinction	0	0		0	0	0		0	1									
Taste of saline	0		0	0	0	0	0	0	1	0	0	0	0	0	0	0	0	0
Removal of reward	0		1	1	1	0	1	0	1	1	1	1	1	1	1	1	1	1
Visual arousal	1		1	0	0	0	0	0	1	0	0	0	0	0	1	0	0	0

Table 4.3 Proportion of different types of neuron recorded in the macaque orbitofrontal cortex during sensory testing and visual discrimination reversal and related tasks. (After Thorpe, Rolls and Maddison 1983)

Sensory testing:

Visual, non-selective	10.7%
Visual, selective (i.e. responding to some objects or images)	13.2%
Visual, food-selective	5.3%
Visual, aversive objects	3.2%
Taste	7.3%
Visual and taste	2.6%
Removal of a food reward	6.3%
Extinction of ad lib licking for juice reward	7.5%

Visual discrimination reversal task:

Visual, reversing in the visual discrimination task	5.3%
Visual, conditional discrimination in the visual discrimination task	2.5%
Visual, stimulus-related (not reversing) in the visual discrimination task	0.8%
Non-reward in the visual discrimination task	0.9%
Auditory tone cue signalling the start of a trial of the visual discrimination task	15.1%

The number of neurons analysed was 463.

signals (Waelti, Dickinson and Schultz 2001) (see Section 8.3.4), one might ask where the error information comes from, given that the dopamine neurons themselves may not receive information about expected rewards (e.g. a visual stimulus associated with the sight of food), obtained rewards (e.g. taste), and would have to compute an error from these signals. On the other hand, the orbitofrontal cortex does have all three types of neuron and the required neuroanatomically defined inputs, and this is an important site in the brain for computing error signals.

It is interesting to note the proportions of different types of neuron recorded in the orbito-frontal cortex in relation to what might or might not be seen in a human brain imaging study. The proportions of different types of neuron in the study by Thorpe, Rolls and Maddison (1983) are shown in Table 4.3. It is seen that only a relatively small percentage convey in-formation about, for example, which of two visual stimuli is currently reward-associated in a visual discrimination task. An even smaller proportion (3.5%) responds in relation to non-reward, and in any particular non-reward task, the proportion is very small, that is, just a fraction of the 3.5%. The implication is that an imaging study might not reveal really what is happening in a brain structure such as the orbitofrontal cortex where quite small proportions of neurons respond to any particular condition; and, especially, one would need to be very careful not to place much weight on a failure to find activation in a particular task, as the proportion of neurons responding may be small, and the time period for which they respond may be small too. For example, non-reward neurons typically respond for 2–8 s on the first two non-reward trials of extinction or reversal (Thorpe, Rolls and Maddison 1983).

In that most neurons in the macaque orbitofrontal cortex respond to reinforcers and pun-ishers, or to stimuli associated with rewards and punishers, and do not respond in relation to responses, the orbitofrontal cortex is closely related to stimulus processing, including the stim-uli that give rise to affective states. When it computes errors, it computes mismatches between stimuli that are expected, and stimuli that are obtained, and in this sense the errors are closely related to those required to correct affective states. This type of error representation may thus be different from that represented in the cingulate cortex, in which behavioural responses are

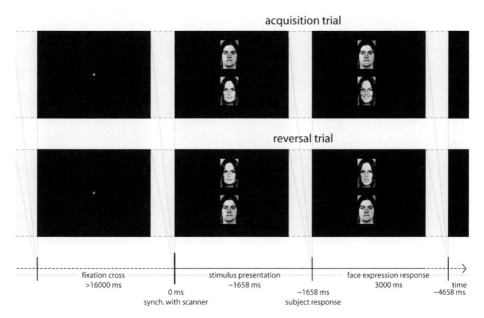

Fig. 4.37 Social reversal task: The trial starts synchronised with the scanner and two people with neutral face expressions are presented to the subject. The subject has to select one of the people by pressing the corresponding button, and the person will then either smile or show an angry face expression for 3000 ms depending on the current mood of the person. The task for the subject is to keep track of the mood of each person and choose the 'happy' person as much as possible (upper row). Over time (after between 4 and 8 correct trials) this will change so that the 'happy' person becomes 'angry' and vice versa, and the subject has to learn to adapt her choices accordingly (bottom row). Randomly intermixed trials with either two men, or two women, were used to control for possible gender and identification effects, and a fixation cross was presented between trials for at least 16000 ms. (After Kringelbach and Rolls, 2003.)

represented, where the errors may be more closely related to errors that arise when action–outcome expectations are not met, and where action–outcome rather than stimulus–reinforcer representations need to be corrected (see Section 4.7).

We have also been able to obtain evidence that non-reward used as a signal to reverse behavioural choice is represented in the human orbitofrontal cortex. Kringelbach and Rolls (2003) used the faces of two different people, and if one face was selected then that face smiled, and if the other was selected, the face showed an angry expression. After good performance was acquired, there were repeated reversals of the visual discrimination task (see Fig. 4.37). Kringelbach and Rolls (2003) found that activation of a lateral part of the orbitofrontal cortex in the fMRI study was produced on the error trials, that is when the human chose a face, and did not obtain the expected reward (see Fig. 4.38). Control tasks showed that the response was related to the error, and the mismatch between what was expected and what was obtained, in that just showing an angry face expression did not selectively activate this part of the lateral orbitofrontal cortex. An interesting aspect of this study that makes it relevant to human social behaviour is that the conditioned stimuli were faces of particular individuals, and the unconditioned stimuli were face expressions. Moreover, the study reveals

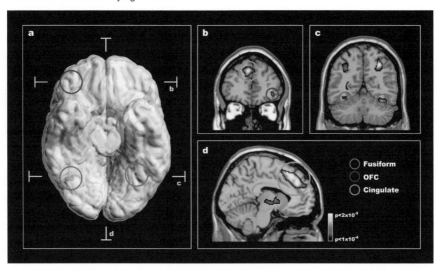

Fig. 4.38 Social reversal: Composite figure showing that changing behaviour based on face expression is correlated with increased brain activity in the human orbitofrontal cortex. a) The figure is based on two different group statistical contrasts from the neuroimaging data which are superimposed on a ventral view of the human brain with the cerebellum removed, and with indication of the location of the two coronal slices (b,c) and the transverse slice (d). The red activations in the orbitofrontal cortex (denoted OFC, maximal activation: z=4.94: 42,42,–8; and z=5.51; X,Y,Z=–46,30,–8) shown on the rendered brain arise from a comparison of reversal events with stable acquisition events, while the blue activations in the fusiform gyrus (denoted Fusiform, maximal activation: z>8; 36,–60,–20 and z=7.80; –30,–56,–16) arise from the main effects of face expression. b) The coronal slice through the frontal part of the brain shows the cluster in the right orbitofrontal cortex across all nine subjects when comparing reversal events with stable acquisition events. Significant activity was also seen in an extended area of the anterior cingulate/paracingulate cortex (denoted Cingulate, maximal activation: z=6.88; –8,22,52; green circle). c) The coronal slice through the posterior part of the brain shows the brain response to the main effects of face expression with significant activation in the fusiform gyrus and the cortex in the intraparietal sulcus (maximal activation: z>8; 32,–60, 46; and z>8: –32,–60,44). d) The transverse slice shows the extent of the activation in the anterior cingulate/paracingulate cortex when comparing reversal events with stable acquisition events. Group statistical results are superimposed on a ventral view of the human brain with the cerebellum removed, and on coronal and transverse slices of the same template brain (activations are thresholded at p=0.0001 for purposes of illustration to show their extent). (After Kringelbach and Rolls 2003.) (See colour plates section.)

that the human orbitofrontal cortex is very sensitive to social feedback when it must be used to change behaviour (Kringelbach and Rolls 2003, Kringelbach and Rolls 2004).

4.5.5.6 A representation of faces in the orbitofrontal cortex

Another type of information represented in the orbitofrontal cortex is information about faces. There is a population of orbitofrontal cortex face-selective neurons that respond in many ways similarly to those in the temporal cortical visual areas (see Rolls (1984b), Rolls (1992a), Rolls (2000a), and Rolls and Deco (2002) for a description of their properties). The orbitofrontal face-responsive neurons, first observed by Thorpe, Rolls and Maddison (1983), then by Rolls, Critchley, Browning and Inoue (2006a), tend to respond with longer latencies than temporal lobe neurons (140–200 ms typically, compared with 80–100 ms); they also

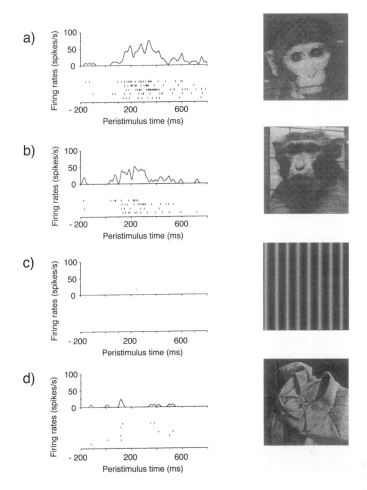

Fig. 4.39 Orbitofrontal cortex face-selective neuron as found in macaques. Peristimulus rastergrams and time histograms are shown. Each trial is a row in the rastergram. Several trials for each stimulus are shown. The ordinate is in spikes/s. The neuron responded best to face (a), also responded, though less to face (b), had different responses to other faces (not shown), and did not respond to non-face stimuli (e.g. (c) and (d)). The stimulus appeared at time 0 on a video monitor. (From Rolls, Critchley, Browning, and Inoue, 2006a.)

convey information about which face is being seen, by having different responses to different faces (see Fig. 4.39); and are typically rather harder to activate strongly than temporal cortical face-selective neurons, in that many of them respond much better to real faces than to two-dimensional images of faces on a video monitor (cf. Rolls and Baylis (1986)). Some of the orbitofrontal cortex face-selective neurons are responsive to face gesture or movement. The findings are consistent with the likelihood that these neurons are activated via the inputs from the temporal cortical visual areas in which face-selective neurons are found (see Fig. 4.2). The significance of the neurons is likely to be related to the fact that faces convey information that is important in social reinforcement, both by conveying face expression (cf. Hasselmo, Rolls

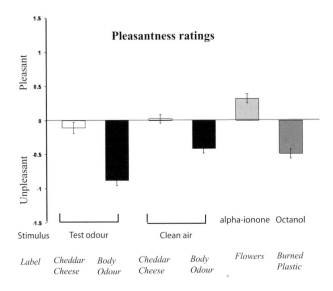

Fig. 4.40 Cognition and emotion. Subjective pleasantness ratings (mean ± s.e.m. across subjects) to odours labelled with words. The corresponding stimulus and label to each bar are listed in the lower part of the figure. The test odour (isovaleric acid) and clean air were paired in different trials with a label of either 'Cheddar cheese' or 'Body odour'. (After DeAraujo, Rolls, Velazco, Margot and Cayeux 2005.)

and Baylis (1989a), which can indicate reinforcement, and by encoding information about which individual is present, also important in evaluating and utilizing reinforcing inputs in social situations (Rolls et al. 2006a).

Consistent with these findings in macaques, and as described above, in humans, activation of the lateral orbitofrontal cortex occurs when a rewarding smile expression is expected, but an angry face expression is obtained, in a visual discrimination reversal task (Kringelbach and Rolls 2003). This is an example of the operation of a social reinforcer, and, consistent with these results, Farrow, Zheng, Wilkinson, Spence, Deakin, Tarrier, Griffiths and Woodruff (2001) have found that activation of the orbitofrontal cortex is found when humans are making social judgements. In addition, activation of the medial orbitofrontal cortex is correlated with face attractiveness (O'Doherty et al. 2003b).

Auditory stimuli may have similar representations in the orbitofrontal cortex related to their affective value. For example, Blood, Zatorre, Bermudez and Evans (1999) found a correlation between subjective ratings of dissonance and consonance of musical chords and the activations produced in the orbitofrontal cortex (see also Blood (2001)). Further evidence on activation by auditory stimuli was found by Frey, Kostopoulos and Petrides (2000).

4.5.5.7 Cognitive influences on the orbitofrontal cortex

Affective states, moods, can influence cognitive processing, including perception and memory (see Section 4.10). But cognition can also influence emotional states. This is not only in the sense that cognitively processed events, if decoded as being rewarding or punishing, can

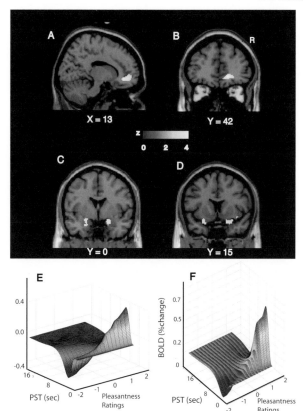

Fig. 4.41 Cognition and emotion. Group (random) effects analysis showing the brain regions where the BOLD signal was correlated with pleasantness ratings given to the test odour. The pleasantness ratings were being modulated by the word labels. A) Activations in the rostral anterior cingulate cortex, in the region adjoining the medial OFC, shown in a sagittal slice. B) The same activation shown coronally. C) Bilateral activations in the amygdala. D) These activations extended anteriorly to the primary olfactory cortex. The image was thresholded at $p<0.0001$ uncorrected in order to show the extent of the activation. E) Parametric plots of the data averaged across all subjects showing that the percentage BOLD change (fitted) correlates with the pleasantness ratings in the region shown in A and B. The parametric plots were very similar for the primary olfactory region shown in D. PST - Post-stimulus time (s). F) Parametric plots for the amygdala region shown in C. (After DeAraujo, Rolls, Velazco, Margot and Cayeux 2005.) (See colour plates section.)

produce emotional states (see Section 2.8), but also in the sense described here that a cognitive input can bias emotional states in different directions. The modulation is rather like the top-down effects of attention on perception (Rolls and Deco 2002, Deco and Rolls 2003, Deco and Rolls 2005b), not only phenomenologically, but also probably computationally. An example of such cognitive influences on the reward/aversive states that are elicited by stimuli was revealed in a study of olfaction described by De Araujo et al. (2005).

In this investigation, a standard test odour, isovaleric acid (with a small amount of cheddar cheese flavour added to make it more pleasant), was used as the test olfactory stimulus delivered with an olfactometer during functional neuroimaging with fMRI (De Araujo et

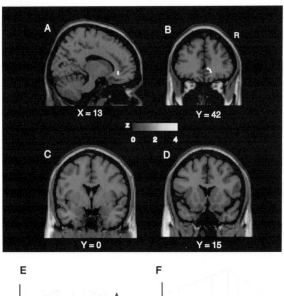

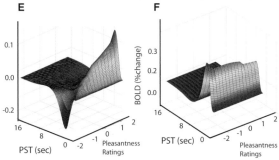

Fig. 4.42 Cognition and emotion. Group (random) effects analysis showing the brain regions where the BOLD signal was correlated with pleasantness ratings given to the clean air. The pleasantness ratings were being modulated by the word labels. A) Activations in the rostral anterior cingulate cortex, in the region adjoining the medial OFC, shown in a sagittal slice. B) The same activation shown coronally. No significant correlations were found with clean air in the amygdala (C) or primary olfactory cortex (D). The image was thresholded at $p<0.0001$ uncorrected in order to show the extent of the activation. E) Parametric plots of the data averaged across all subjects showing that the percentage BOLD change (fitted) correlates with the pleasantness ratings in the region shown in A and B. PST - Post-stimulus time (s). F) Parametric plots showing activation related to stimulus presentation but not related to the pleasantness ratings for the amygdala region shown in C. (After DeAraujo, Rolls, Velazco, Margot and Cayeux 2005.) (See colour plates section.)

al. 2005). This odour is somewhat ambiguous, and might be interpreted as the odour emitted by a cheese-like odour (rather like brie), or might be interpreted as a rather pungent and unpleasant body odour. A word was shown during the 8 s odour delivery. On some trials, the test odour was accompanied by the visually presented word 'Cheddar cheese'. On other trials, the test odour was accompanied by the visually presented word 'Body odour'. A word label was used rather than a picture label to make the modulating input very abstract and cognitive. First, it was found (consistent with psychophysical results of Herz and von Clef (2001)) that the word labels influenced the pleasantness ratings of the test odour, as shown in Fig. 4.40.

However, very interestingly, it was found that the word label modulated the activation to the odour in brain regions activated by odours such as the orbitofrontal cortex (secondary olfactory cortex), cingulate cortex, and amygdala. For example, in the medial orbitofrontal cortex the word label 'Cheddar cheese' caused a larger activation to be produced to the test odour than when the word label 'Body odour' was being presented. In these medial orbito-frontal cortex regions and the amygdala, and even possibly in some parts of the primary ol-factory cortical areas, the activations were correlated with the pleasantness ratings, as shown in Fig. 4.41. This is consistent with the finding that the pleasantness of odours is represented in the medial orbitofrontal cortex (Rolls, Kringelbach and De Araujo 2003c).

The effects of the word were smaller when clean air was the stimulus, as shown in Figs. 4.42 and 4.43, indicating that the effects being imaged were not just effects of a word to influence representations by a top-down recall process, but were instead cognitive top-down effects on states elicited by odours. This type of modulation is typical of a top-down mod-ulatory process such as has been analysed quantitatively in the case of attention (Deco and Rolls 2005b), and indeed no significant effect of the word was found in the amygdala and earlier olfactory cortical areas (see Figs. 4.42 and 4.43). A further implication is that the activations in the human amygdala and primary olfactory cortical areas are more closely bound to the eliciting stimulus and are less influenced by cognition than are activations in the orbitofrontal and cingulate cortices.

These findings show that cognition can influence and indeed modulate reward-related (affective) processing as far down the human olfactory system as the secondary olfactory cortex (in the orbitofrontal cortex), and in the amygdala. This emphasizes the importance of cognitive influences on emotion, and shows how, in situations that might range from enjoying food to a romantic evening, the cognitive top-down influences can play an important role in influencing affective representations in the brain. Indeed, these findings lend support to the hypothesis that an interesting role for cognitive systems in emotion is to help set up the optimal conditions in terms of the reinforcers available and contextual surroundings for reinforcers to produce affective states, as treated further in the dual route hypothesis described in Chapter 10.

Another dramatic example of what could be a similar phenomenon is that colour can have a strong influence on olfactory judgements. This was demonstrated when a white wine was artificially coloured red with an odourless dye, and it was found that participants (undergrad-uates at the Faculty of Oenology of the University of Bordeaux) described the wine using the descriptors normally used for red wine (Morrot, Brochet and Dubourdieu 2001). In this case it is possible that cognitive states elicited by the sight of what was believed to be red wine modulated the olfactory representation. Another possibility is that in a multimodal region such as the orbitofrontal cortex where the sight, smell, taste and texture are brought together onto individual neurons (see Section 4.5.5), the visual input makes a strong contribution to the convergence, and the resulting representation then is available to cognition for verbal description.

The mechanisms by which cognitive states have top-down effects on emotion are probably similar to the biased competition mechanisms that subserve top-down attentional effects (Rolls and Deco 2002, Deco and Rolls 2003, Deco and Rolls 2005b, Rolls and Stringer 2001b, Deco and Rolls 2005a) (see also Section 4.10). In such systems, it is important that the top-down influence does not determine the activity in the system, otherwise stimuli and events would be imagined, and would not represent what was happening in the world. But by having a weak influence, facilitated by the fact that the top-down backprojection connections are relatively

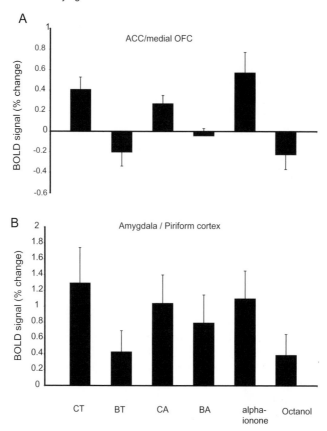

Fig. 4.43 Cognition and emotion. The BOLD signal (% change from control ± s.e.m.) in different brain regions when word labels were presented simultaneously with the test odour (T) or clean air (A). C= 'cheddar cheese' label; B= 'body odour' label. The responses to a reference pleasant odour (alpha-ionone) and unpleasant odour (octanol) are also shown. (After DeAraujo, Rolls, Velazco, Margot and Cayeux 2005.)

weak (Rolls 1989a, Rolls and Treves 1998, Renart, Parga and Rolls 1999b, Renart, Parga and Rolls 1999a, Renart, Moreno, Rocha, Parga and Rolls 2001, Rolls and Stringer 2001b, Rolls and Deco 2002, Deco and Rolls 2005b, Deco and Rolls 2005a), cognition and attention can have beneficial effects in directing sensory and emotional processing towards stimuli and events that the cognitive system has determined are relevant.

Part of the interest and importance of the study by De Araujo, Rolls, Velazco, Margot and Cayeux (2005) is that it shows that cognitive influences, originating from as high in processing as linguistic representations, can reach down into the first part of the brain in which emotion, affective, hedonic or reward value is made explicit in the representation, the orbitofrontal cortex, to modulate the responses there to affective stimuli. The experiment thus shows that linguistic representations can influence how emotional states are represented and thus experienced. It is in this very direct way that cognition can have a powerful effect on emotional states, emotional behaviour, and emotional experience, because the emotional representations are altered.

4.5.5.8 The topology of the functional neuroimaging activations in the orbitofrontal cortex

Kringelbach and Rolls (2004) have reviewed evidence that the activations found in functional neuroimaging studies by many types of reward appear to involve relatively medial parts of the human orbitofrontal cortex, and unpleasant stimuli or non-reward more lateral parts of the human orbitofrontal cortex. For example, we have obtained evidence from an experiment using pleasant, painful and neutral somatosensory stimulation that there is some spatial segregation of the representation of rewards and punishers, where the effects of pleasant somatosensory stimulation are spatially dissociable from the effects of painful stimulation in the human orbitofrontal cortex (Rolls, O'Doherty, Kringelbach, Francis, Bowtell and McGlone 2003d). Further, pleasant odours activate medial, and unpleasant odours lateral, regions of the human orbitofrontal cortex (Rolls, Kringelbach and De Araujo 2003c). Another example comes from the finding that the administration of amphetamine to naive human subjects activated the medial prefrontal cortex (Voellm, De Araujo, Cowen, Rolls, Kringelbach, Smith, Jezzard, Heal and Matthews 2004). An indication that a rewarding effect is being produced by the amphetamine in part because of an action in the orbitofrontal cortex is that macaques will self-administer amphetamine to the orbitofrontal cortex (Phillips, Mora and Rolls 1981). A clear indication of a differentiation in function between medial versus lateral areas of the human orbitofrontal cortex was found in our study investigating visual discrimination reversal learning, which showed a clear dissociation between the medial orbitofrontal areas correlating with monetary gain, and the lateral areas correlating with monetary loss (O'Doherty, Kringelbach, Rolls, Hornak and Andrews 2001a). This result, and some of the other studies included in the meta-analysis (Kringelbach and Rolls 2004), can be interpreted as evidence for a difference between medial orbitofrontal cortex areas involved in decoding and monitoring the reward value of reinforcers, and lateral areas involved in evaluating punishers that when detected may lead to a change in current behaviour. A good example of a study showing the latter involved a visual discrimination reversal task in which face identity was associated with a face expression (Kringelbach and Rolls 2003). When the face expression associated with one of the faces reversed and the face expression was being interpreted as a punisher and indicated that behaviour should change, then lateral parts of the orbitofrontal cortex became activated.

Although our study on abstract reward found that monetary reward and punishment are correlated with activations in different regions of the orbitofrontal cortex (O'Doherty, Kringelbach, Rolls, Hornak and Andrews 2001a), even this evidence does not show that rewards and punishers have totally separate representations in the human brain. In particular, the medial regions of the orbitofrontal cortex that had activations correlating with the magnitude of monetary reward (area 11) also reflected monetary punishers in the sense that the activations in these medial regions correlated positively with the magnitude of monetary wins and negatively with losses (see Fig. 4.33). Similarly, the more lateral regions (area 10) had activations that correlated negatively with the magnitudes of monetary wins and gains, and positively with monetary loss/punishment. This means that in this experiment the medial and lateral regions were apparently coding for both monetary reward and punishment (albeit in opposite ways). The evidence from this experiment would therefore suggest that the segregation between rewards and punishers is not purely spatial but rather encoded in the neuronal responses, which the studies in macaques described above show can be exquisitely tuned differently not only to reinforcers in different sensory modalities (taste, smell, touch etc), but also to combinations of these, and even within any one modality (e.g. with neurons tuned to different tastes). The functional imaging thus provides a very blurred picture of what is really happening at the neuronal and information representation level in the orbitofrontal cortex. Although it is true that similar neurons may tend to cluster together as a result of a self-organizing competitive network with short range excitatory connections (see Rolls and Treves (1998) and Rolls and Deco (2002)), and this may lead to somewhat localized blobs of activity in the cortex, the presence of such blobs should not be taken as more than a gross reflection of the underlying neuronal representations and computations. Integrating over all this heterogeneous neuronal activity is what leads to an fMRI signal (see Appendix 2, Section B.7).

What account might we give for why so many different types of reward are represented in the human medial orbitofrontal cortex? The types of reward include, as described above and in Chapter 5, food reward as shown in sensory-specific satiety experiments (Kringelbach, O'Doherty, Rolls and Andrews 2003), pleasant odours (Rolls, Kringelbach and De Araujo 2003c), pleasant touch (Rolls, O'Doherty, Kringelbach, Francis, Bowtell and McGlone 2003d), face attractiveness (O'Doherty et al. 2003b), monetary reward (O'Doherty, Kringelbach, Rolls, Hornak and Andrews 2001a), conditioned stimuli associated with drug self-administration in addicts (Childress, Mozley, McElgin, Fitzgerald, Reivich and O'Brien 1999), and also the administration of amphetamine to drug-naive human subjects (Voellm, De Araujo, Cowen, Rolls, Kringelbach, Smith, Jezzard, Heal and Matthews 2004). The neuronal recording studies described above in macaques show clearly that there is an exquisite representation of the detailed properties of these different stimuli, with different neurons by virtue of their different tuning to each of these properties and to combinations of these properties providing information about all the individual properties of each particular stimulus. For example, as a population, different orbitofrontal cortex neurons in macaques have different responses to the following properties of oral stimuli, with some neurons encoding each property independently, and others responding to different combinations of them: taste, fat texture, viscosity, astringency, grittiness, capsaicin content, odour, and sight (see above and Chapter 5).

So why are so many of the reward-related properties of stimuli represented in the same medial part of the orbitofrontal cortex? I suggest that part of the functional utility of this is that there can be comparison of the magnitudes of what may be quite different types of reward, implemented by the local lateral inhibition mediated via the inhibitory interneurons.

The architecture required for the implementation is that which is standard for the cerebral cortex: the excitatory pyramidal cells, which are the neurons with the types of often quite selective response just described, connect to inhibitory neurons, which are relatively fewer in number (perhaps 15% of the number of excitatory neurons). The inhibitory neurons receive from random sets of neurons in the vicinity, and project back their summed effects as inhibition to random collections of pyramidal cells. This lateral inhibition system has the effect of controlling the activity of the excitatory neurons, and importantly, the effect of ensuring that the most strongly activated excitatory neurons reduce the activity of less strongly activated excitatory neurons. Contrast enhancement may occur between the competing inputs, and also local scaling of the overall activity of the neurons so that they operate within their working range to reflect in their output firing the inputs being received, in processes that are quantitatively understood and are used in competitive networks (Grossberg 1988, Rolls and Treves 1998, Rolls and Deco 2002, Deco and Rolls 2005b). The result of the mutual inhibition is that the relative magnitude of the different rewards available can be compared, and the most strongly firing neurons after the competition reflect the strongest reward.

This type of comparison would be difficult to implement if each type of reward was represented in a different location in the brain, and may be a useful computational outcome of the fact that different types of reward are represented (by different neurons of course) in the same general brain region, the medial orbitofrontal cortex. This computation would provide scaling of different rewards, both relative to each other when presented simultaneously as in a choice situation, and relative to a fixed maximum if only one reward is present. This would thus implement relative reward preference encoding (Rolls, Sienkiewicz and Yaxley 1989b, Tremblay and Schultz 1999).

It may be useful to note that the human medial orbitofrontal cortex region activated by many types of reward may have shifted medially somewhat with respect to its location in macaques. Spurred by the human neuroimaging studies just described, we (Rolls, Kadohisa and Verhagen) have been making recordings in the topologically most medial part of the macaque orbitofrontal cortex, to determine whether there is a previously undescribed set of reward / taste / olfactory / visual / somatosensory representations in this region. We have not found such neurons in the part of the macaque orbitofrontal cortex that is less than 3–4 mm from the midline. We do find that neurons that respond to the taste, odour, texture, and sight of food start at approximately this laterality, and then extend out laterally from this paramedial orbitofrontal cortex region, through the mid to the far lateral orbitofrontal cortex, at sites that have been illustrated in a number of papers (e.g. Rolls and Baylis (1994), Critchley and Rolls (1996c), and Rolls, Critchley, Wakeman and Mason (1996c)). Indeed, some of these more medial sites in which taste neurons are common are illustrated in Fig. 4.27 on page 107 from Rolls and Baylis (1994). It is quite clear from a retrograde neuronal tracing study with horseradish peroxidase administered to a region containing taste neurons in the macaque lateral orbitofrontal cortex that the lateral part of the orbitofrontal cortex receives direct inputs from the primary taste cortex in the insula (see Fig. 4.44 and Baylis, Rolls and Baylis (1994)). (The location of the macaque primary taste cortex was described by Pritchard, Hamilton, Morse and Norgren (1986).) More medial orbitofrontal cortex areas may also receive inputs directly from the insular and frontal opercular primary taste cortical areas, for, as illustrated in Fig. 4.27, taste neurons are also common in this more medial part of the orbitofrontal cortex (see further Rolls and Baylis (1994) and Critchley and Rolls (1996c)). The more middle / medial part of the orbitofrontal cortex (close to the region indicated in Fig. 4.27) also has neurons that decrease their taste responses in relation to sensory-specific satiety, and a few that do not (Critchley and Rolls 1996a). Thus the macaque posterior orbitofrontal cortex contains taste, and also olfactory and visual, neurons throughout its mediolateral extent, apart from the most medial 3–4 mm. In contrast, the taste and olfactory reward areas in humans appear to reach to the midline, and probably do not extend as far lateral as in non-human primates (see e.g. Figs. 4.25, 4.26, 4.29 and 4.41).

I suggest that as the frontal lobes have developed from macaques to humans, more cortex has been added to the dorsolateral prefrontal cortex areas so important in working memory and hence in attention and executive function (Rolls and Deco 2002, Deco and Rolls 2003), thus displacing the inferior convexity prefrontal cortex more medially in humans, and displacing the main orbitofrontal cortex areas of macaques more medially in humans, so that they reach as far as the midline. This would be the same trend that occurs in the temporal lobes of macaques vs humans, in which the enormous development of language areas in the left hemisphere (and corresponding high order processing areas in the right hemisphere) appear

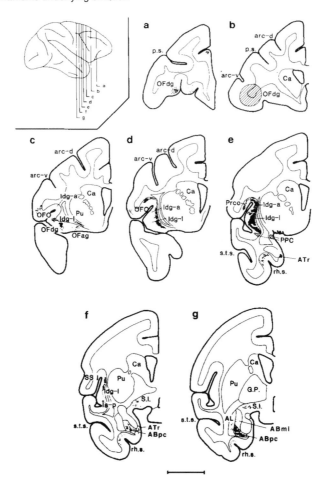

Fig. 4.44 Projections from the primary taste cortex in the upper part of the dysgranular insula and frontal operculum to the orbitofrontal cortex. The horseradish peroxidase injection site into the lateral orbitofrontal cortex where taste neurons were recorded is shown shaded in (b). Filled neurons are shown in e.g.(e) as black circles in the primary taste cortex in the upper part of areas Idg-a (Insula dysgranular area, anterior part: the insular primary taste cortex) and the area labelled Prco in (e) the frontal opercular taste cortex. Abbreviations: AB: basal nucleus of the amygdala with mc magnocellular and pc parvocellular parts; AL: lateral nucleus of the amygdala; arc-d: dorsal limb of the arcuate sulcus; arc-v: ventral limb of the arcuate sulcus; Ca: caudate nucleus; GP: globus pallidus; Idg-l: liminal part of the dysgranular field of the insula; OF: orbitofrontal cortex (with ag agranular and dg dysgranular fields); OFO: orbitofrontal opercular area; PPC: prepyriform cortex (olfactory); Prco: precentral operculum; ps: principal sulcus; Pu: putamen; rh s: rhinal sulcus; SI: substantia innominata; SS 1: primary somaesthetic cortex; sts: superior temporal sulcus. (After Baylis, Rolls and Baylis 1994.)

to have displaced at least parts of the inferior temporal visual cortex to be much more ventrally and medially represented in for example the human fusiform face and related areas (Rolls and Deco 2002, Baylis, Rolls and Leonard 1987, Dolan, Fink, Rolls, Booth, Holmes,

Frackowiak and Friston 1997, Tovee, Rolls and Ramachandran 1996, Kanwisher, McDermott and Chun 1997, Ishai, Ungerleider, Martin and Haxby 2000).

Another possible topological trend in the human orbitofrontal cortex appears to be present in the posterior to anterior direction, with the possibility of some hierarchy (Kringelbach and Rolls 2004). Very abstract reinforcers such as loss of money appear to be represented further anterior towards the frontal pole (e.g. O'Doherty, Kringelbach, Rolls, Hornak and Andrews (2001a)) than in posterior areas representing simple reinforcers such as taste (e.g. De Araujo, Kringelbach, Rolls and Hobden (2003a); De Araujo, Kringelbach, Rolls and McGlone (2003b)) or thermal intensity (Craig, Chen, Bandy and Reiman 2000). This posterior–anterior trend is clearly demonstrated in the statistical results from the meta-analysis (Kringelbach and Rolls 2004) and is likely to reflect some kind of hierarchical processing in the orbitofrontal cortex. Relatively far forward in the orbitofrontal cortex, in area 11, another, memory-related, rather than emotion-related, type of representation is present, for here neurons are activated by novel visual stimuli (Rolls, Browning, Inoue and Hernadi 2005a), and activations in humans are produced by novel visual stimuli (Frey and Petrides 2002).

Another trend is that the main or simple effects in neuroimaging studies of primary reinforcers such as odour and taste tend to be located in relatively more posterior areas of the orbitofrontal cortex, whereas correlations with subjective pleasantness and unpleasantness ratings for frequently the same stimuli tend to be more anterior (Blood, Zatorre, Bermudez and Evans 1999, Blood 2001, De Araujo, Kringelbach, Rolls and Hobden 2003a, De Araujo, Kringelbach, Rolls and McGlone 2003b, Kringelbach, O'Doherty, Rolls and Andrews 2003, O'Doherty, Kringelbach, Rolls, Hornak and Andrews 2001a, O'Doherty, Winston, Critchley, Perrett, Burt and Dolan 2003b, Rolls, Kringelbach and De Araujo 2003c, Voellm, De Araujo, Cowen, Rolls, Kringelbach, Smith, Jezzard, Heal and Matthews 2004). This is consistent with higher level processing more anteriorly which is on a route to parts of the brain involved in making processing available to conscious experience (Rolls 1999a).

Another finding is that areas that have supralinear responses to combinations of sensory inputs, for example taste and smell (De Araujo, Rolls, Kringelbach, McGlone and Phillips 2003c), or the umami taste stimuli monosodium glutamate (MSG) and inosine 5'-monophosphate (De Araujo, Kringelbach, Rolls and Hobden 2003a), tend to be more anterior than the areas where the components of the combinations are represented in the orbitofrontal cortex. This could easily reflect hierarchy in the system, with convergence tending to increase from more posterior to more anterior orbitofrontal cortex areas, and thus effects of combinations of inputs becoming more evident anteriorly.

4.5.6 The human orbitofrontal cortex

In Section 4.5.5 we have considered evidence from neuroimaging on the functions of the human orbitofrontal cortex in emotion and motivation. In this Section we consider complementary evidence from the effects of damage to the human orbitofrontal cortex.

It is of interest that a number of the symptoms of frontal lobe damage in humans appear to be related to the functions described above of representing primary reinforcers, and of altering behaviour when stimulus–reinforcement associations alter, as described next. Thus, humans with frontal lobe damage can show impairments in a number of tasks in which an alteration of behavioural strategy is required in response to a change in environmental reinforcement contingencies (Goodglass and Kaplan 1979, Jouandet and Gazzaniga 1979, Kolb and Whishaw 2003, Zald and Rauch 2006). For example, Milner (1963) showed that in the Wisconsin card sorting task (in which cards are to be sorted according to the colour, shape, or number of items on each card depending on whether the examiner says 'right' or 'wrong' to each placement), frontal patients either had difficulty in determining the first sorting principle, or in shifting to a second principle when required to. Also, in stylus mazes frontal patients have difficulty in changing direction when a sound indicates that the correct path has been left (Milner 1982). It is of interest that, in both types of test, frontal patients may be able to verbalize the correct rules yet may be unable to correct their behavioural sets or strategies appropriately.

Some of the personality changes that can follow frontal lobe damage may be related to a similar type of dysfunction. For example, the euphoria, irresponsibility, lack of affect, and lack of concern for the present or future that can follow frontal lobe damage (see Zald and Rauch (2006) and Section 4.5.1 on page 91) may also be related to a dysfunction in altering behaviour appropriately in response to a change in reinforcement contingencies. Indeed, in so far as the orbitofrontal cortex is involved in the disconnection of stimulus–reinforcer associations, and such associations are important in learned emotional responses (see above), then it follows that the orbitofrontal cortex is involved in emotional responses by correcting stimulus–reinforcer associations when they become inappropriate (see below).

The hypotheses about the role of the orbitofrontal cortex in the rapid alteration of stimulus–reinforcer associations, and the functions more generally of the orbitofrontal cortex in human behaviour, have been investigated in recent studies in humans with damage to the ventral parts of the frontal lobe. (The description ventral is given to indicate that there was pathology in the orbitofrontal or related parts of the frontal lobe, and not in the more dorso-lateral parts of the frontal lobe.) A task that was directed at assessing the rapid alteration of stimulus–reinforcer associations was used, because the findings above indicate that the orbitofrontal cortex is involved in this type of learning. This was used instead of the Wisconsin card sorting task, which requires patients to shift from category (or dimension) to category, e.g. from colour to shape. The task used was visual discrimination reversal, in which patients could learn to obtain points by touching one stimulus when it appeared on a video monitor, but had to withhold a response when a different visual stimulus appeared, otherwise a point was lost. After the subjects had acquired the visual discrimination, the reinforcement contingencies unexpectedly reversed. The patients with ventral frontal lesions made more errors in the reversal (or in a similar extinction) task, and completed fewer reversals, than control patients with damage elsewhere in the frontal lobes or in other brain regions (Rolls, Hornak, Wade and McGrath 1994a) (see Fig. 4.45). A reversal deficit in a similar task in patients with ventromedial frontal cortex damage was also reported by Fellows and Farah (2003).

An important aspect of the findings of Rolls, Hornak, Wade and McGrath (1994a) was that the reversal learning impairment correlated highly with the socially inappropriate or disinhibited behaviour of the patients, and also with their subjective evaluation of the changes in their emotional state since the brain damage. The patients were not impaired at other types of memory task, such as paired associate learning. It is of interest that the patients can often verbalize the correct response, yet commit the incorrect action. This is consistent with the hypothesis that the orbitofrontal cortex is normally involved in executing behaviour when the behaviour is performed by evaluating the reinforcement associations of environmental stimuli (see below). The orbitofrontal cortex seems to be involved in this in both humans and non-human primates, when the learning must be performed rapidly, in, for example, acquisition, and during reversal.

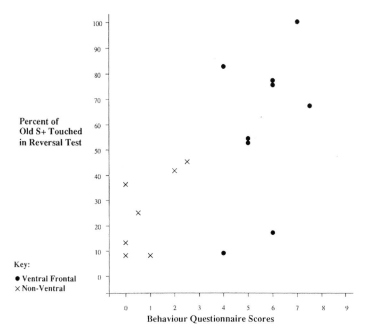

Fig. 4.45 Visual discrimination reversal performance in humans with damage to the ventral part of the frontal lobe. The task was to touch the screen when one image, the S+, was shown in order to obtain a point; and to refrain from touching the screen when a different visual stimulus, the S−, was shown in order to obtain a point. The scattergraph shows that during the reversal the group with ventral damage were more likely to touch the previously rewarded stimulus (Old S+), and that this was related to the score on a Behaviour Questionnaire. Each point represents one patient in the ventral frontal group or in a control group. The Behaviour Questionnaire rating reflected high ratings on at least some of the following: disinhibited or socially inappropriate behaviour; misinterpretation of other people's moods; impulsiveness; unconcern about or underestimation of the seriousness of his condition; and lack of initiative. (From Rolls, Hornak, Rolls and McGrath 1994a.)

To seek positive confirmation that effects on stimulus–reinforcer association learning and reversal were related to orbitofrontal cortex damage rather than to any other associated pathology, a new reversal-learning task was used with a group of patients with discrete, surgically produced, lesions of the orbitofrontal cortex. In the new visual discrimination task (the same as that used in our monetary reward functional neuroimaging task, O'Doherty, Kringelbach, Rolls, Hornak and Andrews (2001a)), two stimuli are always present on the video monitor and the patient obtains 'monetary' reward by touching the correct stimulus, and loses 'money' by touching the incorrect stimulus. This design controls for an effect of the lesion in simply increasing the probability that any response will be made (cf. Aron, Fletcher, Bullmore, Sahakian and Robbins (2003) and Clark, Cools and Robbins (2004)). The new task also uses probabilistic amounts of reward and punishment on each trial, to make it harder to use a verbal strategy with an explicit rule. The task also had the advantage that it was the same as that used in our human functional neuroimaging study that had showed activation of the orbitofrontal cortex by monetary gain or loss (O'Doherty et al. 2001a). It was found that a group of patients with bilateral orbitofrontal cortex lesions were severely impaired at

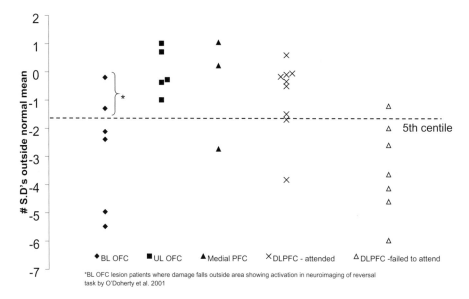

Fig. 4.46 Visual discrimination reversal performance on the probabilistic reversal task in humans with damage to different parts of the ventral part of the frontal lobe. Lesion groups: BL OFC: Bilateral Orbito-frontal cortex; UL OFC: Unilateral Orbitofrontal cortex; Medial PFC: Medial prefrontal cortex; DLPFC: Dorsolateral prefrontal cortex. The patients with bilateral damage to the orbitofrontal cortex performed poorly at the task. Patients with lesions of the dorsolateral prefrontal cortex performed poorly only if they had an attention deficit and failed to pay attention to the part of the display that informed them whether they had won on the current trial of the task. (Attended/Failed to attend: The patient attended/failed to attend to the crucial feedback during the reversal test, namely the amount won or lost on each trial.) (After Hornak, O'Doherty, Bramham, Rolls et al, 2004)

the reversal task, in that they accumulated less money (Hornak, O'Doherty, Bramham, Rolls, Morris, Bullock and Polkey 2004) (see Fig. 4.46). These patients often failed to switch their choice of stimulus after a large loss; and often did switch their choice even though they had just received a reward, and this has been quantified in a more recent study (Berlin, Rolls and Kischka 2004). The investigation showed that the impairment was only obtained with bilateral orbitofrontal cortex damage, in that patients with unilateral orbitofrontal cortex (or medial prefrontal cortex) lesions were not impaired in the reversal task (see Fig. 4.46).

It is of interest that the patients with bilateral orbitofrontal cortex damage who were impaired at the visual discrimination reversal task had high scores on parts of a Social Behaviour Questionnaire in which the patients were rated on behaviours such as emotion recognition in others (e.g. their sad, angry, or disgusted mood); in interpersonal relationships (such as not caring what others think, and not being close to the family); emotional empathy (e.g. when others are happy, is not happy for them); interpersonal relationships (e.g. does not care what others think, and is not close to his family); public behaviour (is uncooperative); an-tisocial behaviour (is critical of and impatient with others); impulsivity (does things without thinking); and sociability (is not sociable, and has difficulty making or maintaining close relationships) (Hornak, Bramham, Rolls, Morris, O'Doherty, Bullock and Polkey 2003), all of which could reflect less behavioural sensitivity to different types of punishment and reward.

Further, in a Subjective Emotional Change Questionnaire in which the patients reported on any changes in the intensity and/or frequency of their own experience of emotions, the bilateral orbitofrontal cortex lesion patients with deficits in the visual discrimination reversal task reported a number of changes, including changes in sadness, anger, fear and happiness (Hornak et al. 2003).

As described above, these results are complemented by neuroimaging results with fMRI in normal subjects, which showed that in the same task, activation of the medial orbitofrontal cortex was correlated with how much money was won on single trials, and activation of the lateral orbitofrontal cortex was correlated with how much money was lost on single trials (O'Doherty et al. 2001a). Together, these results on the effects of brain damage to the orbitofrontal cortex, and these and other complementary neuroimaging results described later, provide evidence that at least part of the function of the orbitofrontal cortex in emotion, social behaviour, and decision making is related to representing reinforcers, detecting changes in the reinforcers being received, using these changes to rapidly reset stimulus–reinforcer associations, and rapidly changing behaviour as a result.

An idea of how such stimulus–reinforcer learning may play an important role in normal human behaviour, and may be related to the behavioural changes seen clinically in the patients of Rolls, Hornak, Wade and McGrath (1994a) with ventral frontal lobe damage, can be provided by summarizing the behavioural ratings given by the carers of these patients (Rolls et al. 1994a). The patients were rated high on at least some of the following: disinhibition or socially inappropriate behaviour; violence, verbal abusiveness; lack of initiative; misinterpretation of other people's behaviour; anger or irritability; and lack of concern for their own condition. Such behavioural changes correlated with the stimulus–reinforcer reversal and extinction learning impairment (Rolls et al. 1994a). The suggestion thus is that the insensitivity to reinforcement changes in the learning task may be at least part of what produces the changes in behaviour found in these patients with ventral frontal lobe damage.

The more general impact on the behaviour of these patients is that their irresponsibility tended to affect their everyday lives. For example, if such patients had received their brain damage in a road traffic accident, and compensation had been awarded, the patients often tended to spend their money without appropriate concern for the future, sometimes, for example, buying a very expensive car. Such patients often find it difficult to invest in relationships too, and are sometimes described by their family as having changed personalities, in that they care less about a wide range of factors than before the brain damage. The suggestion that follows from this is that the orbitofrontal cortex may normally be involved in much social behaviour, and the ability to respond rapidly and appropriately to social reinforcers is, of course, an important aspect of primate social behaviour. When Goleman (1995) writes about emotional intelligence (see Section 2.7), the functions being performed may be those that we are now discussing, and also those concerned with face-expression decoding which are described in this Chapter.

Bechara and colleagues also have findings that are consistent with those described above in patients with frontal lobe damage when they perform a gambling task (Bechara et al. 1994, Bechara et al. 1996, Bechara et al. 1997, Damasio 1994, Bechara et al. 2005). In the Iowa gambling task subjects were asked to select cards from four decks of cards and maximize their winnings. During the task electrodermal activity (Skin Conductance Responses, SCR) of the subject was measured as an index of somatic activation. After each selection of a card, facsimile money is lost or won. Two of the four decks produce large payouts with larger penalties (and can thus be considered high-risk), while the other two decks produce small payouts but smaller penalties (low-risk). The most profitable strategy is therefore to consistently select cards from the two low-risk decks, which is the strategy adopted by normal control subjects. Patients with damage to the ventromedial part of the orbitofrontal cortex, but not the dorsolateral prefrontal cortex, would persistently draw cards from the high-risk packs, and lack anticipatory SCRs while they pondered risky choices. The task was designed to mimic aspects of real-life decision-making that patients with orbitofrontal cortex lesions find difficult. Such decisions typically involve choices between actions associated with differing magnitudes of reward and punishment where the underlying contingencies relating actions to relevant outcomes remain hidden.

Bechara, Damasio, Tranel and Anderson (1998) have since reported a dissociation between subjects with different frontal lobe lesions. All subjects with orbitofrontal cortex lesions were impaired on the gambling task, while only those with the most anteriorly placed lesions were normal on working memory tasks. Other subjects with right dorsolateral/high mesial lesions were impaired on working memory tasks but not on the gambling task. Bechara, Damasio, Damasio and Lee (1999) went on to compare subjects with bilateral amygdala but not orbitofrontal cortex lesions, and subjects with orbitofrontal cortex but not amygdala lesions, and found that all subjects were impaired in the gambling task and all failed to develop anticipatory SCRs. However, while subjects with orbitofrontal cortex lesions still, in general, produced SCRs when receiving a monetary reward or punishment, the subjects with bilateral amygdala lesions failed to do so. Fellows and Farah (2005) found that patients with ventromedial prefrontal or with dorsolateral frontal lobe damage were impaired on the Iowa gambling task, yet only the ventromedial frontal damage group had a reversal deficit. (This reversal deficit can be produced in patients with small bilateral lesions of the orbitofrontal cortex, as shown by Hornak et al. (2004)). Moreover the deficit on the gambling task of the ventromedial prefrontal patients was related to the fact that in the Iowa gambling task the first few choices of a high-risk deck are rewarded, and that later, when a large loss is received from a high-risk deck, an implicit reversal is required. Thus the deficit of patients with orbitofrontal cortex / ventromedial prefrontal cortex damage in the task may be related at least in part to their failure to perform stimulus-reinforcer association reversal learning, rather than for other reasons.

Most known cases of human orbitofrontal damage have occurred in adulthood, but two cases of damage acquired in early life have been reported (Anderson, Bechara, Damasio, Tranel and Damasio 1999). The two patients showed lifelong behavioural problems, which were resistant to corrective influences. But more importantly, the patients appeared completely to lack knowledge about moral and societal conventions. Interestingly, other patients with late acquired orbitofrontal lesions have retained knowledge of such matters, even if they do not always act in accordance with this explicit knowledge. The lack of this moral knowledge and subsequent reckless behaviour in the two patients with early life damage to the orbitofrontal cortex is consistent with the hypothesis that the orbitofrontal cortex is crucial for stimulus–reinforcer association learning (Rolls 1990d, Rolls 1999a). The implication would seem to be that the orbitofrontal cortex is necessary for the development of personal moral-based knowledge based on the processing of rewards and punishers (Dolan 1999).

To investigate the possible significance of face-related inputs to orbitofrontal visual neu-rons described above, we also tested the responses of these patients to faces. We included tests of face (and also voice) expression decoding, because these are ways in which the reinforcing quality of individuals is often indicated. Impairments in the identification of facial and vocal emotional expression were demonstrated in a group of patients with ventral frontal lobe damage who had socially inappropriate behaviour (Hornak, Rolls and Wade 1996, Rolls 1999b) (see Fig. 4.47). The expression identification impairments could occur independently of perceptual impairments in facial recognition, voice discrimination, or environmental sound recognition. The face and voice expression problems did not necessarily occur together in the same patients, providing an indication of separate processing. Poor performance on both expression tests was correlated with the degree of alteration of emotional experience reported by the patients. There was also a strong positive correlation between the degree of altered emotional experience and the severity of the behavioural problems (e.g. disinhibition) found in these patients. A comparison group of patients with brain damage outside the ventral frontal lobe region, without these behavioural problems, was unimpaired on the face expression identification test, was significantly less impaired at vocal expression identification, and reported little subjective emotional change (Hornak et al. 1996, Rolls 1999b).

These findings have been extended, and it has been found that patients with face expression decoding problems do not necessarily have impairments at visual discrimination reversal, and vice versa (Hornak, Bramham, Rolls, Morris, O'Doherty, Bullock and Polkey 2003, Hornak, O'Doherty, Bramham, Rolls, Morris, Bullock and Polkey 2004). This is consistent with some topography in the orbitofrontal cortex (see Section 4.5.5.8 and Rolls and Baylis (1994)).

To obtain clear evidence that the changes in face and voice expression identification, emotional behaviour, and subjective emotional state were related to orbitofrontal cortex damage itself, and not to damage to surrounding areas which is present in many closed head injury patients, we performed these assessments in patients with circumscribed lesions made surgically in the course of treatment (Hornak, Bramham, Rolls, Morris, O'Doherty, Bullock and Polkey 2003). This study also enabled us to determine whether there was functional specialization within the orbitofrontal cortex, and whether damage to nearby and connected areas (such as the anterior cingulate cortex) in which some of the patients had lesions could produce similar effects. We found that some patients with bilateral lesions of the orbitofrontal cortex had deficits in voice and face expression identification, and the group had impairments in social behaviour, and significant changes in their subjective emotional state (Hornak et al. 2003). The same group of patients had deficits on the probabilistic monetary reward task (Hornak et al. 2004). Some patients with unilateral damage restricted to the orbitofrontal cortex also had deficits in voice expression identification, and the group did not have significant changes in social behaviour, or in their subjective emotional state. Patients with unilateral lesions of the antero-ventral part of the anterior cingulate cortex and/or medial prefrontal cortex area BA9 were in some cases impaired on voice and face expression identification, had some change in social behaviour, and had significant changes in their subjective emotional state. Patients with dorsolateral prefrontal cortex lesions or with medial lesions outside the anterior cingulate cortex and medial prefrontal BA9 areas were unimpaired on any of these measures of emotion. In all cases in which voice expression identification was impaired, there were no deficits in control tests of the discrimination of unfamiliar voices and the recognition of environmental sounds.

These results (Hornak, Bramham, Rolls, Morris, O'Doherty, Bullock and Polkey 2003) thus confirm that damage restricted to the orbitofrontal cortex can produce impairments in face and voice expression identification, which may be primary reinforcers. The system is sensitive, in that even patients with unilateral orbitofrontal cortex lesions may be impaired.

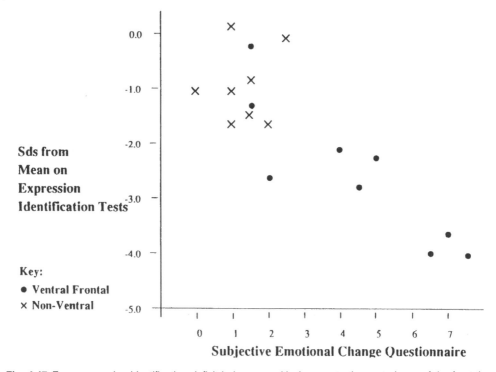

Fig. 4.47 Face expression identification deficit in humans with damage to the ventral part of the frontal lobe, and its relation to the patient's own rating of Subjective Emotional Change since the brain damage, based on sadness (or regret), anger (or frustration), fear (or anxiety), disgust, and excitement or enjoyment. (From Hornak, Rolls and Wade 1996.)

The impairment is not a generic impairment of the ability to recognize any emotions in others, in that frequently voice but not face expression identification was impaired, and vice versa. This implies some functional specialization for visual vs auditory emotion-related processing in the human orbitofrontal cortex. The results also show that the changes in social behaviour can be produced by damage restricted to the orbitofrontal cortex. The patients were particularly likely to be impaired on emotion recognition (they were less likely to notice when others were sad, or happy, or disgusted); on emotional empathy (they were less likely to comfort those who are sad, or afraid, or to feel happy for others who are happy); on interpersonal relationships (not caring what others think, and not being close to his/her family); and were less likely to cooperate with others; were impatient and impulsive; and had difficulty in making and keeping close relationships. The results also show that changes in subjective emotional state (including frequently sadness, anger and happiness) can be produced by damage restricted to the orbitofrontal cortex (Hornak et al. 2003). In addition, the patients with bilateral orbitofrontal cortex lesions were impaired on the probabilistic reversal learning task (Hornak et al. 2004). The findings overall thus make clear the types of deficit found in humans with orbitofrontal cortex damage, and can be easily related to underlying fundamental processes in which the orbitofrontal cortex is involved as described throughout Section 4.5, including decoding and representing primary reinforcers, being sensitive to changes in reinforcers, and rapidly readjusting behaviour to stimuli when the reinforcers available change.

The results (Hornak et al. 2003) also extend these investigations to the anterior cingulate cortex (including some of medial prefrontal cortex area BA9) by showing that lesions in these regions can produce voice and/or face expression identification deficits, and marked changes in subjective emotional state (see Section 4.7).

It is also becoming possible to relate the functions of the orbitofrontal cortex to some psychiatric symptoms. Berlin, Rolls and Kischka (2004), Berlin and Rolls (2004) and Berlin, Rolls and Iversen (2005) compared the symptoms of patients with a personality disorder syndrome, Borderline Personality Disorder (BPD), with those of patients with lesions of the orbitofrontal cortex. The symptoms of the self-harming Borderline Personality Disorder patients include high impulsivity, affective instability, and emotionality; and low extraversion. It was found that orbitofrontal cortex and Borderline Personality Disorder patients performed similarly in that they were more impulsive, reported more inappropriate behaviours in the Frontal Behaviour Questionnaire, and had more Borderline Personality Disorder characteristics, and anger, and less happiness, than control groups (either normals, or patients with lesions outside the orbitofrontal cortex).

One of the measures of impulsiveness was the Matching Familiar Figures Test. In this standard cognitive behavioural measure of impulsivity, created by Kagan (1966), a participant selects (points to), from a set of highly similar pictures, the one that is exactly the same as the standard reference picture. High impulsiveness is reflected in short latencies to make a choice (which are typically 55 s in control subjects), and errors in the choices made. The other measure of impulsiveness was the Barratt Impulsiveness Scale (Patton, Stanford and Barratt 1995) which is a 30-item questionnaire that assesses non-planning impulsivity (attention to details), motor impulsivity (acting without thinking), and cognitive impulsivity (future oriented thinking and coping stability). Both the orbitofrontal and BPD groups were impaired at both measures of impulsiveness.

Both the orbitofrontal and BPD groups also had a faster perception of time (i.e. they underproduced time) than normal controls. This may be one factor underlying their increased impulsiveness, in that they feel that sufficient time has elapsed to initiate action.

It was of considerable interest that the BPD group, as well as the orbitofrontal group, scored highly on the Frontal Behaviour Questionnaire which assessed inappropriate behaviours typical of orbitofrontal cortex patients including disinhibition, social inappropriateness, perseveration, and uncooperativeness. Both groups were also less open to experience (i.e. less open-minded), a personality characteristic.

The orbitofrontal and BPD patients performed differently on other tasks: BPD patients were less extraverted and conscientious, and more neurotic and emotional, than all other groups. Patients with orbitofrontal cortex lesions had more severe deficits in reversing stimulus–reinforcer associations compared to all other groups and had a faster perception of time (overestimated time) than normal controls. These deficits were not related to spatial working memory functions which are impaired by dorsolateral prefrontal cortex damage.

Thus some but not other symptoms of self-harming Borderline Personality Disorder patients are similar to those of patients with orbitofrontal cortex damage. The symptoms the groups have in common include impulsiveness and the inappropriate behaviours typical of 'frontal' patients. This could imply that in BPD patients some aspects of the operation of the orbitofrontal cortex are occurring (whatever their aetiology, which could include innate or acquired changes, and might involve different expression or operation of neurotransmitters) differently to the way they operate in normal control subjects. Part of the interest of this is that it may help to point towards new concepts that may be useful in the treatment of some of the symptoms of patients with Borderline Personality Disorder. On the other hand, other aspects of Borderline Personality Disorder do not appear to be related to orbitofrontal cortex functions, including the more neurotic and more emotional personality characteristics of the BPD group together with their lower extraversion and conscientious (Berlin, Rolls and Kischka 2004, Berlin and Rolls 2004, Berlin, Rolls and Iversen 2005).

Another case in which it is possible to relate psychiatric types of symptom to orbitofrontal cortex function is frontotemporal dementia, which is a progressive neurodegenerative disorder attacking the frontal lobes and producing major and pervasive behavioural changes in personality and social conduct resembling those produced by orbitofrontal lesions (Rahman, Sahakian, Hodges, Rogers and Robbins 1997). Patients appear either socially disinhibited with facetiousness and inappropriate jocularity, or apathetic and withdrawn. Many patients show mental rigidity and inability to appreciate irony or other subtle aspects of language. They tend to engage in ritualistic and stereotypical behaviour, and their planning skills are invariably impaired. The dementia is accompanied by gradual withdrawal from all social interactions. Memory is usually intact but patients have difficulties with working memory and concentration. Interestingly, given the anatomy and physiology of the orbitofrontal cortex, frontotemporal dementia causes profound changes in eating habits, with escalating desire for sweet food coupled with reduced satiety, which is often followed by enormous weight gain.

4.5.7 A neurophysiological and computational basis for stimulus–reinforcer association learning and reversal in the orbitofrontal cortex

The neurophysiological and lesion evidence described suggests that one function implemented by the orbitofrontal cortex is rapid stimulus–reinforcer association learning, and the correction of these associations when reinforcement contingencies in the environment change. To implement this, the orbitofrontal cortex has the necessary representation of primary reinforcers, such as taste and somatosensory inputs (see Section 4.3 and Chapter 5). It also receives information about objects, e.g. visual information, and can associate this very rapidly at the neuronal level with primary reinforcers such as taste, and reverse these associations. Another type of stimulus that can be conditioned in this way in the orbitofrontal cortex is olfactory, although here the learning is slower. It is likely that auditory stimuli can be associated with primary reinforcers in the orbitofrontal cortex, though there is less direct evidence of this yet.

The orbitofrontal cortex neurons that detect non-reward in a context-specific manner are likely to be used in behavioural extinction and reversal. Such non-reward neurons may help behaviour in situations in which stimulus–reinforcer associations must be disconnected, not only by helping to reset the reinforcer association of neurons in the orbitofrontal cortex, but also by sending a signal to the striatum which could be routed by the striatum to produce appropriate behaviours for non-reward (Rolls and Johnstone 1992, Williams, Rolls, Leonard and Stern 1993, Rolls 1994b, Rolls 1999a) (see Chapter 8). Indeed, it is via this route, the striatal, that the orbitofrontal cortex may directly influence behaviour when the orbitofrontal cortex is decoding reinforcement contingencies in the environment, and is altering behaviour in response to altering reinforcement contingencies. Some of the evidence for this is that neurons with responses that reflect these orbitofrontal neuronal responses are found in the ventral part of the head of the caudate nucleus and the ventral striatum, which receive from the orbitofrontal cortex (Rolls, Thorpe and Maddison 1983c, Williams, Rolls, Leonard and Stern 1993); and lesions of the ventral part of the head of the caudate nucleus impair visual discrimination reversal (Divac, Rosvold and Szwarcbart 1967) (see further Chapter 8).

Decoding the reinforcement value of stimuli, which involves for previously neutral (e.g. visual) stimuli learning their association with a primary reinforcer, often rapidly, and which may involve not only rapid learning but also rapid relearning and alteration of responses when reinforcement contingencies change, is then a function proposed for the orbitofrontal cortex. This way of producing behavioural responses would be important in, for example, motivational and emotional behaviour. It would be important in motivational behaviour such as feeding and drinking by enabling primates to learn rapidly about the food reinforcement to be expected from visual stimuli (see Rolls (1999a) and Chapter 5). This is important, for primates frequently eat more than 100 varieties of food; vision by visual-taste association learning can be used to identify when foods are ripe; and during the course of a meal, the pleasantness of the sight of a food eaten in the meal decreases in a sensory-specific way (Rolls, Rolls and Rowe 1983b), a function that is probably implemented by the sensory-specific satiety-related responses of orbitofrontal visual neurons (Critchley and Rolls 1996a).

With regard to emotional behaviour, decoding and rapidly readjusting the reinforcement value of visual signals is likely to be crucial, for emotions can be described as responses elicited by reinforcing signals (Rolls 1986c, Rolls 1986a, Rolls 1990d, Rolls 1995b, Rolls 1999a) (see Chapter 2). The ability to perform this learning very rapidly is probably very important in social situations in primates, in which reinforcing stimuli are continually being exchanged, and the reinforcement value of these must be continually updated (relearned), based on the actual reinforcers received and given. Although the operation of reinforcers such as taste, smell, and faces are best understood in terms of orbitofrontal cortex operation, there are tactile inputs that are likely to be concerned with reward evaluation, and in humans the rewards processed in the orbitofrontal cortex include quite general rewards such as working for 'points' (Rolls et al. 1994a) or for 'monetary' rewards (O'Doherty, Kringelbach, Rolls, Hornak and Andrews 2001a, Hornak, O'Doherty, Bramham, Rolls, Morris, Bullock and Polkey 2004).

Although the amygdala is concerned with some of the same functions as the orbitofrontal cortex, and receives similar inputs (see Figs. 4.2, 4.18 and 4.51), there is evidence that it may function less effectively in the very rapid learning and reversal of stimulus–reinforcer associations, as indicated by the greater difficulty in obtaining reversal from amygdala neurons (see, e.g., Rolls (2000d)), and by the greater effect of orbitofrontal lesions in leading to continuing behavioural responses to previously rewarded stimuli (see Sections 4.5.4 and 4.5.6). In primates the necessity for very rapid stimulus–reinforcement re-evaluation, and the development of powerful cortical learning systems, may result in the orbitofrontal cortex effectively taking over this aspect of amygdala functions (Rolls 1992b, Rolls 1999a, Rolls 2000d) (see Appendix B). The mechanism of rapid reversal learning that may be implemented in the orbitofrontal cortex may utilize a working memory of which rule is currently active, which may depend on a highly developed recurrent collateral set of synaptic connections present in the orbitofrontal cortex but not the amygdala, as described in Appendix 2 and by Deco and Rolls (2005d). This offers a more computational account of the different functions of the orbitofrontal cortex and amygdala in emotion than previous accounts (e.g. Pickens, Saddoris, Setlow, Gallagher, Holland and Schoenbaum (2003), and Holland and Gallagher

A model for how the very rapid, one-trial, reversal could be implemented has now been developed (see Deco and Rolls (2005d) and Appendix 2 for a full description). The model uses a short term memory autoassociation attractor network with associatively modifiable synaptic connections (see Appendix 2) to hold the neurons representing the current rule active (see Fig. 4.48). Rule one might correspond to 'stimulus 1 (e.g. a triangle) is associated with reward, and stimulus 2 (e.g. a square) is associated with punishment'. Rule 2 might correspond to the opposite contingency. A small, very biologically plausible, modification of the standard one-layer autoassociation network is that there is a small amount of adaptation in the recurrent collateral synapses that keep the neurons representing the current rule firing. Now consider the case when the neurons representing rule one are firing. How does the rule module reverse? The proposal is that when the non-reward or error neurons described above (Section 4.5.5.5) fire, this additional set of firing neurons destabilizes the rule attractor module, by for example producing extra firing of the inhibitory neurons in the orbitofrontal cortex, which in turn inhibit the excitatory neurons in the rule autoassociation network, thus quenching its attractor state. This error input to the rule attractor network is shown in Fig. 4.48. After neuronal firing in the network has stopped and the error signal, which may last for 10 s as illustrated in Fig. 4.36 on page 117, is no longer present, then firing gradually can build up again in the rule attractor network. (This build-up may be assisted by non-specific inputs from other neurons in the area, as illustrated in Appendix 2.) However, with the competitive processes operating within the rule attractor network between the populations of neurons representing rule 1 and those representing rule 2, and the fact that the neurons or synapses that are part of the rule 1 attractor are partly adapted, the neurons that win the competition and become active are those representing rule 2, and the rule attractor has reversed its state. This process is illustrated in Fig. 4.49, and takes one trial. Reversal learning set takes a number of reversals to acquire because the correct attractors for the relevant rules, and their connections to other 'mapping' neurons, have to be learned.

To achieve the correct 'mapping' from stimuli to their reinforcer association, and thus emotional state, the rule neurons bias the competition in a mapping module, illustrated in Fig. 4.48. The mapping module has sensory input neurons, intermediate 'conditional reward' neurons (of the type described in Section 4.5.5.4 and illustrated in Fig. 4.32) which respond to combinations of stimuli and whether they are currently associated with reward (or for other neurons to a punisher), and output neurons which represent the reinforcement association of the stimulus currently being viewed. (In the case described there are four populations or pools of neurons at the intermediate level, two for the direct rewarding context: object 1-rewarding, object 2-punishing, and two for the reversal condition: object 1-punishing, object 2-rewarding). These intermediate pools or populations of neurons respond to combinations of the sensory stimuli and the expected reward, e.g. to object1 and an expected reward (glucose obtained after licking), and are the conditional reward neurons described in Section 4.5.5.4 and illustrated in Fig. 4.32 on page 112. The sensory – intermediate – reward module thus consists of three hierarchically organised levels of attractor network, with stronger synaptic connections in the forward direction from input to output than the backprojection direction. The rule module acts as a biasing input to bias the competition between the object–reward combination neurons at the intermediate level of the sensory – intermediate – reward module. This biasing is achieved because rule 1 has associatively strengthened connections to object 1–rewarding and object 2–punishing neurons. (The whole network could be set up by simple associative learning operating to strengthen connections made with low probability between

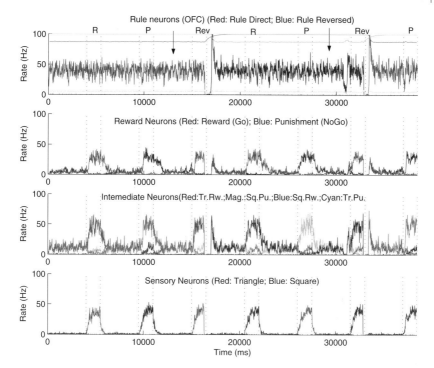

Fig. 4.49 Reward reversal model: Temporal evolution of the averaged population activity for all neural pools (sensory, intermediate (stimulus–reward), and Reward/Punishment) in the stimulus – intermediate – reward module and the rule module, during the execution and the reversal of the Go/NoGo visual discrimination task with a pseudorandom trial sequence after Thorpe, Rolls and Maddison (1983) and Rolls, Critchley, Mason and Wakeman (1996). Bottom row: the sensory neuronal populations, one of which responds to Object 1, a triangle (red), and the other to Object 2, a square (blue). The intermediate conditional stimulus–reward and stimulus–punishment neurons respond to for example Object 1 (Tr) when it is associated with reward (Rw) (e.g. on trial 1, corresponding to O1R in Fig. 4.48), or to Object 2 (Sq) when it is associated with punishment (Pu) (e.g. on trial 2, O2P). The top row shows the firing rate activity in the rule module, with the thin line at the top of this graph showing the mean probability of release P_{rel} of transmitter from the synapses of each population of neurons. The arrows show when the contingencies reversed. R: Reward trial; P: Punishment Trial; Rev: Reversal trial, i.e. the first trial after the reward contingency was reversed when Reward was expected but Punishment was obtained. The intertrial interval was 4 s. The yellow line shows the average activity of the inhibitory neurons. (See text for further details.) (After Deco and Rolls, 2005d.) (See colour plates section.)

different neurons that are conjunctively active during the task in the network – see Deco and Rolls (2005d).)

Thus when object 1, e.g. the triangle, is being presented and rule one for direct mapping is in the rule module and biasing the intermediate neurons of the sensory – intermediate – reward module, then the intermediate neurons that fire are the object 1-reward neurons (O1R in Fig. 4.48), and these in turn through associative connections activate the reward neurons (Rwd in Fig. 4.48) at the third, reward/punishment, level of the hierarchy. If on the other hand object 1, e.g. the triangle, is being presented and rule two for reversed mapping is in the rule module and biasing the intermediate neurons of the sensory – intermediate – reward module, then the intermediate neurons that fire are the object 1–punishment (O1P) neurons, and these in turn through associative connections activate the punishment neurons (Pun) at the third, reward/punishment, level of the hierarchy. This model can thus account for one-trial reversal learning, and provides an account for the presence of the conditional reward and conditional punishment neurons found by Thorpe, Rolls and Maddison (1983) and Rolls, Critchley, Mason and Wakeman (1996b) in the orbitofrontal cortex (Section 4.5.5.4).

It is an important part of the architecture that at the intermediate level of the sensory – intermediate – reward module one set of neurons fire if an object being presented is currently associated with reward, and a different set if the object being presented is currently associated with punishment. This representation means that these neurons can be used for different functions, such as the elicitation of emotional or autonomic responses, which can occur for example to particular stimuli associated with particular reinforcers (Rolls 1999a). For example, particular emotions might arise if a particular cognitively processed input such as a particular person is associated with a particular type of reinforcer or reinforcement contingency.

It is also an interesting part of the architecture that associative synaptic modifiability (LTP, and LTD if present) is needed only to set up the functional architecture of the network while the reversal learning set is being acquired. However, once the correct synaptic connections have been set up to implement the architecture illustrated in Fig. 4.48, then no further synaptic modifiability is needed each time reversal occurs, as reversal is achieved just by the error signal quenching the current rule attractor, and the attractor for the other rule then starting up because its synapses are not adapted. This is an interesting prediction of the model. If tested by NMDA receptor blockers, which can block LTP, then it would be important to ensure that non-specific factors produced by the NMDA blockade such as less overall activity in the network, and the stabilizing effects of the long time constants of NMDA receptors, do not contribute to any result obtained. For this reason, use of a procedure for impairing synaptic modifiability other than NMDA receptor blockade would be useful in testing this prediction.

The network just described uses biased competition from a rule module to bias the mapping from sensory stimuli to the representation of a reward vs a punisher. An analogous rule network reversed in the same way by error signals quenching the current rule attractor, can be used to reverse the mapping from stimuli via intermediate stimulus–response neurons to response neurons, and thus to switch the stimulus-to-motor response being mapped in a model of conditional response learning (Deco and Rolls 2003, Deco and Rolls 2005d) (see Appendix 2). While reward rule neurons have not been described yet for the orbitofrontal cortex, neurons which may correspond to stimulus–response rule neurons have been found in the dorsolateral prefrontal cortex (Wallis, Anderson and Miller 2001).

This model also provides a computational account of why the orbitofrontal cortex may play a more important role in rapid reversal learning than the amygdala. The account is based on the fact that a feature of cortical architecture is a highly developed set of local (within 1–2 mm) recurrent collateral excitatory associatively modifiable connections between pyramidal cells (Rolls and Deco 2002, Rolls and Treves 1998). These provide the basis for short term memory attractor networks, and thus the basis for the rule attractor model which is at the heart of my suggestion for how rapid reversal learning is implemented (Deco and Rolls 2005d). In contrast, the amygdala is thought to have a much less well developed set of recurrent collateral excitatory connections, and thus may not be able to implement rapid reversal learning in the way described using competition biased by a rule module. Instead, the amygdala would need to rely on synaptic relearning as described in the first approach above, and this would be likely to be a slower process, and would certainly not lead to correct choice of the new S+ the first time it is presented after a punishment trial when the reversal contingency changes. Of course, in addition it is possible that the rapidity of LTP, and the efficacy of LTD, both of which would also facilitate rapid reversal, may be enhanced in the orbitofrontal cortex compared to the amygdala. Thus, the cortical neuronal reversal mechanism in the orbitofrontal cortex may be effectively a faster implementation in two ways than what is implemented in the amygdala. The cortical (in this case orbitofrontal cortex) mechanism may have evolved particularly to enable rapid updating by received reinforcers in social and other situations in primates. This hypothesis, that the orbitofrontal cortex, as a rapid learning mechanism, effectively provides an additional route for some of the functions performed by the amygdala, and is very important when this stimulus–reinforcer learning must be rapidly readjusted, has been developed elsewhere (Rolls 1990d, Rolls 1992b, Rolls 1996a, Rolls 1999a, Rolls 2000d).

Another feature of the rule attractor model of rapid reversal learning (Deco and Rolls 2005d) is that it does utilize a set of coupled attractor networks in the orbitofrontal cortex. Consistent with this, Hikosaka and Watanabe (2000) have shown that a short term memory for reward, such as the flavour of a food, is represented by continuing firing in orbitofrontal cortex neurons in a reward delayed match-to-sample short term memory task. This could be implemented by associatively modified synaptic connections between taste reward neurons (see Section 4.3) in the orbitofrontal cortex.

Although the mechanism has been described so far for visual-to-taste association learning, this is because neurophysiological experiments on this are most direct. It is likely, given the evidence from the effects of lesions, that taste is only one type of primary reinforcer about which such learning occurs in the orbitofrontal cortex, and is likely to be an example of a much more general type of stimulus–reinforcer learning system. Some of the evidence for this is that humans with orbitofrontal cortex damage are impaired at visual discrimination reversal when working for a reward that consists of points (Rolls, Hornak, Wade and McGrath 1994a) or money (Hornak, Bramham, Rolls, Morris, O'Doherty, Bullock and Polkey 2003) (see Section 4.5.6). Moreover, as described above, there is now evidence that the representation of the affective aspects of touch are represented in the human orbitofrontal cortex (Rolls et al. 2003d), and learning about what stimuli are associated with this class of primary reinforcer is also likely to be an important aspect of the stimulus–reinforcer association learning performed by the orbitofrontal cortex.

4.5.8 Executive functions of the orbitofrontal cortex

The research described indicates that the orbitofrontal cortex is involved in the execution of behavioural responses when these are computed by reward or punisher association learning, a function for which the orbitofrontal cortex is specialized, in terms of representations of primary (unlearned) reinforcers, and in rapidly learning and readjusting associations of stimuli with these primary reinforcers. The fact that patients with ventral frontal lesions often can express verbally what the correct responses should be, yet cannot follow what previously obtained rewards and punishers indicate is appropriate behaviour, is an indication that when primates (including humans) normally execute behavioural responses on the basis of reinforcement evaluation, they do so using the orbitofrontal cortex. Eliciting behaviour on the basis of rewards and punishers obtained previously in similar situations is of course a simple and adaptive way to control behavioural responses that has been studied and accepted for very many years (throughout the history of psychology; and in terms of brain mechanisms, see, e.g., Rolls (1975), Rolls (1986c), Rolls (1986a), Rolls (1990d), Rolls (1995b), Rolls (1999a), Rolls (2004b) and Cardinal, Parkinson, Hall and Everitt (2002)).

The particular utility of one of the alternative routes to behaviour (there are, of course, many routes to behaviour) made possible by language is that this enables long-term planning, where the plan involves many syntactic arrangements of symbols (e.g. many 'if ... then' statements). It is suggested that when this linguistic (in terms of syntactic manipulation of symbols) system needs correction, being able to think about the plans (higher-order thoughts), enables the plans to be corrected, and that this process is closely related to explicit, conscious, processing (Rolls 1995b, Rolls 1997b, Rolls 1999a, Rolls 2004c, Rosenthal 1993) (see Chapter 10). It follows that the functions performed by the orbitofrontal cortex need not be performed with explicit (conscious) processing, but can be performed with implicit processing. It is in this way that it is suggested that the orbitofrontal cortex is involved in some, but certainly not all, types of executive function.

In that the orbitofrontal cortex may retain as a result of synaptic modification in a pattern associator (see Appendix 1, Rolls and Treves (1990), and Rolls and Treves (1998)) the most recent reinforcer associations for large numbers of different stimuli, it could perhaps be fitted into a view that the frontal cortical areas are in general concerned with different types of working memory. However, the term working memory is normally used in neurophysiology to refer to a memory in which the memoranda are held in the memory by continuing neuronal activity, as in an autoassociator or attractor network which has recurrent collateral connections (see, e.g., Rolls and Treves (1998), Rolls and Deco (2002), and Appendix 1). It should be realized that although there may be a functional similarity between such a working memory and the ability of the orbitofrontal cortex to retain the most recent reinforcer association of many stimuli, the implementations are very different. The different implementations do in fact have strong functional consequences: it is difficult to retain more than a few items active in an autoassociative memory, and hence in practice individual items are retained typically only for short periods in such working memories (Deco and Rolls 2005c); whereas in pattern associators, because synaptic modification has taken place, the last reinforcement association of a very large number of stimuli can be stored for long periods, and recalled whenever each stimulus is seen again in the future, without any ongoing neuronal firing to hold the representation active (see, e.g., Rolls and Treves (1998)).

It is perhaps useful to note how the orbitofrontal cortex may link to output systems to control behaviour, for the occasions when the orbitofrontal cortex does control behaviour. Rolls has proposed (Rolls 1984a, Rolls 1994b, Rolls and Johnstone 1992, Rolls and Treves 1998, Rolls 1999a) (see Chapter 8) the outline of a theory of striatal function according to which all areas of the cerebral cortex gain access to the striatum, and compete within the striatum and the rest of the basal ganglia system for behavioural output depending on how strongly each part of the cerebral cortex is calling for output. The striatum then maps (as a result of slow previous habit or stimulus–response learning) each particular type of input to the striatum to the appropriate behavioural output (implemented via the return basal ganglia connections to premotor/prefrontal parts of the cerebral cortex). This is one of the ways in which reinforcing stimuli can exert their influence relatively directly on behavioural output. The importance of this route is attested to by the fact that restricted striatal lesions impair functions implemented by the part of the cortex that projects to the lesioned part of the striatum (Rolls 1984a, Rolls 1994b, Rolls and Johnstone 1992, Rolls and Treves 1998) (see Section 8.4).

Another set of outputs from the orbitofrontal cortex enables it to influence autonomic function. The fact that ventral prefrontal lesions block autonomic responses to learned re-inforcers (Damasio 1994) [actually known since at least the 1950s, e.g. Elithorn, Piercy and Crosskey (1955) in humans; Grueninger, Kimble, Grueninger and Levine (1965) in macaques], is of course consistent with the hypothesis that learned reinforcers elicit autonomic responses via the orbitofrontal cortex and amygdala (see, e.g., Rolls (1986c), Rolls (1986a) and Rolls (1990d)). It is worth emphasizing here that this does not prove the hypothesis that behavioural responses elicited by conditioned reinforcers are mediated via peripheral changes, themselves used as 'somatic markers' to determine which response to make. The question of whether there is any returning information from the periphery which is necessary for emotion, as the somatic marker hypothesis postulates, has been considered in Section 2.6.1. The present hypothesis is, in contrast, that somatic markers are not part of the route by which emotions are felt or emotional decisions are taken, but that instead the much more direct neural route from the orbitofrontal cortex and amygdala to the basal ganglia provides a pathway that is much more efficient, and is directly implicated in producing, the behavioural responses to learned incentives (Divac et al. 1967, Everitt and Robbins 1992, Williams et al. 1993, Rolls 1994b) (see Chapter 8, and for explicit verbal outputs see Chapter 10 also). Another potentially important output route from the orbitofrontal cortex is to the cingulate cortex (see Section 4.7).

4.6   The amygdala

Bilateral damage to the amygdala produces a deficit in learning to associate visual and other stimuli with a primary (i.e. unlearned) reward or punisher. For example, monkeys with damage to the amygdala when shown foods and non-foods pick up both and place them in their mouths. When such visual or auditory discrimination learning and learned emotional responses to stimuli are tested more formally, it is found that animals have difficulty in associating the sight or sound of a stimulus with whether it produces a reward, or is noxious and should be avoided (see Rolls (1990d), Rolls (1992b), Rolls (2000d) and Aggleton (2000)). Similar changes in behaviour have been seen in humans with extensive damage to the temporal lobe. The primate amygdala also contains a population of neurons specialized to respond to faces, and damage to the human amygdala can alter the ability to discriminate between different facial expressions.

Because the amygdala is implicated in some but not other learning processes involved in emotion, Section 4.6.1 provides a description of some of the different associative processes involved in emotion-related learning, as part of the background for considering the functions of the amygdala in emotion, and more generally, for understanding the types of learning that influence decision processes involved in emotional behaviours (see further Section 11.2).

4.6.1   Associative processes involved in emotion-related learning

When a conditioned stimulus (CS) (such as a tone) is paired with a primary reinforcer or unconditioned stimulus (US) (such as a painful stimulus), then there are opportunities for a number of types of association to be formed.

Some of these involve 'classical conditioning' or 'Pavlovian conditioning', in which no action is performed that affects the contingency between the conditioned stimulus and the unconditioned stimulus. Typically an unconditioned response (UR), for example an alteration of heart rate, is produced by the US, and will come to be elicited by the CS as a conditioned response (CR). These responses are typically autonomic (such as the heart beating faster), or endocrine (for example the release of adrenaline (epinephrine in American usage) by the adrenal gland).

In addition, the organism may learn to perform an instrumental response with the skeletal muscles in order to alter the probability that the primary reinforcer will be obtained. In our example, the experimenter might alter the contingencies so that when the tone sounded, if the organism performed an action such as pressing a lever, then the painful stimulus could be avoided. This is confirmed to be instrumental learning if the response learned is arbitrary, for example performing the opposite response, such as raising the lever to avoid the painful stimulus.

In the instrumental learning situation there are still opportunities for many classically conditioned responses including emotional states such as fear to occur, and, as different neural subsystems appear to contribute differently to these different types of learning that occur in emotional situations produced by reinforcers, I will next separate out some of the different associative processes that can occur, to provide a basis for understanding the roles of different neural subsystems in the different emotion-related responses and states, following the general approach reviewed by Cardinal, Parkinson, Hall and Everitt (2002).

4.6.1.1   Pavlovian or classical conditioning

As shown in Fig. 4.50, Pavlovian conditioning has the potential to create multiple associative representations in the brain, as described next (Cardinal et al. 2002, Mackintosh 1983, Gewirtz and Davis 1998, Dickinson 1980, Cardinal and Everitt 2004).

Stimulus–Response association. First, the CS may become directly associated with the UR, a simple stimulus–response association that carries no information about the identity of the US (Kandel 2000) (pathway 1 in Fig. 4.50). Such US-elicited responses include preparatory responses which are not specific to the type of US involved (e.g. orienting to a stimulus, or increased arousal), and 'consummatory' responses which are specific to the US such as salivation to food, or blinking to an air puff applied to the eye, or approach to a food. A single US may elicit both preparatory and consummatory responses, and thus the CS may enter into simple S–R associations with several types of response. The nature of the CS can influence which response is evoked; for example if a poorly localized CS such as a tone is paired with food, it may not elicit conditioned approach, while a localized light does. It is notable in this last example that the approach response is skeletal, so that we are going beyond the concept that Pavlovian conditioning applies only to autonomic responses.

A representation of affect, i.e. an emotional state. Second, the CS can evoke a representation of affect, i.e. an emotional state, such as fear or the expectation of reward (pathway 2 in Fig. 4.50). It is demonstrated operationally by the phenomenon of transreinforcer blocking. Blocking is a feature of Pavlovian conditioning in which an animal does not learn about one CS in the presence of another CS that already predicts the same US (Dickinson 1980). In *transreinforcer blocking*, the presence of a CS previously paired with shock can block or prevent conditioning to a CS paired with the absence of otherwise expected food reward (Dickinson and Dearing 1979). These two reinforcers share no common properties other than their aversiveness, and therefore the blocking effect must depend on an association between the CS and

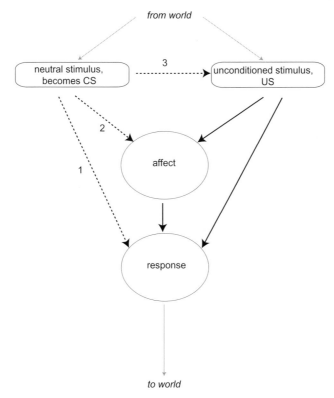

Fig. 4.50 Pavlovian conditioning has the potential to create associations between a conditioned stimulus (CS) and representations of the unconditioned stimulus (US), central affective or emotional states such as fear, and unconditioned responses. Dashed lines represent associatively learned links. Several different types of response may be involved, including preparatory responses which are not specific to the type of US involved (e.g. orienting to a stimulus, or increased arousal), and 'consummatory' responses which are specific to the US such as salivation to food, or blinking to an air puff applied to the eye. (After Cardinal, Parkinson, Hall and Everitt, 2002).

affect. Affective states, it is argued (Dickinson and Dearing 1979, Konorski 1967, Cardinal et al. 2002), can therefore be independent of the specific reinforcer and response – they are pure 'value' states. However, I note that, at least in humans, affective states normally have content, that is they are about particular reinforcers (such as feeling happy because I am seeing a friend, or feeling happy because I am receiving a gift), and these states are better described by the third type of association, described next.

Conditioned-Stimulus (CS)–Unconditioned Stimulus (US) associations. Third, the CS can become associated with the specific sensory properties of the US including its visual appearance, sound, and smell and its 'consummatory' (primary reinforcing) properties such as its taste, nutritive value, and feel (pathway 3 in Fig. 4.50). An operational demonstration of this type of representation is sensory preconditioning, in which two neutral stimuli are first associated; one neutral stimulus is then paired with a primary reinforcer, and the other stimulus can subsequently evoke a CR (Dickinson 1980). Further evidence for the US specificity of

Pavlovian associations comes from the effect of post-conditioning changes in the value of the US. If a CS is paired with a rewarding food, and the food is subsequently devalued by pairing it with a lithium chloride (LiCl) injection to induce nausea, not only does the animal reject the food US, but its reaction to the CS changes (Mackintosh 1983, Holland and Straub 1979). Therefore the CS could not have been associated just with an abstract affective representation, as it was able to retrieve, by association, the new value of the US. As the LiCl pairing does not affect the reaction to a second CS predicting a different food, each CS must have been associated with some specific aspect of its US.

We will see later that different pathways in the brain are involved in the Pavlovian learned autonomic and skeletal responses to a CS, and in the affective representation or state (e.g. fear), which may itself enter into associations and influence choice.

4.6.1.2 Instrumental learning

In instrumental learning, there is a contingency between the behaviour and the reinforcing outcome. A number of different learning processes may operate during this procedure (Cardinal et al. 2002, Dickinson 1994, Dickinson and Balleine 1994). These learning processes are summarized next as they help to understand some of the different brain mechanisms that become engaged and affect behaviour when emotion-provoking stimuli are delivered. These learning processes are closely related to emotion, for as argued in Chapter 2 emotions are states elicited by instrumental reinforcers. Moreover, as argued in Chapter 3, an important part of the evolutionary adaptive value of emotions is that genes can influence our behaviour efficiently by specifying the goals for our actions, and then instrumental learning in life leads us to learn appropriate behaviours to obtain those gene-specified goals. This of course leads to selection of the genes that specify the goals (rewards and punishers), and thereby promote their own survival into the next generation. Part of the adaptive value of emotional states, as argued in Chapter 3, is that they persist for some time after the reinforcer has gone, and this continuation enables the reinforcers to influence our behaviour (by unconditioned, classically conditioned, and instrumentally learned, processes) for often a considerable time.

An example of a goal-directed behaviour is when an organism presses a lever for food because it knows that lever-pressing produces food and that it wants the food. More formally, behaviour may be said to be goal-directed if it depends on both (1) the instrumental contingency between the action and a particular outcome (A–O contingency), and (2) a representation of the outcome as a goal (Dickinson and Balleine 1994, Cardinal et al. 2002). As two representations must interact, the knowledge required may be called declarative.

Instrumental (Action–Outcome) contingency. Vertebrates, and some invertebrates, can learn the instrumental contingency between an action and its consequence. For example rats can be arbitrarily trained to press a lever down or pull it up in order to obtain a goal. (This is a bidirectional control assay to show that the action is arbitrary.) Not all behaviours can be trained in this way, and in this sense there is some preparedness to learn. For example, locomotor approach to a visual stimulus in rats is predominantly under the control of Pavlovian and not instrumental processes, in that rats could not learn to withhold an approach response to a visual CS in order to be rewarded (Bussey and Everitt 1997).

Incentive value. Rats also fulfil the second requirement for instrumental learning: they demonstrate that they want the outcomes for which they work. The goal status (or *incentive value*) of an instrumental outcome can be demonstrated by devaluing it (Dickinson and

Balleine 1994). For example, if rats are trained to lever-press for food, and then receive pairings of that food with LiCl (lithium chloride, which induces a conditioned taste aversion), they will subsequently work less for that food – even if the test is conducted in extinction, when there is no opportunity to learn a new relationship between a response and the less pleasant outcome (Adams and Dickinson 1981, Colwill and Rescorla 1985). A surprising point is that although after the LiCl conditioning the rats reject the taste of the conditioned food, they may nevertheless initially perform the instrumental response for the food, until they have had the opportunity to re-experience the food by consuming it (Balleine and Dickinson 1991). Thus the incentive value that controls instrumental performance can be dissociated in a short initial period from the hedonic value that can influence rejection or acceptance of a taste. When the rat re-experiences the food and its new hedonic impact, the instrumental incentive value is updated by a process referred to as *incentive learning* (Balleine and Dickinson 1991, Dickinson and Balleine 1994). A similar phenomenon has been demonstrated for the control of behaviour by motivational state. For example, if a hungry rat is trained to respond for food, and then satiated before being tested in extinction (i.e. with no food available), it will perform the instrumental response as much as a hungry rat, until it experiences the reduced value of the food when satiated (Balleine 1992). One factor that may lead to this paradoxical behaviour is that if a rat has been highly trained in an instrumental learning task, then that behaviour becomes a stimulus–response habit that is not under normal control by goal availability and even normal stimuli (see below). For example, a rat well trained in a T maze runway task to turn left at the end to obtain food will turn left and bump into the wall if the length of the runway is increased.

Hedonic assessment. Hedonic assessment may be measured directly by questions such as 'How pleasant does the food taste?' (see Section 5.3.1). In monkeys, one can show the monkey a food, and obtain clear evidence on a defined rating scale of how rewarding the food is to the monkey (Burton, Rolls and Mora 1976, Rolls, Judge and Sanghera 1977, Rolls, Sienkiewicz and Yaxley 1989b), by measuring whether he will reach for the food to place it in his mouth (+2), whether he will not reach but will open the mouth readily to accept the food (+1), whether he will swallow the food if it is placed in the mouth (0, neutral), whether he will close his mouth to prevent the food being placed in his mouth (–1), or whether he will use his hand to push away the food to prevent it approaching the mouth (–2). These appear to correspond approximately to the human subjective ratings of very pleasant (+2), pleasant (+1), neutral (0), unpleasant (–1), and very unpleasant (–2) (Rolls, Rolls, Rowe and Sweeney 1981a).

In rodents, it is apparently more difficult to measure hedonic responses to food (Cardinal, Parkinson, Hall and Everitt 2002). The suggestion that orofacial responses such as gaping to a bitter taste placed in the mouth measure hedonics (Cardinal et al. 2002, Garcia 1989) does not appear to be relevant to primates including humans, in that we know from the effects of decerebration that these responses can be reflexes organized in the brain stem (Grill and Norgren 1978) (with consistent evidence from anencephalic humans (Steiner, Glaser, Hawilo and Berridge 2001)). Further, in primates including humans it is found that flavour processing proceeds as far as the primary taste and olfactory cortex without any modulation by hunger, so that hedonics cannot be represented before these primary cortical areas in primates including humans (Rolls, Scott, Sienkiewicz and Yaxley 1988, Yaxley, Rolls and Sienkiewicz 1988, Kringelbach, O'Doherty, Rolls and Andrews 2003, De Araujo, Kringelbach, Rolls and McGlone 2003b, De Araujo, Rolls, Kringelbach, McGlone and Phillips

2003c). In addition, in the secondary but not primary olfactory cortex in humans activations in fMRI experiments are correlated with the pleasantness of the smell, whereas in the primary olfactory cortex activations are correlated with the intensity of the odour (Rolls, Kringelbach and De Araujo 2003c) (see Section 4.5.5.2 and Chapter 5).

Discriminative stimuli. When instrumental responding is rewarded in the presence of a stimulus but not in its absence, that stimulus is established as a discriminative stimulus S^D. For example, in a visual discrimination task, the visual stimulus (e.g. a triangle) that is shown to indicate that a lick response will be rewarded with fruit juice is an S^D. The visual stimulus that indicates that if a response is made it will be punished with salt taste is an S^Δ. This is a Go/NoGo visual discrimination task which we have frequently used to study brain mechanisms involved in processing reward-related visual and olfactory stimuli (Rolls, Judge and Sanghera 1977, Rolls, Sanghera and Roper-Hall 1979a, Thorpe, Rolls and Maddison 1983, Critchley and Rolls 1996b, Rolls, Critchley, Mason and Wakeman 1996b). Although an S^D can serve as a Pavlovian CS (Colwill and Rescorla 1988), S^Ds have effects that can not be explained in this manner (Holman and Mackintosh 1981): there is a conditional relationship in which an S^D signals the operation of a particular response-reinforcer (instrumental, action–outcome) contingency (Colwill and Rescorla 1990, Rescorla 1990b, Rescorla 1990a).

Stimulus–Response habits. Overtraining in an instrumental task results in instrumental behaviour that becomes performed as a fixed inflexible habit. Under these circumstances, behaviour is under automatic response control, and not under direct control of the goal, in that if the reinforcer is devalued (by for example pairing with LiCl or by satiation), instrumental behaviour may continue for a few trials until the animal obtains the reinforcer, and then the instrumental behaviour stops (Adams 1982, Dickinson 1994, Dickinson 1985, Dickinson, Balleine, Watt, Gonzalez and Boakes 1995, Dickinson, Nicholas and Adams 1983). The interest here is that early on in training the learning and the behaviour are directly guided by the hedonic or reward value of the reinforcer or goal, and if the reinforcer is devalued, the behaviour stops. These processes are implemented in brain regions such as the amygdala and orbitofrontal cortex, as described in this Chapter (see also for reinforcer devaluation studies in primates (Malkova, Gaffan and Murray 1997, Baxter and Murray 2000, Baylis and Gaffan 1991)). During this training period, the conditions are in fact set up for habit, stimulus–response, learned associations, perhaps implemented in the basal ganglia (see Section 8.4), to be learned. Once the stimulus comes automatically and rapidly to produce the response, then behaviour is not being performed in a so literally goal-directed manner.

Pavlovian–instrumental transfer (PIT). If a stimulus that predicts the arrival of sucrose as a result of Pavlovian conditioning is provided during an instrumental task such as working to obtain sucrose, the responding (e.g. lever pressing) can be enhanced (Lovibond 1983, Estes 1948, Dickinson 1994, Dickinson and Balleine 1994). There is an outcome- or response-specific form in which only instrumental performance for sucrose reward is facilitated, and a non-specific form in which performance for other rewards such as food pellets is enhanced (Balleine 1994, Dickinson and Dawson 1987a, Dickinson and Dawson 1987b, Colwill and Rescorla 1988). The effect is sometimes termed conditioned motivation (Rescorla and Solomon 1967), and is an example of the *incentive motivation* effect described by Donald Hebb (Hebb 1949), in which giving a few free salted nuts in a market place will increase the probability that humans will buy some peanuts (the 'salted nut effect'). A similar phenomenon is the release of the pleasant smell of bread cooking near bakeries, which increases motivation to buy bread.

Pavlovian–instrumental transfer is optimal when motivation for the US (e.g. hunger making the taste of bread pleasant) is present, and thus it is argued that the 'Pavlovian value' depends directly on the motivational state in a way in which instrumental incentive value does not (at least when assessed after overtraining using devaluation procedures). It is thus suggested that the Pavlovian CS accesses the US (Cardinal et al. 2002, Dickinson and Dawson 1987a, Dickinson and Dawson 1987b, Dickinson 1986) (in our example, the taste of food), which is a motivation-dependent representation. Pavlovian–instrumental transfer may be involved in cue-induced relapse in drug addiction (Gawin 1991, Tiffany and Drobes 1990, O'Brien, Childress, Ehrman and Robbins 1998).

Summary of instrumental learning. This survey shows that multiple processes, which it turns out may have somewhat different brain implementations as described below, are involved in instrumental learning. One key process is action–outcome learning. The outcome is represented as reward or affective value, such as I suggest is implemented by the firing of orbitofrontal cortex neurons that respond to the taste of food only if hunger is present. The orbitofrontal cortex appears to be involved in the representation of the reward, and in the processes that learn which stimuli are associated with rewards, but not with forming associations between behavioural responses (actions) and rewards (outcomes), in that orbitofrontal cortex neurons in primates do not respond to motor responses or actions.

Other processes influence instrumental learning including Pavlovian processes that can facilitate performance (as in Pavlovian-instrumental transfer, PIT). Further, approach to a food may be under Pavlovian rather than instrumental control. Finally, we must beware of the facts that after overtraining, responses may become inflexibly linked to stimuli, and that the goals, and the reward value of the goals, may no longer be directly influencing behaviour in an ongoing way.

4.6.2 Connections of the amygdala

The amygdala is a subcortical region in the anterior part of the temporal lobe. It receives massive projections in the primate from the overlying temporal lobe cortex (see Amaral, Price, Pitkanen and Carmichael (1992); Van Hoesen (1981)) (see Fig. 4.51). These come in the monkey to overlapping but partly separate regions of the lateral and basal amygdala from the inferior temporal visual cortex, the superior temporal auditory cortex, the cortex of the temporal pole, and the cortex in the superior temporal sulcus. These inputs thus come from the higher stages of sensory processing in the visual and auditory modalities, and not from early cortical processing areas. Via these inputs, the amygdala receives inputs about objects that could become secondary reinforcers, as a result of pattern association in the amygdala with primary reinforcers. The amygdala also receives inputs that are potentially about primary reinforcers, e.g. taste inputs (from the secondary taste cortex, via connections from the orbitofrontal cortex to the amygdala), and somatosensory inputs, potentially about the rewarding or painful aspects of touch (from the somatosensory cortex via the insula) (Mesulam and Mufson 1982a, Mesulam and Mufson 1982b, Friedman, Murray, O'Neill and Mishkin 1986). The amygdala also receives projections from the posterior orbitofrontal cortex (Carmichael and Price 1995a) (see Fig. 4.51, areas 12 and 13).

Subcortical inputs to the amygdala include projections from the midline thalamic nuclei,

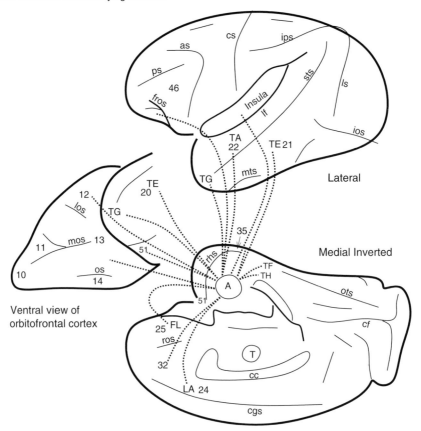

Fig. 4.51 Connections of the amygdala shown on lateral, ventral, and medial inverted views of the monkey brain (after Van Hoesen 1981). Abbreviations: as, arcuate sulcus; cc, corpus callosum; cf, calcarine fissure; cgs, cingulate sulcus; cs, central sulcus; ls, lunate sulcus; ios, inferior occipital sulcus; mos, medial orbital sulcus; os, orbital sulcus; ots, occipito-temporal sulcus; ps, principal sulcus; rhs, rhinal sulcus; sts, superior temporal sulcus; lf, lateral (or Sylvian) fissure (which has been opened to reveal the insula); A, amygdala; INS, insula; T, thalamus; TE (21), inferior temporal visual cortex; TA (22), superior temporal auditory association cortex; TF and TH, parahippocampal cortex; TG, temporal pole cortex; 12, 13, 11, orbitofrontal cortex; 24, part of the cingulate cortex; 35, perirhinal cortex; 51, olfactory (prepyriform and periamygdaloid) cortex. The cortical connections shown provide afferents to the amygdala, but are reciprocated.

the subiculum, and CA1 parts of the hippocampal formation, the hypothalamus and substantia innominata, the nucleus of the solitary tract (which receives gustatory and visceral inputs), and from olfactory structures (Amaral et al. 1992, Pitkanen 2000). Although there are some inputs from early on in some sensory pathways, for example auditory inputs from the medial geniculate nucleus (LeDoux 1987, LeDoux 1992), this route is unlikely to be involved in most emotions, for which cortical analysis of the stimulus is likely to be required. Emotions are usually elicited to environmental stimuli analysed to the object level (including other organisms), and not to retinal arrays of spots or the frequency (tone) of a sound as represented in the cochlea. Consistent with this view (that neural systems involved in emotion in primates generally receive from sensory systems where analysis of the identity of the stimulus as an object is performed), neurons in the inferior temporal visual cortex do not have responses related to the association with reinforcement of visual stimuli (Rolls, Judge and Sanghera 1977); whereas such neurons are found in the amygdala and orbitofrontal cortex (see below; cf. Fig. 4.2). Similarly, processing in the taste system of primates up to and including the primary taste cortex reflects the identity of the tastant, whereas its hedonic value as influenced by hunger is reflected in the responses of neurons in the secondary taste cortex (Rolls 1989c, Rolls 1995a, Rolls and Scott 2003) (see Fig. 4.2).

The outputs of the amygdala (Amaral et al. 1992) include the well-known projections to the hypothalamus, from the lateral amygdala via the ventral amygdalofugal pathway to the lateral hypothalamus; and from the medial amygdala, which is relatively small in the primate, via the stria terminalis to the medial hypothalamus. The ventral amygdalofugal pathway includes some long descending fibres that project to the autonomic centres in the medulla oblongata, and provides a route for cortically processed signals to reach the brainstem. A further interesting output of the amygdala is to the ventral striatum (Heimer, Switzer and Van Hoesen 1982) including the nucleus accumbens, for via this route information processed in the amygdala could gain access to the basal ganglia and thus influence motor output. (The output of the amygdala also reaches more dorsal parts of the striatum such as the head of the caudate nucleus.) The amygdala also projects to the medial part of the mediodorsal nucleus of the thalamus, which projects to the orbitofrontal cortex, providing another output pathway for the amygdala. In addition, the amygdala has direct projections back to many areas of the temporal, orbitofrontal, and insular cortices from which it receives inputs (Amaral et al. 1992). It is suggested elsewhere (Rolls 1989c, Rolls 1989a, Treves and Rolls 1994, Rolls 1996b, Rolls and Treves 1998, Rolls 2000b) that the functions of these backprojections include the guidance of information representation and storage in the neocortex, and recall (when this is related to reinforcing stimuli). Another interesting set of output pathways of the amygdala are the projections to the entorhinal cortex, which provides the major input to the hippocampus and dentate gyrus, and to the ventral subiculum, which provides a major output of the hippocampus (Amaral et al. 1992). Via these pathways, reward influences may be introduced into the hippocampal memory system, and provide for associations to be formed between viewed places 'out there' and the rewards at those places (Rolls and Xiang 2005, Rolls and Kesner 2006) (see Section 4.10).

These anatomical connections of the amygdala indicate that it is strategically placed to receive highly processed information from the cortex and to influence motor systems, autonomic systems, some of the cortical areas from which it receives inputs, and other limbic areas. The functions mediated through these connections will now be considered, using information available from the effects of damage to the amygdala and from the activity of neurons in the amygdala.

4.6.3   Effects of amygdala lesions

Bilateral removal of the amygdala in monkeys produces striking behavioural changes which include tameness, a lack of emotional responsiveness, excessive examination of objects, often with the mouth, and eating of previously rejected items such as meat (Weiskrantz 1956). These behavioural changes comprise much of the Kluver-Bucy syndrome which is produced in monkeys by bilateral anterior temporal lobectomy (Kluver and Bucy 1939). In analyses of the bases of these behavioural changes, it has been observed that there are deficits in some types of learning. For example, Weiskrantz (1956) found that bilateral ablation of the amygdala in the monkey produced a deficit on learning an active avoidance task. The monkeys failed to learn to make a response when a light signalled that shock would follow unless the response was made. He was perhaps the first to suggest that these monkeys had difficulty with forming associations between stimuli and reinforcers, when he suggested that "the effect of amygdalectomy is to make it difficult for reinforcing stimuli, whether positive or negative, to become established or to be recognized as such" (Weiskrantz 1956). In this avoidance task, associations between a stimulus and punishers were impaired.

Evidence soon became available that associations between stimuli and positive reinforcers (reward) were also impaired in, for example, serial reversals of a visual discrimination made to obtain food (Jones and Mishkin 1972, Spiegler and Mishkin 1981). In this task the monkey must learn that food is under one of two objects, and after he has learned this, he must then relearn (reverse) the association as the food is then placed under the other object. Jones and Mishkin (1972) showed that the stages of this task that are particularly affected by damage to this region are those when the monkeys are responding at chance to the two visual stimuli or are starting to respond more to the currently rewarded stimuli, rather than the stage when the monkeys are continuing to make perseverative responses to the previously rewarded visual stimulus. They thus argued that the difficulty produced by this anterior temporal lobe damage is in learning to associate stimuli with reinforcers, in this case with food reward.

There is evidence from lesion studies in monkeys that the amygdala is involved in learning associations between visual stimuli and rewards (Gaffan 1992, Gaffan and Harrison 1987, Gaffan, Gaffan and Harrison 1988, Gaffan, Gaffan and Harrison 1989, Baylis and Gaffan 1991). However, lesion studies are subject to the criticism that the effects of a lesion could be due to inadvertent damage to other brain structures or pathways close to the intended lesion site. For this reason, many of the older lesion studies are being repeated and extended with lesions in which instead of an ablation (removal) or electrolytic lesion (which can damage axons passing through a brain region), a neurotoxin is used to damage cells in a localized region, but to leave intact fibres of passage.

Using such lesions (made with ibotenic acid) in monkeys, Malkova et al. (1997) showed that amygdala lesions did not impair visual discrimination learning when the reinforcer was an auditory secondary reinforcer learned as being positively reinforcing preoperatively. This was in contrast to an earlier study by Gaffan and Harrison (1987) (see also Gaffan (1992)). In the study by Malkova et al. (1997) the animals with amygdala lesions were somewhat slower to learn a visual discrimination task for food reward, and made more errors, but with the small numbers of animals (the numbers in the groups were 3 and 4), the difference did not reach statistical significance. It would be interesting to test such animals when the association was directly between a visual stimulus and a primary reinforcer such as taste. (In most such studies, the reward being given is usually solid food, which is seen before it is tasted, and for which the food delivery mechanism makes a noise. These factors mean that the reward for which the animal is working includes secondary reinforcing components, the sight and sound). However, in the study by Malkova et al. (1997) it was shown that amygdala lesions made with ibotenic acid did impair the processing of reward-related stimuli, in that when the reward value of one set of foods was devalued by feeding it to satiety (i.e. sensory-specific satiety, a reward devaluation procedure, see also Section 4.6.1.2), the monkeys still chose the visual stimuli associated with the foods with which they had been satiated (Malkova et al. 1997, Baxter and Murray 2000). Further evidence that neurotoxic lesions of the amygdala in primates affect behaviour to stimuli learned as being reward-related as well as punishment-related is that monkeys with neurotoxic lesions of the amygdala showed abnormal patterns of food choice, picking up and eating foods not normally eaten such as meat, and picking up and placing in their mouths inedible objects (Murray, Gaffan and Flint 1996, Baxter and Murray 2000, Baxter and Murray 2002). These symptoms produced by selective amygdala lesions are classical Kluver-Bucy symptoms. Thus in primates, there is evidence that selective amygdala lesions impair some types of behaviour to learned reward-related stimuli as well as to learned punisher-related stimuli. However, we should not conclude that this is the only brain structure involved in this type of learning, for especially when rapid stimulus–reinforcer association learning is performed in primates, the orbitofrontal cortex is involved, as shown in Section 4.5. Further, studies in macaques with neurotoxic (ibotenic acid) lesions of the amygdala reveal relatively mild deficits in social behaviour (Amaral 2003, Amaral, Bauman, Capitanio, Lavenex, Mason, Mauldin-Jourdain and Mendoza 2003, Bauman, Lavenex, Mason, Capitanio and Amaral 2004), and this is consistent with the trend for the orbitofrontal cortex to become relatively more important in emotion and social behaviour in primates including humans. This is shown for example by the findings that damage to the human orbitofrontal cortex does produce large changes in social and emotional behaviour (see Section 4.5.6).

Another type of evidence linking the amygdala to reinforcement mechanisms is that monkeys will work in order to obtain electrical stimulation of the amygdala, and that single neurons in the amygdala are activated by brain-stimulation reward of a number of different sites (Rolls 1975, Rolls, Burton and Mora 1980c).

The symptoms of the Kluver-Bucy syndrome, including the emotional changes, could be a result of this type of deficit in learning stimulus–reinforcer associations (Jones and Mishkin 1972, Mishkin and Aggleton 1981, Rolls 1986c, Rolls 1986a, Rolls 1990d, Rolls 1992b, Rolls 2000d). For example, the tameness, the hypoemotionality, the increased orality, and the altered responses to food would arise because of damage to the normal mechanism by which stimuli become associated with a reward or punisher. Other evidence is also consistent with the hypothesis that there is a close relationship between the learning deficit and the emotion-related and other symptoms of the Kluver-Bucy syndrome. For example, in a study of subtotal lesions of the amygdala, Aggleton and Passingham (1981) found that in only those monkeys in which the lesions produced a serial reversal learning deficit was hypoemotionality present.

In rats, there is also evidence that the amygdala is involved in behaviour to stimuli learned as being associated with reward as well as with punishers. In studies to investigate the role of the amygdala in reward-related learning in the rat, Cador, Robbins and Everitt (1989) obtained evidence consistent with the hypothesis that the learned incentive (conditioned reinforcing) effects of previously neutral stimuli paired with rewards are mediated by the amygdala acting through the ventral striatum, in that amphetamine injections into the ventral striatum enhanced the effects of a conditioned reinforcing stimulus only if the amygdala was intact (see further Everitt and Robbins (1992); Robbins, Cador, Taylor and Everitt (1989); Everitt, Cardinal, Hall, Parkinson and Robbins (2000)). In another study, Everitt, Cador and Robbins (1989) showed that excitotoxic lesions of the basolateral amygdala disrupted appetitive sexual responses maintained by a visual conditioned reinforcer, but not the behaviour to the primary reinforcer for the male rats, copulation with a female rat in heat (see further Everitt and Robbins (1992)). (The details of the study were that the learned reinforcer or conditioned stimulus was a light for which the male rats worked on a Fixed Ratio 10 schedule (i.e. 10 responses made to obtain a presentation of the light), with access to the female being allowed for the first FR10 completed after a fixed period of 15 min. This is a second order schedule of reinforcement. For comparison, and this is relevant to Chapter 9, medial preoptic area lesions eliminated the copulatory behaviour of mounting, intromission and ejaculation to the primary reinforcer, the female rat, but did not affect the learned appetitive responding for the conditioned or secondary reinforcing stimulus, the light.) In another study demonstrating the role of the amygdala in responses to learned positive reinforcers in rats, Everitt, Morris, O'Brien and Robbins (1991) showed that a conditioned place preference to a place where rats were given 10% sucrose was abolished by bilateral excitotoxic lesions of the basolateral amygdala. Moreover, the output of the amygdala for this learned reinforcement effect on behaviour appears to be via the ventral striatum, for a unilateral lesion of the amygdala and a contralateral lesion of the nucleus accumbens also impaired the conditioned place preference for the place where sucrose was made available (Everitt et al. 1991, Everitt and Robbins 1992). In another study showing the importance of the basolateral amygdala for effects of learned rewards on behaviour, Whitelaw, Markou, Robbins and Everitt (1996) showed that excitotoxic lesions of the basolateral amygdala in rats impaired behavioural responses to a light associated with intravenous administration of cocaine, but not to the primary reinforcer of the cocaine itself. (A second order schedule comparable to that described above was used to show the impairment of drug-seeking behaviour, that is responses made to obtain the light associated with delivery of the drug. Self-administration of the drug in a continuous reinforcement schedule was not impaired, showing that the amygdala is not necessary for the primary reinforcing effects of cocaine.)

It has long been known that rats with lesions of the amygdala display altered fear responses. For example, Rolls and Rolls (1973b) showed that rats with amygdala lesions showed less neophobia to new foods. In a model of fear conditioning in the rat, LeDoux and colleagues (see LeDoux (1994), LeDoux (1995), LeDoux (1996); Quirk, Armony, Repa, Li and LeDoux (1996); LeDoux (2000); and Pare, Quirk and LeDoux (2004)) have shown that lesions of the amygdala attenuate fear responses learned when pure tones are associated with footshock. The learned responses include typical classically conditioned responses such as heart-rate changes and freezing to fear-inducing stimuli (see, e.g., LeDoux (1994)), and also operant responses (see, e.g., Gallagher and Holland (1994)). The deficits typically involve particularly the learned (emotional) responses, e.g. fear to the conditioned stimuli, rather than changes in behavioural responses to the unconditioned stimuli such as altered responses to pain per se (but see Hebert, Ardid, Henrie, Tamashiro, Blanchard and Blanchard (1999)). In another type of paradigm, it has been shown that amygdala lesions impair the devaluing effect of pairing a food reward with (aversive) lithium chloride, in that amygdala lesions reduced the classically conditioned responses of the rats to a light previously paired with the food (Hatfield, Han, Conley, Gallagher and Holland 1996).

In a different model of fear-conditioning in the rat, Davis and colleagues (Davis 1992, Davis 1994, Davis, Campeau, Kim and Falls 1995, Davis 2000), have used the fear-potentiated startle test, in which the amplitude of the acoustic startle reflex is increased when elicited in the presence of a stimulus previously paired with shock. The conditioned stimulus can be visual or a low-frequency auditory stimulus. Chemical or electrolytic lesions of either the central nucleus or the lateral and basolateral nuclei of the amygdala block the expression of fear-potentiated startle. These latter amygdala nuclei may be the site of plasticity for fear conditioning, because local infusion of the NMDA (N-methyl-d-aspartate) receptor antagonist AP5 (which blocks long-term potentiation, an index of synaptic plasticity) blocks the

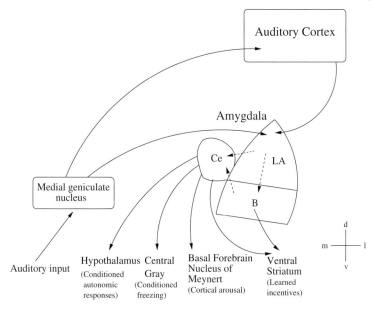

Fig. 4.52 The pathways for fear-conditioning to pure-tone auditory stimuli associated with footshock in the rat (after Quirk, Armony, Repa, Li and LeDoux 1996). The lateral amygdala (LA) receives auditory information directly from the medial part of the medial geniculate nucleus (the auditory thalamic nucleus), and from the auditory cortex. Intra-amygdala projections (directly and via the basal and basal accessory nuclei, B) end in the central nucleus (Ce) of the amygdala. Different output pathways from the central nucleus and the basal nucleus mediate different conditioned fear-related effects. d, dorsal; v, ventral; m, medial; l, lateral.

acquisition but not the maintenance of fear-potentiated startle (Davis 1992, Davis 1994, Davis et al. 1995, Davis 2000).

There are separate output pathways for the amygdala for different fear-related responses (see Fig. 4.52). Lesions of the lateral hypothalamus (which receives from the central nucleus of the amygdala) blocked conditioned heart rate (autonomic) responses. Lesions of the central gray of the midbrain (which also receives from the central nucleus of the amygdala) blocked the conditioned freezing but not the conditioned autonomic response (LeDoux, Iwata, Cicchetti and Reis 1988), and lesions of the stria terminalis blocked the neuroendocrine responses (Gray, Piechowski, Yracheta, Rittenhouse, Betha and Van der Kar 1993). In addition, cortical arousal may be produced by the conditioned stimuli via the central nucleus of the amygdala outputs to the cholinergic basal forebrain magnocellular nuclei of Meynert (see Section 4.9.5; Kapp, Whalen, Supple and Pascoe (1992); Wilson and Rolls (1990c), Wilson and Rolls (1990b), Wilson and Rolls (1990a); and Rolls and Treves (1998) Section 7.1.5).

The different output routes for different effects mediated by the amygdala are complemented by separate roles of different nuclei within the amygdala in conditioned fear responses (see Cardinal et al. (2002)). In a study by Killcross, Robbins and Everitt (1997), rats with lesions of the central nucleus exhibited a reduction in the suppression of behaviour (i.e. a reduction in freezing) elicited by a conditioned fear stimulus, but were simultaneously able to direct their actions to avoid further presentations of this aversive stimulus. In contrast, animals with lesions of the basolateral amygdala were unable to avoid the conditioned aversive stimulus by their choice behaviour, but exhibited normal conditioned suppression to this stimulus. This double dissociation indicates separable contributions of different amygdaloid nuclei to different types of conditioned fear behaviour, with the central nuclei especially involved in Pavlovian processes such as conditioned suppression of behaviour, and the basolateral amygdala more involved in instrumental, action–outcome, learning (Cardinal et al. 2002).

Different nuclei of the amygdala correspondingly have different functions in reward-related (or appetitive) learning in rats (Cardinal et al. 2002, Everitt, Cardinal, Parkinson and Robbins 2003, Holland and Gallagher 2003, Holland and Gallagher 2004, Everitt et al. 2000, Gallagher 2000). For example, the basolateral amygdala (BLA) nuclei are involved in some motivational aspects of the classically or Pavlovian conditioned effects of rewards (also known as appetitive reinforcers), in that BLA lesions impair the ability of conditioned stimuli (such as a tone) paired with food in associative learning to influence instrumental behaviour (such as bar pressing to earn food) (Holland and Gallagher 2003), perhaps reflecting impaired outputs to feeding systems in the lateral hypothalamus (see Fig. 4.52). (The BLA lesions also impair the learning of second-order associative conditioning, in that the lesioned rats cannot learn an association of an auditory stimulus with a previously conditioned visual stimulus (Setlow, Gallagher and Holland 2002)). In monkeys (Malkova et al. 1997) as well as rats (Cardinal et al. 2002), BLA lesions also impair reinforcer devaluation effects on actions. *The implication is that BLA lesioned animals cannot use a CS to gain access to the current value of its specific US, and in turn use this US representation as a goal for instrumental action, for freezing, or for fear-potentiated startle.* In this sense, BLA lesions may impair the elicitation of learned affective states used to influence these three types of behaviour. The fact that amygdala lesions do not affect food preferences per se (Rolls and Rolls 1973b, Murray et al. 1996) suggests that affective states elicited by primary reinforcers are not impaired. In contrast, lesions of the central nucleus of the amygdala impaired the ability of conditioned stimuli (such as a tone) paired with food in associative learning to influence food consumption (Holland and Gallagher 2003), which could reflect a reduction in Pavlovian conditioned arousal produced by output pathways from the central nuclei (see Fig. 4.52 and also Everitt, Cardinal, Parkinson and Robbins (2003)).

We may summarize these investigations performed primarily in the rat by stating that the central nuclei of the amygdala encode or express Pavlovian S–R (stimulus–response, CS–UR) associations (including conditioned suppression, conditioned orienting, conditioned autonomic and endocrine responses, and Pavlovian–instrumental transfer); and modulate perhaps by arousal the associability of representations stored elsewhere in the brain (Gallagher and Holland 1994, Gallagher and Holland 1992, Holland and Gallagher 1999). In contrast, the basolateral amygdala (BLA) encodes or retrieves the affective value of the predicted US, and can use this to influence action–outcome learning via pathways to brain regions such as the nucleus accumbens and prefrontal cortex including the orbitofrontal cortex (Cardinal et al. 2002). We shall see below that the nucleus accumbens is not involved in action–outcome learning itself, but does allow the affective states retrieved by the BLA to conditioned stimuli to influence instrumental behaviour by for example Pavlovian–instrumental transfer, and facilitating locomotor approach to food which appears to be in rats a Pavlovian process (Cardinal et al. 2002, Cardinal and Everitt 2004). This leaves parts of the prefrontal and cingulate cortices as strong candidates for action–outcome learning.

This may be an appropriate place to consider the issue of 'wanting' vs 'liking' discussed by Berridge and Robinson (1998). 'Wanting' or conditioned 'incentive salience' effects are used to describe classically conditioned approach behaviours to rewards (Berridge and Robinson 1998, Berridge and Robinson 2003), and this learning is implemented via the amygdala and ventral striatum, is under control of dopamine (Cardinal et al. 2002), and contributes to addiction (Robinson and Berridge 2003). Conditioned 'incentive salience' effects can influence instrumental responses, made for example to obtain food. Berridge and Robinson (1998) suggest that 'liking' can be measured by orofacial reflexes such as ingesting sweet solutions or rejecting bitter solutions. There is evidence that brain opioid systems are involved in influencing the palatability of and hedonic reactions to foods, in that humans report a reduction in the pleasantness of sucrose solution following administration of naltrexone which blocks opiate receptors, but can still discriminate between sucrose solutions (Bertino, Beauchamp and Engelman 1991, Levine and Billington 2004) (see further Section 8.5). One problem here is that orofacial reflexes may reflect brainstem mechanisms that are not at all closely related to the reward value of food as reflected in instrumental actions performed to obtain food. Some of the evidence for this is that these responses occur after decerebration, in which the brainstem is all that remains to control behaviour (Grill and Norgren 1978) (with consistent evidence from anencephalic humans, Steiner et al. (2001)) (see further Section 4.6.1.2 on page 153). A second point is that normally the rated reward value or pleasantness given in humans to food is closely related to instrumental actions performed to obtain food, as shown by the close relation between pleasantness ratings ('liking') by humans given to a food in a sensory-specific satiety experiment, and whether that food is subsequently eaten in a meal ('wanting') (Rolls, Rowe, Rolls, Kingston, Megson and Gunary 1981b). Third, a confusion may arise when a stimulus–response habit is formed by overlearning, and persists even when the reward is devalued by for example feeding to satiety. This persistence of stimulus–response habits after reward devaluation should not necessarily be interpreted as 'wanting' when not 'liking', for it may just reflect the operation of a stimulus–response habit system that produces responses after overlearning without any guidance from reward, pleasantness, and liking (see further Section 10.3 and Cardinal et al. (2002)). I believe that normally liking, defined by pleasantness ratings of stimuli, is very closely related to wanting, that is being willing to perform behaviours (instrumental actions) to obtain a reward of the pleasant stimulus. Thus motivational behaviour is normally controlled by reward stimuli or goals (unless the behaviour is overlearned, see Section 4.6.1.2), and motivational state (e.g. hunger) modulates the reward value of unconditioned and conditioned stimuli such as the taste and sight of food, as described in Chapter 5. Thus normally, liking a goal object and wanting it are different aspects of how reward systems control instrumental behaviour. Nevertheless, it is possible to dissociate the brain mechanisms involved in 'wanting' and 'liking' experimentally, with the classically conditioned 'incentive salience' stimuli that influence approach and instrumental actions and which influence 'appetitive' behaviour implemented in part separately from the reward systems that are activated by a primary reinforcer such as the taste of food during 'consummatory' behaviour. In a sense, the 'incentive salience' effects require learning to predict primary rewards and punishers, and then to influence behaviours, and thus require additional brain mechanisms to those involved in representing primary rewards and punishers.

One output system of the amygdala is the nucleus accumbens, a part of the striatum (see Section 8.4). The core part of the nucleus accumbens is part of the pathway for approach responses to conditioned stimuli ('autoshaping'), and for Pavlovian–instrumental transfer, but not for the learning of new goal-directed instrumental actions (action–outcome learning) (Cardinal et al. 2002, Cardinal and Everitt 2004). Consistently, dopamine release in the core part of the nucleus accumbens is increased by conditioned emotional stimuli, both appetitive and aversive (Cardinal et al. 2002), and this part of the accumbens may be involved in preparatory aspects of rewarded behaviour, including behaviour when there is a reward delay period (Cardinal, Pennicott, Sugathapala, Robbins and Everitt 2001). In contrast, the release of dopamine in the shell part of the nucleus accumbens is produced by primary (i.e. unconditioned) rewards and punishers such as food, and this part of the accumbens may be involved in consummatory behaviour such as eating (Kelley 1999, Cardinal et al. 2002) (see further Section 8.4). Psychostimulant drugs such as amphetamine may operate in part by sensitizing the process by which non-contingent Pavlovian conditioned stimuli increase the probability of instrumental behaviour and Pavlovian conditioned approach to rewards (Cardinal et al. 2002), an effect related to 'conditioned salience' or 'wanting' (Berridge and Robinson 1998, Robinson and Berridge 1993).

In summary, there is thus much evidence from the effects of lesions that the amygdala is involved in responses made to stimuli that are associated by learning with primary reinforcers, including rewards as well as punishers. The evidence is consistent with the hypothesis that the amygdala is a brain region for stimulus–reinforcer association learning, and has partly dissociable systems for Pavlovian effects implemented via the central nucleus, and for effects of affective representations implemented via the basolateral amygdala. There is also evidence that it may be involved in whether novel stimuli are approached, for monkeys with amygdala lesions place novel foods and non-food objects in their mouths, and rats with amygdala lesions have decreased neophobia, in that they more quickly accept new foods (Rolls and Rolls 1973b) (see also Dunn and Everitt (1988); Rolls (1992b); Rolls (2000d); Wilson and Rolls (1993)).

4.6.4 Neuronal activity in the primate amygdala to reinforcing stimuli

There is now clear evidence that some neurons in the primate amygdala respond to stimuli that are potentially primary reinforcers. For example, Sanghera, Rolls and Roper-Hall (1979) found some amygdala neurons with taste responses, and these were investigated by Scott, Karadi, Oomura, Nishino, Plata-Salaman, Lenard, Giza and Aou (1993). In an extensive study of 1416 macaque amygdala neurons, Kadohisa, Rolls and Verhagen (2005b) showed that a very rich and detailed representation of the stimulus (such as food) that is in the mouth is provided by neurons that respond to oral stimuli. An example of a macaque single amygdala orally-responsive neuron is shown in Fig. 4.53. The neuron had different responses to different tastes, different temperatures of what was in the mouth, and different viscosities, but had no response to the texture of fatty oils. Other amygdala neurons were selective for even one modality, responding for example only to the oral texture of fat (Kadohisa, Rolls and Verhagen 2005b). 3.1% of the recorded amygdala neurons responded to oral stimuli. Of the orally responsive neurons, some (39%) represent the viscosity of oral stimuli, tested using carboxymethyl-cellulose in the range 1–10,000 centiPoise. Other neurons (5%) responded to fat in the mouth by encoding its texture (shown by the responses of these neurons to a range of fats, and also to non-fat oils such as silicone oil ($Si(CH_3)_2O)_n$) and mineral oil (pure hydrocarbon), but no or small responses to the cellulose viscosity series or to the fatty acids linoleic acid and lauric acid). Some neurons (7%) responded to gritty texture (produced by microspheres suspended in carboxymethyl cellulose). Some neurons (41%) responded to the temperature of the liquid in the mouth. Some amygdala neurons responded to capsaicin, and some to fatty acids (but not to fats in the mouth). Some amygdala neurons respond to taste, texture and temperature unimodally, but others combine these inputs. 66% (29/44) had taste

bo217

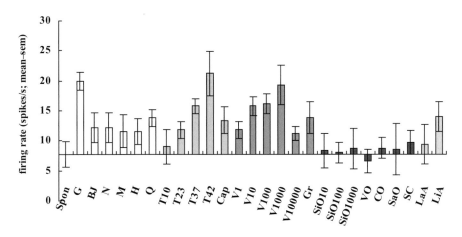

Fig. 4.53 The responses of an amygdala neuron (bo217) with differential responses to taste, temperature and viscosity. The neuron did not respond to fat texture. The mean ($\pm$ the standard error of the mean, sem) firing rate responses to each stimulus calculated in a 1 s period over 4–6 trials are shown. The spontaneous (Spon) firing rate is shown. G, N, M, H and Q are the taste stimuli. T10–T42 are the temperature stimuli. V1 - V10,000 are the CMC viscosity series with the viscosity in cP. The fat texture stimuli were SiO10, SiO100, SiO1000 (silicone oil with the viscosity indicated), vegetable oil (VO), coconut oil (CO) and safflower oil (SaO). BJ is fruit juice; Cap is 10 μM capsaicin; LaA is 0.1 mM lauric acid; LiA is 0.1 mM linoleic acid; Gr is the gritty stimulus. After Kadohisa, Rolls and Verhagen, 2005b.

responses. An interesting difference is that in terms of best responses to different tastes, 57% of the orbitofrontal cortex taste neurons had their best responses to glucose, whereas 21% of the amygdala neurons had their best response to glucose (χ^2=12.5, df=5, P<0.03) (Kadohisa, Rolls and Verhagen 2005a). (More amygdala neurons had their best responses to sour (HCl) (18%) and monosodium glutamate (14%) (Kadohisa, Rolls and Verhagen 2005a)).

These results show that a very detailed representation of substances in the mouth, which are likely to be primary reinforcers, is present in the primate amygdala (Kadohisa, Rolls and Verhagen 2005b). Less is known about whether it is though the reinforcer value of the stimuli that is represented. It has previously been shown that satiety produces a rather modest (on average 58%) reduction in the responses of amygdala neurons to taste (Yan and Scott 1996, Rolls and Scott 2003), in comparison to the essentially complete reduction of responsiveness found in orbitofrontal cortex taste neurons (Rolls, Sienkiewicz and Yaxley 1989b). Further, the representation in the amygdala of these oral stimuli does not appear to be on any simple hedonic basis, in that no direction in the multidimensional taste space in Fig. 7 of Kadohisa, Rolls and Verhagen (2005b) reflected the measured preference of the monkeys for the stimuli, nor were the response profiles of the neurons to the set of stimuli closely related to the preferences of the macaques for the stimuli (Kadohisa, Rolls and Verhagen 2005b). The failure to find very strong effects of satiety on the responsiveness of amygdala taste neurons mirrors the earlier finding of Sanghera, Rolls and Roper-Hall (1979) of inconsistent effects of feeding to satiety on the responses of amygdala visual neurons responding to the sight of

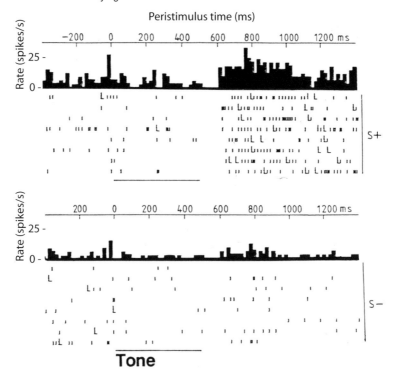

Fig. 4.54 Responses of a primate amygdala neuron in a visual discrimination task. Each tic represents the occurrence of an action potential; each row of tics represents the firing of the neuron on a single trial to the presentation of the S+ visual stimulus (which indicated that a lick could be made to obtain a taste of fruit juice) or of the S– visual stimulus (which indicated that a lick should not be made or (aversive) saline would be delivered. Presentations of the S+ and S- occurred in pseudorandom order but are grouped for clarity. The L indicates the occurrence of the lick response. Bin width = 10 ms. (After Rolls 2000d, and Wilson and Rolls 2005.)

food.

Recordings from single neurons in the amygdala of the monkey have shown that some neurons do respond to visual stimuli, consistent with the inputs from the temporal lobe visual cortex (Sanghera, Rolls and Roper-Hall 1979). Other neurons responded to auditory, gustatory, olfactory, or somatosensory stimuli, or in relation to movements. In tests of whether the neurons responded on the basis of the association of stimuli with reinforcers, it was found that approximately 20% of the neurons with visual responses had responses that occurred primarily to stimuli associated with reinforcers, for example to food and to a range of stimuli which the monkey had learned signified food in a visual discrimination task (Sanghera, Rolls and Roper-Hall 1979, Rolls 1981c, Wilson and Rolls 1993, Wilson and Rolls 2005, Rolls 2000d) (see example in Fig. 4.54). Many of these neurons responded more to the positive discriminative stimulus (S+) than to the negative visual discriminative stimulus (S–) in the Go/NoGo visual discrimination task, as shown in Fig. 4.55 (Rolls 2000d, Wilson and Rolls 2005). However, none of these neurons (in contrast with some neurons in the hypothalamus and orbitofrontal cortex) responded exclusively to rewarded stimuli, in that all responded at least partly to one

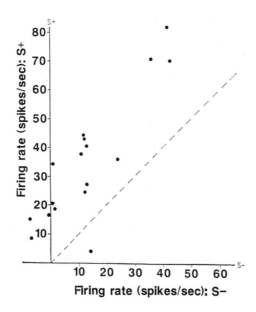

Fig. 4.55 Responses of amygdala neurons that responded more in a visual discrimination task to the reward-related visual stimulus (S+) than to the saline-related visual stimulus (S–). In the task, the macaque monkeys made lick responses to obtain fruit juice when the S+ was the discriminandum, and had to withhold lick responses when the S– was the discriminandum in order to avoid the taste of saline. Each point shows the responses of one neuron to the S+ and to the S– measured in a 0.5 s period starting 100 msec after the visual stimulus was shown. The responses are shown as the change from the spontaneous firing rate. Most of the points lie above the dashed line drawn at 45 degrees, showing that most of these neurons responded more to the S+ than to the S–. (After Rolls 2000d, and Wilson and Rolls 2005.)

or more neutral, novel, or aversive stimuli (see example in Fig. 4.57). Neurons with responses that are probably similar to these have also been described by Ono, Nishino, Sasaki, Fukuda and Muramoto (1980), and by Nishijo, Ono and Nishino (1988) (see Ono and Nishijo (1992)).

The degree to which the visual responses of these amygdala neurons are associated with reinforcers has been assessed in learning tasks. When the association between a visual stimulus and a reinforcer was altered by reversal (so that the visual stimulus formerly associated with juice reward became associated with aversive saline and vice versa), it was found that 10 of 11 neurons did not reverse their responses (and for the other neuron the evidence was not clear) (Sanghera, Rolls and Roper-Hall 1979, Rolls 1992b, Rolls 2000d). On the other hand, in a rather simpler relearning situation in which salt was added to a piece of food such as a water melon (but it was difficult to be sure that the monkey looked at the stimulus as much after it was salted), the responses of four amygdala neurons to the sight of the water melon diminished (Nishijo et al. 1988). To obtain further evidence on this issue, Wilson and Rolls (2005) tested visual discrimination reversal learning further using a similar procedure to that of Sanghera, Rolls and Roper-Hall (1979) in which two stimuli, one rewarded, and the other associated with punishment, were shown in random order and using an electronic shutter, so that it could be confirmed that the monkey performed a visual discrimination on every trial. The results

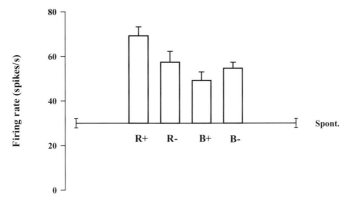

Fig. 4.56 The responses of a macaque amygdala neuron with more activity to a standard rewarded visual stimulus (S+) than to a standard punished visual stimulus (S–) in a Go/NoGo visual discrimination task. The neuron was then tested in a discrimination reversal task with a new pair of stimuli, which were Red and Blue. When the Red stimulus was associated with taste reward (R+), and the blue stimulus was associated with aversive saline if the monkey licked (B–), the neuron did not respond significantly differently to these two stimuli, even though the monkey performed the task correctly. Thus the neuron did not learn the discrimination with the new pair of stimuli. The contingencies were then reversed, and the monkey learned that the Red stimulus was now associated with saline (R–), and the Blue stimulus was associated with taste reward (B+). The neuron did not alter its activity after the reversal. The means and s.e.m. of the neuronal responses based on 4–8 trials for each condition are shown. The spontaneous firing rate of the neuron is also shown (Spont.) (After Wilson and Rolls 2005.)

are illustrated in Fig. 4.56, which shows that the neuron did not reverse its responses when the reinforcement contingency was reversed in the visual discrimination task. This experiment was repeated for two neurons, with identical results. Although more investigations would be useful, the evidence now available indicates that primate amygdala neurons do not alter their activity flexibly and rapidly in relearning visual discrimination reversal learning (see further Rolls (1992b) and Rolls (2000d)). What has been found in contrast is that neurons in the orbitofrontal cortex do show very rapid reversal of their responses in visual discrimination reversal, and it therefore seems likely that the orbitofrontal cortex is especially involved when repeated relearning and re-assessment of stimulus–reinforcer associations are required, as described above, rather than initial learning, in which the amygdala may be involved.

LeDoux and colleagues (see LeDoux (1995); LeDoux (1996); Quirk et al. (1996); LeDoux (2000); and Pare et al. (2004)) have made interesting contributions to understanding the role of the amygdala and related systems in fear-conditioning in the rat. They have shown that for some classes of stimulus, such as pure tones, the association between the tone and an aversive unconditioned stimulus (a footshock) is reflected in the responses of neurons in the amygdala. Some of the circuitry involved is shown in Fig. 4.52. The auditory inputs reach the amygdala both from the subcortical, thalamic, auditory nucleus, the medial geniculate (medial part), and from the auditory cortex. These auditory inputs project to the lateral nucleus of the amygdala (LA), which in turn projects to the central nucleus of the amygdala (Ce) both directly and via the basal (B) and accessory basal nuclei of the amygdala. LeDoux has emphasized the role of the subcortical inputs to the amygdala in this type of conditioning, based on the observations that the conditioning to pure tones can take place without the cortex, and that the shortest latencies of the auditory responses in the amygdala are too short to be mediated via the auditory cortex. (Although some conditioning of auditory responses has been found even in the medial geniculate to these pure tones, this conditioning is not of short latency, and LeDoux suggests that it reflects backprojections from the cortex (in which conditioning is also found) to the thalamus.)

The amygdala is well placed anatomically for learning associations between objects and primary reinforcers, for it receives inputs from the higher parts of the visual system, and from systems processing primary reinforcers such as taste, smell, and touch (see Fig. 4.2). The association learning in the amygdala may be implemented by Hebb-modifiable synapses from visual and auditory neurons on to neurons receiving inputs from taste, olfactory, or somatosensory primary reinforcers (see Figs. 4.3 and 4.5; Rolls (1986c); Rolls (1986a); Rolls (1990d); Rolls (1999a)). Consistent with this, Davis and colleagues (Davis 1992, Davis 1994, Davis et al. 1995, Davis 2000) have shown that the stimulus–reinforcer association learning involved in fear-potentiated startle (see Section 4.6.3) is blocked by local application to the lateral amygdala of the NMDA-receptor blocking agent AP5, which blocks long-term potentiation. The hypothesis (see Figs. 4.3 and 4.5, and Appendix 1) thus is that synaptic modification takes place between potential secondary reinforcers and primary reinforcers which project on to the same neurons in the amygdala. One index of synaptic modification is long-term potentiation (see Appendix 1), and consistent with this hypothesis, the potential evoked in the rat amygdala by a pure tone increased (suggesting long-term potentiation) after the tone was paired with footshock as the unconditioned stimulus (Rogan, Staubli and LeDoux 1997). Further, presentation of a tone paired with application of glutamate iontophoretically to activate a single amygdala neuron produced an increased response later to the tone alone, providing evidence that the site of the synaptic modification was on that neuron in the amygdala (Blair, Schafe, Bauer, Rodrigues and LeDoux 2001, LeDoux 2000, Blair, Tinkelman, Moita and LeDoux 2003).

LeDoux (LeDoux 1992, LeDoux 1995, LeDoux 1996) has described a theory of the neural basis of emotion which is conceptually similar to that of Rolls (Rolls 1975, Rolls 1986c, Rolls 1986a, Rolls 1990d, Rolls 1995b, Rolls 1999a, Rolls 2000f) (and this book), except that he focuses mostly on the role of the amygdala in emotion (and not on other brain regions such as the orbitofrontal cortex, which are poorly developed in the rat); except that he focuses mainly on fear (based on his studies of the role of the amygdala and related structures in fear conditioning in the rat); and except that he suggests from his neurophysiological findings that an important route for conditioned emotional stimuli to influence behaviour is via the subcortical inputs (especially auditory from the medial part of the medial geniculate nucleus of the thalamus) to the amygdala.

This latter issue, of the normal routes for sensory information about potential secondary reinforcers to reach the amygdala via subcortical pathways will now be addressed, because it raises important issues about the stimuli that normally cause emotion, and about brain design. For simple stimuli such as pure tones, there is evidence of subcortical inputs for the conditioned stimuli to the amygdala, and even of the conditioned stimulus–unconditioned stimulus association being learned prior to involvement of the amygdala (see LeDoux (1995); LeDoux (1996); Quirk et al. (1996)). However, as described above in Section 4.4.4 entitled 'Why reward and punishment associations of stimuli are not represented early in information processing in the primate brain', we humans and other animals do not generally want to learn that a particular pure tone is associated with reward or punishment. Instead, it might be a particular complex pattern of sounds such as a vocalization (or, for example, in vision, a face expression) that carries a reinforcement signal, and this may be independent of the exact pitch at which it is uttered. Thus cases in which some modulation of neuronal responses to pure tones in parts of the brain such as the medial geniculate (the thalamic relay for hearing) where tonotopic tuning is found (LeDoux 1994) may be rather special model systems (i.e. simplified systems on which to perform experiments), and not reflect the way in which auditory-to-reinforcer pattern associations are normally learned. (For discrimination of more complex sounds, such as frequency modulated tone sweeps, the auditory cortex is required.) The same is true for vision, in that we do not normally want to associate particular blobs of light at given positions on our retinae (which is what could be represented at the thalamic level in the lateral geniculate nucleus) with a primary reinforcer, but instead we may want to associate an invariant representation of an object, or of a person's face, or of a facial expression, with a primary reinforcer. Such analysis requires cortical processing, and it is in high-order temporal lobe cortical areas (which provide major afferents to the primate amygdala) that invariant representations of these types of stimulus are found (Rolls 1994a, Wallis and Rolls 1997, Rolls 2000a, Rolls and Deco 2002). Moreover, it is crucial that the representation is invariant (with respect to, for example, position on the retina, size, and, for identity, even viewing angle), so that if an association is learned to the object when in one position on the retina, it can generalize correctly to the same object in different positions on the retina, in different sizes, and even with different viewing angles. For this to occur, the invariant representation must be formed before the object–reinforcer association is learned, otherwise generalization to the same object seen on different occasions would not occur, and different inconsistent associations might even be learned to the same object when seen in slightly different positions on the retina, in slightly different sizes, etc. (see Rolls and Treves (1998); Rolls and Deco (2002)). Rolls and Treves (1998) and Rolls and Deco (2002) also show that it is not a simple property of neuronal networks that they generalize correctly across variations of position and size; special mechanisms, which happen to take a great deal of cortical visual processing, are required to perform such computations. Similar points may also be made for touch in so far as one considers associations between objects identified by somatosensory input, and primary reinforcers. An example might be selecting a food object by either hand from a whole collection of objects in the dark. These points make it unlikely that the subcortical route for conditioned stimuli to reach the amygdala, suggested by LeDoux (1992), LeDoux (1995) and LeDoux (1996), is generally relevant to the learning of emotional responses to stimuli.

4.6.5 Responses of these amygdala neurons to novel stimuli that are reinforcing

As described above, some of the amygdala neurons that responded to rewarding visual stimuli also responded to some other stimuli that were not associated with reward. Wilson and Rolls (2005) (see Rolls (2000d)) discovered a possible reason for this. They showed that these neurons with reward-related responses also responded to relatively novel visual stimuli. This was shown in a serial recognition memory task, in which it was found that these neurons responded the first and the second times that visual stimuli were shown in this task (see Fig. 4.57). On the two presentations of each stimulus used in this task, the stimuli were thus either novel or still relatively novel. When the monkeys are given such relatively novel stimuli outside the task, they will reach out for and explore the objects, and in this respect the novel stimuli are reinforcing. Repeated presentation of the stimuli results in habituation of the neuronal response and of behavioural approach, if the stimuli are not associated with a primary reinforcer. It is

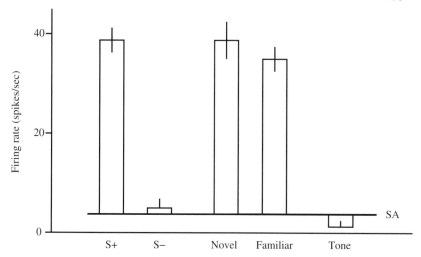

Fig. 4.57 This macaque amygdala neuron responded to the sight of a stimulus associated with food reward (S+), but not to a visual stimulus associated with aversive saline (S–) in a visual discrimination task. The same neuron responded to visual stimuli while they were relatively novel, including here on the first (Novel) and second (Familiar) presentations of new stimuli. The neuron did not respond to the tone that indicated the start of a trial. The visual stimulus appeared when the tone ended, at time=500 ms. SA, spontaneous firing rate of the neuron. The mean responses and the s.e.m. to the different stimuli are shown. (After Rolls 2000d, and Wilson and Rolls 2005.)

thus suggested that the amygdala neurons described operate as filters that provide an output if a stimulus is associated with a positive reinforcer, or is positively reinforcing because of relative unfamiliarity, and that provide no output if a stimulus is familiar and has not been associated with a positive primary reinforcer or is associated with a punisher. The functions of this output may be to influence the interest shown in a stimulus, whether it is approached or avoided, whether an affective response occurs to it, and whether a representation of the stimulus is made or maintained via an action mediated through either the basal forebrain nucleus of Meynert or the backprojections to the cerebral cortex (Rolls 1987, Rolls 1989a, Rolls 1990c, Rolls and Treves 1998, Rolls 2000b). It is an important adaptation to the environment to explore relatively novel objects or situations, for in this way advantage due to gene inheritance can become expressed and selected for. This function appears to be implemented in the amygdala in this way. Lesions of the amygdala impair the operation of this mechanism, in that objects are approached and explored indiscriminately, relatively independently of whether they are associated with reinforcers (including punishers), or are novel or familiar.

An interesting observation on the neurons that respond to rewarding and to relatively novel visual stimuli was made in the recognition memory task used by Wilson and Rolls (2005) (see also Rolls (2000d)). It was found that the neurons responded the first time a stimulus was shown, when the monkey had to use the rule 'Do not make a lick response to a stimulus the first time a stimulus is shown, otherwise aversive saline will be obtained', as well as the second time the stimulus was shown when the monkey had to apply the rule 'If a stimulus has been seen before today, lick to it to obtain glucose reward'. Thus these amygdala neurons do not code for reward value when this is based on a rule (e.g. first presentation aversive; second presentation reward), but instead code for reward value when it is decoded on the basis of previous stimulus–reinforcer associations, or when relatively novel stimuli are shown that are treated as rewarding and to be explored.

The details of the neuronal mechanisms that implement the process by which relatively novel stimuli are treated as rewarding in the amygdala are not currently known, but could be as follows. Cortical visual signals which do not show major habituation with repeated visual stimuli, as shown by recordings in the temporal cortical visual areas (see Rolls, Judge and Sanghera (1977), Rolls and Treves (1998) and Rolls and Deco (2002)) reach the amygdala. In the amygdala, neurons respond to these at first, and have the property that they gradually habituate unless the pattern-association mechanism in the amygdala detects co-occurrence of these stimuli with a primary reinforcer, in which case it strengthens the active synapses for that object, so that it continues to produce an output from amygdala neurons that respond to either rewarding or punishing visual stimuli. Neurophysiologically, the habituation condition would correspond in a pattern associator to long-term depression (LTD) of synapses with high presynaptic activity but low postsynaptic activity, that is to homosynaptic LTD (see Rolls and Treves (1998) and Rolls and Deco (2002)).

4.6.6 Neuronal responses in the amygdala to faces

Another interesting group of neurons in the amygdala responds primarily to faces (Rolls 1981c, Leonard, Rolls, Wilson and Baylis 1985). Each of these neurons responds to some but not all of a set of faces, and thus across an ensemble could convey information about the identity of the face (see Fig. 4.58). These neurons are found especially in the basal accessory nucleus of the amygdala (see Fig. 4.59; Leonard, Rolls, Wilson and Baylis (1985)), a part of the amygdala that develops markedly in primates (Amaral et al. 1992). It will be of interest to investigate whether some of these amygdala face neurons respond on the basis of facial expression. Some neurons in the amygdala do respond during social interactions (Brothers and Ring 1993).

It is probable that the amygdala neurons responsive to faces receive their inputs from a group of neurons in the cortex in the superior temporal sulcus that respond to faces, often on the basis of features present, such as eyes, hair, or mouth (Perrett, Rolls and Caan 1982), and consistent with this, the response latencies of the amygdala neurons tend to be longer than those of neurons in the cortex in the superior temporal sulcus (Leonard, Rolls, Wilson and Baylis 1985, Rolls 1984b). It has been suggested that this is part of a system that has evolved for the rapid and reliable identification of individuals from their faces, because of the importance of this in primate social behaviour (Rolls 1981c, Rolls 1984b, Rolls 1992b, Rolls 1992a, Rolls 1992c, Leonard, Rolls, Wilson and Baylis 1985, Perrett and Rolls 1983, Leonard, Rolls, Wilson and Baylis 1985). The part of this system in the amygdala may be particularly involved in emotional and social responses to faces. According to one possibility, such emotional and social responses would be 'looked up' (in a pattern associator, see Appendix 1) by a 'key' stimulus, which consisted of the face of a particular individual (Rolls 1984b, Rolls 1987, Rolls 1990d, Rolls 1992b, Rolls 1992a, Rolls 1992c, Rolls and Treves 1998, Rolls 1999a). Indeed, it is suggested that the tameness of the Kluver-Bucy syndrome, and the changes in amygdalectomized monkeys in their interactions in a social group (Kling and Steklis 1976, Kling and Brothers 1992) (though these are more subtle after selective amygdala lesions, Amaral (2003)), arise because of damage to this system specialized for processing faces (Rolls 1981b, Rolls 1981c, Rolls 1984b, Rolls 1990d, Rolls 1992b, Rolls 1992a, Rolls 1992c, Rolls 2000a, Rolls and Deco 2002). The amygdala may allow neurons

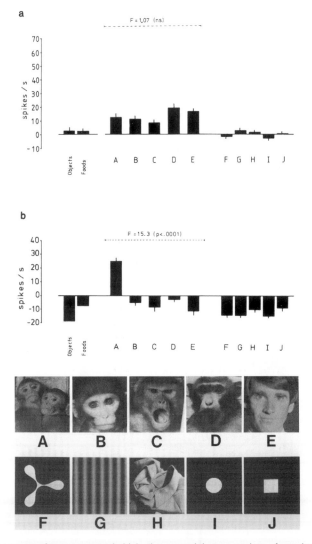

Fig. 4.58 The responses of two neurons (a,b) in the amygdala to a variety of monkey and human face stimuli (A–E), and to non-face stimuli (F–J, objects, and foods). Each bar represents the mean response above baseline with the standard error calculated over 4 to 10 presentations. The F ratio for an analysis of variance calculated over the face sets indicates that the neurons shown range from very selective between faces (neuron b, Y0809) to relatively non-selective (neuron A, Z0264). Some stimuli produced inhibition below the spontaneous firing rate. (After Leonard, Rolls, Wilson and Baylis 1985.)

that reflect the social significance of faces to be formed using face representations received from the temporal cortical areas, and information about primary reinforcers received from, for example, the somatosensory system (via the insula (Mesulam and Mufson 1982a, Mesulam and Mufson 1982b)), and the gustatory system (via, for example, the orbitofrontal cortex) (see Fig. 4.2).

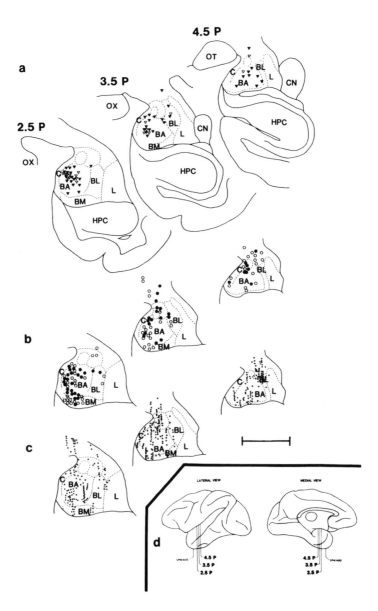

Fig. 4.59 (a) The distribution of neurons responsive to faces in the amygdala of four monkeys. The cells are plotted on three coronal sections at different distances (in mm) posterior (P) to the sphenoid (see inset). Filled triangles: cells selective for faces; open triangles: cells responding to face and hands. (b) Other responsive neurons. Closed circles: cells with other visual responses; open circles: cells responding to cues, movement, or arousal. (c) The locations of non-responsive cells. Abbreviations: BA, basal accessory nucleus of the amygdala; BL, basolateral nucleus of the amygdala; BM, basomedial nucleus of the amygdala; C, cortical nucleus of the amygdala; CN, tail of the caudate nucleus; HPC, hippocampus; L, lateral nucleus of the amygdala; OF, optic tract; OX, optic chiasm. (From Leonard, Rolls, Wilson and Baylis 1985.)

4.6.7 Evidence from humans

The theory described above about the role of the amygdala in emotion, based largely on research in non-human primates, has been followed up by studies in humans which are producing generally consistent results. One type of evidence comes from the effects of brain damage, which though rarely restricted just to the amygdala, and almost never bilateral, does provide some consistent evidence (Aggleton 1992). For example, in some patients alterations in feeding behaviour and emotion might occur after damage to the amygdala (see Aggleton (1992); Halgren (1992)). In relation to neurons in the macaque amygdala with responses selective for faces and social interactions (Leonard, Rolls, Wilson and Baylis 1985, Brothers and Ring 1993), a patient D. R. has been described who has bilateral damage to or disconnection of the amygdala, and has an impairment of face-expression matching and identification, but not of matching face identity or in discrimination (Young, Aggleton, Hellawell, Johnson, Broks and Hanley 1995, Young, Hellawell, Van de Wal and Johnson 1996). This patient is also impaired at detecting whether someone is gazing at the patient, another important social signal (Perrett et al. 1985). The same patient is also impaired at the auditory recognition of fear and anger (Scott, Young, Calder, Hellawell, Aggleton and Johnson 1997).

Adolphs, Tranel, Damasio and Damasio (1994) also found face expression but not face identity impairments in a patient (S. M.) with bilateral damage to the amygdala, and extended this to other patients (Adolphs, Tranel and Baron-Cohen 2002, Adolphs, Tranel, Hamann, Young, Calder, Phelps, Anderson, Lee and Damasio 1999) (see also Calder, Young, Rowland, Perrett, Hodges and Etcoff (1996)). A similar impairment was not found in patients with unilateral amygdala damage (Adolphs, Tranel, Damasio and Damasio 1995). The bilateral amygdala patient SM was especially impaired at recognizing the face expression of fear, and also rated expressions of fear, anger, and surprise as less intense than control subjects. It has been shown that SM's impairment stems from an inability to make normal use of information from the eye region of faces when judging emotions, which in turn is related to a lack of spontaneous fixations on the eyes during free viewing of faces (Adolphs, Gosselin, Buchanan, Tranel, Schyns and Damasio 2005). Although SM fails to look normally at the eye region in all facial expressions, her selective impairment in recognizing fear is explained by the fact that the eyes are the most important feature for identifying this emotion. Indeed, SM's recognition of fearful faces became entirely normal when she was instructed explicitly to look at the eyes. This finding provides a mechanism to explain the amygdala's role in fear recognition, and points to new approaches for the possible rehabilitation of patients with defective emotion perception.

The backprojections to the neocortex from the amygdala may produce larger activations in these cortical areas to visual stimuli which either are fear face expressions, or which occur in association with fear face expressions, for these larger activations are not found in patients with amygdala damage (Phelps 2004, Anderson and Phelps 2001). Patients with amygdala lesions are also impaired at learning conditioned skin conductance responses when a blue square is associated with a shock, and are also impaired in acquiring the same autonomic response to fear by verbally instructed learning or by observational learning (Phelps 2004, Phelps, O'Connor, Gatenby, Gore, Grillon and Davis 2001).

The possibility has been discussed (Blair 2003) that there may be a subcortical pathway to the amygdala which bypasses the temporal cortical visual areas, based partly on evidence that a 'blindsight' patient with a right-sided hemianopia after occipital lobe damage showed some ability to discriminate when guessing between different facial expressions in the blind hemifield (De Gelder, Vroomen, Pourtois and Weiskrantz 1999). Further evidence was that in the same patient activations occurred in the amygdala to fearful vs happy face expressions when these were presented to the blind and seeing hemifields, but only in the fusiform cortex (face) area when the stimuli were presented to the seeing hemifield (Morris, De Gelder, Weiskrantz and Dolan 2001). However, a more relevant cortical area to examine would be the cortex in the anterior part of the superior temporal sulcus, which in macaques as shown by neuronal recording studies (Hasselmo, Rolls and Baylis 1989a) and in human neuroimaging (Haxby, Hoffman and Gobbini 2002) is especially involved in face expression analysis. The evidence from the latency of neuronal responses to faces does not suggest that there is a rapid subcortical pathway for processing faces, for in macaques the latencies of activation of face-selective neurons in the temporal cortex visual areas are typically 80–120 ms (Rolls 1984b, Leonard et al. 1985), in the amygdala are typically 110–180 ms (Leonard, Rolls, Wilson and Baylis 1985), and in the orbitofrontal cortex are typically 130–280 ms (Rolls, Critchley, Browning and Inoue 2006a). These latencies are consistent with cortical processing in the temporal cortical visual areas before neurons become activated by faces in the amygdala and orbitofrontal cortex, both of which receive direct inputs from the temporal cortical visual areas as described above.

Deficits produced by amygdala damage may extend beyond face expression recognition deficits, in that bilateral amygdala patients are impaired not only at 'theory of mind' attributions when these are based on eye gaze, but also when they are related to an inability to recognise 'faux pas' situations in narratives (Stone, Baron-Cohen, Calder, Keane and Young 2003). With respect to autism, in which a 'theory of mind' deficit is a major component (Frith 2001), children with autism have usually been found to be unimpaired in facial affect recognition when the groups are matched on mental age (Baron-Cohen, Wheelwright and Joliffe 1997, Blair 2003). However, some evidence linking the amygdala and autism is that patients with autism or Asperger's syndrome did not activate the amygdala when making mentalistic inferences from the eyes (Baron-Cohen, Ring, Bullmore, Wheelwright, Ashwin and Williams 2000).

There is some evidence that another face expression, disgust, involves special processing by the insula. Not only is there some evidence that the insula can be differentially activated by the face expression of disgust (Phillips 2004, Phillips, Williams, Heining, Herba, Russell, Andrew, Bullmore, Brammer, Williams, Morgan, Young and Gray 2004), but also patient NK with an insular lesion is impaired on disgust face and voice expression identification, and on self-experience of disgust (Calder, Keane, Manes, Antoun and Young 2000). It could be that the involvement of the insula is related to the contribution of part of it to visceral/autonomic responses, and indeed Krolak-Salmon, Henaff, Isnard, Tallon-Baudry, Guenot, Vighetto, Bertrand and Mauguiere (2003) found that electrical stimulation in the antero-ventral insula produced feelings related to disgust, including viscero-autonomic feelings.

In another system with some apparent specificity, there is some evidence that patients with lesions in the ventral putamen (which does receive inputs from the inferior temporal visual cortex and contains visually responsive neurons (Caan, Perrett and Rolls 1984)) may have impaired anger face recognition (Calder, Keane, Lawrence and Manes 2004), and this was related to evidence that the D2 dopamine receptor blocker sulpiride decreases the identification of angry face expressions (Lawrence, Calder, McGowan and Grasby 2002). Insofar as activation of the ventral putamen may be larger to angry face expressions and of the insula to disgust face expressions, we might note that skeletomotor responses (likely to be involved in anger) are functions of much of the putamen, and that visceral responses (likely to occur in disgust) may be produced in part via the anteroventral insula. Thus the activations of both regions by faces may be related to the responses normally produced by different face expressions.

For comparison, in a much more extensive series of patients it has been shown that damage to the orbitofrontal cortex can produce face expression deficits in the absence of face identification deficits, and that some patients with orbitofrontal cortex damage are impaired at the auditory identification of emotional sounds (Hornak, Rolls and Wade 1996, Hornak, Bramham, Rolls, Morris, O'Doherty, Bullock and Polkey 2003, Rolls 1999b) (see Section 4.5.6). Interestingly, the visual face expression and auditory vocal expression impairments are partly dissociable in these orbitofrontal patients, indicating partially separate processing systems in the orbitofrontal cortex, and indicating that a general emotional impairment produced by these lesions is not the simple explanation of the alterations in face and voice expression processing after damage to the orbitofrontal cortex. I note that the most consistent change after orbitofrontal cortex damage in our series of patients (Rolls, Hornak, Wade and McGrath 1994a, Hornak, Rolls and Wade 1996, Hornak, Bramham, Rolls, Morris, O'Doherty, Bullock and Polkey 2003, Rolls 1999b, Hornak, O'Doherty, Bramham, Rolls, Morris, Bullock and Polkey 2004) is an alteration in voice and face expression decoding, and that the amygdala is strongly connected to the orbitofrontal cortex.

Functional brain imaging studies have also shown activation of the amygdala by face expression. For example, Morris, Frith, Perrett, Rowland, Young, Calder and Dolan (1996) found more activation of the left amygdala by face expressions of fear than of happiness in a PET study. They also reported that the activation increased as the intensity of the fear expression increased, and decreased as the intensity of the happy expression increased.

However, although in studies of the effects of amygdala damage in humans greater impairments have been reported to face expressions of fear than to some other expressions (Adolphs et al. 1994, Scott et al. 1997), and in functional brain imaging studies greater activation may be found to certain classes of emotion-provoking stimuli, e.g. to stimuli that provoke fear compared with those that produce happiness (Morris et al. 1996), it is most unlikely that the amygdala is specialized for the decoding of only certain classes of emotional stimulus, such as fear. This emphasis on fear may be related to the research in rats on the role of the amygdala in fear conditioning (LeDoux 1992, LeDoux 1994, LeDoux 1996, Pare et al. 2004). It is quite clear from single-neuron neurophysiological studies in non-human primates that different amygdala neurons are activated by different classes of both rewarding and punishing stimuli (Sanghera, Rolls and Roper-Hall 1979, Rolls 1992b, Ono and Nishijo 1992, Wilson and Rolls 1993, Wilson and Rolls 2005) and by a wide range of different face stimuli (Leonard, Rolls, Wilson and Baylis 1985). Also, lesions of the macaque amygdala impair the learning of both stimulus–reward and stimulus–punisher associations (see Section 4.6.3). Amygdala lesions with ibotenic acid impair the processing of reward-related stimuli, in that when the reward value of a set of foods was reduced by feeding it to satiety (i.e. sensory-specific satiety), the monkeys still chose the visual stimuli associated with the foods with which they had been satiated (Malkova et al. 1997). Further, electrical stimulation of the macaque and human amygdala at some sites is rewarding, and humans report pleasure from stimulation at such sites (Rolls 1975, Rolls et al. 1980c, Sem-Jacobsen 1968, Sem-Jacobsen 1976, Halgren 1992). Further, in a functional neuroimaging study, O'Doherty, Rolls, Francis, Bowtell and McGlone (2001b) showed that activation of the human amygdala was larger and more reliably produced by the pleasant taste of glucose than by the unpleasant taste of salt, both of which are primary reinforcers. Thus any differences in the magnitude of effects between different classes of emotional stimuli that appear in human functional brain imaging studies (Morris et al. 1996) or even after amygdala damage (Adolphs et al. 1994, Scott et al. 1997) should not be taken as showing that the human amygdala is involved in only some emotions, but instead may reflect differences in the efficacy of the stimuli in leading to strong emotional reactions, or differences in the magnitude per se of different emotions, making some effects more apparent for some emotions than others. Consistent with this view, LaBar, Gitelman, Parrish, Kim, Nobre and Mesulam (1999) showed that both pleasant and unpleasant stimuli produced more activation of the human amygdala than neutral stimuli.

A very interesting clarification is provided by the finding that personality interacts with whether particular stimuli activate the human amygdala. For example, happy face expressions are more likely to activate the human amygdala in extraverts than in introverts (Canli et al. 2002). In addition, positively affective pictures interact with extraversion to produce activation of the amygdala (Canli et al. 2001). This supports the conceptually important point described in section 2.7 that part of the basis of personality may be differential sensitivity to different rewards and punishers, and omission and termination of rewards and punishers. The observations just described are consistent with the hypothesis that part of the basis of extraversion is increased reactivity to positively affective (as compared to negatively affective) face expressions and other positively affective stimuli including pictures. The exact mechanisms involved may be revealed in the future by genetic studies, and these might potentially address for example whether genes control responses to positively affective stimuli; or whether some more general personality trait by altering perhaps mood produces differential top-down biasing of face expression decoding systems in the way outlined in Section 4.10. It has additionally been found that negative pictures interact with neuroticism in producing differential activation of the human amygdala (Canli et al. 2001).

Additional factors are that some expressions are much more identifiable than others. For example, we (Hornak, Rolls and Wade 1996, Rolls 1999b) found that happy faces were easier to identify than other face expressions in the Ekman set, and that the orbitofrontal patients we studied were not impaired at identifying the (easy) happy face expression, but showed deficits primarily on the more difficult set of other expressions (fear, surprise, anger, sadness, etc.). Another factor in imaging studies in which the human subjects may be slightly apprehensive is that happy expressions may produce some relaxation in the situation, whereas expressions of fear may do the opposite, and this could contribute to the results found. Thus I suggest caution in interpreting human studies as showing that the amygdala (or orbitofrontal cortex) are involved only in certain emotions. It is much more likely that both are involved in emotions produced to rewarding stimuli as well as to punishers. However, an interesting difference between non-human primates and humans may be found in the degree of lateralization of some types of processing related to emotions in different hemispheres evident in humans. This is discussed in Section 4.11.

4.6.8 Amygdala summary

The evidence described in Section 4.6 implicates the amygdala in the processing of a number of stimuli that are primary reinforcers, including the sight, smell, and taste of food, touch, and pain.

The amygdala also receives information about potential secondary reinforcers, such as visual stimuli, including faces. Many of the deficits produced by amygdala damage are related to impairments in learning associations between stimuli and primary reinforcers, e.g. between visual or auditory stimuli and pain.

The amygdala is not concerned only with aversive reinforcers, in that it receives information about food, and in that amygdala lesions impair the altered behaviour that normally occurs to foods when their reward value is reduced by feeding to satiety.

The associative stimulus–reinforcer learning or conditioning in the amygdala may require NMDA receptor activation for the learning, which appears to occur by a process like long-term potentiation.

We know that autonomic responses learned to conditioned stimuli can depend on outputs from the amygdala to the hypothalamus, and that the effects that learned incentives have on behaviour may involve outputs from the amygdala to the ventral striatum. We also know that there are similar neurons in the ventral striatum to some of those described in the amygdala (Williams, Rolls, Leonard and Stern 1993).

All this evidence is consistent with the hypothesis that there are neuronal networks in the amygdala that perform the required pattern association. Interestingly, there is somewhat of a gap in our knowledge here, for the microcircuitry of the amygdala has been remarkably little studied. It is known from Golgi studies (performed in young rats in which sufficiently few amygdala cells are stained that it is possible to see them individually) that there are pyramidal cells in the amygdala with large dendrites and many synapses (Millhouse and DeOlmos 1983, McDonald 1992, Millhouse 1986). What has not yet been defined is whether visual and taste inputs converge anatomically on to some cells, and whether (as might be predicted) the taste inputs are likely to be strong (e.g. large synapses close to the cell body), whereas the visual inputs are more numerous, and on a part of the dendrite with NMDA receptors. Clearly to bring our understanding fully to the network level, such evidence is required, together with further neurophysiological evidence showing the appropriate convergence at the single neuron level, and evidence that the appropriate synapses on to these single neurons are modifiable by a Hebb-like rule (such as might be implemented using the NMDA receptors, see Appendix 1), in a network of the type shown in Fig. 4.5.

At least part of the importance of the amygdala in emotion appears to be that it is involved in this type of emotional learning. However, the amygdala does not appear to provide such rapid relearning of reward-related emotional responses to stimuli as does the orbitofrontal cortex, as described in Section 4.5. Further, the amygdala does not appear in non-human primates and humans to play such an important role in emotional and social behaviour as the orbitofrontal cortex (see Section 4.5).

4.7 The cingulate cortex

The perigenual cingulate area occupying approximately the anterior one third of the cingulate cortex (see Fig. 4.60) and involved in emotion may be distinguished from a mid-cingulate area (i.e. further back than the perigenual cingulate region and occupying approximately the middle third of the cingulate cortex) which has been termed the cingulate motor area (Vogt, Derbyshire and Jones 1996) and may be involved in response selection (Rushworth, Walton, Kennerley and Bannerman 2004). Both the perigenual and midcingulate areas are part of what anatomically is frequently termed anterior cingulate cortex, but for convenience, when using the term anterior cingulate cortex I will be referring in the following two sections to perigenual

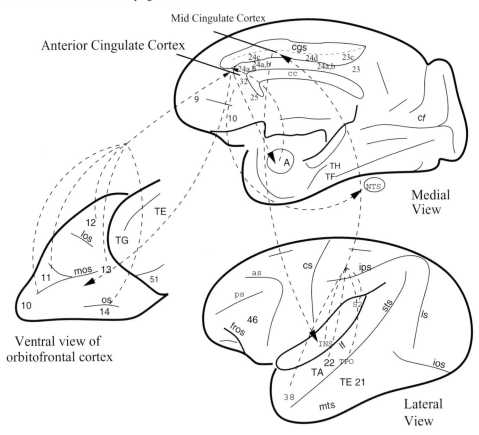

Fig. 4.60 Connections of the perigenual and midcingulate cortical areas (shown on views of the primate brain). The cingulate sulcus (cgs) has been opened to reveal the cortex in the sulcus, with the dashed line indicating the depths (fundus) of the sulcus. The cingulate cortex is in the lower bank of this sulcus, and in the cingulate gyrus which hooks above the corpus callosum and around the corpus callosum at the front and the back. The perigenual cingulate cortex extends from cingulate areas 32, 24a and 24b to subgenual cingulate area 25. (The cortex is called subgenual because it is below the genu (knee) formed by the anterior end of the corpus callosum, cc.) The perigenual cingulate cortex tends to have connections with the amygdala and orbitofrontal cortex, whereas area 24c tends to have connections with the somatosensory insula (INS), the auditory association cortex (22, TA), and with the temporal pole cortex (38). The midcingulate areas include area 24d, which is part of the cingulate motor area. Abbreviations: as, arcuate sulcus; cc, corpus callosum; cf, calcarine fissure; cgs, cingulate sulcus; cs, central sulcus; ls, lunate sulcus; ios, inferior occipital sulcus; mos, medial orbital sulcus; os, orbital sulcus; ps, principal sulcus; sts, superior temporal sulcus; lf, lateral (or Sylvian) fissure (which has been opened to reveal the insula); A, amygdala; INS, insula; NTS, autonomic areas in the medulla, including the nucleus of the solitary tract and the dorsal motor nucleus of the vagus; TE (21), inferior temporal visual cortex; TA (22), superior temporal auditory association cortex; TF and TH, parahippocampal cortex; TPO, multimodal cortical area in the superior temporal sulcus; 38, TG, temporal pole cortex; 12, 13, 11, orbitofrontal cortex; 51, olfactory (prepyriform and periamygdaloid) cortex.

cingulate cortex (see Section 4.7.1), and will distinguish this from the midcingulate cortex described in Section 4.7.2.

Vogt et al. (1996) showed that pain produced an increase in regional cerebral blood flow (rCBF, measured with positron emission tomography, PET) in an area of perigenual cingulate cortex which included parts of areas 25, 32, 24a, 24b and/or 24c. Vogt et al. suggested that activation of the anterior part of the cingulate area is related to the affective aspect of pain. There are direct projections to the cingulate cortex from medial thalamic areas that relay pain inputs, including the parafascicular nucleus. In terms of other connections (see Van Hoesen, Morecraft and Vogt (1993); Vogt, Pandya and Rosene (1987); and Vogt and Pandya (1987)), the anterior cingulate cortex is connected to the medial orbitofrontal areas, parts of lateral orbitofrontal area 12 (Carmichael and Price 1995a), the amygdala (which projects strongly to cingulate subgenual area 25) and the temporal pole cortex, and also receives somatosensory inputs from the insula and other somatosensory cortical areas (see Fig. 4.60). The anterior cingulate cortex has output projections to the periaqueductal gray in the midbrain (which is implicated in pain processing), to the nucleus of the solitary tract and dorsal motor nucleus of the vagus (through which autonomic effects can be elicited), and to the ventral striatum and caudate nucleus (through which behavioural responses could be produced).

Consistent with the anterior cingulate region being involved in affect, it is close to (just above) the area activated by the induction of a sad mood in the study described by Mayberg (1997) and Mayberg, Liotti, Brannan, McGinnis, Mahurin, Jerabek, Silva, Tekell, Martin, Lancaster and Fox (1999). Also consistent with this region being involved in affect, Lane, Fink, Chau and Dolan (1997a) found increased regional blood flow in a PET study in a far anterior part of the cingulate cortex where it adjoins prefrontal cortex when humans paid attention to the affective aspects of pictures they were being shown which contained pleasant images (e.g. flowers) and unpleasant pictures (e.g. a mangled face and a snake). What we will now call the perigenual anterior cingulate cortex, approximately the anterior one third of the cingulate cortex and including parts of areas 32, 24 and 25, is thus related to affect, and will be considered next in Section 4.7.1. The functions of the midcingulate area will be considered in Section 4.7.2.

4.7.1 Perigenual cingulate cortex and affect

The perigenual cingulate cortex may be part of an executive, output, response selection system for some emotional states, where the responses can include autonomic responses. Part of the basis for this suggestion is its inputs from somatosensory cortical areas including the insula, and the orbitofrontal cortex and amygdala (see Fig. 4.60), and its outputs to brainstem areas such as the periaqueductal (or central) gray in the midbrain (which is implicated in pain, see Section 8.5 and Melzack and Wall (1996)), the ventral striatum, and the autonomic brainstem nuclei (see Van Hoesen et al. (1993)). Devinsky, Morrell and Vogt (1995) and Cardinal et al. (2002) review evidence that anterior cingulate lesions in humans produce apathy, autonomic dysregulation, and emotional instability. We ourselves have shown that patients with circumscribed, even unilateral, surgical lesions of the anterior/perigenual cingulate cortex may be impaired at voice and face expression identification, have impaired subjective emotional states, and some changes in social behaviour including being less likely to notice when other people were angry, not being close to his or her family, and doing things without thinking (Hornak, Bramham, Rolls, Morris, O'Doherty, Bullock and Polkey 2003).

In macaques, anterior cingulate cortex lesions can produce a type of social apathy (Hadland, Rushworth, Gaffan and Passingham 2003). Although the exact homology of what is called in rodents anterior cingulate cortex (ACC) is not clear, it is of interest that ACC lesions in rodents impair stimulus–reinforcer association learning, in tasks in which subjects must learn which stimulus to select in each of eight pairs in order to obtain reward (Bussey, Muir, Everitt and Robbins 1997). ACC lesions also impair the Pavlovian associative stimulus–reward learning involved in autoshaping in rodents, but seem to have their effects only when multiple conditioned stimuli must be distinguished, and perhaps when there is some conflict (Cardinal et al. 2002).

Functional neuroimaging studies are now showing that there appear to be separate representations of aversive and positively affective stimuli in the anterior/perigenual cingulate cortex (Rolls 2007a), with the results of one series of studies summarized in Fig. 4.61. The area activated by pain is typically 10–30 mm behind and above the most anterior (i.e. pre- or peri-genual) part of the anterior cingulate cortex (see e.g. Rolls, O'Doherty, Kringelbach, Francis, Bowtell and McGlone (2003d), Fig. 4.4, and Vogt and Sikes (2000)). Pleasant touch was found to activate the most anterior part of the anterior cingulate cortex, just in front of the (genu or knee of the) corpus callosum (i.e. pregenual cingulate cortex) (Rolls, O'Doherty, Kringelbach, Francis, Bowtell and McGlone 2003d) (Fig. 4.4). Oral somatosensory stimuli such as viscosity and fat texture also activate this most anterior part of the anterior cingulate cortex (De Araujo and Rolls 2004). More than just somatosensory stimuli are represented, however, in that (pleasant) sweet taste also activates the most anterior part of the anterior cingulate cortex (De Araujo and Rolls 2004, De Araujo, Kringelbach, Rolls and Hobden 2003a) (Fig. 5.15), as do pleasant odours (Rolls, Kringelbach and De Araujo 2003c) (Figs. 4.25 and 4.26), and cognitive inputs that influence the pleasantness of odours (De Araujo et al. 2005) (Figs. 4.41 and 4.42). Unpleasant odours activate further back in the anterior cingulate cortex (Rolls, Kringelbach and De Araujo 2003c) (Fig. 4.25). Activations in the anterior/perigenual cingulate cortex are also produced by the taste of water when it is rewarding because of thirst (De Araujo, Kringelbach, Rolls and McGlone 2003b) (Fig. 6.7), by the flavour of food (Kringelbach, O'Doherty, Rolls and Andrews 2003), and by monetary reward (O'Doherty, Kringelbach, Rolls, Hornak and Andrews 2001a) (Fig. 4.33). The locations of some of these activations are shown in Fig. 4.61, from which it is clear that many positively affective stimuli are represented in the most anterior part of the perigenual cingulate cortex, with some less positively affective or negatively affective stimuli activating a region of the cingulate cortex which is just posterior to this above the corpus callosum.

In addition to the pregenual cingulate sites which are activated in many of our studies of affective stimuli, it is also frequently found that activation in a region at the intersection of the medial prefrontal cortex, the subgenual cingulate cortex, and the orbitofrontal cortex is activated by positively affective stimuli. The region is illustrated in Figs. 4.25 and 4.26 (lower region) where activations were correlated with the pleasantness of olfactory stimuli (Rolls, Kringelbach and De Araujo 2003c), in Fig. 4.41A and B where cognitive inputs increased activations that were related to the pleasantness of olfactory stimuli (De Araujo, Rolls, Velazco, Margot and Cayeux 2005), in Fig. 5.15 where glucose taste produced activations (De Araujo, Kringelbach, Rolls and Hobden 2003a), and in a similar region in which intraoral fat and sucrose both produced activations (De Araujo and Rolls 2004). This region is also activated by monetary reward (O'Doherty, Kringelbach, Rolls, Hornak and Andrews 2001a). The region is probably part of area 10, and is part of a medial prefrontal network of connected regions that includes the subgenual cingulate cortex (Ongur and Price 2000). The fact that this region is activated by many rewarding stimuli as just summarized, if lesioned affects emotion (Hornak, Bramham, Rolls, Morris, O'Doherty, Bullock and Polkey 2003), and is

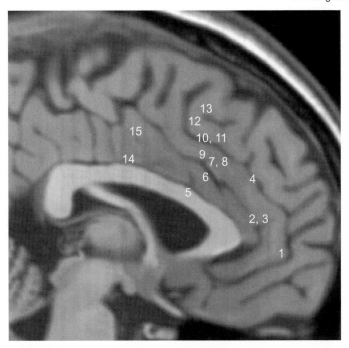

Fig. 4.61 Activations of the most anterior part of the perigenual cingulate cortex by different positively affective stimuli, with less positively affective or negatively affective stimuli producing activations centered just behind this area. Touch: 3 pleasant [10 42 16], 14 unpleasant/pain [10 -6 34], 5 unpleasant/pain [-8 12 22] (from Rolls et al 2003d); Odour: 7 pleasant [2 20 32], 2 correlation with pleasantness ratings [4 42 12], 9 unpleasant [0 18 36] (from Rolls et al 2003c); 8 Monetary loss [2 25 32] (from O'Doherty et al 2001a); Water: 6 correlation with pleasantness [-2 19 28], 15 correlation with pleasantness [-2 -5 43] (from De Araujo et al 2003b); Taste: 10 glucose [9 17 42], 11 salt [15 21 42], 4 salt [-16 39 24] (from O'Doherty et al 2001b); Sucrose and fat: 1 [-10 48 -2] (from De Araujo and Rolls 2004); Non-reward in a social reversal task: 13 [-8 22 52], 12 [-6 18 48] (from Kringelbach and Rolls 2003).

connected with the orbitofrontal cortex, indicates that it is important in emotion, perhaps as a region linking the orbitofrontal cortex to outputs. It is in this context very interesting that chronic electrical stimulation in or close to this region (in the 'subgenual cingulate cortex') relieved symptoms of treatment-resistant depression in some patients (Mayberg, Lozano, Voon, McNeely, Seminowicz, Hamani, Schwalb and Kennedy 2005). This provides a close link between evidence from neuroscience about the functions of this medial region, and the therapeutic potential of these concepts for helping to understand and treat depression.

Overall, it is thus notable that what can be termed an affective part of the anterior cingulate cortex, the perigenual cingulate cortex, appears to have a most anterior part where activations are produced by a number of different pleasant stimuli, while further back towards the junction with the midcingulate area and perhaps sometimes including parts of the midcingulate area several affectively negative stimuli produce activations.

An investigation in patients with selective surgical lesions has shown that patients with unilateral lesions of the antero-ventral part of the anterior cingulate cortex (ACC) and/or medial BA9 were in some cases impaired on voice and face expression identification, had some change in social behaviour, such as inappropriateness, and had significant changes in their subjective emotional state (Hornak, Bramham, Rolls, Morris, O'Doherty, Bullock and Polkey 2003). Unilateral lesions were sufficient to produce these effects, and there were no strong laterality effects. In line with these results in humans, Hadland et al. (2003) found diminished social vocalization in monkeys with anterior cingulate lesions, and also emotional and social changes. Consistent with the effects of the anterior cingulate lesions in humans on recognizing voice (and in some cases face) emotional expression (Hornak et al. 2003), neuroimaging studies concerned with vocal expression identification have reported orbital and medial activation. These include a study by Morris et al. (1996) using non-verbal sounds expressing fear, sadness and happiness that, when compared to a neutral condition, activated BA11 (orbital cortex) bilaterally and Medial BA9 on the left. Fear-related increases in activity were also found on the right only in BA11. In another study Phillips, Young, Scott, Calder, Andrew, Giampetro, Williams, Bullmore, Brammer and Gray (1998) found that fearful sounds activated Medial BA32 and BA24 (anterior cingulate at/below the level of the genu of the corpus callosum) - again on the right side only. More extensive studies of facial expression identification have been conducted, and these report activation in a number of sites within both orbital and medial regions, including Medial BA9 and BA32/24 (anterior cingulate) (Blair, Morris, Frith, Perrett and Dolan 1999, Dolan, Fletcher, Morris, Kapur, Deakin and Frith 1996, Nakamura, Kawashima, Ito, Sugiura, Kato, Nakamura, Hatano, Nagumo, Kubota, Fukuda and Kojima 1999).

There is also neuroimaging evidence that complements the effects of lesions (Hornak, Bramham, Rolls, Morris, O'Doherty, Bullock and Polkey 2003) in suggesting a role for certain medial regions in the subjective experience of emotion. In neuroimaging studies with normal human subjects bilateral activations in Medial BA9 were found as subjects viewed emotion-laden stimuli, and in both Medial BA9 as well as in ventral ACC during self-generated emotional experience (i.e., in the absence of a stimulus) as subjects recalled emotions of sadness or happiness (Lane, Reiman, Ahern, Schwartz and Davidson 1997b, Lane, Reiman, Bradley, Lang, Ahern, Davidson and Schwartz 1997c, Lane et al. 1998, Phillips, Drevets, Rauch and Lane 2003a). On the basis of a review of imaging studies which consistently emphasize the importance of anterior and ventral regions of the anterior cingulate cortex for emotion, Bush, Luu and Posner (2000) argue that the anterior cingulate cortex can be divided into a ventral 'affective' division (which includes the subcallosal region and the part anterior to the corpus callosum), and a dorsal 'cognitive' division, a view strengthened by the demonstration of reciprocally inhibitory interactions between these two regions.

The subgenual part (area 25) of the anterior cingulate cortex is, via its outputs to the hypothalamus and brainstem autonomic regions, involved in the autonomic component of emotion (Koski and Paus 2000, Barbas and Pandya 1989, Ongur and Price 2000, Gabbott, Warner, Jays and Bacon 2003). The anterior cingulate cortex is also activated in relation to autonomic events, and Nagai, Critchley, Featherstone, Trimble and Dolan (2004) have shown that there is a correlation with skin conductance, a measure of autonomic activity related to sympathetic activation, in the anterior cingulate cortex and related areas.

A current working hypothesis is that the affective part of the anterior cingulate cortex receives inputs about expected rewards and punishers, and about the rewards and punishers received, from the orbitofrontal cortex and amygdala. There is some segregation of the areas that receive these inputs. The anterior cingulate cortex may compare these signals, and utilize them in functions such as affective decision-making and in producing autonomic responses.

As such, the perigenual cingulate cortex may act as an output system for emotional responses and actions.

4.7.2 Mid-cingulate cortex, the cingulate motor area, and action–outcome learning

The anterior or perigenual cingulate area may be distinguished from a mid-cingulate area (i.e. further back than the perigenual cingulate region and occupying approximately the middle third of the cingulate cortex) which has been termed the cingulate motor area (Vogt et al. 1996, Vogt, Berger and Derbyshire 2003). (Both may be included in what anatomically is designated as the anterior cingulate cortex.) This area is also activated by pain but, because this area is also activated in response selection tasks such as divided attention and Stroop tasks (which involve cues that cause conflict such as the word red written in green when the task is to make a response to the green colour), it is suggested that activation of this mid-cingulate area by painful stimuli was related to the response selection processes initiated by painful stimuli (Vogt et al. 1996, Derbyshire, Vogt and Jones 1998). Both the perigenual and the mid-cingulate areas may be activated in functional neuroimaging studies not only by physical pain, but also by social pain, for example being excluded from a social group (Eisenberger and Lieberman 2004).

The mid-cingulate area may be divided into an anterior or rostral cingulate motor area (24c′) concerned with skeletomotor control which may be required in avoidance and fear tasks, and a posterior or caudal cingulate motor area (24d) which may be more involved in skeletomotor orientation (Vogt et al. 2003).

In macaques, lesions of the anterior cingulate cortex that include the midcingulate area do not affect working memory (measured by delayed alternation), and are in this respect different from dorsolateral prefrontal cortex lesions, but may affect task switching (Rushworth, Hadland, Gaffan and Passingham 2003, Rushworth et al. 2004).

In human imaging studies it has been found that the anterior/mid-cingulate cortex is activated when there is a change in response set or when there is conflict between possible responses, but it is not activated when only stimulus selection is at issue (van Veen, Cohen, Botvinick, Stenger and Carter 2001, Rushworth, Hadland, Paus and Sipila 2002).

Some anterior/mid-cingulate neurons respond when errors are made (Niki and Watanabe 1979, Gemba, Sasaki and Brooks 1986), or when rewards are reduced (Shima and Tanji 1998) (and activations are found in corresponding imaging studies, Bush, Vogt, Holmes, Dales, Greve, Jenike and Rosen (2002)). In humans, an event-related potential (ERP), called the error related negativity (ERN), may originate in the area 24c′ (Ullsperger and von Cramon 2001), and many studies provide evidence that errors made in many tasks activate the anterior/mid-cingulate cortex, whereas tasks with response conflict activate the superior frontal gyrus (Rushworth et al. 2004).

Anterior cingulate neurons in macaques may also respond to rewards (Ito, Stuphorn, Brown and Schall 2003), and indeed action–outcome associations appear to be represented in the anterior cingulate cortex, in that in tasks in which there were different relations between actions and rewards, it was found that even before a response was made, while the monkey was looking at a visual cue, the activity of ACC neurons depended on the expectation of reward or non-reward (25%), the intention to move or not (25%), or a combination of movement intention and reward expectation (11%) (Matsumoto, Suzuki and Tanaka 2001). Correspondingly, in rodents a part of the medial prefrontal / anterior cingulate cortex termed the prelimbic cortex is involved in learning relations between behavioural responses and reinforcers, that is between actions and outcomes (Balleine and Dickinson 1998, Cardinal et al. 2002, Killcross and Coutureau 2003). Balleine and Dickinson (1998) showed that the sensitivity of instrumental behaviour to whether a particular action was followed by a reward was impaired by prelimbic cortex lesions.

To perform action–outcome learning, the anterior/mid-cingulate cortical area must contain a representation of the behavioural action just performed, and receive information about rewards and punishers being obtained. The reward-related information may come from structures such as the orbitofrontal cortex and amygdala. In addition, the cortical area involved in action–outcome learning must be able to hold the representation of the action just performed in a type of working memory until the reward or punishment is received (or more probably receive delay-related information from the prefrontal cortex, see Rushworth et al. (2004)), as there may be a delay between the action and the outcome.

When making decisions about actions, it is important to take into account the costs as well as the benefits. There is some evidence implicating the rodent anterior cingulate cortex (prelimbic cortex) in this, in that rats with prelimbic cortex lesions were impaired in a task that required decisions about an action with a large reward but a high barrier to climb, vs an action with a lower reward but no barrier (Walton, Bannerman and Rushworth 2002, Walton, Bannerman, Alterescu and Rushworth 2003). An output region from the anterior cingulate cortex for action–outcome learning may be the nucleus accumbens, for neurons in the macaque nucleus accumbens as well as the anterior cingulate cortex appear to encode the position of the monkey in a sequence of actions required to obtain a reward (Shidara and Richmond 2002).

It should be noted that stimulus–response or habit learning, although instrumental, is separate, in that it involves different associations (between stimuli and responses, not between actions and outcomes), and is implemented in different brain regions such as the basal ganglia (see Section 8.4).

Although understanding of the brain mechanisms of action–outcome learning is still at an early stage, it may well involve the anterior cingulate cortex. It is not yet clear whether the perigenual and mid-cingulate regions are involved together in action–outcome learning, but this does appear to be a possibility. There appear to be strong representations of rewards and punishers (see above), and the elicitation of autonomic responses (Nagai et al. 2004), in the perigenual cingulate cortex, accounting for its designation as affective cingulate cortex. This reward and punisher-related information may then reach the mid-cingulate area, where it can be associated with skeletomotor response representations, producing neurons that respond to different combinations of actions and outcomes. Although such neurons may well be a crucial part of the implementation of action–outcome learning, it is not yet clear at the computational level how costs are taken into account, and the correct action is selected. This will be a topic of future interest.

In any case, it is useful to place action–outcome learning in the wider context of emotion. When stimuli are presented, they are decoded to determine whether they are primary rewards or punishers by structures such as the orbitofrontal cortex and amygdala. If the stimulus presented has been associated with a primary reward or punisher, this stimulus–stimulus association is also decoded in the orbitofrontal cortex and amygdala. Affective states, and autonomic responses, can be produced by these processes, subjective states are influenced, and choices of stimuli to select are determined. When reinforcer contingencies change, the orbitofrontal cortex is important in reversing the stimulus–stimulus association, and contains appropriate error neurons. It thus seems to be able to implement stimulus selection. The orbitofrontal cortex is involved in this way in decision-making and executive function. On the other hand, if more complex contingencies are operating so that actions that give rise to particular outcomes must be selected, then this clearly requires a representation of actions, and it may be for these situations that the anterior cingulate cortex is especially important. Much affective computation, including the elicitation of affective states, may thus not computationally require the anterior cingulate cortex; but if to obtain the goal particular responses must be selected, then in those affective situations the anterior cingulate cortex may be especially computationally important. We return to the different types of decision-making in Section 11.2.

4.8 Human brain imaging investigations of mood and depression

Brain regions involved in mood and in depression (which has biological and cognitive aspects, Clark and Beck (1999)) have been investigated by mood induction in normal subjects; and by measuring the changes in activity associated with depression, and its treatment by antidepressant drugs (see Mayberg (1997); Mayberg et al. (1999); Mayberg (2003); Drevets and Raichle (1992); Dolan, Bench, Brown, Scott, Friston and Frackowiak (1992); George, Ketter, Parekh, Herscovitch and Post (1996); Dolan (1997); Phillips et al. (2003a)).

In one example of this approach, Drevets, Price, Simpson, Todd, Reich, Vannier and Raichle (1997) showed that positron emission tomography (PET) measures of regional blood flow and glucose metabolism and magnetic resonance imaging (MRI)-based measures of gray matter volume are abnormally reduced in the 'subgenual prefrontal cortex' in depressed subjects with familial major depressive disorder ('unipolar depression') and bipolar disorder ('manic-depressive illness') (Ongur, Drevets and Price 1998, Torrey, Webster, Knable, Johnson and Yolken 2000). This cortex is situated on the anterior cingulate gyrus lying ventral to the genu of the corpus callosum and may also be described as the subgenual or subcallosal anterior cingulate cortex (see Fig. 4.60).

In other PET imaging studies, which implicate a similar area although apparently in the opposite direction, treatment-resistant depression is associated with metabolic over-activity in the subgenual cingulate cortex; the recovery of depression associated with fluoxetine treatment is associated with a decrease of glucose metabolism (as indicated by fluorodeoxyglucose PET) in the ventral (subgenual) cingulate area 25; and the induction of a mood of sadness in normal subjects increases glucose metabolism in the same area (Mayberg 1997, Mayberg, Brannan, Mahurin, Jerabek, Brickman, Tekell, Silva, McGinnis, Glass, Martin and Fox 1997, Mayberg et al. 1999, Mayberg 2003, Mayberg et al. 2005) (see Fig. 4.62). At the same time, the induced sadness was associated with reduced glucose metabolism in more dorsal areas such as the dorsal prefrontal cortex (labelled F9 in Fig. 4.62), the inferior parietal cortex, and the dorsal anterior cingulate and the posterior cingulate cortex (Mayberg 1997). These dorsal cingulate areas are involved in processing sensory and spatial stimuli, in spatial attention, and in sensori-motor responses (see Rolls and Treves (1998) and Koski and Paus (2000)), and the reduced metabolism in these dorsal areas during sadness might reflect less interaction with the environment and less activity which normally accompanies such a change of mood. In contrast, the changes in the more ventral areas such as the ventral (i.e. subgenual) cingulate cortex may be more closely related to the changes in mood per se. Further evidence that the subgenual cingulate cortex is a brain area with activity related to depression is that chronic

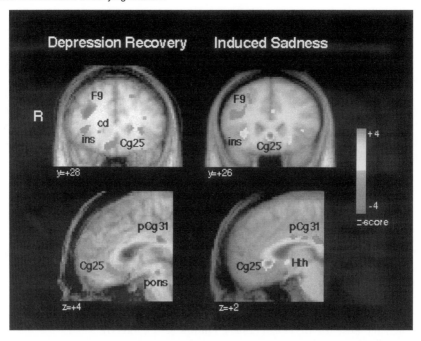

Fig. 4.62 Changes in the subgenual cingulate area (Cg25) associated with the recovery from depression (left), and with the induction of a mood state of sadness (right). Left images: Z-score maps demonstrating changes in regional glucose metabolism (fluorodeoxyglucose PET) in depressed patients following 6 weeks of treatment with the antidepressant fluoxetine. Upper: coronal view; lower, sagittal view). Green indicates that the change is a decrease, and red or yellow an increase (see calibration bar on far right). Right images: changes in regional cerebral blood flow (oxygen-15 water PET) in healthy volunteers 10 min after induction of acute sadness. The recovery from depression and the induction of sadness produce opposite changes in Cg25. Reciprocal changes were seen in a dorsal part of the prefrontal cortex, labelled F9. F, frontal; cd, caudate nucleus; ins, anterior insula; Cg25, subgenual cingulate; Hth, hypothalamus; pCG31, posterior cingulate; R, right. (After Mayberg et al. 1999.) (See colour plates section.)

electrical stimulation in this region has been found to relieve symptoms of treatment-resistant depression in some patients (Mayberg et al. 2005).

Further, anatomical abnormalities of the orbitofrontal cortex are found in patients with depression (Bremner, Vythilingam, Vermetten, Nazeer, Adil, Khan, Staib and Charney 2002, Rajkowska 2000), in whom anhedonia is a key feature, and the orbitofrontal cortex provides inputs to the anterior and subgenual cingulate cortex.

Pharmacological investigations of depression and the effects these have on different brain systems are described in Section 8.6.

4.9 Output pathways for emotional responses

4.9.1 The autonomic and endocrine systems

The first output system introduced above in Section 4.2 is the autonomic and endocrine system. Through it changes such as increased heart rate and the release of adrenaline, which prepare the body for action, are produced by emotional stimuli. There are brainstem routes through which peripheral stimuli can produce reflex autonomic responses. In addition, there are outputs from the hypothalamus to the autonomic brainstem centres (Schwaber, Kapp, Higgins and Rapp 1982).

Structures such as the amygdala and orbitofrontal cortex can produce autonomic responses to secondary reinforcing (or classically conditioned) stimuli both directly, for example by direct connections from the amygdala to the dorsal motor nucleus of the vagus (Schwaber et al. 1982), and via the lateral hypothalamus. For example, LeDoux et al. (1988) showed that lesions of the lateral hypothalamus (which receives from the central nucleus of the amygdala) blocked conditioned heart rate (autonomic) responses (see also Kapp et al. (1992)). The outputs of the orbitofrontal cortex are also involved in learned autonomic responses, in that ventral prefrontal lesions block autonomic responses to learned reinforcers (Elithorn, Piercy and Crosskey (1955) and Damasio (1994) in humans; Grueninger, Kimble, Grueninger and Levine (1965) in macaques).

Further, activation of the anterior cingulate cortex in humans is correlated with autonomic states (Nagai et al. 2004), and the subgenual cingulate cortex has strong projections to brainstem structures that control autonomic activity (Gabbott et al. 2003).

4.9.2 Motor systems for implicit responses, including the basal ganglia

The second type of output is to brain systems concerned with performing actions unconsciously or implicitly, in order to obtain rewards or avoid punishers. These brain systems include the basal ganglia. For example, Cador, Robbins and Everitt (1989) obtained evidence consistent with the hypothesis that the learned incentive (conditioned reinforcing) effects of previously neutral stimuli paired with rewards are mediated by the amygdala acting through the ventral striatum (which includes the nucleus accumbens), in that amphetamine injections into the ventral striatum enhanced the effects of a conditioned reinforcing stimulus only if the amygdala was intact (see further Everitt and Robbins (1992), Everitt et al. (2000), and Cardinal et al. (2002)).

To analyse the functions of the ventral striatum, the responses of more than 1000 single neurons were recorded in a region that included the nucleus accumbens and olfactory tubercle in five macaque monkeys in test situations in which lesions of the amygdala, hippocampus and inferior temporal cortex produce deficits, and in which neurons in these structures respond (Rolls and Williams 1987a, Rolls 1990a, Williams, Rolls, Leonard and Stern 1993). While the monkeys performed visual discrimination and related feeding tasks, the different populations of neurons found included neurons that responded to novel visual stimuli; to reinforcer-related visual stimuli such as (for different neurons) food-related stimuli, aversive stimuli, or faces; to other visual stimuli; in relation to somatosensory stimulation and movement; or to cues that signalled the start of a task (see Section 8.4.3.1 on page 325). The neurons with responses to reinforcing or novel visual stimuli may reflect the inputs to the ventral striatum from the amygdala and hippocampus, and are consistent with the hypothesis that the ventral striatum provides a route for learned reinforcing and novel visual stimuli to influence behaviour.

The output for the shell, limbic-related, part of the nucleus accumbens is directed towards the ventral pallidum, and thus to the mediodorsal nucleus of the thalamus, which in turn projects to the prefrontal cortex. In primates, the outputs from brain regions such as the amygdala and orbitofrontal cortex spread though much beyond the ventral striatum, to the ventral parts of the head of the caudate nucleus (Kemp and Powell 1970). This other part of the striatum is important as an output route to behaviour for the amygdala and orbitofrontal cortex, in that damage to the head of the caudate nucleus can impair the performance of monkeys on tasks also affected by lesions of, for example, the orbitofrontal cortex, such as visual discrimination reversal (Divac et al. 1967, Divac and Oberg 1979, Oberg and Divac 1979, Iversen 1984). For example, in the monkey, lesions of the ventrolateral part of the head of the caudate nucleus (as of the orbitofrontal cortex which projects to it) impaired object reversal performance, which measures the ability to reverse stimulus–reinforcement associations. In contrast, lesions of the anterodorsal part of the head of the caudate nucleus disrupted delayed spatial alternation performance, a task that requires spatial short-term memory, which is also impaired by lesions of the corresponding cortical region, the dorsolateral prefrontal cortex. Lastly, lesions of the tail of the caudate nucleus (as of the inferior temporal visual cortex which projects to this part of the caudate) produced a visual pattern discrimination deficit (Divac et al. 1967). A fuller description of the functions of the ventral striatum as an output system for the effects of learned incentives decoded by the amygdala and orbitofrontal cortex to influence behaviour is provided in Chapter 8.

Other outputs for learned implicit behavioural responses may proceed from the amygdala through the midbrain, in that lesions of the central gray of the midbrain (which also receives from the central nucleus of the amygdala) blocked the conditioned freezing but not the conditioned autonomic response to the aversive conditioned stimulus (LeDoux et al. 1988, Pare et al. 2004).

action–outcome (or response-reinforcer association) learning itself may be implemented in parts of the prefrontal and cingulate cortex (Cardinal et al. 2002, Matsumoto et al. 2001, Rushworth et al. 2004). In the rat, the prelimbic cortex, which is part of the medial prefrontal cortex, appears to be involved in action–outcome contingency learning. For example, rats may be trained to perform two actions concurrently for two different food rewards. In addition, one of those reinforcers may be delivered non-contingently with respect to the subject's behaviour, so that the degree of action–outcome contingency is selectively degraded for this reinforcer. Balleine and Dickinson (1998) found that prelimbic lesions did make the rats insensitive to this contingency manipulation (although the lesions did not impair instrumental learning, which may have occurred using a habit, Stimulus–Response, system). The prelimbic cortex may receive information about the reward or affective value of the rewards from the orbitofrontal cortex and amygdala, in both of which it is represented, as described above.

4.9.3   Output systems for explicit responses to emotional stimuli

The third type of output is to a system capable of planning many steps ahead and, for example, deferring short-term rewards in order to execute a long-term plan. This system may use syntactic processing in order to perform the planning, and is therefore part of a linguistic system that performs explicit processing. This system, discussed in Chapter 10, is the one in which explicit, declarative, processing occurs. Processing in this system is frequently associated with reason and rationality, in that many of the consequences of possible actions can be taken into account. The actual computation of how rewarding a particular stimulus or situation is, or will be, probably still depends on activity in the orbitofrontal cortex and amygdala, in that the reward value of stimuli is computed and represented in these regions, and in that it is found that verbalized expressions of the reward (or punishment) value of stimuli are dampened by damage to these systems. (For example, damage to the orbitofrontal cortex renders painful input still identifiable as pain, but without the strong affective, 'unpleasant', reaction to it.)

4.9.4 Basal forebrain and hypothalamus

It was suggested above that the hypothalamus and basal forebrain may provide one output system for the amygdala and orbitofrontal cortex for autonomic and other responses to emotional stimuli. Consistent with this, there are neurons in the lateral hypothalamus and basal forebrain of monkeys that respond to visual stimuli associated with rewards such as food (Rolls 1975, Rolls 1981b, Rolls 1981a, Rolls 1982, Rolls 1986c, Rolls 1986a, Rolls 1986b, Rolls 1990d, Rolls 1993, Rolls 1999a, Rolls, Burton and Mora 1976, Burton, Rolls and Mora 1976, Mora, Rolls and Burton 1976b, Wilson and Rolls 1990b, Wilson and Rolls 1990a). These neurons show rapid reversal of their responses during the reversal of stimulus–reinforcer associations. Other neurons in the hypothalamus responded only to stimuli associated with punishment, that is to aversive visual stimuli (Rolls, Sanghera and Roper-Hall 1979a). The responses of these neurons with reinforcement-related activity would be appropriate for producing autonomic responses to emotional stimuli, via pathways that descend from the hypothalamus towards the brainstem autonomic motor nuclei (Saper, Loewy, Swanson and Cowan 1976, Schwaber et al. 1982). It is also possible that these outputs could influence emotional behaviour, through, for example, the connections from the hypothalamus to the amygdala (Aggleton, Burton and Passingham 1980), to the substantia nigra (Nauta and Domesick 1978), or even by the connections to the neocortex (Divac 1975, Kievit and Kuypers 1975). Indeed, it is suggested that the latter projection, by releasing acetylcholine in the cerebral cortex when emotional stimuli (including reinforcing and novel stimuli) are seen, provides one way in which emotion can influence the storage of memories in the cerebral cortex (Rolls 1987, Wilson and Rolls 1990c, Wilson and Rolls 1990b, Wilson and Rolls 1990a). In this case, the basal forebrain magnocellular neurons may act as a 'cortical strobe' which facilitates memory storage and processing when the neurons are firing fast.

4.9.5 Basal forebrain cholinergic neurons

Before leaving the learning systems in the amygdala and orbitofrontal cortex, it is useful to consider the role in memory of one of the systems to which they project, the basal forebrain magnocellular nuclei of Meynert. The cells in these nuclei lie just lateral to the lateral hypothalamus in the substantia innominata, and extend forward through the preoptic area into the diagonal band of Broca (Mesulam 1990). These cells, many of which are cholinergic, project directly to the cerebral cortex (Divac 1975, Kievit and Kuypers 1975, Mesulam 1990). These cells provide the major cholinergic input to the cerebral cortex, in that if they are lesioned the cortex is depleted of acetylcholine (Mesulam 1990). Loss of these cells does occur in Alzheimer's disease, and there is consequently a reduction in cortical acetylcholine in this disease (Mesulam 1990). This loss of cortical acetylcholine may contribute to the memory loss in Alzheimer's disease, although it may well not be the primary factor in the aetiology.

In order to investigate the role of the basal forebrain nuclei in memory, Aigner, Mitchell, Aggleton, DeLong, Struble, Price, Wenk, Pettigrew and Mishkin (1991) made neurotoxic lesions of them in monkeys. Some impairments on a simple test of recognition memory, delayed non-match-to-sample, were found. Analysis of the effects of similar lesions in rats showed that performance on memory tasks was impaired, perhaps because of failure to attend properly (Muir, Everitt and Robbins 1994). Damage to the cholinergic neurons in this region in monkeys with a selective neurotoxin was also shown to impair memory (Easton and Gaffan 2000, Easton, Ridley, Baker and Gaffan 2002).

There are quite limited numbers of these basal forebrain neurons (in the order of thousands). Given that there are relatively few of these neurons, it is not likely that they carry the information to be stored in cortical memory circuits, for the number of different patterns that could be represented and stored is so small. (The number of different patterns that could be stored is dependent in a leading way on the number of input connections on to each neuron in a pattern associator, see Appendix 1.) With this few neurons distributed throughout the cerebral cortex, the memory capacity of the whole system would be impractically small. This argument alone indicates that they are unlikely to carry the information to be stored in cortical memory systems. Instead, they could modulate information storage in the cortex of information derived from what provides the numerically major input to cortical neurons, the glutamatergic terminals of other cortical neurons. This modulation may operate by setting thresholds for cortical cells to the appropriate value, or by more directly influencing the cascade of processes involved in long-term potentiation (see Appendix 1). There is indeed evidence that acetylcholine is necessary for cortical synaptic modifiability, as shown by studies in which depletion of acetylcholine and noradrenaline impaired cortical LTP/synaptic modifiability (Bear and Singer 1986). However, non-specific effects of damage to the basal forebrain cholinergic neurons are also likely, with cortical neurons becoming much more sluggish in their responses, and showing much more adaptation, in the absence of cholinergic inputs (Markram and Tsodyks 1996, Abbott, Varela, Sen and Nelson 1996b) (see below).

The question then arises of whether the basal forebrain cholinergic neurons tonically release acetylcholine, or whether they release it particularly in response to some external influence. To examine this, recordings have been made from basal forebrain neurons, at least some of which project to the cortex (see Section 5.4.1.2) and will have been the cholinergic neurons just described. It has been found that some of these neurons respond to visual stimuli associated with rewards such as food (Rolls 1975, Rolls 1981b, Rolls 1981a, Rolls 1982, Rolls 1986c, Rolls 1986a, Rolls 1986b, Rolls 1990d, Rolls 1993, Rolls 1999a, Rolls, Burton and Mora 1976, Burton, Rolls and Mora 1976, Mora, Rolls and Burton 1976b, Wilson and Rolls 1990b, Wilson and Rolls 1990a) (see example in Fig. 5.10 on page 236), or with punishment (Rolls, Sanghera and Roper-Hall 1979a), that others respond to novel visual stimuli (Wilson and Rolls 1990c), and that others respond to a range of visual stimuli. For example, in one set of recordings, one group of these neurons (1.5%) responded to novel visual stimuli while monkeys performed recognition or visual discrimination tasks (Wilson and Rolls 1990c). A complementary group of neurons more anteriorly responded to familiar visual stimuli in the same tasks (Rolls, Perrett, Caan and Wilson 1982c, Wilson and Rolls 1990c). A third group of neurons (5.7%) responded to positively reinforcing visual stimuli in visual discrimination and in recognition memory tasks (Wilson and Rolls 1990b, Wilson and Rolls 1990a). In addition, a considerable proportion of these neurons (21.8%) responded to any visual stimuli shown in the tasks, and some (13.1%) responded to the tone cue that preceded the presentation of the visual stimuli in the task, and was provided to enable the monkey to alert to the visual stimuli (Wilson and Rolls 1990c). These neurons did not respond to touch to the leg which induced arousal, so their responses did not simply reflect arousal. Neurons in this region receive inputs from the amygdala (see Mesulam (1990); Amaral et al. (1992); Russchen, Amaral and

Price (1985)) and orbitofrontal cortex, and it is probably via the amygdala (and orbitofrontal cortex) that the information described here reaches the basal forebrain neurons, for neurons with similar response properties have been found in the amygdala, and the amygdala appears to be involved in decoding visual stimuli that are associated with reinforcers, or are novel (Rolls 1990d, Rolls 1992b, Rolls 2000d, Wilson and Rolls 1993, Wilson and Rolls 2005).

It is therefore suggested that the normal physiological function of these basal forebrain neurons is to send a general activation signal to the cortex when certain classes of environmental stimulus occur. These stimuli are often stimuli to which behavioural activation is appropriate or required, such as positively or negatively reinforcing visual stimuli, or novel visual stimuli. The effect of the firing of these neurons on the cortex is excitatory, and in this way produces activation. This cortical activation may produce behavioural arousal, and may thus facilitate concentration and attention, which are both impaired in Alzheimer's disease. The reduced arousal and concentration may themselves contribute to the memory disorders. But the acetylcholine released from these basal magnocellular neurons may in addition be more directly necessary for memory formation, for Bear and Singer (1986) showed that long-term potentiation, used as an indicator of the synaptic modification which underlies learning, requires the presence in the cortex of acetylcholine as well as noradrenaline. For comparison, acetylcholine in the hippocampus makes it more likely that LTP will occur, probably through activation of an inositol phosphate second messenger cascade (Markram and Siegel 1992, Seigel and Auerbach 1996, Hasselmo and Bower 1993, Hasselmo, Schnell and Barkai 1995).

The adaptive value of the cortical strobe provided by the basal magnocellular neurons may thus be that it facilitates memory storage especially when significant (e.g. reinforcing) environmental stimuli are detected. This means that memory storage is likely to be conserved (new memories are less likely to be laid down) when significant environmental stimuli are not present. In that the basal forebrain projection spreads widely to many areas of the cerebral cortex, and in that there are relatively few basal forebrain neurons (in the order of thousands), the basal forebrain neurons do not determine the actual memories that are stored. Instead the actual memories stored are determined by the active subset of the thousands of cortical afferents on to a strongly activated cortical neuron (Treves and Rolls 1994, Rolls and Treves 1998). The basal forebrain magnocellular neurons would then according to this analysis simply when activated increase the probability that a memory would be stored. Impairment of the normal operation of the basal forebrain magnocellular neurons would be expected to interfere with normal memory by interfering with this function, and this interference could contribute in this way to the memory disorder in Alzheimer's disease.

Another property of cortical neurons (Markram and Tsodyks 1996, Abbott et al. 1996b) is that they tend to adapt with repeated input. However, this adaptation is most marked in slices, in which there is no acetylcholine. One effect of acetylcholine is to reduce this adaptation. When recordings are made from single neurons operating in physiological conditions in the awake behaving monkey, peristimulus time histograms of inferior temporal cortex neurons to visual stimuli show only limited adaptation. There is typically an onset of the neuronal response at 80–100 ms after the stimulus, followed within 50 ms by the highest firing rate. There is after that some reduction in the firing rate, but the firing rate is still typically more than half maximal 500 ms later (see example in Fig. 4.11 on page 85). Thus under normal physiological conditions, firing rate adaptation can occur, but does not involve a major adaptation, even when cells are responding fast (at e.g. 100 spikes/s) to a visual stimulus. One of the factors that keeps the response relatively maintained may however be the presence of acetylcholine. Its depletion in some disease states could lead to less sustained neuronal responses (i.e. more adaptation), and this may contribute to the symptoms found.

4.9.6 Noradrenergic neurons

The source of the noradrenergic projection to the neocortex is the locus coeruleus (noradrenergic cell group A6) in the pons (Cooper, Bloom and Roth 2003). (Note that noradrenaline is the same as norepinephrine.) There are a few thousand of these neurons that innervate the whole of the cerebral cortex, as well as the amygdala and other structures, so it is unlikely that the noradrenergic neurons convey the specific information stored in synapses that specifies each memory. Instead, to the extent that the noradrenergic neurons are involved in memory (including pattern association), it is likely that they would have a modulatory role on cell excitability, which would influence the extent to which the voltage-dependent NMDA receptors are activated, and thus the likelihood that information carried on specific afferents would be stored (Seigel and Auerbach 1996). Evidence that this may be the case comes from a study in which it was shown that neocortical LTP is impaired if noradrenergic and simultaneously cholinergic inputs to cortical cells are blocked pharmacologically (Bear and Singer 1986).

Further, in a study designed to show whether the noradrenergic modulation is necessary for memory, Borsini and Rolls (1984) showed that intra-amygdaloid injections of noradrenergic receptor blockers did impair the type of learning in which rats gradually learned to accept novel foods.

The function implemented by this noradrenergic input may more be general activation, rather than a signal that carries information about whether reward vs punishment has been given, for noradrenergic neurons in rats respond to both rewarding and punishing stimuli, and one of the more effective stimuli for producing release of noradrenaline is placing the feet in cool water (McGinty and Szymusiak 1988).

4.10 Effects of emotion on cognitive processing and memory

The analyses above of the neural mechanisms of emotion have been concerned primarily with how stimuli are decoded to produce emotional states, and with how these states can influence behaviour. In addition, current mood state can affect the cognitive evaluation of events or memories (Blaney 1986). For example, happy memories are more likely to be recalled when happy. Another example is that when people are in a depressed mood, they tend to recall memories that were stored when they were depressed. The recall of depressing memories when depressed can have the effect of perpetuating the depression, and this may be a factor with relevance to the aetiology and treatment of depression.

A normal function of the effects of mood state on memory recall might be to facilitate continuity in the interpretation of the reinforcing value of events in the environment, or in the interpretation of an individual's behaviour by others, or simply to keep behaviour motivated to a particular goal. Another possibility is that the effects of mood on memory do not have adaptive value, but are a consequence of having a general cortical architecture with backprojections. According to the latter hypothesis, the selection pressure is great for leaving the general architecture operational, rather than trying to find a genetic way to switch off

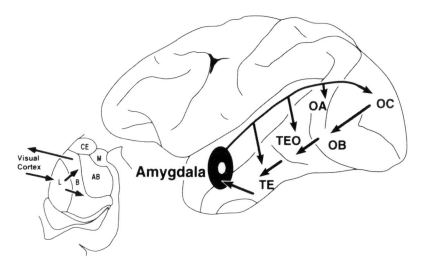

Fig. 4.63 The backprojections from the primate amygdala to the cortex spread more widely than the afferent connections, which for vision come mainly from the inferior temporal visual cortical areas, e.g. area TE. OC, striate cortex; OB, OA, prestriate visual cortical areas; TEO, posterior inferior temporal visual cortex. The insert to the left shows a coronal section of the primate amygdala, with lateral on the left, to indicate that many of the visual cortical afferents reach the lateral nucleus of the amygdala (L), and that many of the backprojections arise from the basal nucleus of the amygdala (B). CE, central nucleus of the amygdala; AB, accessory basal nucleus; M, medial nucleus. (Reproduced with permission from Amaral et al. 1992.)

backprojections just for the projections of mood systems back to perceptual systems, some of which are illustrated in Fig. 4.63 (cf. Rolls and Stringer (2000)).

How does mood affect memory?

It is suggested that whenever memories are stored, part of the context is stored with the memory. This is very likely to happen in associative neuronal networks such as those in the hippocampus (Rolls 1989a, Rolls 2000c, Rolls 1990c, Rolls 1996b, Treves and Rolls 1994, Rolls and Treves 1998, Rolls, Stringer and Trappenberg 2002, Rolls 2004f, Rolls and Kesner 2006). The CA3 part of the hippocampus may operate as a single autoassociative memory capable of linking together almost arbitrary co-occurrences of inputs, including inputs about emotional state that reach the entorhinal cortex from, for example, the amygdala. Recall of a memory occurs best in such networks when the input key to the memory is nearest to the original input pattern of activity that was stored (Rolls and Treves 1990, Treves and Rolls 1991, Treves and Rolls 1992, Treves and Rolls 1994, Rolls, Treves, Foster and Perez-Vicente 1997c, Rolls and Treves 1998, Rolls and Deco 2002) (see Appendix 1). It thus follows that a memory of, for example, a happy episode is recalled best when in a happy mood state. This is a special case of a general theory of how context is stored with a memory, and of how context influences recall (Treves and Rolls 1994, Rolls 1996b). The recall itself from the hippocampus is likely to use the highly developed backprojections from the hippocampus to the neocortex shown in Fig. 10.1 on page 402 (Treves and Rolls 1994, Rolls 1996b). The effect of emotional state on cognitive processing and memory is thus suggested to be a particular case of a more general way in which context can affect the storage and retrieval of memories,

a. Neuronal responses to rewards at locations in 3 scenes

c. Spatial arrangement

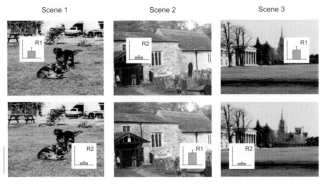

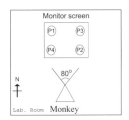

b. Place-Reward firing

d. Recording site

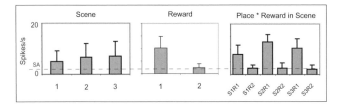

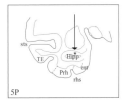

Fig. 4.64 A hippocampal neuron that encoded the particular rewards available at different locations in different scenes. On each trial the monkey could touch a circled location in the scene, and, depending on the location, received either a preferred juice reward or a less preferred juice reward. a. Firing rate inserts to show the firing in 3 different scenes (S1–S3) of the locations associated with reward 1 (R1, preferred) and reward 2 (R2, less preferred). The mean responses ± s.e.m. are shown. SA, spontaneous firing rate. b. The firing rates sorted by scene, by reward (1 vs 2), and by scene–reward combinations (e.g. scene 1 reward 1 = S1R1). c. The spatial arrangement on the screen of the 4 spatial locations (P1–P4). d. The recording site of the neuron. ent, entorhinal cortex; Hipp, hippocampal pyramidal cell field CA3/CA1 and dentate gyrus; Prh, perirhinal cortex; rhs, rhinal sulcus; sts, superior temporal sulcus; TE, inferior temporal visual cortex. (After Rolls and Xiang 2005a.)

or can affect cognitive processing.

There is now direct evidence that the hippocampus, which is implicated in the memory for past episodes (Rolls and Treves 1998, Rolls 1999c, Rolls et al. 2002), contains neurons in primates that respond to combinations of spatial information and reward information (Rolls and Xiang 2005), as described next. The ability to form associations between events including where they occur and what is present is a fundamental property of episodic memory (Treves and Rolls 1994, Rolls 1996b, Rolls and Kesner 2006), and this new neurophysiological evidence shows that reward-related information, relevant to affect and mood, is associated with other events in the representations in the primate hippocampus. The primate anterior hippocampus (which corresponds to the rodent ventral hippocampus) receives inputs from brain regions involved in reward processing such as the amygdala and orbitofrontal cortex (Amaral et al. 1992, Suzuki and Amaral 1994, Pitkanen, Kelly and Amaral 2002, Stefanacci, Suzuki and Amaral 1996).

To investigate how this affective input may be incorporated into primate hippocampal function, Rolls and Xiang (2005) recorded neuronal activity while macaques performed a reward–place association task in which each spatial scene shown on a video monitor had one location that if touched yielded a preferred fruit juice reward, and a second location that yielded a less preferred juice reward. Each scene had different locations for the different rewards. An example of a hippocampal neuron recorded in this task is shown in Fig. 4.64 on page 196. The neuron responded more to the location in each scene at which the preferred reward was available.

Of 409 neurons analysed, 16% responded more to the location of the preferred reward in different scenes, and 4% to the location of the less preferred reward (Rolls and Xiang 2005). When the locations of the preferred rewards in the scenes were reversed, 70% of 50 neurons tested reversed the location to which they responded, showing that the reward–place associations could be altered by new learning in a few trials. The majority (80%) of these 50 reward–place neurons tested did not respond to object-reward associations in a visual discrimination object–reward association task. Thus the primate hippocampus contains a representation of the reward associations of places 'out there' being viewed, and this is a way in which affective information can be stored as part of an episodic memory, and how the current mood state may influence the retrieval of episodic memories. There is consistent recent evidence that rewards available in a spatial environment can influence the responsiveness of rodent place neurons (Hölscher, Jacob and Mallot 2003a, Tabuchi, Mulder and Wiener 2003) which respond to the place where the animal is located, not to the view of a place 'out there' (Rolls 1999c, De Araujo, Rolls and Stringer 2001).

This discovery of reward–spatial view neurons built on findings that some hippocampal neurons in primates respond to the place at which the monkey is looking. These spatial view neurons (Rolls, Robertson and Georges-François 1997a, Rolls, Treves, Robertson, Georges-François and Panzeri 1998b, Robertson, Rolls and Georges-François 1998, Rolls 1999c) code for particular locations at which the monkey is looking in allocentric (world-based rather than egocentric) space, and do not encode the place where the monkey is located (Georges-François, Rolls and Robertson 1999, Rolls, Treves, Robertson, Georges-François and Panzeri 1998b). Part of the interest of spatial view cells is that they could provide the spatial representation required to enable primates to perform object–place memory, for example remembering where they saw a person or object, which is an example of an episodic memory. Consistent with this, some hippocampal neurons respond in object-place memory tasks to combinations of the object being shown and where it is being shown in space (Rolls, Miyashita, Cahusac, Kesner, Niki, Feigenbaum and Bach 1989a, Rolls, Xiang and Franco 2005c). Further evidence for this convergence of spatial and object information in the hippocampus is that in another memory task for which the hippocampus is needed, learning where to make spatial responses conditional on which picture is shown, some primate hippocampal neurons respond to a combination of which picture is shown, and where the response must be made (Miyashita, Rolls, Cahusac, Niki and Feigenbaum 1989, Cahusac, Rolls, Miyashita and Niki 1993). Thus the primate hippocampus contains a representation of places 'out there', and can combine this information by associative learning not only with which object is present at the viewed location (Rolls, Xiang and Franco 2005c, Rolls and Xiang 2006), but also with which reward is present at the viewed location (Rolls and Xiang 2005).

The general principle here then is that the hippocampus may store information about where emotion-related (e.g. rewarding) events happened; may take part in the recall of emotions when particular places are seen again; and may provide a system in which the current mood can influence which memories are recalled.

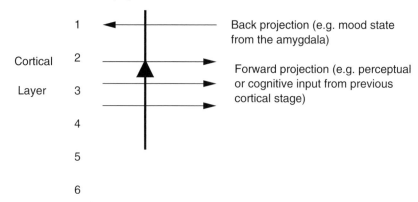

Fig. 4.65 Pyramidal cells in, for example, layers 2 and 3 of the temporal lobe association cortex receive forward inputs from preceding cortical stages of processing, and also backprojections from the amygdala. It is suggested that the backprojections from the amygdala make modifiable synapses on the apical dendrites of cortical pyramidal cells during learning when amygdala neurons are active in relation to a mood state; and that the backprojections from the amygdala via these modified synapses allow mood state to influence later cognitive processing, for example by facilitating some perceptual representations.

Another brain system where effects of mood on storage and recall could be instantiated is in the backprojection system from structures important in emotion such as the amygdala and orbitofrontal cortex to parts of the cerebral cortex important in the representation of objects, such as the inferior temporal visual cortex (see Fig. 4.63), and more generally, to parts of the cerebral cortex involved in storing memories. It is suggested (Rolls 1989a, Rolls 1989d, Rolls 1990b, Treves and Rolls 1994, Rolls and Treves 1998, Rolls 2000b) that co-activity between forward inputs and backprojecting inputs to strongly activated cortical pyramidal cells would lead to both sets of synapses being modified (see Fig. 4.65). This could result in facilitation or recall of cortical representations (for example of particular faces) that had become associated with emotional states, represented by activity in the amygdala (see further Rolls (1990d)).

Rolls and Stringer (2001b) (see also Rolls (1989a) and Rolls (1999a)) have developed a theory of how the effects of mood on memory and perception could be implemented in the brain. The architecture, shown in Fig. 4.66, uses the massive backprojections from parts of the brain where mood is represented, such as the orbitofrontal cortex and amygdala, to the cortical areas such as the inferior temporal visual cortex and hippocampus-related areas (labelled IT in Fig. 4.66) that project into these mood-representing areas (Amaral, Price, Pitkanen and Carmichael 1992, Amaral and Price 1984). The model uses an attractor network (see Appendix 1 Section A.3) in the mood module (labelled amygdala in Fig. 4.66), which helps the mood to be an enduring state, and also an attractor in the inferior temporal visual cortex (IT) (or any other cortical area that receives backprojections from the amygdala or orbitofrontal cortex). The system is treated as a system of coupled attractors (see Appendix 1 Section A.4), but with an odd twist: many different perceptual states are associated with any one mood state. Overall, there is a large number of perceptual/ memory states, and only a few mood states, so that there is a many-to-one relation between perceptual/memory states and the associated mood states. The network displays the properties that one would expect (provided that the coupling parameters g (see Appendix 1, Section A.4) are weak). These include the ability of a perceptual input to trigger a mood state in the 'amygdala' module if

Memory or Perceptual state

Mood state

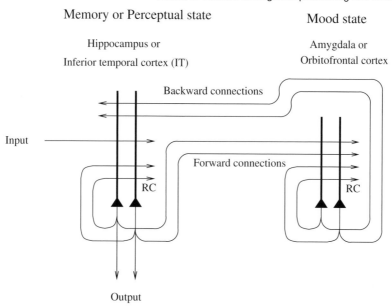

Hippocampus or
Inferior temporal cortex (IT)

Amygdala or
Orbitofrontal cortex

Fig. 4.66 Architecture used to investigate how mood can affect perception and memory. The IT module represents brain areas such as the inferior temporal cortex involved in perception and hippocampus-related cortical areas that have forward connections to regions such as the amygdala and orbitofrontal cortex involved in mood. (After Rolls and Stringer 2001.)

there is not an existing mood, but greater difficulty to induce a new mood if there is already a strong mood attractor present; and the ability of the mood to affect via the backprojections which memories or perceptual states are triggered.

Another interesting finding was that the forward connections to the mood module from the memory module must be relatively strong, if new inputs to the memory module are to alter the firing in the mood module by overcoming an existing mood state being kept active by the recurrent collateral connections. These results are consistent with the general effects needed for forward and backward projections in the brain, namely that forward projections must be relatively strong in order to produce new firing in a module when a new (forward) input is received, and backward projections must be relatively weak, if they are to mildly implement 'top-down' constraints without dominating the activity of earlier modules (Renart, Parga and Rolls 1999b, Renart, Parga and Rolls 1999a, Renart, Moreno, Rocha, Parga and Rolls 2001, Rolls and Deco 2002, Deco and Rolls 2004, Deco and Rolls 2005b). Consistent with this, forward projections terminate on cortical neurons closer to the cell body (where they can have a stronger influence) than backprojections (which typically terminate on the distal extremities of the apical dendrite of cortical neurons, in layer 1, the top layer of the cortex (see Rolls and Treves (1998), Chapter 10).

An interesting property that was revealed by the model is that because of the many-to-few mapping of perceptual to mood states, an effect of a mood was that it tended to make all the perceptual or memory states associated with a particular mood more similar then they would otherwise have been (Rolls and Stringer 2001b). The implication is that the coupling parameter g for the backprojections must be quite weak, as otherwise interference increases in the perceptual/memory module (IT in Fig. 4.66).

In conclusion, emotional states may affect whether or how strongly memories are stored using the basal forebrain memory strobe (see Section 4.9.5); be stored as part of many memories in for example the hippocampus; and may influence both the recall of such memories, and the operation of cognitive processing, using backprojections in the way described in the preceding paragraphs. In turn, cognitive inputs can influence affective states, as described in Chapter 2 and Section 4.5.5.7.

4.11   Laterality effects in human emotional processing

In humans, there is some lateralization of function of emotional processing, with the right hemisphere frequently being implicated in processing face expressions. Some of the evidence for this is reviewed next.

A first type of evidence comes from the effects of brain damage in humans. Damage to the left hemisphere (in right handed people) is more likely to affect language, and to the right hemisphere is more likely to affect emotional processing. This may be evident, for example, in the greater probability of impairments in recognizing facial expressions after right rather than left hemisphere damage (see Etcoff (1989)). Further, patients are more likely to be depressed by a stroke if it is to the left than to the right hemisphere (see Starkstein and Robinson (1991)). This may indicate that to feel depressed, the right hemisphere is normally involved.

A second type of evidence comes from split brain patients (with the corpus callosum sectioned to prevent epilepsy on one side affecting the other side of the brain). These patients may respond behaviourally to an emotion-provoking stimulus which reaches the right hemisphere, even though they cannot specify verbally (with the left hemisphere) what they saw (Gazzaniga 1988). This is clear evidence for separate processing of implicit information about emotion in humans that can be dissociated from explicit, language-based, systems (see Section 10.3).

Third, when faces are flashed rapidly on a screen, there may be better performance in identifying the expression on the face when the stimulus is projected to the right than to the left hemisphere (Strauss and Moscowitsch 1981). These effects on face expression identification are not produced just because face-processing modules are lateralized to the right hemisphere: face identification deficits are not necessarily associated with face expression identification impairments.

Fourth, emotions may be more clearly expressed on the left side than the right side of the face, suggesting some specialization of the right hemisphere in controlling face expression (Nicholls, Ellis, Clement and Yoshino 2004). There may further be a weak specialization of the right hemisphere for negative emotions, as there is a trend for left-sided face expression to occur more for negative than positive emotions. Further, a left-sided view of the face was judged as being sadder and a right-sided view was rated as being happier (Nicholls et al. 2004). Consistent with a valence effect whereby the right hemisphere may be more related to negative (e.g. sad) emotions, Davidson, Ekman, Saron, Senulis and Friesen (1990) and Davidson (1992) have some evidence from EEG recording that for negative emotional episodes there is more activation of the right side of the brain; and for positive episodes there is more activation of the left side of the brain. However, there may be individual differences in the activation of prefrontal areas that are related to the affective reactivity of the individual (Davidson 2003).

Why should there be some lateralization of emotional processing in humans? One argument is that whenever a function does not need to be represented bilaterally due to the topology of the body (e.g. we have left and right hands, and separate representations of each hand are needed), then it is more efficient to place the group of neurons concerned with that processing close together. One advantage of placing neurons concerned with similar processing close together is that the length of the connections between the neurons will be minimized. This is important for minimizing brain size and weight, which is a significant factor in evolution. If half the neurons concerned with a particular function were on one side of the brain, and the other half were on the contralateral side, then the total length of the connections between the neurons would be large (see further Rolls and Deco (2002) Section 7.4.6).

Neurons concerned with the same function are frequently interconnected for a number of reasons. One is that there are recurrent collateral axons between nearby cortical neurons concerned with the same function. One of the functions performed by these excitatory recurrent collaterals is to enable the network to act as a local attractor or autoassociation memory, so that the output of the module can take into account not only the activation produced in any one neuron, but also the activations received by the other connected neurons (see Appendix 1, Section A.3). Another way in which this is performed is by using feedback inhibitory interneurons, which are activated by many of the cortical pyramidal cells in a region. This helps not only autoassociation (and pattern association) networks to remain stable, but also is important for competitive networks, in which categorization of stimuli occurs, by effectively allowing the neurons in a population with the strongest activation by a particular stimulus to remain active (see Rolls and Treves (1998), Chapter 4, and Rolls and Deco (2002), Chapter 7).

A second advantage of placing neurons concerned with the same function close together is that this may simplify the wiring rules between neurons which must be implemented genetically (see further Rolls and Deco (2002) Section 7.4.6). Given that there are in the order of 35,000 genes in the human genome, and more than 10^{14} synapses, it is clearly impossible for genes to specify all the connections between every neuron. Instead, the genetic rules may specify, for example, that neurons of type y receive approximately 12,000 excitatory synapses with associative long-term potentiation and heterosynaptic long-term depression from other neurons of type y in the surrounding 2 mm (this forms a recurrent collateral pathway); make approximately 12,000 excitatory synapses with associative long-term potentiation and heterosynaptic long-term depression with neurons of type z up to 4 mm away (which might be the next cortical area); receive approximately 500 synapses from neurons of type I within 2 mm (which might be GABA-containing inhibitory feedback neurons); and receive approximately 6000 inputs from neurons of type x up to 4 mm away (which might be the pyramidal cells in the preceding cortical area). This type of specification would build many of the networks found in different brain regions (see Rolls and Stringer (2000) and Rolls and Treves (1998)).

An advantage of this type of genetic specification of connectivity between neuron types, and of keeping neurons concerned with the same computation close together, is that this minimizes the problems of guidance of axons towards their targets. If neurons concerned with the same function were randomly distributed in the brain, then finding the distant correct neurons with which to connect would be an impossible guidance problem. (As it is, some distant parts of the brain that are connected in adults are connected because the connections can be made early in development, before the different brain regions have migrated to become possibly distant.)

All these constraints imply that wherever possible neurons performing the same computation should be close together. Where there is no body-symmetry reason to have separate representations for each side of the body, then the representation would optimally be lateralized. This appears to be the case for certain aspects of emotional processing.

However, it is of interest that this lateralization of function may itself give rise to lateralization of performance. It may be because the brain mechanisms concerned with face expression identification are better represented in the right hemisphere that expression identification is better for the left half of the visual field (which might correspond to the left half of a centrally fixated face). Another possible reason for partial lateralization of human emotion may be that language is predominantly in the left hemisphere (for right-handed people). The result of this may be that although explicit (conscious, verbal) processing related to emotion (see Chapter 10) may take place in the left hemisphere, the implicit type of processing may take place preferentially where there is room in the brain, that is with a bias for the right hemisphere. The suggestion that there are these two types of output route for emotional behaviour is made in Section 4.9, and in Chapter 10. The fact that they are to some extent separate types of output processing may account for the fact that they can be placed in different modules, which happen to be to some extent in different hemispheres.

4.12 Summary

Some of the fundamental architectural and design principles of the brain for sensory, reward, and punishment information processing relevant to emotion in primates *including humans* include the following:

1. For primary reinforcers, the reward decoding may occur after several stages of processing, as in the primate taste system in which reward is decoded only after the primary taste cortex. The architectural principle here is that in primates there is one main taste information-processing stream in the brain, via the thalamus to the primary taste cortex, and the information about the identity of the taste is not biased with modulation by how good the taste is before this. Thus the taste representation in the primary taste cortex can be used for purposes that are not reward-dependent. For example, it may be important to learn about a particular taste, even if one is not hungry. Even for the primary reinforcers of pleasant touch and pain, although there are different peripheral nerve fibres for pain and touch, it appears that the affective component in primates involves especially the activation of higher cortical areas such as the orbitofrontal cortex, as shown by functional neuroimaging studies and by the effects of damage to the orbitofrontal cortex.

2. For potential secondary reinforcers, analysis is to the stage of invariant object identification in structures such as the inferior temporal visual cortex before reward and punisher associations are learned. The reason for this is to enable correct generalization to other instances of the same or similar objects, when a reward or punisher has been associated with as little as one instance (e.g. one view of an object) previously.

3. The representation of the object provided at the end of 'what' processing streams (e.g. the inferior temporal visual cortex) is (appropriately) in a form which is ideal as an input to pattern associators which allow the associations with primary reinforcers to be learned at the next stage of processing. The representations are appropriately encoded in that they can be decoded by dot product decoding of the type that is very neuronally plausible; are distributed so allowing excellent generalization and graceful degradation; have relatively independent information conveyed by different neurons in the ensemble thus allowing very high capacity; and allow much of the information to be read off very quickly, in periods of 20–50 ms.

4. Especially in primates, the visual processing in emotional and social behaviour requires sophisticated representation of individuals, and for this there are many neurons devoted to face processing. In addition, there is a separate system that encodes face gesture, movement, and view, as all are important in social behaviour, for interpreting whether a particular individual, with his or her own reinforcement associations, is producing threats or appeasements.

5. After mainly unimodal processing to the object level, sensory systems then project into convergence zones. Those especially important for reward and punishment, emotion and motivation, are the orbitofrontal cortex and amygdala, where primary reinforcers are represented. These parts of the brain appear to be especially important in emotion and motivation not only because they are the parts of the brain where in primates the primary (unlearned) reinforcing value of stimuli is represented, but also because they are the parts of the brain that perform pattern-association learning between potential secondary reinforcers and primary reinforcers. They are thus the parts of the brain involved in learning the emotional and motivational value of stimuli.

6. The orbitofrontal cortex is involved in the rapid, one-trial, reversal of emotional behaviour when the reinforcement contingencies change, and this may be implemented by switching a rule. The rapid reversal which is provided by the orbitofrontal cortex much more than the amygdala may be facilitated by the recurrent collateral connections between neurons in the orbitofrontal cortex, which provide for a short term memory of the current rule. The orbitofrontal cortex thus allows flexibility of emotional behaviour, and rapid sensitivity to the changes in the reinforcers being received. This is very important in primates (including humans), in which it is important in social situations to change behaviour rapidly to what may be subtle cues, such as changes in face expression.

7. Cognitive inputs and states that are decoded as reinforcing and thus lead to emotions are represented in the orbitofrontal cortex. An example is monetary reward or loss. Modulation by cognition of the reinforcement or subjective affective value of stimuli also is expressed in the orbitofrontal cortex. An example is the modulating effect that a word can have on the pleasantness vs unpleasantness of a test odour, which is represented in the orbitofrontal cortex.

8. Damage to the orbitofrontal cortex in humans can affect subjective emotional states, can impair emotional behaviour (producing for example some disinhibition and uncooperativeness), can be associated with personality changes including increased impulsiveness, and can impair the ability to identify correctly face and voice expressions.

9. The outputs of the amygdala are involved in many Pavlovian (conditioned) effects of stimuli on behaviour, including the elicitation of autonomic responses, and via the ventral striatum of Pavlovian effects on instrumental behaviour, such as Pavlovian-instrumental transfer (PIT).

10. The outputs of the orbitofrontal cortex may be used in structures such as the anterior cingulate cortex for action–outcome learning; in the basal ganglia for stimulus–response (habit) learning; and via the anterior cingulate cortex and lateral hypothalamus for autonomic responses to emotion-provoking stimuli.

11. A separate route to action is provided by an explicit, language-based system, for humans can sometimes state verbally what action they should have taken to a reinforcer, even though after orbitofrontal cortex damage they may not have made the appropriate choice when reinforcement contingencies change.

12. In non-primates including, for example, rodents, the design principles may involve less sophisticated design features, partly because the stimuli being processed are simpler. For example, view-invariant object recognition is probably much less developed in non-primates, with the recognition that is possible being based more on physical similarity in terms of texture, colour, simple features, etc. It may be because there is less sophisticated cortical processing of visual stimuli in this way that other sensory systems are also organized more simply, with, for example, some (but not total, only perhaps 30%) modulation of taste processing by hunger early in sensory processing in rodents (Rolls and Scott 2003), and even connectivity of the taste system that allows brainstem taste processing to gain direct access to the amygdala without cortical processing. Further, while it is appropriate usually to have emotional responses to well-processed objects or individuals (e.g. the sight of a particular person), there are instances, such as a loud noise or a pure tone associated with punishment, where it may be possible to tap off a sensory representation early in sensory information processing that can be used to produce emotional responses, and this may occur, for example, in rodents, where the subcortical auditory system provides afferents to the amygdala.

4.13 Colour plates

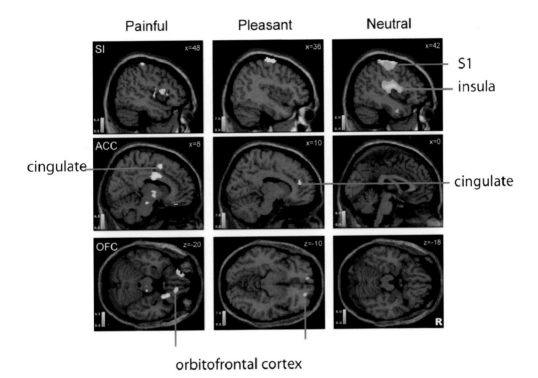

Fig. 4.4. Brain activation to painful, pleasant and neutral touch of the human brain. The top row shows strongest activation of the somatosensory cortex S1/insula by the neutral touch, on sagittal sections (parallel to the midline). The middle row shows activation of the most anterior part of the anterior cingulate cortex by the pleasant touch, and of a more posterior part by the painful touch, on sagittal sections. The bottom row shows activation of the orbitofrontal cortex by the pleasant and by the painful touch, on axial sections (in the horizontal plane). The activations were thresholded at p<0.0001 to show the extent of the activations. (After Rolls, O'Doherty et al., 2003d.)

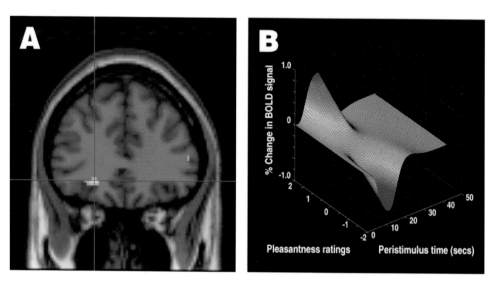

Fig. 4.22. Areas of the human orbitofrontal cortex with activations correlating with pleasantness ratings for food in the mouth. (A) Coronal section through the region of the orbitofrontal cortex from the random effects group analysis showing the peak in the left orbitofrontal cortex (Talairach co-ordinates X,Y,Z=–22,34,–8, z-score=4.06), in which the BOLD signal in the voxels shown in yellow was significantly correlated with the subjects' subjective pleasantness ratings of the foods throughout an experiment in which the subjects were hungry and found the food pleasant, and were then fed to satiety with the food, after which the pleasantness of the food decreased to neutral or slightly unpleasant. The design was a sensory-specific satiety design, and the pleasantness of the food not eaten in the meal, and the BOLD activation in the orbitofrontal cortex, were not altered by eating the other food to satiety. The two foods were tomato juice and chocolate milk. (B) Plot of the magnitude of the fitted haemodynamic response from a representative single subject against the subjective pleasantness ratings (on a scale from –2 to +2) and peristimulus time in seconds. (After Kringelbach, O'Doherty, Rolls and Andrews, 2003.)

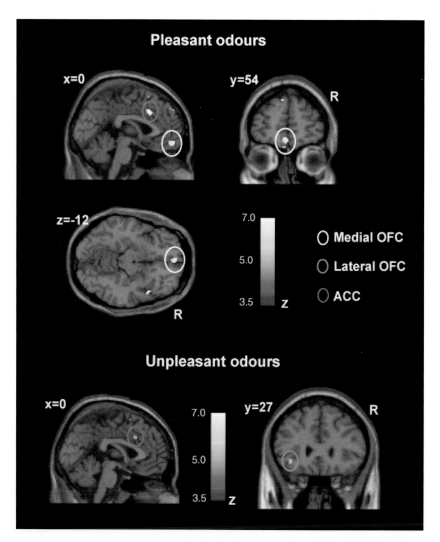

Fig. 4.25 The representation of pleasant and unpleasant odours in the human brain. Above : Group conjunction results for the 3 pleasant odours. Sagittal, horizontal and coronal views are shown at the levels indicated, all including the same activation in the medial orbitofrontal cortex, OFC (X,Y,Z = 0,54,–12; z=5.23). Also shown is activation for the 3 pleasant odours in the anterior cingulate cortex, ACC (X,Y,Z= 2,20,32; z=5.44). These activations were significant at p<0.05 fully corrected for multiple comparisons. Below : Group conjunction results for the 3 unpleasant odours. The sagittal view (left) shows an activated region of the anterior cingulate cortex (X,Y,Z= 0,18,36; z=4.42, p<0.05, S.V.C.). The coronal view (right) shows an activated region of the lateral orbitofrontal cortex (–36,27,–8; z=4.23, p<0.05 S.V.C.). All the activations were thresholded at p<0.00001 to show the extent of the activations. (After Rolls, Kringelbach and De Araujo, 2003c.)

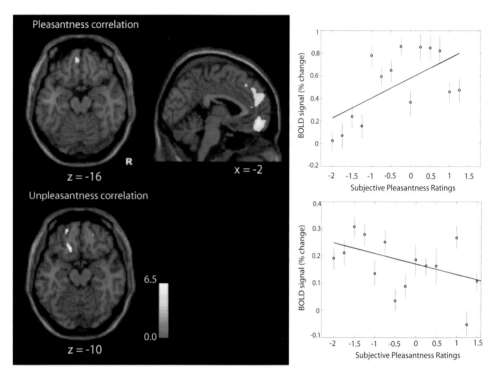

Fig. 4.26 The representation of pleasant and unpleasant odours in the human brain. Random effects group analysis correlation analysis of the BOLD signal with the subjective pleasantness ratings. On the top left is shown the region of the medio-rostral orbitofrontal (peak at [−2,52,−10]; z=4.28) correlating positively with pleasantness ratings, as well as the region of the anterior cingulate cortex in the top middle. On the far top-right of the figure is shown the relation between the subjective pleasantness ratings and the BOLD signal from this cluster (in the medial orbitofrontal cortex at Y = 52), together with the regression line. The means and s.e.m. across subjects are shown. At the bottom of the figure are shown the regions of left more lateral orbitofrontal cortex (peaks at [−20,54,−14]; z=4.26 and [−16,28,−18]; z=4.08) correlating negatively with pleasantness ratings. On the far bottom-right of the figure is shown the relation between the subjective pleasantness ratings and the BOLD signal from the first cluster (in the lateral orbitofrontal cortex at Y = 54), together with the regression line. The means and s.e.m. across subjects are shown. The activations were thresholded at p<0.0001 for extent. (After Rolls, Kringelbach and De Araujo, 2003c.)

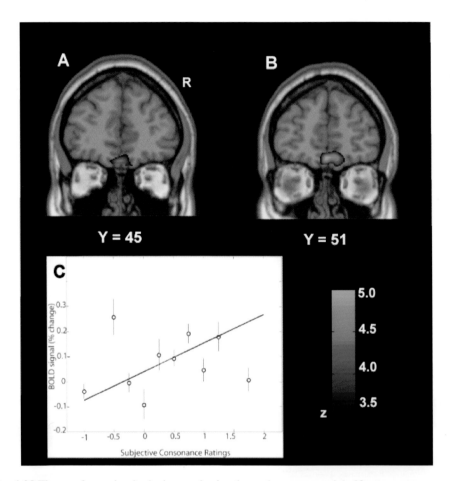

Fig. 4.29 Flavour formation in the human brain, shown by cross-modal olfactory–taste conver-gence. Brain areas where activations were correlated with the subjective ratings for stimulus (taste–odour) consonance and pleasantness. (A) A second-level, random effects analysis based on individual contrasts (the consonance ratings being the only effect of interest) revealed a significant activation in a medial part of the anterior orbitofrontal cortex. (B) Random effects analysis based on the pleasantness ratings showed a significant cluster of activation located in a (nearby) medial part of the anterior orbitofrontal cortex. The images were thresholded at p<0.0001 for illustration. (C) The relation between the BOLD signal from the cluster of voxels in the medial orbitofrontal cortex shown in (A) and the subjective consonance ratings. The analyses shown included all the stimuli included in this investigation. The means and standard errors of the mean across subjects are shown, together with the regression line, for which r=0.52. (After DeAraujo, Rolls, Kringelbach, McGlone and Phillips, 2003c.)

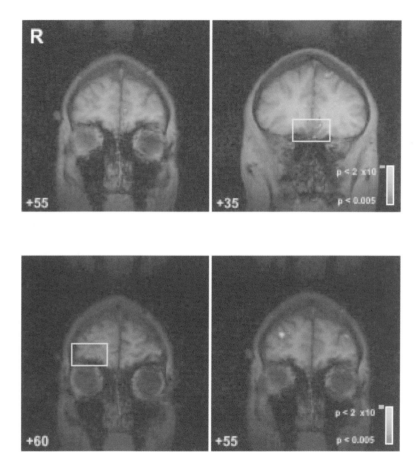

Fig. 4.33 Correlation of brain activations with the amount of money won (upper) or lost (lower)in a visual discrimination reversal task with probabilistic monetary reward and loss. Voxels in the OFC and other regions whose activity increases relative to the increasing magnitude of Reward or of Punishment obtained. Voxels in an area of left medial OFC (Talairach coordinates [X,Y,Z] : [−6,34,−28]) correlated positively with Reward, and voxels in an area of right lateral OFC (Talairach co-ordinates [X,Y,Z] : [28,60,−6]) correlated positively with Punishment. (After O'Doherty, Kringelbach, Rolls, Hornak and Andrews, 2001a.)

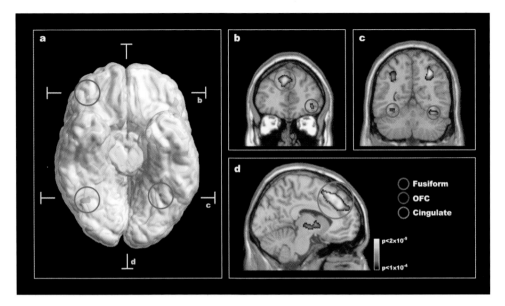

Fig. 4.38 Social reversal: Composite figure showing that changing behaviour based on face expression is correlated with increased brain activity in the human orbitofrontal cortex. a) The figure is based on two different group statistical contrasts from the neuroimaging data which are superimposed on a ventral view of the human brain with the cerebellum removed, and with indication of the location of the two coronal slices (b,c) and the transverse slice (d). The red activations in the orbitofrontal cortex (denoted OFC, maximal activation: z=4.94: 42,42,–8; and z=5.51; X,Y,Z=–46,30,–8) shown on the rendered brain arise from a comparison of reversal events with stable acquisition events, while the blue activations in the fusiform gyrus (denoted Fusiform, maximal activation: z>8; 36,–60,–20 and Z=7.80; –30,–56,–16) arise from the main effects of face expression. b) The coronal slice through the frontal part of the brain shows the cluster in the right orbitofrontal cortex across all nine subjects when comparing reversal events with stable acquisition events. Significant activity was also seen in an extended area of the anterior cingulate/paracingulate cortex (denoted Cingulate, maximal activation: z=6.88; –8,22,52; green circle). c) The coronal slice through the posterior part of the brain shows the brain response to the main effects of face expression with significant activation in the fusiform gyrus and the cortex in the intraparietal sulcus (maximal activation: z>8; 32,–60,46; and z>8: –32,–60,44). d) The transverse slice shows the extent of the activation in the anterior cingulate/paracingulate cortex when comparing reversal events with stable acquisition events. Group statistical results are superimposed on a ventral view of the human brain with the cerebellum removed, and on coronal and transverse slices of the same template brain (activations are thresholded at P=0.0001 for purposes of illustration to show their extent). (After Kringelbach and Rolls 2003.)

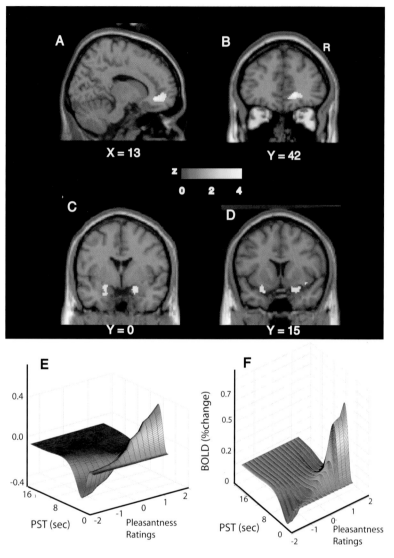

Fig. 4.41 Cognition and emotion. Group (random) effects analysis showing the brain regions where the BOLD signal was correlated with pleasantness ratings given to the test odour. The pleasantness ratings were being modulated by the word labels. A) Activations in the rostral anterior cingulate cortex, in the region adjoining the medial OFC, shown in a sagittal slice. B) The same activation shown coronally. C) Bilateral activations in the amygdala. D) These activations extended anteriorly to the primary olfactory cortex. The image was thresholded at $p<0.0001$ uncorrected in order to show the extent of the activation. E) Parametric plots of the data averaged across all subjects showing that the percentage BOLD change (fitted) correlates with the pleasantness ratings in the region shown in A and B. The parametric plots were very similar for the primary olfactory region shown in D. PST - Post-stimulus time (s). F) Parametric plots for the amygdala region shown in C. (After DeAraujo, Rolls, Velazco, Margot and Cayeux 2005.)

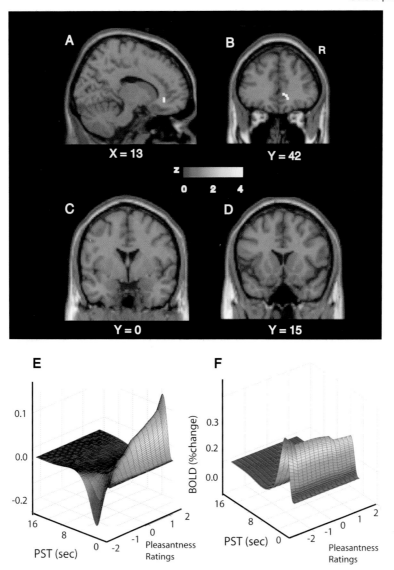

Fig. 4.42 Cognition and emotion. Group (random) effects analysis showing the brain regions where the BOLD signal was correlated with pleasantness ratings given to the clean air. The pleasantness ratings were being modulated by the word labels. A) Activations in the rostral anterior cingulate cortex, in the region adjoining the medial OFC, shown in a sagittal slice. B) The same activation shown coronally. No significant correlations were found with clean air in the amygdala (C) or primary olfactory cortex (D). The image was thresholded at p<0.0001 uncorrected in order to show the extent of the activation. E) Parametric plots of the data averaged across all subjects showing that the percentage BOLD change (fitted) correlates with the pleasantness ratings in the region shown in A and B. PST - Post-stimulus time (s). F) Parametric plots showing activation related to stimulus presentation but not related to the pleasantness ratings for the amygdala region shown in C. (After DeAraujo, Rolls, Velazco, Margot and Cayeux 2005.)

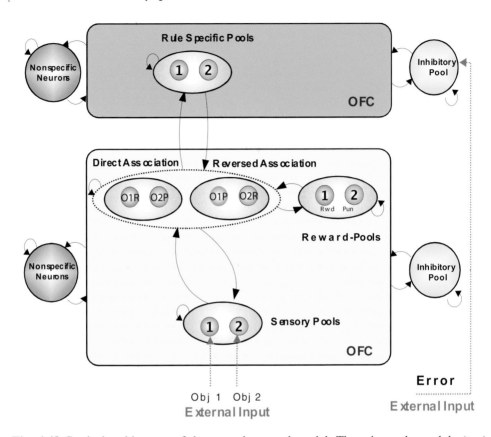

Fig. 4.48 Cortical architecture of the reward reversal model. There is a rule module (top) and a sensory – intermediate neuron – reward module (below). Neurons within each module are fully connected, and form attractor states. The sensory – intermediate neuron – reward module consists of three hierarchically organized levels of attractor network, with stronger synaptic connections in the forward than the backprojection direction. The intermediate level of the sensory – intermediate neuron – reward module contains neurons that respond to combinations of an object and its association with reward or punishment, e.g. object 1–reward (O1R, in the direct association set of pools), and object 1–punishment (O1P in the reversed association set of pools). The rule module acts as a biasing input to bias the competition between the object-reward combination neurons at the intermediate level of the sensory – intermediate neuron – reward module. The synaptic current flows into the cells are mediated by four different families of receptors. The recurrent excitatory postsynaptic currents are given by two different types of EPSP (excitatory post-synaptic potentials), respectively mediated by AMPA and NMDA receptors. These two glutamatergic excitatory synapses are on the pyramidal cells and interneurons. The external background is mediated by AMPA synapses on pyramidal cells and interneurons. Each neuron receives N_{ext} excitatory AMPA synaptic connections from outside the network. The visual input is also introduced by AMPA synapses on specific pyramidal cells. Inhibitory GABAergic synapses on pyramidal cells and interneurons yield corresponding IPSPs (inhibitory post-synaptic potentials). (See text and Appendix 2 for details.) OFC, orbitofrontal cortex. (After Deco and Rolls, 2005d.)

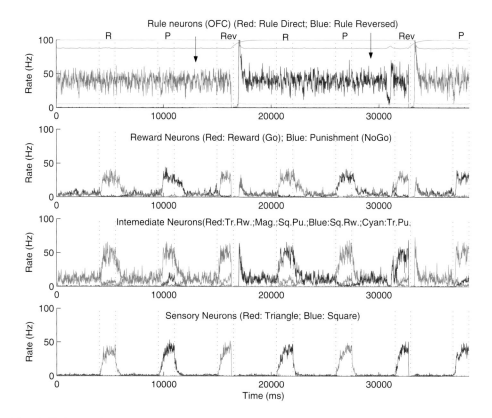

Fig. 4.49 Reward reversal model: Temporal evolution of the averaged population activity for all neural pools (sensory, intermediate (stimulus–reward), and Reward/Punishment) in the stimulus – intermediate – reward module and the rule module, during the execution and the reversal of the Go/NoGo visual discrimination task with a pseudorandom trial sequence after Thorpe, Rolls and Maddison (1983) and Rolls, Critchley, Mason and Wakeman (1996). Bottom row: the sensory neuronal populations, one of which responds to Object 1, a triangle (red), and the other to Object 2, a square (blue). The intermediate conditional stimulus–reward and stimulus-punishment neurons respond to for example Object 1 (Tr) when it is associated with reward (Rw) (e.g. on trial 1, corresponding to O1R in Fig. 4.48), or to Object 2 (Sq) when it is associated with punishment (Pu) (e.g. on trial 2, O2P). The top row shows the firing rate activity in the rule module, with the thin line at the top of this graph showing the mean probability of release P_{rel} of transmitter from the synapses of each population of neurons. The arrows show when the contingencies reversed. R: Reward trial; P: Punishment Trial; Rev: Reversal trial, i.e. the first trial after the reward contingency was reversed when Reward was expected but Punishment was obtained. The intertrial interval was 4 sec. The yellow line shows the average activity of the inhibitory neurons. (See text for further details.) (After Deco and Rolls, 2005d.)

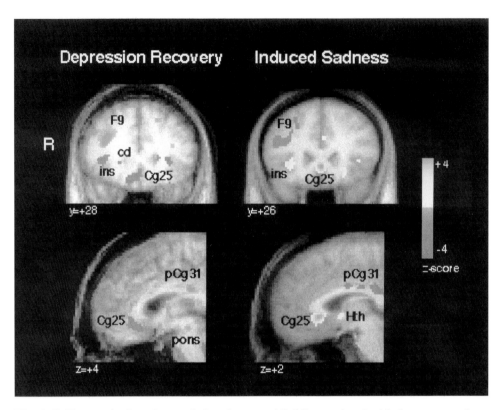

Fig. 4.62 Changes in the subgenual cingulate area (Cg25) associated with the recovery from depression (left), and with the induction of a mood state of sadness (right). Left images: Z-score maps demonstrating changes in regional glucose metabolism (fluorodeoxyglucose PET) in depressed patients following 6 weeks of treatment with the antidepressant fluoxetine. Upper: coronal view; lower, sagittal view). Green indicates that the change is a decrease, and red or yellow an increase (see calibration bar on far right). Right images: changes in regional cerebral blood flow (oxygen-15 water PET) in healthy volunteers 10 min after induction of acute sadness. The recovery from depression and the induction of sadness produce opposite changes in Cg25. Reciprocal changes were seen in a dorsal part of the prefrontal cortex, labelled F9. F, frontal; cd, caudate nucleus; ins, anterior insula; Cg25, subgenual cingulate; Hth, hypothalamus; pCG31, posterior cingulate; R, right. (After Mayberg et al 1999.)

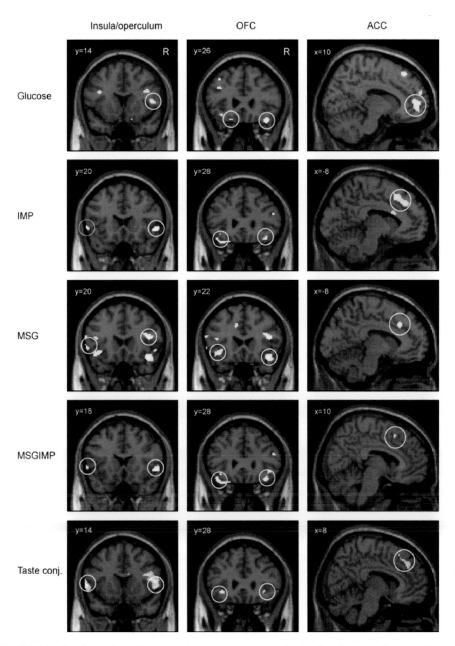

Fig. 5.15 Activation of the human primary taste cortex in the insula/frontal operculum; the orbitofrontal cortex (OFC); and the anterior cingulate cortex (ACC) by taste. The stimuli used included glucose, two umami taste stimuli (monosodium glutamate (MSG) and inosine monophosphate (IMP)), and a mixture of the two umami stimuli. Taste conj. refers to a conjunction analysis over all the taste stimuli. (After DeAraujo, Kringelbach, Rolls and Hobden 2003.)

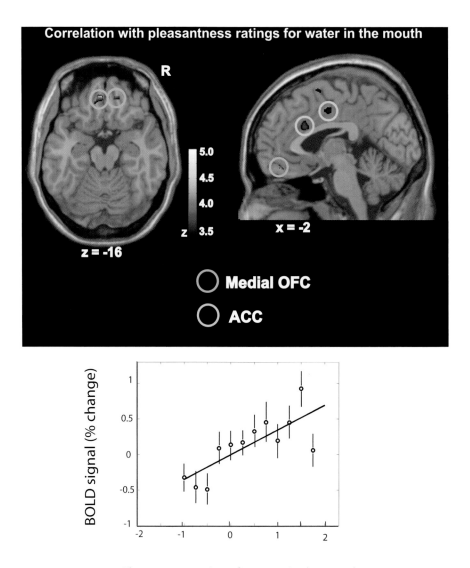

Fig. 6.7 Representation of the pleasantness of the taste of water in the human brain. Correlations with the pleasantness of the taste of water in a group random effects analysis. Top left: Regions of the medial caudal orbitofrontal where the activation was correlated with the subjective pleasantness ratings of water throughout the experiment. Bottom: A scatter plot showing the values of the BOLD signal in the medial orbitofrontal cortex (mean across subjects, ± s.e.m.), with the regression line shown. Top right: The regions of anterior cingulate cortex (ACC) where activation was correlated with the subjective pleasantness ratings of water given throughout the experiment. (After DeAraujo, Kringelbach, Rolls and McGlone, 2003.)

TD error signal in the ventral striatum
in a probabilistic monetary decision-making task

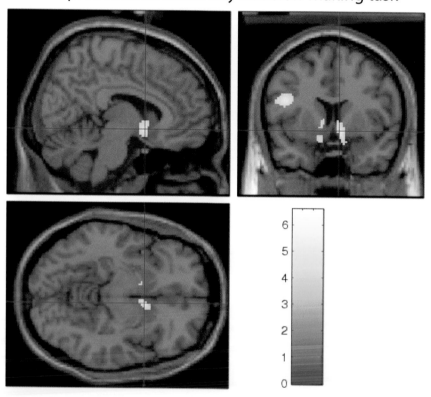

Fig. 8.10 Temporal Difference (TD) error signal in the ventral striatum in a probabilistic monetary decision-making task. The correlation between the TD error and the activation in the nucleus accumbens was significant in a group random effects analysis fully corrected at the cluster level with p<0.048 (voxel z=3.84) at MNI coordinates [8,8,–8]. (From Rolls, McCabe and Redoute, 2007.)

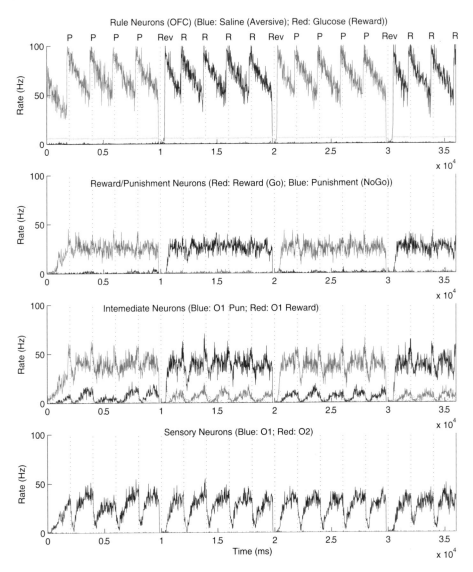

Fig. B.3 Temporal evolution of the averaged population activity for all neural pools (sensory, intermediate (stimulus–reward/punishment), and Reward/Punishment) in the stimulus – intermediate – reward module and the rule module during the execution of the reversal of the Go/NoGo visual discrimination task shown in Fig. 4.31. Each vertical line indicates a new trial. The yellow curve in the top graph shows the average activity of the inhibitory interneurons in the rule module. O1 was the syringe used to present the stimuli in Fig. 4.31. R: Reward trial; P: Punishment Trial; Rev: Reversal trial, i.e. the first trial after the reward contingency was reversed when Reward was expected but Punishment was obtained. (After Deco and Rolls 2005d.)

5 Hunger

5.1 Introduction

In this Chapter we consider the rewards and affective states relevant to eating, and in Chapter 6 for drinking. In these cases there are internal signals which indicate that there is a need for food or water. The food or water are rewards, in that the organism will work to obtain the food or water. The signals that make the food or water rewarding originate internally. In the case of hunger, the internal signals reflect the state of energy balance, reflecting stimuli such as plasma glucose and gastric distension. In the case of thirst, the internal signals reflect the volumes of the cellular and extracellular fluids. In both cases the hunger and thirst operate to maintain the constancy of the internal milieu. The signals operate to alter the reward value that food or water has for the hungry or thirsty organism. The reward signals are conveyed primarily by the taste, texture, smell, and sight of food or water.

In this Chapter we will consider where in information processing in these sensory systems the sensory stimulation produced by food is decoded not just as a physical stimulus, but is coded in terms of its reward and affective value. An important aspect of brain organization is that these two aspects of information processing, representing the identity of objects, and representing their affective value, are kept separate, at least in primates including humans. Another important aspect of brain organization for these types of reward is that the learning of which visual stimuli are food or water, or are associated with food or water, takes places in specialized parts of the brain for this type of learning. This learning takes place in the brain after analysis of what the stimulus is.

The study of hunger and thirst allows precise analysis of the relation between motivational states (e.g. hunger and thirst), and emotional states including affective reactions to sensory stimuli such as food. It is also important to understand dysfunctions of the eating control systems that lead to obesity, which is now a major health issue in many countries.

5.2 Peripheral signals for hunger and satiety

To understand how food intake is controlled, we first consider the functions of the different peripheral factors (i.e. factors outside the brain) such as taste, smell, and gastric distension, and the control signals, such as the amount of glucose in the blood. We focus particularly on which sensory inputs produce reward, and on which inputs act as hunger or satiety signals to modulate the reward value of the sensory inputs. Then we consider how the brain integrates these different signals, learns about which stimuli in the environment provide food, and how the brain initiates behaviour to obtain the correct variety and amount of food.

The functions of some different peripheral signals in the control of eating can be revealed with the sham feeding preparation shown in Fig. 5.1. In this situation, the animal can taste, smell, and eat the food normally, but the food drains from the stomach, so that no distension

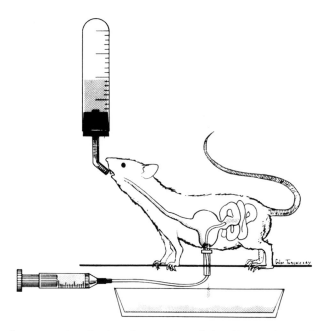

Fig. 5.1 Sham feeding preparation. Food can be tasted, smelled and ingested normally, but then it drains from the stomach so that gastric distension and other gastrointestinal factors are not produced. The diagram also shows a cannula entering the duodenum, so that the role of intestinal factors in eating can be studied by infusions of for example potential satiety-producing substances.

of the stomach occurs, and nor does any food enter the intestine for absorption. It is found that rats, monkeys, and humans will work to obtain food when they are sham feeding. This finding for primates is demonstrated in Fig. 5.2. This shows that it is the taste and smell of food which provide the immediate reward for food-motivated behaviour. Consistent with this, humans rate the taste and smell of food as being pleasant when they are hungry (see Section 5.3.1).

A second important aspect of sham feeding is that satiety (reduction of appetite) does not occur – instead rats and monkeys continue to eat for often more than an hour when they can taste and smell food normally, but food drains from the stomach, so that it does not accumulate in the stomach and enter the intestine (see e.g. Fig. 5.2, the classical literature reviewed by Grossman (1967), and Gibbs, Maddison and Rolls (1981)). We can conclude that taste and smell, and even swallowing food, do not produce satiety.

There is an important psychological point here – **reward itself does not produce satiety**. Instead, the satiety for feeding is produced by food accumulating in the stomach, and entering the intestine. Evidence that gastric distension is an important satiety signal is that if an animal is allowed to eat to normal satiety, and then the food is drained through a cannula from the stomach, then the animal starts eating again immediately (Gibbs, Maddison and Rolls 1981). Evidence that food entering the intestine can produce satiety is that small infusions of food into the duodenum (the first part of the intestine) reduce sham feeding (Gibbs, Maddison and Rolls 1981). It is also interesting that food delivered directly into the stomach, or even glucose intravenously, is not very rewarding, in that animals learn only with difficulty to perform a response to obtain an intragastric or intravenous infusion of food or fluid (Nicolaidis and

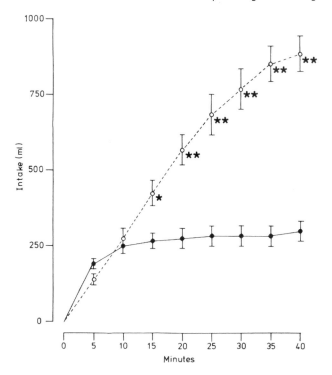

Fig. 5.2 Sham feeding in the monkey. The cumulative intakes of food with normal feeding (gastric cannula closed, closed circles), and with the gastric cannula open (open circles) allowing drainage of food from the stomach, are shown. The stars indicate significant differences between the open and closed gastric cannula conditions. (From Gibbs, Maddison and Rolls 1981).

Rowland 1976, Nicolaidis and Rowland 1977, Nicolaidis and Rowland 1975).

This evidence, summarized in Table 5.1, emphasizes the point that the taste, smell, and sight of food are what normally provide the reward, and correspondingly the pleasant sensation, associated with eating.

Table 5.1 Summary of functions of peripheral signals in feeding

	Reinforcement	Satiety
Oropharyngeal factors	Yes	No (though contribute to sensory-specific satiety)
Gastric and intestinal factors	No	Yes

Important conclusions about reward and its relation to hunger and satiety signals follow from what has just been described. First, reward and satiety are different processes. Second, reward is produced by oropharyngeal sensory signals such as the taste and smell of food. Third, satiety is produced by gastric, intestinal, and eventually other signals after the food is absorbed from the intestine. Fourth, hunger and satiety signals modulate the reward value of food (in that the taste and smell of food are rewarding when hunger signals are present and satiety signals are not present). In more general and psychological terminology, motivational state modulates the reward or reinforcement value of sensory stimuli. Fifth, given that reward and satiety are produced by different peripheral signals, one function of brain (i.e. central) processes in the control of feeding is to bring together satiety and reward signals in such a way that satiety modulates the reward value of food.

One of the aims of this Chapter is to show how the brain processes sensory stimuli that can produce rewards for animals, where in the brain the reward value of such sensory stimuli is represented, and where and how the motivational signals that reflect hunger modulate this processing as part of the reward-decoding process. Of crucial interest in understanding the rules of operation of this reward system will therefore be where and how in the brain gastric and other satiety signals are brought together with taste and smell signals of food, to produce a taste/smell reward signal that is modulated by satiety.

5.3   The control signals for hunger and satiety

There is a set of different signals that each plays a role in determining the level of hunger vs satiety. These signals must all be integrated by the brain, and must then modulate how rewarding the sensory inputs such as the sight, taste, and smell of food are. These signals that influence hunger and satiety are summarized next, taken to some extent in the order in which they are activated in a meal.

5.3.1   Sensory-specific satiety

During experiments on brain mechanisms of reward and satiety, E. T. Rolls and colleagues observed in 1974 that if a lateral hypothalamic neuron had ceased to respond to a food on which the monkey had been fed to satiety, then the neuron might still respond to a different food (see examples in Figs. 5.3 and 5.11, and Section 5.4.1.2). This occurred for neurons with responses associated with the taste (Rolls 1981a, Rolls 1981b, Rolls, Murzi, Yaxley, Thorpe and Simpson 1986) or sight (Rolls 1981a, Rolls and Rolls 1982b, Rolls, Murzi, Yaxley, Thorpe and Simpson 1986) of food. Corresponding to this neuronal specificity of the effects of feeding to satiety, the monkey rejected the food on which he had been fed to satiety, but accepted other foods that he had not been fed. I well remember the occasion on which we discovered sensory-specific satiety in 1974 when we were recording from a lateral hypothalamic neuron in the monkey that responded to the sight of glucose (fed to the monkey from a syringe) and other foods. We fed the monkey to satiety with glucose, and observed the neuronal response to the glucose fall to zero, as illustrated for one such neuron in Fig. 5.3. I then showed the monkey a peanut, and heard a large response of the neuron, which was confirmed by the high firing rate printed out on the teletype (ASR33) by the PDP11 computer. I was disconcerted at first because the monkey was supposed to be satiated, having drunk as much glucose as it wanted. However, I had the presence of mind to offer the peanut to the monkey, and found that the monkey reached out for the peanut, and avidly consumed it. I realised that something interesting was happening in terms of the brain mechanisms that implement satiety, and repeated the observations a number of times, confirming that the lateral hypothalamic neuron did not respond to the sight of the glucose and that the monkey did not accept the glucose, whereas the neuron did respond vigorously to the sight of the peanut, which the monkey avidly reached for and ate. The fact that quantitative firing rates were being printed out on the teletype helped to impress on me the fact that this was a strong effect,

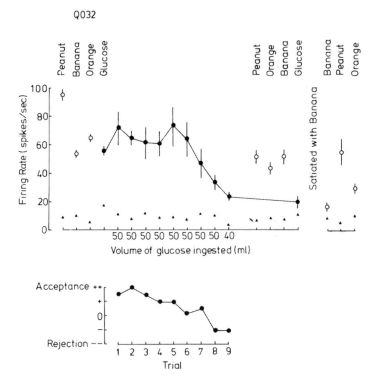

Fig. 5.3 The effect of feeding the monkey to satiety with 20% glucose solution on the responses of a lateral hypothalamic neuron to the sight the glucose (filled circles) and to the sight of other foods (open circles). After the monkey had fed to satiety with glucose, the neuron responded much less to the sight of glucose, but still responded to the other foods. The mean responses of the neuron ($\pm$ s.e.m.) are shown to the stimuli at different stages of the experiment. The satiety of the monkey, shown below, was measured by whether he accepted or rejected the glucose. After satiety with glucose, a second satiety experiment was performed in which banana was fed to satiety, and after this, the responses of the neuron decreased to the sight of the banana, but remained to the sight of peanut and orange, for which he still had an appetite. (From Rolls, Murzi, Yaxley, Thorpe and Simpson 1986, after Rolls 1981a.)

which we termed sensory-specific satiety. The neurophysiological finding was published for example in Rolls (1981a) and Rolls et al. (1986).

I lectured on the result to my Oxford undergraduate class, and proposed an experiment to explore the effect in humans. The experiment was performed as an undergraduate practical (with Barbara Rolls as a co-organiser) in which humans rated the pleasantness and intensity of 6 foods, and then ate one of the foods to satiety. Whichever food was eaten to satiety showed a large decrease in the pleasantness rating, whereas other foods that had not been eaten to satiety showed a much smaller decrease, or in some cases even a small increase in pleasantness (e.g. for a sweet food after a savory food had been eaten to satiety), as shown in Fig. 5.4. The result was published by Rolls, Rolls, Rowe and Sweeney (1981a), and led to a series of other investigations on sensory-specific satiety described below.

We performed further experiments to determine whether satiety in humans is specific to foods eaten. These experiments were performed as a result of the neurophysiological and

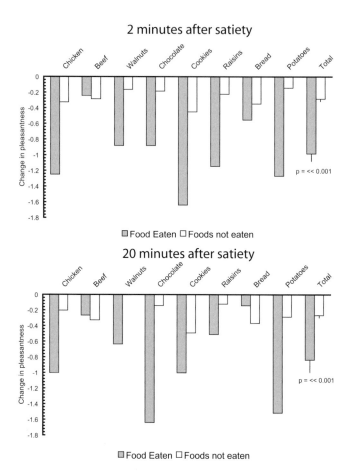

Fig. 5.4 Sensory-specific satiety for the flavour of a food. The change in the pleasantness of the flavour of food after eating one to satiety. For each food, the change of pleasantness after eating that food to satiety is shown (food eaten), compared to the average change of pleasantness of the other foods not eaten in the meal. The ratings are on a scale from +2 very pleasant to −2 very unpleasant, and the change of pleasantness rating from before until after eating one of the foods to satiety is shown. The ratings were made by a group of participants 2 min and 20 min after eating one of the foods to satiety for lunch. (After Rolls, Rolls, Rowe and Sweeney, 1981a.)

behavioural observations showing the specificity of satiety in the monkey (Rolls 1981a, Rolls 1981b, Rolls, Murzi, Yaxley, Thorpe and Simpson 1986), and the experiment illustrated in Fig. 5.4[13]. In the further experiments, it was found that the pleasantness of the taste of food eaten to satiety decreased more than for foods that had not been eaten (Rolls, Rolls, Rowe and Sweeney 1981a). The results of an experiment of this type are shown in Fig. 5.5.

One implication of this finding is that if one food is eaten to satiety, appetite reduction for other foods is often incomplete, and this should mean that in humans also at least some of the other foods will be eaten. This has been confirmed by an experiment in which either sausages

[13]LeMagnen (1956) had also shown that rats drank more water if several tubes of water each had a different odour added to the water.

Banana Eaten Chicken Eaten

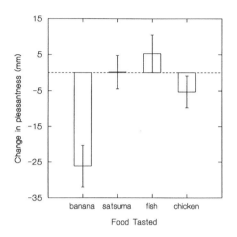

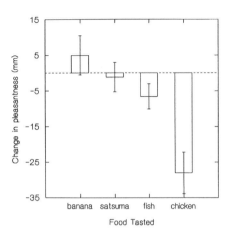

Fig. 5.5 Sensory-specific satiety for the flavour of a food: the changes in the pleasantness of the taste of four different foods after eating banana (left) or chicken (right) to satiety are shown. The change is shown as mm difference ($\pm$ the standard error of the mean, s.e.m.) on a 100 mm visual analogue rating scale marked at one end 'very pleasant' and at the other end 'very unpleasant'. The decrease of pleasantness of the taste of a food was greater for the food eaten to satiety. (From Rolls,E.T. and Rolls,J.H. 1997).

or cheese with crackers were eaten for lunch. The liking for the food eaten decreased more than for the food not eaten and, when an unexpected second course was offered, more was eaten if a subject had not been given that food in the first course than if he had been given that food in the first course (98% vs 40% of the first course intake eaten in the second courses, p < 0.01, Rolls, Rolls, Rowe and Sweeney (1981a)).

A further implication of these findings is that if a variety of foods is available, the total amount consumed will be more than when only one food is offered repeatedly. This prediction has been confirmed in a study in which humans ate more when offered a variety of sandwich fillings than one filling or a variety of types of yoghurt which differed in taste, texture, and colour (Rolls, Rowe, Rolls, Kingston, Megson and Gunary 1981b). It has also been confirmed in a study in which humans were offered a relatively normal meal of four courses, and it was found that the change of food at each course significantly enhanced intake (Rolls, Van Duijen-voorde and Rolls 1984a). Because sensory factors such as similarity of colour, shape, flavour, and texture are usually more important than metabolic equivalence in terms of protein, carbohydrate, and fat content in influencing how foods interact in this type of satiety, it has been termed 'sensory-specific satiety' (Rolls and Rolls 1977, Rolls and Rolls 1982b, Rolls, Rolls, Rowe and Sweeney 1981a, Rolls, Rowe, Rolls, Kingston, Megson and Gunary 1981b, Rolls, Rowe and Rolls 1982b, Rolls, Rowe and Rolls 1982a, Rolls and Rolls 1997, Rolls 1999a).

It should be noted that sensory-specific satiety is distinct from alliesthesia, in that alliesthesia is a change in the pleasantness of sensory inputs produced by internal signals (such as glucose in the gut) (Cabanac and Duclaux 1970, Cabanac 1971, Cabanac and Fantino 1977), whereas sensory-specific satiety is a change in the pleasantness of sensory inputs which is

Banana Chewed

Chicken Chewed

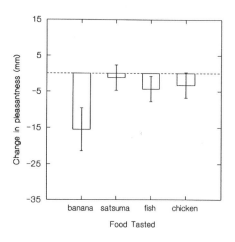
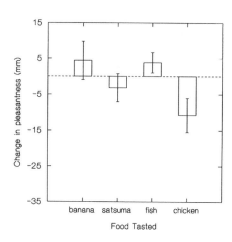

Fig. 5.6 Sensory-specific satiety for the flavour of a food: the change in the pleasantness of the taste of four different foods after chewing but not swallowing banana (left) or chicken (right) for five minutes. Conventions as in Fig. 5.5. The decrease of pleasantness of the taste of a food was greater for the food chewed. (From Rolls, E.T. and Rolls, J.H. 1997.)

accounted for at least partly by the external sensory stimulation received (such as the taste of a particular food), in that as shown above it is at least partly specific to the external sensory stimulation received.

The parallel between these studies of feeding in humans and of the neurophysiology of hypothalamic neurons in the monkey has been extended by the observations that in humans, sensory-specific satiety occurs for the sight (Rolls, Rowe and Rolls 1982b) and smell (Rolls and Rolls 1997) as well as for the taste and even texture (Rolls, Rowe and Rolls 1982b) of food. Further, to complement the finding that in the hypothalamus neurons are found that respond differently to food and to water (see Fig. 5.12, Rolls and colleagues, unpublished observations), and that satiety with water can reduce the responsiveness of hypothalamic neurons that respond to water, it has been shown that in humans motivation-specific satiety can also be detected. For example, satiety with water reduces the pleasantness of the sight and taste of water but not of food (Rolls, Rolls and Rowe 1983b).

Some sensory-specific satiety can be produced just by tasting or even smelling a food for a few minutes, without swallowing any of it (Rolls and Rolls 1997) (see Fig. 5.6). This shows that just the presence of neuronal activity produced by the taste or the smell of food is sufficient to reduce the firing of neurons which represent the pleasantness of the taste or smell of food. This can occur to some extent even without gastric and post-gastric factors such as gastric distension and intestinal stimulation by food. This indicates that this aspect of sensory-specific satiety can be produced by firing that is sustained for a few minutes in neurons in the pathway. Moreover, the decline in neuronal responsiveness must be at a late stage of the processing of the taste and probably the olfactory signals, in that just smelling the food for several minutes produces much more of a reduction in the pleasantness than in the intensity of the odour, and just tasting the food for several minutes produces much more of a decrease in the pleasantness than in the intensity of the taste (Rolls and Rolls 1997).

It is a general finding with sensory-specific satiety that the decrease is pleasantness is much greater than any decrease in intensity of the food eaten to satiety. Indeed, Rolls, Rolls and Rowe (1983b) specifically addressed this using different concentrations of glucose and salt (NaCl), and showed that the subjective intensity but much less the subjective pleasantness of the tastes was related to the concentrations. Conversely, feeding to satiety produced a much greater decrease in pleasantness than in intensity. The neurophysiological basis for this is that processing as far as the primary taste cortex (Rolls, Scott, Sienkiewicz and Yaxley 1988, Yaxley, Rolls and Sienkiewicz 1988), the primary olfactory cortex (Rolls, Kringelbach and De Araujo 2003c), and the inferior temporal visual cortex is related to the identity and intensity of the stimulus (Rolls, Judge and Sanghera 1977); whereas in the orbitofrontal cortex it is the pleasantness of the taste (Rolls, Sienkiewicz and Yaxley 1989b), smell, and sight of food which is represented (Critchley and Rolls 1996a, Rolls, Kringelbach and De Araujo 2003c, De Araujo, Rolls, Kringelbach, McGlone and Phillips 2003c, Kringelbach, O'Doherty, Rolls and Andrews 2003, De Araujo, Rolls, Velazco, Margot and Cayeux 2005). The adaptive value of this is that it is important that we do not go 'blind' to the taste or sight of food after we have eaten it to satiety, for it is important to be able to learn about the food (e.g. where food has been seen), even when we are not hungry.

It should be noticed that this decrease in the pleasantness of the sensory stimulation produced by a food only occurs if the sensory stimulation is repeated for several minutes. It has the adaptive value of changing the behaviour after a significant amount of that behaviour has been performed. In contrast, the reward value of sensory stimulation may increase over the first short period (of the order of a minute). This is called *incentive motivation* or the salted-nut phenomenon. It has the adaptive value that once a behaviour has been initiated, it will tend to continue for at least a little while. This is much more adaptive than continually switching behaviour, which has at least some cost in terms of efficiency, and might have a high cost if the different rewards are located far apart. The increase in the rate of behaviour, for example in the rate of feeding in the first part of a meal, probably reflects this effect. It was observed that this typical increase in the rate of working for a reward early on in a meal was not found in rats with amygdala lesions (Rolls and Rolls 1973b), and this implies that part of the mechanism for the increasing hedonic value of a food reward is implemented, at least in the rat, in the amygdala. Associated with this lack of increase in the rate of feeding early on in the meal, in the rat the meal pattern was disturbed. Instead of short rapid meals following by a bout of drinking and then other activity, the rats had long periods in which slow feeding and drinking were interspersed. This emphasizes the suggested function of the reward facilitation normally seen at the start of a period of rewarding sensory stimulation.

The enhanced eating when a variety of foods is available, as a result of the operation of sensory-specific satiety, may have been advantageous in evolution in ensuring that different foods with important different nutrients were consumed, but today in humans, when a wide variety of foods is readily available, it may be a factor which can lead to overeating and obesity. In a test of this in the rat, it has been found that variety itself can lead to obesity (Rolls, Van Duijenvoorde and Rowe 1983a, Rolls and Hetherington 1989).

Advances in understanding the neurophysiological mechanisms of sensory-specific satiety are being made in analyses of information processing in the taste and olfactory systems, as described below.

In addition to the sensory-specific satiety described above which operates primarily during the meal (see above) and during the post-meal period (Rolls, Van Duijenvoorde and Rolls 1984a), there is now evidence for a long-term form of sensory-specific satiety (Rolls and de Waal 1985). This was shown in a study in an Ethiopian refugee camp, in which it was found that refugees who had been in the camp for 6 months found the taste of their three regular foods less pleasant than that of three comparable foods which they had not been eating. The effect was a long-term form of sensory-specific satiety in that it was not found in refugees who had been in the camp and eaten the regular foods for two days (Rolls and de Waal 1985). It is suggested that it is important to recognize the operation of long-term sensory-specific satiety in conditions such as these, for it may enhance malnutrition if the regular foods become less acceptable and so are rejected, exchanged for other less nutritionally effective foods or goods, or are inadequately prepared. It may be advantageous in these circumstances to attempt to minimize the operation of long-term sensory-specific satiety by providing some variety, perhaps even with spices (Rolls and de Waal 1985).

5.3.2 Gastric distension

This is one of the signals that is normally necessary for satiety, as shown by the experiment in which gastric drainage of food after a meal leads to the immediate resumption of eating (Gibbs, Maddison and Rolls 1981). Gastric distension only builds up if the pyloric sphincter closes. The pyloric sphincter controls the emptying of the stomach into the next part of the gastrointestinal tract, the duodenum. The sphincter closes only when food reaches the duodenum, stimulating chemosensors and osmosensors to regulate the action of the sphincter, by both local neural circuits and by hormones, in what is called the enterogastric loop (Gibbs, Maddison and Rolls 1981, Gibbs, Fauser, Rowe, Rolls, Rolls and Maddison 1979).

5.3.3 Duodenal chemosensors

The duodenum contains receptors sensitive to the chemical composition of the food draining from the stomach. One set of receptors responds to glucose, and can contribute to satiety via the vagus nerve, which carries signals to the brain. The evidence that the vagus is the pathway is that cutting the vagus nerve (vagotomy) abolishes the satiating effects of glucose infusions into the duodenum. Fats infused into the duodenum can also produce satiety, but in this case the link to the brain may be hormonal (a hormone is a blood-borne signal), for vagotomy does not abolish the satiating effect of fat infusions into the duodenum (Greenberg, Smith and Gibbs 1990, Mei 1993).

5.3.4 Glucostatic hypothesis

There are many lines of evidence, summarized next, that one signal that controls appetite is the concentration of glucose circulating in the plasma – we eat in order to maintain glucostasis, i.e. constancy of glucose in the internal milieu (Woods, Schwartz, Baskin and Seeley 2000). More accurately, the actual signal appears to be the utilization of glucose by the body and brain – if the arterial minus the venous concentration is low, indicating that the body is not extracting much glucose from the bloodstream, then we feel hungry and eat; and if the utilization measured in this way is high, we feel satiated. Consistent with this correlation between glucose and eating, there is a small reduction in plasma glucose concentration just before the onset of meals in rats, suggesting that the decreasing glucose concentration initiates a meal

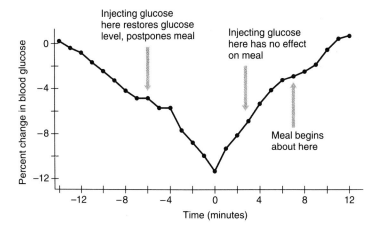

Fig. 5.7 Alterations in plasma glucose concentration that occur just before the onset of a meal in rats. (After Campfield and Smith 1990)

(Campfield and Smith 1990) (see Fig. 5.7). At the end of a meal, plasma glucose concentrations (and insulin, which helps the glucose to be used by cells) increase. A second line of evidence is that injections of insulin, which reduce the concentration of glucose in the plasma (by facilitating its entry to cells and storage as fat), provoke food intake. Third, 2-deoxyglucose, a competitive inhibitor of glucose metabolism, elicits feeding. Fourth, infusions of glucose and insulin can reduce feeding. Fifth, the brain's monitoring system for glucose availability seems to be in the area postrema in the medulla (part of the brainstem), for infusions there of a competitive inhibitor of glucose, 5-thioglucose, elicit feeding (Ritter 1986).

It is worth noting that in diabetes (that is, diabetes mellitus), the cells can become insulin-resistant, so that in this condition it is difficult to interpret whatever plasma levels of glucose are present in terms of their possible role in hunger and satiety.

5.3.5 Body fat regulation – leptin or OB protein

The signals described so far would be appropriate for regulation on the meal-to-meal timescale, but might not be adequate for the longer term regulation of body weight, and in particular of body fat. So the search has been on for another signal that might affect appetite based on, for example, the amount of fat in the body. Recent research has uncovered a candidate hormone that performs this function. Some of the evidence is as follows (Campfield, Smith, Guisez, Devos and Burn 1995, Cummings and Schwartz 2003):

1. OB protein or leptin is the hormone encoded by the mouse ob gene (here ob stands for obesity).

2. Genetically obese mice that are double recessive for the ob gene (i.e. obob mice) produce no leptin.

3. Leptin reduces food intake in wild type (lean) mice (who have genes which are OBOB or OBob so that they produce leptin) and in obob mice (showing that obob mice have receptors sensitive to leptin).

4. The satiety effect of leptin can be produced by injections into the brain.

5. Leptin does not produce satiety (reduce food intake) in another type of genetically obese mouse designated dbdb. These mice may be obese because they lack the leptin receptor, or mechanisms associated with it.

6. Leptin has a long time-course: it fluctuates over 24 h, but not in relation to individual meals. Thus it might be appropriate for the longer-term regulation of appetite.

7. Leptin could play a role in humans, for leptin is found in humans.

8. Leptin concentration may correlate with body weight/adiposity, consistent with the possibility that it is produced by fat cells, and can signal the total amount of body fat.

A hypothesis consistent with these findings is that a hormone, leptin, is produced in proportion to the amount of body fat, and that this is normally one of the signals that controls how much food is eaten (see further Fig. 5.14). Although this is an interesting mechanism implicated in the long term control of body weight, it appears that most obesity in humans cannot be accounted for by malfunction of the leptin system, for even though genetic malfunction of this system can produce obesity in humans, such genetic malfunctions are very rare (Farooqi, Keogh, Kamath, Jones, Gibson, Trussell, Jebb, Lip and O'Rahilly 2001) (see Section 5.4.1.2 on page 234). It is found that obese people generally have high levels of leptin, so leptin production is not the problem, and instead leptin resistance (i.e. insensitivity) may be somewhat related to obesity, with the resistance perhaps related in part to smaller effects of leptin on arcuate nucleus NPY/AGRP neurons (Munzberg and Myers 2005), as described below.

In parallel with the leptin mechanism, it is possible that the hypothalamus senses long-chain fatty acids as an indicator of ongoing metabolic state, and uses this to influence appetite (Lam, Schwartz and Rossetti 2005).

5.3.6 Conditioned appetite and satiety

If we eat food containing much energy (e.g. rich in fat) for a few days, we gradually eat less of it. If we eat food containing little energy, we gradually, over days, ingest more of it. This regulation involves learning, learning to associate the sight, taste, smell, texture, etc., of the food with the energy that is released from it in the hours after it is eaten. This form of learning was demonstrated by Booth (1985) who, after several days of offering sandwiches with different energy content and flavours, on a test day offered subjects medium-energy sandwiches (so that the subjects could not select by the amount of energy in the food). The subjects ate few of the sandwiches if they had the flavour of the high-energy sandwiches eaten previously, and many of the sandwiches if they had the flavour of the low-energy sandwiches eaten previously.

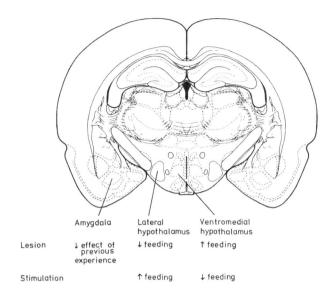

	Amygdala	Lateral hypothalamus	Ventromedial hypothalamus
Lesion	↓ effect of previous experience	↓ feeding	↑ feeding
Stimulation		↑ feeding	↓ feeding

Fig. 5.8 Coronal section through the rat hypothalamus showing the effects of lesions and stimulation of different hypothalamic regions on feeding.

5.4 The brain control of eating and reward

5.4.1 The hypothalamus

5.4.1.1 Effects of damage to the hypothalamus

From clinical evidence it has been known since early this century that damage to the base of the brain can influence food intake and body weight. Later it was demonstrated that one critical region is the ventromedial hypothalamus, for bilateral lesions here in animals led to hyperphagia and obesity (Grossman 1967, Grossman 1973) (see Fig. 5.8). Then Anand and Brobeck (1951) discovered that bilateral lesions of the lateral hypothalamus can produce a reduction in feeding and body weight. Evidence of this type led in the 1950s and 1960s to the view that food intake is controlled by two interacting 'centres', a feeding centre in the lateral hypothalamus and a satiety centre in the ventromedial hypothalamus (Stellar 1954, Grossman 1967, Grossman 1973) (see Fig. 5.8).

Soon, problems with this evidence for a dual-centre hypothesis of the control of food intake appeared. It appears that lesions of the ventromedial hypothalamus act indirectly to increase feeding. These lesions increase the secretion of insulin by the pancreas, this reduces plasma glucose concentration, and then feeding results. This mechanism is demonstrated by the finding that cutting the vagus nerve, which disconnects the brain from the pancreas, prevents ventromedial hypothalamic lesions from causing hypoglycemia, and also prevents the overeating that otherwise occurs after ventromedial hypothalamic lesions (Bray, Inoue and Nishizawa 1981). The ventromedial nucleus of the hypothalamus is thus thought of as a region that can influence the secretion of insulin and thus can indirectly influence body weight, but not as a satiety centre (Woods et al. 2000) (see though Fig. 5.14 for evidence on the functions of the arcuate nucleus).

With regard to the lateral hypothalamus, a contribution to the reduced eating that follows lateral hypothalamic lesions arises from damage to fibre pathways coursing nearby, such as the dopaminergic nigro-striatal bundle. Damage to this pathway leads to motor and sensory deficits because it impairs the normal operation of the basal ganglia (striatum, globus pallidus and substantia nigra), brain structures involved in the initiation and control of movement (Marshall, Richardson and Teitelbaum 1974). Thus by the middle 1970s it was clear that the lesion evidence for a lateral hypothalamic feeding centre was not straightforward, for at least part of the effect of the lesions was due to damage to fibres of passage travelling through or near the lateral hypothalamus (Stricker and Zigmond 1976). It was thus not clear by this time what role the hypothalamus played in feeding.

However, in more recent investigations it has been possible to damage the cells in the lateral hypothalamus without damaging fibres of passage, using locally injected neurotoxins such as ibotenic acid or N-methyl-D-aspartate (NMDA) (Winn, Tarbuck and Dunnett 1984, Dunnett, Lane and Winn 1985, Winn, Clark, Hastings, Clark, Latimer, Rugg and Brownlee 1990, Clark, Clark, Bartle and Winn 1991). With these techniques, it has been shown that damage to lateral hypothalamic cells does produce a lasting decrease in food intake and body weight, and that this is not associated with dopamine depletion as a result of damage to dopamine pathways, or with the akinesia and sensorimotor deficits that are produced by damage to the dopamine systems (Winn et al. 1984, Dunnett et al. 1985, Winn et al. 1990, Clark et al. 1991). Moreover, the lesioned rats do not respond normally to experimental interventions which normally cause eating by reducing the availability of glucose (Clark et al. 1991). Thus the more recent lesion evidence does indicate that the lateral hypothalamus is involved in the control of feeding and body weight.

The evidence just described implicates the hypothalamus in the control of food intake and body weight, but does not show what functions important in feeding are being performed by the hypothalamus and by other brain areas. More direct evidence on the neural processing involved in feeding, based on recordings of the activity of single neurons in the hypothalamus and other brain regions, is described next. These other brain systems include systems that perform sensory analysis involved in the control of feeding such as the taste and olfactory pathways; brain systems involved in learning about foods including the amygdala and orbitofrontal cortex; and brain systems involved in the initiation of feeding behaviour such as the striatum. Some of the brain regions and pathways described in the text are shown in Fig. 4.1 on a lateral view of the brain of the macaque monkey, and some of the connections are shown schematically in Fig. 4.2. Some of the findings described have been made in monkeys, because neuronal activity in non-human primates is especially relevant to understanding brain function and its disorders in humans.

5.4.1.2   Neuronal activity in the lateral hypothalamus during feeding

Hypothalamic neurons responsive to the sight, smell, and taste of food

It has been found that there is a population of neurons in the lateral hypothalamus and substantia innominata of the monkey with responses that are related to feeding (see Rolls (1981b), Rolls (1981a) and Rolls (1986b)). These neurons, which comprised 13.6% in one sample of 764 hypothalamic neurons, respond to the taste and/or sight of food (Rolls, Burton and Mora 1976). The neurons respond to taste in that they respond only when certain substances, such as glucose solution but not water or saline, are in the mouth, and in that their firing rates are related to the concentration of the substance to which they respond (Rolls, Burton and Mora 1980c). These neurons did not respond simply in relation to mouth movements, and comprised 4.3% of the sample of 764 neurons. An example of a primate lateral

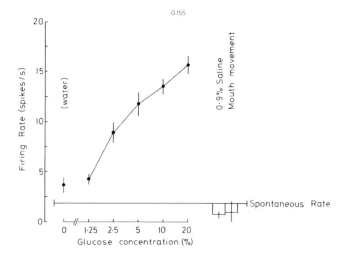

Fig. 5.9 Lateral hypothalamic neuron responding to the taste of food. The firing rate of the neuron depended on the concentration of glucose in the mouth. The neuron did not respond to isotonic saline in the mouth, or in relation to mouth movements. (From Rolls, Murzi, Yaxley, Thorpe and Simpson, 1986).

hypothalamic neuron responding to the taste of food is shown in Fig. 5.9.

The responses of the neurons associated with the sight of food occurred as soon as the monkey saw the food, before the food was in his mouth, and occurred only to foods and not to non-food objects (Rolls, Sanghera and Roper-Hall 1979a, Mora, Rolls and Burton 1976b) (see example in Fig. 5.10). These neurons comprised 11.8% of the sample of 764 neurons (Rolls, Burton and Mora 1976, Rolls, Burton and Mora 1980c). Some of these neurons (2.5% of the total sample) responded to both the sight and taste of food (Rolls, Burton and Mora 1976, Rolls, Burton and Mora 1980c). The finding that there are neurons in the lateral hypothalamus of the monkey that respond to the sight of food was confirmed by Ono et al. (1980).

The discovery that there are neurons in the lateral hypothalamus that respond to the sight of food was an interesting discovery, for it emphasizes the importance in primates of vision, and not just generally, but for motivational behaviour in the selection of a goal object such as food. Indeed, the sight of what we eat conveys important information that can influence not only whether we select the food but also how the food tastes to us (see Section 4.5.5.7). The hypothesis that the lateral hypothalamic neurons were involved in reward effects which the sight and taste of food might produce by activating lateral hypothalamic neurons led to the next experiments, which investigated whether these neurons only responded to the sight and taste of food when it was rewarding. The experiments involved reducing the reward value of the food by feeding as much of the food as was wanted, and then measuring whether the neurons still responded to the sight and taste of the food when it was no longer rewarding.

Effect of hunger

When Rolls and colleagues fed monkeys to satiety, they found that gradually the lateral hypothalamic neurons reduced the magnitude of their responses, until when the monkey was satiated the neurons did not respond at all to the sight and taste of food (Burton, Rolls and

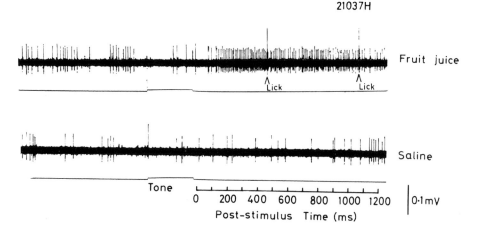

Fig. 5.10 Lateral hypothalamic neuron responding to the sight of food in a visual discrimination task. The neuron increased its firing above the spontaneous rate when a triangle was shown at time 0 which indicated that the monkey could lick a tube in front of his mouth to obtain fruit juice (top trace). The action potentials of the single neuron are the vertical spikes. The neuron did not respond when a square was shown which indicated that if the monkey licked, he would obtain aversive hypertonic saline from the lick tube (bottom trace). The latency of activation of different hypothalamic neurons by the sight of food was 150–200 ms, and compared with a latency of 250–300 ms for the earliest electrical activity associated with the motor responses of a lick made to obtain food when the food-related visual stimulus was shown. (From Rolls, Sanghera and Roper-Hall 1979).

Mora 1976, Rolls 1981a, Rolls, Murzi, Yaxley, Thorpe and Simpson 1986). An example is shown in Fig. 5.3 of a neuron that stopped responding to the sight of glucose after feeding to satiety with glucose, but which still responded to the sight of other foods. A sensory-specific satiety experiment for a lateral hypothalamic neuron with responses to the taste of food is illustrated in Fig. 5.11. These findings provide evidence that these neurons have activity that is closely related to either or both autonomic responses (such as salivation to the sight of food) and behavioural responses (such as approach to a food reward) to the sight and taste of food, which only occur to food if hunger is present.

The signals that reflect the motivational state and perform this modulation probably include many of those described in Section 5.3, such as gastric distension and duodenal stimulation by food (e.g. Gibbs, Maddison and Rolls (1981)), and reach the nucleus of the solitary tract via the vagus nerve as in rats (Ewart 1993, Mei 1993, Mei 1994). The plasma glucose level may be sensed by cells in the hindbrain near the area postrema in the rat (Ritter 1986). In the monkey there is less evidence about the location of the crucial sites for glucose sensing that control food intake. It is known that there are glucose-sensitive neurons in a number of hindbrain and hypothalamic sites, as shown by micro-electro-osmotic experiments in which glucose is applied locally to a neuron being recorded by using a small current to draw out sodium ion which then drags glucose with it (Oomura and Yoshimatsu 1984, Aou, Oomura, Lenard, Nishino, Inokuchi, Minami and Misaki 1984).

The hypothalamus is not necessarily the first stage at which processing of food-related stimuli is modulated by hunger. Evidence on which is the first stage of processing where modulation by hunger occurs in primates is considered for the taste system below. To investigate

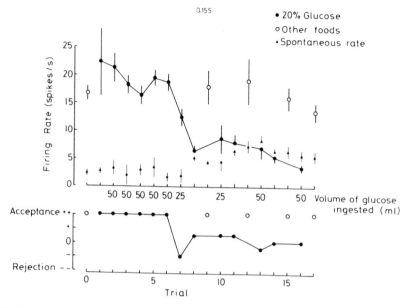

Fig. 5.11 The effect of feeding the monkey to satiety with 20% glucose solution on the responses of a lateral hypothalamic neuron to the taste of the glucose (filled circles) and to the taste of other foods (open circles). After the monkey had fed to satiety with glucose, the neuron responded much less to the taste of glucose, but still responded to the other foods. The mean responses of the neuron ($\pm$ s.e.m.) are shown to the stimuli at different stages of the experiment. The satiety of the monkey, shown below, was measured by whether he accepted or rejected the glucose. (From Rolls, Murzi, Yaxley, Thorpe and Simpson 1986, after Rolls 1981a.)

whether hunger modulates neuronal responses in parts of the visual system through which visual information is likely to reach the hypothalamus (see below), the activity of neurons in the visual inferior temporal cortex was recorded in the same testing situations. It was found that the neuronal responses here to visual stimuli were not dependent on hunger (Rolls, Judge and Sanghera 1977). Nor were the responses of an initial sample of neurons in the amygdala, which connects the inferior temporal visual cortex to the hypothalamus (see below), found to depend on hunger (Sanghera, Rolls and Roper-Hall 1979, Rolls 1992b). However, in the orbitofrontal cortex, which receives inputs from the inferior temporal visual cortex, and projects into the hypothalamus (see below and Russchen et al. (1985)), neurons with visual responses to food are found, and neuronal responses to food in this region are modulated by hunger (Thorpe, Rolls and Maddison 1983, Critchley and Rolls 1996a) (see Sections 5.4.2.3, 5.4.4.2 and 5.4.5).

Thus for visual processing, hunger modulates neuronal responsiveness only at late stages of sensory processing and in the hypothalamus. The adaptive value of modulation of sensory processing only at late stages of processing, which occurs also in the taste system of primates, is discussed when food-related taste processing is described below.

Sensory-specific modulation of the responsiveness of lateral hypothalamic neurons and of appetite

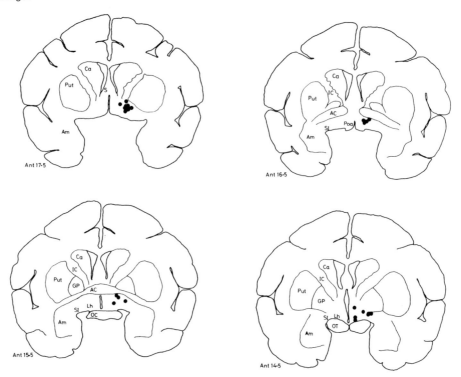

Fig. 5.13 Sites in the lateral hypothalamus and basal forebrain of the macaque at which neurons were recorded that responded to the sight of food. Abbreviations: AC, anterior commissure; Am, amygdala; Ca, caudate nucleus; GP, globus pallidus; IC, internal capsule; Lh, lateral hypothalamus; OC, optic chiasm; OT, optic tract; Poa, preoptic area; Put, putamen; S, septal region; SI, substantia innominata. (From Rolls, Sanghera and Roper-Hall 1979)

these neurons by food, and that this is what makes food rewarding. At the same time this accounts for self-stimulation of some brain sites, which is understood as the animal seeking to activate the neurons that he normally seeks to activate by food when he is hungry. This and other evidence (Rolls 1975, Rolls 1999a) indicates that feeding normally occurs in order to obtain the sensory input produced by food which is rewarding if the animal is hungry.

Sites in the hypothalamus and basal forebrain of neurons that respond to food

These neurons are found as a relatively small proportion of cells in a region which includes the lateral hypothalamus and substantia innominata and extends from the lateral hypothalamus posteriorly through the anterior hypothalamus and lateral preoptic area to a region ventral to and anterior to the anterior commissure (Rolls, Sanghera and Roper-Hall 1979a)) (see Fig. 5.13).

Useful further information about the particular populations of neurons in these regions with feeding-related activity, and about the functions of these neurons in feeding, could be provided by evidence on their output connections. It is known that some hypothalamic neurons project to brainstem autonomic regions such as the dorsal motor nucleus of the vagus (Saper et al. 1976, Saper, Swanson and Cowan 1979). If some of the hypothalamic neurons with feeding-related activity projected in this way, it would be very likely that their functions would include the generation of autonomic responses to the sight of food. Some hypothalamic neurons project to the substantia nigra (Nauta and Domesick 1978), and some neurons in the lateral hypothalamus and basal magnocellular forebrain nuclei of Meynert project directly to the cerebral cortex (Kievit and Kuypers 1975, Divac 1975, Heimer and Alheid 1991). If some of these were feeding-related neurons, then by such routes they could influence whether feeding is initiated.

To determine to which regions hypothalamic neurons with feeding-related activity project, electrical stimulation was applied to these different regions, to determine from which regions hypothalamic neurons with feeding-related activity can be antidromically activated. It was found in such experiments by E. T. Rolls and E. Murzi that some of these feeding-related neurons in the lateral hypothalamus and substantia innominata project directly to the cerebral cortex, to such areas as the prefrontal cortex in the sulcus principalis and the supplementary motor cortex. This provides evidence that at least some of these neurons with feeding-related activity project this information to the cerebral cortex, where it could be used in such processes as the initiation of feeding behaviour. It also indicates that at least some of these feeding-related neurons are in the basal magnocellular forebrain nuclei of Meynert, which is quite consistent with the reconstructions of the recording sites (Fig. 5.13) (see also Section 4.9.5).

In addition to a role in food reward and thus in the control of feeding, it seems quite likely that at least some of the hypothalamic feeding-related neurons influence brainstem autonomic motor neurons. Consistent with this, it is known that there are projections from the lateral hypothalamus to the brainstem autonomic motor nuclei, and that lesions of the lateral hypothalamus disrupt conditioned autonomic responses (LeDoux et al. 1988).

Effects of signals related to hunger and satiety on hypothalamic neurons

We have seen that external signals such as the taste, smell, and sight of food influence lateral hypothalamic neurons only if hunger is present. The question then arises of how hunger and satiety-related signals such as peripherally produced leptin, insulin, and glucose influence hypothalamic neurons, to provide a potential source of the signals that help to modulate sensory neuronal responses to food. It is now known (see Carlson (2004), Woods et al. (2000), and Cummings and Schwartz (2003)) that there are melanin-concentrating hormone (MCH) and orexin producing neurons in the lateral hypothalamus, and that an increase in their activity increases food intake and decreases metabolic rate (see Fig. 5.14). These neurons are activated by neuropeptide Y (NPY), itself a potent stimulator of food intake, produced by neurons in the arcuate nucleus, a hypothalamic nucleus in the ventromedial hypothalamic region. The arcuate NPY neurons also release agouti-related peptide (AGRP), itself a potent stimulator of food intake. One of the signals that activates NPY/AGRP neurons is ghrelin, a hunger-producing hormone produced by the stomach (Cummings, Frayo, Marmonier, Aubert and Chapolet 2004) (see Fig. 5.14). NPY/AGRP neurons increase their firing rates during fasting, and are inhibited by leptin (Cone 2005, Horvath 2005). Obese people generally have high levels of leptin, so leptin production is not the problem, and instead leptin resistance (i.e. insensitivity) may be somewhat related to obesity, with the resistance perhaps related in part to smaller effects of leptin on arcuate nucleus NPY/AGRP neurons (Munzberg and Myers 2005).

Leptin not only inhibits the production of NPY and AGRP by the arcuate NPY/AGRP neurons, but also inhibits the lateral hypothalamic orexin-producing neurons, and these are

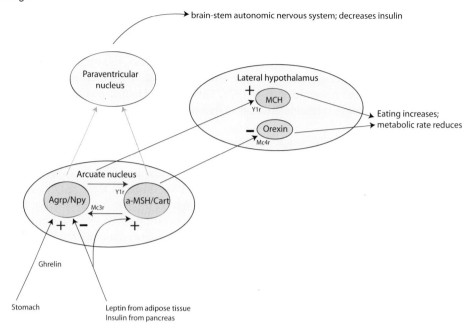

Fig. 5.14 Effects of peripheral hunger and satiety-related signals on some of the neurochemically identified feeding-related neurons of the arcuate and lateral hypothalamic nuclei. (See text for abbreviations and description)

two ways in which leptin may decrease feeding (Pinto, Roseberry, Liu, Diano, Shanabrough, Cai, Friedman and Horvath 2004). CART (cocaine- and amphetamine-regulated transcript), produced by the α-MSH/CART/POMC neurons in the arcuate nucleus shown in Fig. 5.14[14], reduces hunger (i.e. is anorexigenic), so does α-melanocyte-stimulating hormone (α-MSH) produced by the same neurons, and these neurons are also activated by leptin, providing more ways in which leptin may act to reduce feeding (Elmquist, Elias and Saper 1999, Carlson 2004, Cone 2005, Horvath 2005) (see Fig. 5.14). Consistent with this, the (very rare) humans with clear genetic dysfunctions of the leptin receptor systems may show overeating and obesity which is treatable by leptin (Farooqi et al. 2001), and approximately 4% of obese people have deficient (MC4) receptors for melanocyte stimulating hormone (MSH) (Barsh, Farooqi and O'Rahilly 2000, Cummings and Schwartz 2003, Cone 2005). Also consistently, a very rare mutation in the gene encoding POMC in humans results in low MSH levels and obesity (and red hair due to the absence of melanin) (Cone 2005).

It is also known that cannabinoids (see Section 8.8) can increase appetite and body weight (Di Marzo and Matias 2005).

Functions of the hypothalamus in feeding

The functions of the hypothalamus in feeding are thus related at least in part to the inputs that it receives from the forebrain, in that it contains neurons that respond to the sight of food, and that are influenced by learning. (Such pattern-specific visual responses,

---

[14]POMC is pro-opiomelanocortin

and their modification by learning, require forebrain areas such as the inferior temporal visual cortex and the amygdala, as described below.) This conclusion is consistent with the anatomy of the hypothalamus and substantia innominata, which receive projections from limbic structures such as the amygdala which in turn receive projections from the association cortex (Nauta 1961, Herzog and Van Hoesen 1976). The conclusion is also consistent with the evidence that decerebrate rats retain simple controls of feeding, but do not show normal learning about foods (Grill and Norgren 1978). These rats accept sweet solutions placed in their mouths when hungry and reject them when satiated, so some control of responses to gustatory stimuli which depends on hunger can occur caudal to the level of the hypothalamus. However, these rats are unable to feed themselves, and do not learn to avoid poisoned solutions.

The importance of visual inputs and learning to feeding, in relation to which some hypothalamic neurons respond, is that animals, and especially primates, may eat many foods every day, and must be able to select foods from other visual stimuli, as well as produce appropriate preparative responses to them such as salivation and the release of insulin. They must also be able to initiate appropriate actions in the environment to obtain food. Before any activation of motor neurons, such as those that innervate the masticatory muscles, involved in feeding, it is normally necessary to select which reinforcer in the environment should be the object of action, and then to select an appropriate (arbitrary) action to obtain the selected reinforcer. This indicates that direct connections from food reward systems or feeding control systems in the brain directly to motor neurons are likely to be involved only in the lowest level (in the sense of Hughlings Jackson, see Swash (1989)) of the control of behaviour. Instead, food reward systems might be expected to project to an action-control system, and connections therefore from the lateral hypothalamus, amygdala, and orbitofrontal cortex to systems such as the basal ganglia are likely to be more important as routes for the initiation of normal feeding (see Section 8.4 on the striatum and basal ganglia).

5.4.2   Brain mechanisms for the reward produced by the taste of food

5.4.2.1   Taste processing up to and including the primary taste cortex of primates is related to the identity of the tastant, and not to its reward value

Given that there are neurons in the hypothalamus that can respond to the taste (and/or sight) of foods but not of non-foods, and that modulation of this sensory input by motivation is seen when recordings are made from these hypothalamic neurons, it may be asked whether these are special properties of hypothalamic neurons which they show because they are specially involved in the control of motivational responses, or whether this degree of specificity and type of modulation are general properties which are evident throughout sensory systems. In one respect it would be inefficient if motivational modulation were present far peripherally, because this would imply that sensory information was being discarded without the possibility for central processing. A subjective correspondent of such a situation might be that it might not be possible to taste food, or even to see food, when satiated! It is perhaps more efficient for most of the system to function similarly whether hungry or satiated, and to have a special system (such as the hypothalamus) following sensory processing where motivational state influences responsiveness. Evidence on the actual state of affairs that exists for visual processing in primates in relation to feeding has been summarized above. In contrast, apparently there is at least some peripheral modulation of taste processing in rats (in the nucleus of the solitary tract)

(Scott and Giza 1992, Rolls and Scott 2003). Evidence is now being obtained for primates on the tuning of neurons in the gustatory pathways, and on whether responsiveness at different stages is influenced by motivation, as follows. These investigations on the gustatory pathways have also been able to show where flavour, that is a combination of taste and olfactory input, is computed in the primate brain. The gustatory and olfactory pathways, and some of their onward connections, are shown in Fig. 4.2.

The first central synapse of the gustatory system is in the rostral part of the nucleus of the solitary tract (Beckstead and Norgren 1979, Beckstead, Morse and Norgren 1980, Rolls and Scott 2003). The caudal half of this nucleus receives visceral afferents, and it is a possibility that such visceral information, reflecting, for example, gastric distension, is used to modulate gustatory processing even at this early stage of the gustatory system.

In order to investigate the tuning of neurons in the nucleus of the solitary tract, and whether hunger does influence processing at this first central opportunity in the gustatory system of primates, we recorded the activity of single neurons in the nucleus of the solitary tract. To ensure that our results were relevant to the normal control of feeding (and were not, for example, because of abnormally high levels of artificially administered putative satiety signals), we allowed the monkeys to feed until they were satiated, and determined whether this normal and physiological induction of satiety influenced the responsiveness of neurons in the nucleus of the solitary tract, which were recorded throughout the feeding, until satiety was reached. It was found that in the nucleus of the solitary tract, the first central relay in the gustatory system, neurons are relatively broadly tuned to the prototypical taste stimuli (sweet, salt, bitter, and sour) (Scott, Yaxley, Sienkiewicz and Rolls 1986b). It was also found that neuronal responses in the nucleus of the solitary tract to the taste of food are not influenced by whether the monkey is hungry or satiated (Yaxley, Rolls, Sienkiewicz and Scott 1985).

To investigate whether there are neurons in the primary gustatory cortex in the primate that are more closely tuned to respond to foods as compared to non-foods, and whether hunger modulates the responsiveness of these neurons, we have recorded the activity of single neurons in the primary gustatory cortex during feeding in the monkey. In the primary gustatory cortex in the frontal operculum and insula, neurons are more sharply tuned to gustatory stimuli than in the nucleus of the solitary tract, with some neurons responding primarily, for example, to sweet, and much less to salt, bitter, or sour stimuli (Scott, Yaxley, Sienkiewicz and Rolls 1986a, Yaxley, Rolls and Sienkiewicz 1990). However, here also, hunger does not influence the magnitude of neuronal responses to gustatory stimuli (Rolls, Scott, Sienkiewicz and Yaxley 1988, Yaxley, Rolls and Sienkiewicz 1988).

5.4.2.2 Taste and taste-related processing in the secondary taste cortex, including umami taste, astringency, fat, viscosity, temperature and capsaicin

A secondary cortical taste area has been discovered in the caudolateral orbitofrontal taste cortex of the primate in which gustatory neurons can be even more finely tuned to particular taste stimuli (Rolls, Yaxley and Sienkiewicz 1990, Rolls and Treves 1990) (see Fig. 4.19). In addition to representations of the 'prototypical' taste stimuli sweet, salt, bitter, and sour, different neurons in this region respond to other taste and taste-related stimuli that provide information about the reward value of a potential food (Rolls 2007b, Rolls 2006b, Kadohisa, Rolls and Verhagen 2005a). One example of this additional taste information is a set of neurons that respond to umami taste, as described next.

Umami taste. An important food taste which appears to be different from that produced by sweet, salt, bitter, or sour is the taste of protein. At least part of this taste is captured by the Japanese word 'umami', which is a taste common to a diversity of food sources including fish, meats, mushrooms, cheese, and some vegetables such as tomatoes. Within these food sources, it is glutamates and $5'$ nucleotides, sometimes in a synergistic combination, that create the umami taste (Ikeda 1909, Yamaguchi 1967, Yamaguchi and Kimizuka 1979, Kawamura and Kare 1992). Monosodium L-glutamate (MSG), and the $5'$ nucleotides guanosine $5'$-monophosphate (GMP), and inosine $5'$-monophosphate (IMP), are examples of umami stimuli.

These findings raise the question of whether umami taste operates through information channels in the primate taste system which are separable from those for the 'prototypical' tastes sweet, salt, bitter, and sour. (Although the concept of four prototypical tastes has been used by tradition, there is increasing discussion about the utility of the concept, and increasing evidence that the taste system is more diverse than this – see, e.g., Kawamura and Kare (1992)). To investigate the neural encoding of glutamate in the primate, Baylis and Rolls (1991) made recordings from 190 taste-responsive neurons in the primary taste cortex and adjoining orbitofrontal cortex taste area in macaques. Single neurons were found that were tuned to respond best to monosodium glutamate (umami taste), just as other cells were found with best responses to glucose (sweet), sodium chloride (salty), HCl (sour), and quinine HCl (bitter). Across the population of neurons, the responsiveness to glutamate was poorly correlated with the responsiveness to NaCl, so that the representation of glutamate was clearly different from that of NaCl. Further, the representation of glutamate was shown to be approximately as different from each of the other four tastants as they are from each other, as shown by multidimensional scaling and cluster analysis. Moreover, it was found that glutamate is approximately as well represented in terms of mean evoked neural activity and the number of cells with best responses to it as the other four stimuli glucose, NaCl, HCl and quinine. It was concluded that in primate taste cortical areas, glutamate, which produces umami taste in humans, is approximately as well represented as are the tastes produced by: glucose (sweet), NaCl (salty), HCl (sour) and quinine HCl (bitter) (Baylis and Rolls 1991).

In a further investigation, these findings have been extended beyond the sodium salt of glutamate to other umami tastants which have the glutamate ion but which do not introduce sodium ion into the experiment; and to a nucleotide umami tastant (Rolls, Critchley, Wakeman and Mason 1996c). In recordings made mainly from neurons in the orbitofrontal cortex taste area, it was shown that single neurons that had their best responses to sodium glutamate also had good responses to glutamic acid. The correlation between the responses to these two tastants was higher than between any other pair which included in addition a prototypical set including glucose (sweet), sodium chloride (salty), HCl (sour), and quinine HCl (bitter). Moreover, the responsiveness to glutamic acid clustered with the response to monosodium glutamate in a cluster analysis with this set of stimuli, and glutamic acid was close to sodium glutamate in a space created by multidimensional scaling. It was also shown that the responses of these neurons to the nucleotide umami tastant inosine $5'$-monophosphate were more correlated with their responses to monosodium glutamate than to any prototypical tastant.

Thus neurophysiological evidence in primates does indicate that there is a representation of umami flavour in the cortical areas which is separable from that to the prototypical tastants sweet, salt, bitter, and sour (see further (Rolls, Critchley, Browning and Hernadi 1998a). This

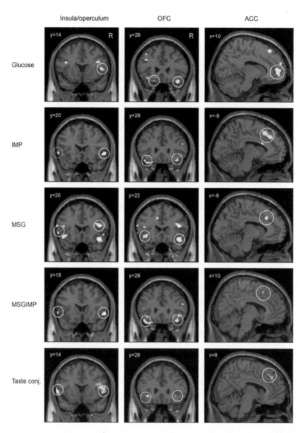

Fig. 5.15 Activation of the human primary taste cortex in the insula/frontal operculum; the orbitofrontal cortex (OFC); and the anterior cingulate cortex (ACC) by taste. The stimuli used included glucose, two umami taste stimuli (monosodium glutamate (MSG) and inosine monophosphate (IMP)), and a mixture of the two umami stimuli. Taste conj. refers to a conjunction analysis over all the taste stimuli. (After DeAraujo, Kringelbach, Rolls and Hobden 2003.) (See colour plates section.)

representation is probably important in the taste produced by proteins (cf. Chaudhari, Yang, Lamp, Delay, Cartford, Than and Roper (1996) and Chaudhari, Landin and Roper (2000). These neurons are found not only in the orbitofrontal cortex taste areas, but also in the primary taste cortex (Baylis and Rolls 1991).

Recently, evidence has started to accumulate that there may be taste receptors on the tongue specialized for umami taste (Chaudhari, Yang, Lamp, Delay, Cartford, Than and Roper 1996, Chaudhari and Roper 1998, Chaudhari, Landin and Roper 2000, Zhao, Zhang, Hoon, Chandrashekar, Erlenbach, Ryba and Zucker 2003, Lin, Ogura and Kinnamon 2003).

In addition, we have recently shown that the umami tastants monosodium glutamate and inosine monophosphate activate the human primary taste cortex in the insula/operculum, the secondary taste cortex in the orbitofrontal cortex, and the cingulate cortex (De Araujo, Kringelbach, Rolls and Hobden 2003a), as shown in Fig. 5.15.

This evidence shows that umami taste, an indicator of the presence of protein, is implemented by neurons in the primary and secondary taste cortex that are tuned to umami stimuli.

Umami is a component of many foods which helps to make them taste pleasant, especially when the umami taste is paired with a consonant savoury odour (Rolls, Critchley, Browning and Hernadi 1998a).

Astringency. Another taste-related stimulus quality that provides important information about the reward value of a potential food source is astringency. In humans, tannic acid elicits a characteristic astringent taste. Oral astringency is perceived as the feeling of long-lasting puckering and drying sensations on the tongue and membranes of the oral cavity. High levels of tannic acid in some potential foods makes them unpalatable without preparative techniques to reduce its presence (Johns and Duquette 1991), yet in small quantities it is commonly used to enhance the flavour of food. In this context tannic acid is a constituent of a large range of spices and condiments, such as ginger, chillies, and black pepper (Uma-Pradeep, Geervani and Eggum 1993). (Tannic acid itself is not present in tea, yet a range of related polyphenol compounds are, particularly in green tea (Graham 1992)). Tannic acid is a natural antioxidant by virtue of its chemical structure (see Critchley and Rolls (1996c)).

The evolutionary adaptive value of the ability to detect astringency may be related to some of the properties of tannic acid. Tannic acid is a member of the class of compounds known as polyphenols, which are present in a wide spectrum of plant matter, particularly in foliage, the skin and husks of fruit and nuts, and the bark of trees. The tannic acid in leaves is produced as a defence against insects. There is less tannic acid in young leaves than in old leaves. Large monkeys cannot obtain the whole of their protein intake from small animals, insects etc., and thus obtain some of their protein from leaves. Tannic acid binds protein (hence its use in tanning) and amino acids, and thus prevents their absorption. Thus it is adaptive for monkeys to be able to taste tannic acid, so that they can select food sources without too much tannic acid (Hladik 1978).

In order to investigate whether astringency is represented in the cortical taste areas concerned with taste, Critchley and Rolls (1996c) recorded from taste-responsive neurons in the orbitofrontal cortex and adjacent insula. Single neurons were found that were tuned to respond to tannic acid (0.001 M), and represented a subpopulation of neurons that was distinct from neurons responsive to the tastes of glucose (sweet), NaCl (salty), HCl (sour), quinine (bitter) and monosodium glutamate (umami). In addition, across the population of taste-responsive neurons, tannic acid was as well represented as the tastes of NaCl, HCl, quinine, or monosodium glutamate. Multidimensional scaling analysis of the neuronal responses to the tastants indicates that tannic acid lies outside the boundaries of the four conventional taste qualities (sweet, sour, bitter, and salty). Taken together these data indicate that the astringent taste of tannic acid should be considered as a distinct 'taste' quality, which receives a separate representation from sweet, salt, bitter, and sour in the primate cortical taste areas. Tannic acid may produce its 'taste' effects not through the taste nerves, but through the somatosensory inputs conveyed through the trigeminal nerve. Astringency is thus strictly not a sixth taste in the sense that umami is a fifth taste. However, what has been shown in these studies is that the orosensory, probably somatosensory, sensations produced by tannic acid do converge with effects produced through taste inputs, to result in neurons in the orbitofrontal cortex responding to both taste stimuli and to astringent stimuli.

Food texture: viscosity. Another important type of input to the same region of the orbitofrontal cortex that is concerned with detecting the reward value of a potential food is an input

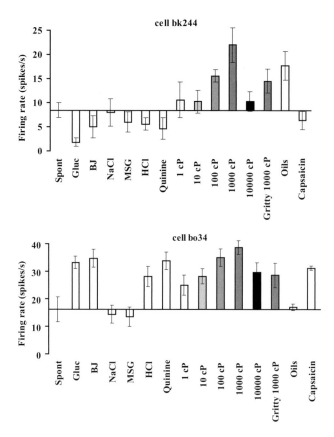

Fig. 5.16 Above. Firing rates (mean ± s.e.m.) of orbitofrontal cortex viscosity-sensitive neuron bk244 which did not have taste responses. The firing rates are shown to the viscosity series (carboxymethylcellulose in the range 1–10,000 centiPoise), to the gritty stimulus (carboxymethylcellulose with Fillite microspheres), to the taste stimuli 1 M glucose (Gluc), 0.1 M NaCl, 0.1 M MSG , 0.01 M HCl and 0.001 M QuinineHCl, and to fruit juice (BJ). Spont = spontaneous firing rate. Below. Firing rates (mean ± s.e.m.) of viscosity-sensitive neuron bo34 which had no response to the oils (mineral oil, vegetable oil, safflower oil and coconut oil, which have viscosities which are all close to 50 cP). The neuron did not respond to the gritty stimulus in a way that was unexpected given the viscosity of the stimulus, was taste tuned, and did respond to capsaicin. (After Rolls, Verhagen and Kadohisa 2003.)

produced by the texture of food in the mouth. We have shown for example in recent recordings that single neurons influenced by taste in this region can in some cases have their responses modulated by the texture of the food. This was shown in experiments in which the texture of food was manipulated by the addition of methyl cellulose or gelatine, or by puréeing a semi-solid food (Rolls and Critchley, in preparation). We have been able to show that some of these neurons respond to the viscosity of the food in the mouth, as altered parametrically using the standard food thickening agent carboxymethylcellulose made up in viscosities of 1–10,000 cPoise (Rolls, Verhagen and Kadohisa 2003e). (10,000 cP is approximately the viscosity of toothpaste.) Some of these neurons are unimodal, responding just to texture and not to taste (see Fig. 5.16 upper). Others respond to different combinations of texture and

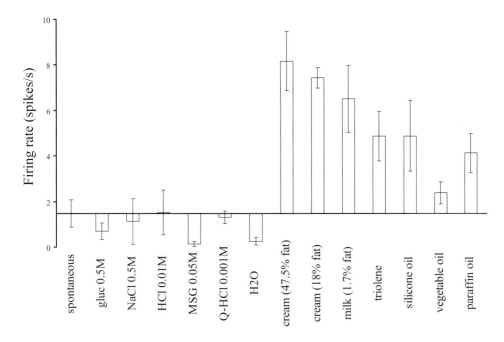

Fig. 5.17 A neuron in the primate orbitofrontal cortex responding to the texture of fat in the mouth. The neuron increased its firing rate to cream (double and single cream, with the fat proportions shown), and responded to texture rather than the chemical structure of the fat in that it also responded to 0.5 ml of silicone oil ($Si(CH_3)_2O)_n$) or paraffin oil (hydrocarbon). The neuron did not have a taste input. Gluc, glucose; NaCl, salt; HCl, sour; Q-HCl, quinine, bitter. The spontaneous firing rate of the cell is also shown. (After Rolls, Critchley et al, 1999.)

taste, as illustrated in Fig. 5.16 (lower). These recordings provide unique evidence about the texture channels that convey information from the mouth to the cortex, for they show that the system can potentially have responses to texture separately from the other sensory attributes of food, as well as to particular combinations of taste, texture, and other sensory properties of food.

The somatosensory inputs may reach the orbitofrontal cortex via the primary taste cortex in the rostral insula and adjoining frontal operculum, which we have shown does project into this region (Baylis, Rolls and Baylis 1994), and which also contains a representation of the viscosity of what is in the mouth (Verhagen, Kadohisa and Rolls 2004). A number of parts of the insula are known to receive somatosensory inputs (Mesulam and Mufson 1982a, Mesulam and Mufson 1982b, Mufson and Mesulam 1982). The texture of food is an important cue about the quality of the food, for example about the ripeness of fruit.

These findings have recently been extended to the human, with the finding with fMRI that the activation of the primary taste cortex is proportional to the logarithm of the viscosity of the stimulus in the mouth (De Araujo and Rolls 2004).

Food texture: fat. Texture in the mouth is also an important indicator of whether fat is present in the food, which is important not only as a high value energy source, but also as a potential source of essential fatty acids. In the orbitofrontal cortex, Rolls, Critchley, Browning, Hernadi and Lenard (1999a) have found a population of neurons that responds when fat is in the mouth. An example of such a neuron is shown in Fig. 5.17. This neuron had no response to taste, but some other neurons had convergence of fat texture and taste inputs. The fat-related responses of these neurons are produced at least in part by the texture of the food rather than by chemical receptors sensitive to certain chemicals, in that such neurons typically respond not only to foods such as cream and milk containing fat, but also to paraffin oil (which is a pure hydrocarbon) and to silicone oil (which contains $(Si(CH_3)_2O)_n$).

Some of the fat-related neurons do though have multimodal convergent inputs from the chemical senses, in that in addition to taste inputs some of these neurons respond to the odour associated with a fat, such as the odour of cream (Rolls, Critchley, Browning, Hernadi and Lenard 1999a). The texture-related responses of these oral fat-sensitive neurons are independent of the viscosity of what is in the mouth and of fatty acids in the mouth (Verhagen, Rolls and Kadohisa 2003), so that fat in food can be detected orally by a specialized fat/oil texture channel.

This type of discovery can be made only at the single neuron level, and paves the way for further studies of the transducing mechanism, understanding of which could be important in the design of foods with pleasant textures which do not bring with them high caloric content with its implications for obesity.

These findings have recently been extended to the human, with the finding with fMRI that activation of the orbitofrontal cortex and perigenual cingulate cortex is produced by the texture of fat in the mouth (De Araujo and Rolls 2004).

5.4.2.3 The reward value of taste is represented in the orbitofrontal cortex

In the primate orbitofrontal cortex, it is found that the responses of taste neurons to the particular food with which a monkey is fed to satiety decrease to zero (Rolls, Sienkiewicz and Yaxley 1989b). An example is shown in Fig. 4.21. This neuron reduced its responses to the taste of glucose during the course of feeding as much glucose as the monkey wanted to drink. When the monkey was fully satiated, and did not want to drink any more glucose, the neuron no longer responded to the taste of glucose. Thus the responses of these neurons decrease to zero when the reward value of the food decreases to zero. Interestingly the neuron still responded to other foods, and the monkey was willing to eat these other foods. Thus the modulation of the responses of these orbitofrontal cortex taste neurons occurs in a sensory-specific way.

The orbitofrontal cortex is the first stage of the primate taste system in which this modulation of the responses of neurons to the taste of food is affected by hunger, in that this modulation is not found in the nucleus of the solitary tract, or in the frontal opercular or insular primary gustatory cortices (Yaxley, Rolls, Sienkiewicz and Scott 1985, Rolls, Scott, Sienkiewicz and Yaxley 1988, Yaxley, Rolls and Sienkiewicz 1988). It is of course only when hungry that the taste of food is rewarding. This is an indication that the responses of these orbitofrontal cortex taste neurons reflect the reward value of food. The firing of these orbitofrontal neurons may actually implement the reward value of a food. The hypothesis is that primates work to obtain firing of these neurons, by eating food when they are hungry.

Further evidence that the firing of these orbitofrontal cortex taste neurons does actually implement the primary reward value of food is that in another experiment we showed that monkeys would work to obtain electrical stimulation of this area of the brain (Rolls, Burton and Mora 1980c, Mora, Avrith, Phillips and Rolls 1979, Mora, Avrith and Rolls 1980). Moreover, the reward value of the electrical stimulation was dependent on hunger being present. If the monkey was fed to satiety, the monkey no longer found electrical stimulation at this site so rewarding, and stopped working for the electrical stimulation. Indeed, of all the brain sites tested, this orbitofrontal cortex region was the part of the brain in which the reward value of the electrical stimulation was most affected by feeding to satiety (Mora, Avrith, Phillips and Rolls 1979, Mora, Avrith and Rolls 1980, Rolls, Burton and Mora 1980c). Thus all this evidence indicates that the reward value of taste is decoded in the secondary taste cortex, and that primates work to obtain food in order to activate these neurons, the activation of which actually mediates reward. This is probably an innate reward system, in that taste can act as a reward in rats without prior training (Berridge, Flynn, Schulkin and Grill 1984).

The neurophysiological discoveries that feeding to satiety reduces the responses of secondary taste cortex neurons, but not neurons earlier in taste processing, are relevant to what normally produces satiety, in that in these experiments the neurons were recorded while the monkeys were fed to normal satiety. It could be that later in satiety there is some modulation of responsiveness earlier in the taste pathways, occurring perhaps as food is absorbed. But even if this does occur, such modulation would not then account for the change in acceptability of food, which of course is seen as the satiety develops, and is used to define satiety. Nor would this modulation be relevant to the decrease in the pleasantness in the taste of a food which occurs when it is eaten to satiety (Cabanac 1971, Rolls, Rolls, Rowe and Sweeney 1981a, Rolls, Rowe, Rolls, Kingston, Megson and Gunary 1981b, Rolls, Rolls and Rowe 1983b, Rolls and Rolls 1977, Rolls and Rolls 1982b).

Thus it appears that the reduced acceptance of food as satiety develops, and the reduction in its pleasantness, are not produced by a reduction in the responses of neurons in the nucleus of the solitary tract or frontal opercular or insular gustatory cortices to gustatory stimuli. (As described above, the responses of gustatory neurons in these areas do not decrease as satiety develops.) Indeed, after feeding to satiety, humans reported that the taste of the food on which they had been satiated tasted almost as intense as when they were hungry, though much less pleasant (Rolls, Rolls and Rowe 1983b). This comparison is consistent with the possibility that activity in the frontal opercular and insular taste cortices as well as the nucleus of the solitary tract does not reflect the pleasantness of the taste of a food, but rather its sensory qualities independently of motivational state. On the other hand, the responses of the neurons in the orbitofrontal taste area and in the lateral hypothalamus are modulated by satiety, and it is presumably in areas such as these that neuronal activity may be related to whether a food tastes pleasant, and to whether the human or animal will work to obtain and then eat the food, that is to whether the food is rewarding. The situation is not necessarily the same in non-primates, in that in the rat some reduction in the responses of taste neurons in the nucleus of the solitary tract was produced by glucose infusions (Scott and Giza 1992, Scott et al. 1995, Rolls and Scott 2003).

The present results also provide evidence on the nature of the mechanisms that underlie sensory-specific satiety. Sensory-specific satiety, as noted above in Section 5.3.1, is the phenomenon in which the decrease in the palatability and acceptability of a food that has been eaten to satiety are partly specific to the particular food that has been eaten. The results just described suggest that such sensory-specific satiety for taste cannot be largely accounted for by adaptation at the receptor level, in the nucleus of the solitary tract, or in the frontal opercular or insular gustatory cortices, to the food which has been eaten to satiety, otherwise modulation of neuronal responsiveness should have been apparent in the recordings made in these regions. Indeed, the findings suggest that sensory-specific satiety is not represented in

Critchley, Mason and Wakeman 1996b). In the task, if one odour was delivered through an olfactometer tube close to the nose, then the monkey could lick to obtain glucose (Reward trials). If a different odour was delivered, the monkey had to avoid licking, otherwise he obtained saline (Saline trials). The neuron shown in Fig. 4.28 responded well to the smell of onion (the discriminative stimulus on saline trials), and much less to the odour of fruit juice (the stimulus on Reward trials). The neuron had a selective and specific response to odour, and did not respond non-specifically in the discrimination task, as shown by the absence of neuronal activity while the monkey performed a visual discrimination task. The different types of neuron (unimodal in different modalities, and multimodal) were frequently found close to one another in tracks made into this region (see Fig. 4.27), consistent with the hypothesis that the multimodal representations are actually being formed from unimodal inputs to this region.

These results show that there are regions in the orbitofrontal cortex of primates where the sensory modalities of taste, vision, and olfaction converge; and that in many cases the neurons have corresponding sensitivities across modalities. It appears to be in these areas that flavour representations are built, where flavour is taken to mean a representation that is evoked best by a combination of gustatory and olfactory input. This orbitofrontal region does appear to be an important region for convergence, for there is only a very low proportion of bimodal taste and olfactory neurons in the primary taste cortex (Rolls and Baylis 1994), and in general primary taste cortex neurons do not respond to olfactory or visual stimuli even if they are associated with the taste of food (Verhagen, Kadohisa and Rolls 2004).

To investigate where flavour is formed in humans by olfactory and taste convergence, De Araujo, Rolls, Kringelbach, McGlone and Phillips (2003c) performed an fMRI investigation with unimodal taste (sucrose), unimodal olfactory (strawberry odour), and a mixture of both. They found that a part of the human insular taste cortex was unimodal for taste, and that both olfactory and taste stimuli activated the orbitofrontal cortex and its posterior extension into the agranular insula. Moreover, supralinear additivity of the olfactory and taste components was found in a part of the orbitofrontal cortex. Further, the consonance and pleasantness subjective ratings of the olfactory and taste mixtures (which included some non-consonant mixtures such as sucrose and savory odour) were correlated with activations in the medial orbitofrontal cortex (see Fig. 4.29). Thus the processing that it is possible to analyse in detail at the neuronal level in primates appears to provide a good model for how taste and odour combine to produce pleasant flavour in humans (Rolls 2004g, Rolls 2004h).

5.4.4 Brain mechanisms for the reward produced by the odour of food

5.4.4.1 The rules underlying the formation of olfactory representations in the primate cortex

A schematic diagram of the olfactory pathways in primates is shown in Fig. 4.2 on page 65. There are direct connections from the olfactory bulb to the primary olfactory cortex, pyriform cortex, and from there a connection to a caudal part of the mid (in terms of medial and lateral) orbitofrontal cortex, area 13a, which in turn has onward projections to the lateral orbitofrontal cortex area which we have shown is secondary taste cortex, and to more rostral parts of the orbitofrontal cortex (area 11) (Price et al. 1991, Carmichael and Price 1994, Carmichael et al. 1994) (see Figs. 5.18 and 4.2).

There is evidence that in the olfactory bulb, a coding principle is that in many cases each glomerulus (of which there are approximately 1000) is tuned to respond to its own characteris-

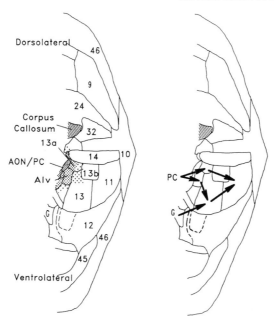

Fig. 5.18 The progression of olfactory inputs to the orbitofrontal cortex in the monkey, drawn on unfolded maps of the frontal lobe. The cortex was unfolded by splitting it along the principal sulcus, which is therefore located at the top and bottom of each map. (Reference to Figs. 4.1 and 4.2 may help to show how the map was constructed.) Left: inputs from the primary olfactory (pyriform) cortex (PC) terminate in the shaded region, that is in the caudal medial part of area 13, i.e. 13a, and in the ventral agranular insular cortex (AIv), which could therefore be termed secondary olfactory cortex. Right: the secondary olfactory cortices then project into the caudolateral orbitofrontal cortex, that is into the secondary taste cortex in that it receives from the primary taste cortex (G); and there are further projections into more anterior and medial parts of the orbitofrontal cortex. (After Price et al. 1991, with permission).

tic hydrocarbon chain length of odourant (Mori, Mataga and Imamura 1992, Imamura, Mataga and Mori 1992, Mori, Nagao and Yoshihara 1999). Evidence for this is that each mitral/tufted cell in the olfactory bulb can be quite sharply tuned, responding for example best to a 5-C length aliphatic odourant (e.g. acid or aldehyde), and being inhibited by nearby hydrocarbon chain-length aliphatic odourants. An effect of this coding might appear to be to spread out the olfactory stimulus space in this early part of the olfactory system, based on the stereochemical structure of the odourant. The code would be spread out in that different parts of chemical space would be relatively evenly represented, in that each part would be represented independently of the presence of other odourants, and in that the code would be relatively sparse, leading to low correlations between the representations of different odours. (Such a coding principle might be facilitated by the presence of in the order of 1000 different genes to code for different olfactory receptor molecules (Buck and Axel 1991, Buck 2000, Mombaerts 1999, Zhang and Firestein 2002, Zou, Horowitz, Montmayeur, Snapper and Buck 2001)).

Is this same coding principle, based on simple physico-chemical properties, used later on in the (primate) olfactory system, or do other principles operate? One example of another coding principle is that representations may be built that represent the co-occurrence of pairs or groups of odourants, so that particular smells in the environment, which typically are produced by combinations of chemical stimuli, are reflected in the responses of neurons. Another coding principle is that olfactory coding might represent in some sense the biological significance of an odour, for example whether it is a food odour that is normally associated with a particular taste. Another principle is that at some stage of olfactory processing the reward or hedonic value of the odourant is represented (whether the odourant smells good), rather than purely the identity of the odourant. For example, whether a food-related odour smells good depends on hunger, and this hedonic representation of odours must be represented in some part of the olfactory system. To elucidate these issues, and thus to provide principles by which the primate olfactory system may operate, the following investigations have been performed.

To investigate how olfactory information is encoded in the orbitofrontal cortex, the responses of single neurons in the orbitofrontal cortex and surrounding areas were recorded during the performance of an olfactory discrimination task (Critchley and Rolls 1996b). The task was designed to show whether there are neurons in this region that categorize odours based on the taste with which the odour is associated. In the task, the delivery of one of eight different odours indicated that the monkey could lick to obtain a taste of sucrose. If one of two other odours was delivered from the olfactometer, the monkey had to refrain from licking, otherwise he received a taste of saline. It was found that 3.1% (48) of the 1580 neurons recorded had olfactory responses, and 34 (2.2%) responded differently to the different odours in the task. The neurons responded with a typical latency of 180 ms from the onset of odourant delivery. 35% of the olfactory neurons with differential responses in the task responded on the basis of the taste reward association of the odourants. Such neurons responded either to all the rewarded stimuli, and to none of the saline-associated stimuli, or vice versa. The remaining 65% of these neurons showed differential selectivity for the stimuli based on the odour quality, and not on the taste reward association of the odour.

The findings thus show that the olfactory representation within the primate orbitofrontal cortex reflects for some neurons (65%) which odour is present independently of its association with taste reward, and that for other neurons (35%), the olfactory response reflects (and encodes) the taste association of the odour (Critchley and Rolls 1996b). The additional finding that some of the odour-responsive neurons were also responsive to taste stimuli supports the hypothesis that odour–taste association learning at the level of single neurons in the orbitofrontal cortex enables such cells to show olfactory responses that reflect the taste association of the odour.

The neurons that classify odours based on the taste with which the odour is associated are likely to respond in this way as a result of learning. Repeated pairing of an odour with a taste (especially if it is a neuron with a taste input) may by pattern-association learning lead it to respond to that odour in future. To investigate whether the responses of neurons to odours could be affected depending on the taste with which the odour was paired, we have performed a series of experiments in which the associations of odours and tastes in the olfactory discrimination task have been reversed (Rolls, Critchley, Mason and Wakeman 1996b). For example, the monkey might learn that when amyl acetate was delivered, a lick response would result in the delivery of a drop of glucose, and that when cineole was delivered, a lick would result in the delivery of a drop of saline. After this had been learned, the contingency was then reversed, so that cineole might after the reversal be associated with the taste of glucose. Rolls, Critchley, Mason and Wakeman (1996b) found that 68% of the odour-responsive neurons analysed modified their responses following the changes in the taste reward associations of the odourants. Full reversal of the neuronal responses was seen in 25% of the neurons analysed (see example in Fig. 4.23). (In full reversal, the odour to which the neuron responded reversed when the taste with which it was associated reversed.) Extinction of the differential neuronal responses after task reversal was seen in 43% of these neurons. (These neurons simply stopped discriminating between the two odours after the reversal.)

These findings demonstrate directly a coding principle in primate olfaction whereby the responses of some orbitofrontal cortex olfactory neurons are modified by and depend upon the taste with which the odour is associated. This modification is likely to be important for setting the motivational or reward value of olfactory stimuli for feeding and other rewarded behaviour. It was of interest however that this modification was less complete, and much slower, than the modifications found for orbitofrontal visual neurons during visual-taste reversal (Rolls, Critchley, Mason and Wakeman 1996b). This relative inflexibility of olfactory responses is consistent with the need for some stability in odour–taste associations to facilitate the formation and perception of flavours.

5.4.4.2 The effects of hunger on olfactory processing in the orbitofrontal cortex: evidence that the reward value of odour is represented

It has also been possible to investigate whether the olfactory representation in the orbitofrontal cortex is affected by hunger. In satiety experiments, Critchley and Rolls (1996a) have been able to show that the responses of some olfactory neurons to a food odour are reduced when the monkey is fed to satiety with a food (e.g. fruit juice) with that odour. In particular, seven of nine olfactory neurons that were responsive to the odours of foods, such as blackcurrant juice, were found to reduce their responses to the odour of the satiating food. The decrease was typically at least partly specific to the odour of the food that had been eaten to satiety, potentially providing part of the basis for sensory-specific satiety. (It was also found for eight of nine neurons that had selective responses to the sight of food that they demonstrated a sensory-specific reduction in their visual responses to foods following satiation.) These findings show that the olfactory and visual representations of food, as well as the taste representation of food, in the primate orbitofrontal cortex are modulated by hunger. Usually a component related to sensory-specific satiety can be demonstrated. The findings link at least part of the processing of olfactory and visual information in this brain region to the control of feeding-related behaviour. This is further evidence that part of the olfactory representation in this region is related to the hedonic value of the olfactory stimulus, and in particular that at this level of the olfactory system in primates, the pleasure elicited by the food odour is at least part of what is represented.

To investigate whether the sensory-specific reduction in the responsiveness of the orbito-frontal olfactory neurons might be related to a sensory-specific reduction in the pleasure produced by the odour of a food when it is eaten to satiety, Rolls and Rolls (1997) measured humans' responses to the smell of a food that was eaten to satiety. It was found that the pleasantness of the odour of a food, but much less significantly its intensity, was reduced when the subjects ate it to satiety. It was also found that the pleasantness of the smell of other foods (i.e. not foods eaten in the meal) showed much less decrease. This finding has clear implications for the control of food intake; for ways to keep foods presented in a meal appetitive; and for effects on odour pleasantness ratings that could occur following meals.

In an investigation of the mechanisms of this odour-specific sensory-specific satiety, Rolls and Rolls (1997) allowed humans to chew a food without swallowing, for approximately as long as the food is normally in the mouth during eating. They demonstrated a sensory-specific satiety with this procedure, showing that the sensory-specific satiety does not depend on food reaching the stomach. Thus at least part of the mechanism is likely to be produced by a change in processing in the olfactory pathways. It is not yet known which is the earliest stage of olfactory processing at which this modulation occurs. It is unlikely to be in the receptors of early stages of olfactory processing in the brain, because the change in pleasantness found was much more significant than the change in the intensity (Rolls and Rolls 1997). Consistent with this, activations in the primary olfactory cortical areas are related to the intensity of odours, and in the orbitofrontal cortex to the pleasantness of odours (Rolls, Kringelbach and De Araujo 2003c).

In humans, it has been shown that the modulation of the pleasantness of odour by satiety is represented in the orbitofrontal cortex, in that there is a sensory-specific reduction of the fMRI BOLD signal in the orbitofrontal cortex to the odour of a food eaten to satiety, but not to the odour of another food not eaten in a meal (O'Doherty, Rolls, Francis, Bowtell, McGlone, Kobal, Renner and Ahne 2000).

In addition to this modulation of neuronal responses to the taste and smell of foods eaten, there will be effects of the energy ingested on taste and smell responses to food. These are likely to depend on factors such as gastric distension, and the concentration of glucose and other indicators of hunger/satiety in the systemic circulation (Karadi, Oomura, Nishino, Scott, Lenard and Aou 1990, Karadi, Oomura, Nishino, Scott, Lenard and Aou 1992, Oomura, Nishino, Karadi, Aou and Scott 1991, LeMagnen 1992, Rolls 1999a, Campfield et al. 1995).

5.4.4.3 The representation of information about odours by populations of neurons in the orbitofrontal cortex

To investigate how information about odours is represented by the responses of neurons in the primate orbitofrontal cortex, Rolls, Critchley and Treves (1996a) applied information theoretic analyses to the responses of these neurons recorded to 7–9 odours in an olfactory discrimination task. The information reflected by the firing rate of the response accounted for the majority of the information present (86%) when compared with that which was decodable if temporal encoding in the spike train was taken into account. This indicated that temporal encoding had a very minor role in the encoding of olfactory information by orbitofrontal cortex olfactory neurons. The average information about which odourant was presented, averaged across the 38 neurons, was 0.09 bits, a figure that is low when compared with the information values previously published for the responses of temporal lobe face-selective neurons.

However, it was shown that the information available from the population as a whole of these neurons increased approximately linearly with the number of neurons in the population (Rolls and Critchley 2007). Given that information is a log measure, the number of stimuli that can be encoded increases exponentially with the number of neurons in the sample. Thus the principle of encoding by the populations of neurons is that the combinatorial potential of distributed encoding is used. The significance of this is that with relatively limited numbers of neurons, information about a large number of stimuli can be represented. This means that receiving neurons need only receive from limited numbers of neurons of the type described here, and can nevertheless reflect the information about many stimuli. This type of combinatorial encoding makes brain connectivity possible. The fact that the information can largely be read out from the firing rates of a population of these neurons also makes the decoding of this information (by other neurons) relatively simple (see Rolls and Treves (1998) and Rolls and Deco (2002)).

5.4.5 The responses of orbitofrontal cortex taste and olfactory neurons to the sight of food

Many of the neurons with visual responses in this region also show olfactory or taste re- sponses (Rolls and Baylis 1994), reverse rapidly in visual discrimination reversal (Rolls, Critchley, Mason and Wakeman 1996b), and only respond to the sight of food if hunger is present (Critchley and Rolls 1996a). This part of the orbitofrontal cortex thus seems to implement a mechanism that can flexibly alter the responses to visual stimuli depending on the reinforcement (e.g. the taste) associated with the visual stimulus (Thorpe, Rolls and Maddison 1983, Rolls 2000e, Rolls 2004b) (see Section 4.5.5.4). This enables prediction of the taste associated with ingestion of what is seen, and thus in the visual selection of foods.

This cortical region is implicated more generally in a certain type of learning, namely in extinction and in the reversal of visual discriminations. It is suggested that the taste neurons in this region are important for these functions, for they provide information about whether a reward has been obtained (Thorpe, Rolls and Maddison 1983, Rolls 1999a, Rolls 2000e, Rolls 2004b). These taste neurons represent a number of important primary reinforcers. The ability of this part of the cortex to perform rapid learning of associations between visual stimuli and primary reinforcers such as taste provides the basis for the importance of this part of the brain in food-related and emotion-related learning (Rolls 1986a, Rolls 1990d, Rolls 1999a, Rolls 2000e, Rolls 2004b) (see Chapter 4). Consistent with this function, parts of the orbitofrontal cortex receive direct projections from the inferior temporal visual cortex (Barbas 1988, Seltzer and Pandya 1989), a region important in high-order visual information processing (Rolls 1992a, Rolls 2000a, Rolls and Deco 2002).

The convergence of visual information onto neurons in this region not only enables associations to be learned between the sight of a food and its taste and smell, but also may provide the neural basis for the well-known effect which the sight of a food has on its perceived taste (see Section 4.5.5.7).

5.4.6 Functions of the amygdala and temporal cortex in feeding

5.4.6.1 Effects of lesions

Bilateral damage to the temporal lobes of primates leads to the Kluver-Bucy syndrome, in which lesioned monkeys, for example, select and place in their mouths non-food as well as food items shown to them, and repeatedly fail to avoid noxious stimuli (Kluver and Bucy 1939, Jones and Mishkin 1972, Aggleton and Passingham 1982, Baylis and Gaffan 1991) (see Section 4.6.3). Rats with lesions in the basolateral amygdala also display altered food selection, in that they ingest relatively novel foods (Rolls and Rolls 1973b, Borsini and Rolls 1984), and do not normally learn to avoid to ingest a solution that has previously resulted in sickness (Rolls and Rolls 1973a). (The deficit in learned taste avoidance in rats may be because of damage to the insular taste cortex, which has projections through and to the amygdala, see Dunn and Everitt (1988).) The basis for these alterations in food selection and in food-related learning are considered next (see also Rolls (2000d) and Section 4.6.3).

The monkeys with temporal lobe damage have a visual discrimination deficit, in that they are impaired in learning to select one of two objects under which food is found, and thus fail to form correctly an association between the visual stimulus and reinforcement (Jones and Mishkin 1972, Gaffan 1992) (see Section 4.6.3). In the study by Malkova et al. (1997) it was shown that amygdala lesions made with ibotenic acid did impair the processing of reward-related stimuli, in that when the reward value of one set of foods was devalued by feeding it to satiety (i.e. sensory-specific satiety, a reward devaluation procedure, see also Section 4.6.1.2), the monkeys still chose the visual stimuli associated with the foods with which they had been satiated (Malkova et al. 1997, Baxter and Murray 2000). Further evidence that neurotoxic lesions of the amygdala in primates affect behaviour to stimuli learned as being reward-related as well as punishment-related is that monkeys with neurotoxic lesions of the amygdala showed abnormal patterns of food choice, picking up and eating foods not normally eaten such as meat, and picking up and placing in their mouths inedible objects (Murray et al. 1996, Baxter and Murray 2000). These symptoms produced by selective amygdala lesions are classical Kluver-Bucy symptoms. Thus in primates, there is evidence that selective amygdala lesions impair some types of behaviour to learned reward-related stimuli such as the sight of food.

Further evidence linking the amygdala to reinforcement mechanisms is that monkeys will work in order to obtain electrical stimulation of the amygdala, and that single neurons in the amygdala are activated by brain-stimulation reward of a number of different sites (Rolls 1975, Rolls et al. 1980c) (see Chapter 7).

The Kluver-Bucy syndrome is produced by lesions which damage the cortical areas in the anterior part of the temporal lobe and the underlying amygdala (Jones and Mishkin 1972), or by lesions of the amygdala (Weiskrantz 1956, Aggleton and Passingham 1981, Gaffan 1992), or (for the visual aspects) of the temporal lobe neocortex (Akert, Gruesen, Woolsey and Meyer 1961). Lesions to part of the temporal lobe neocortex, damaging the inferior temporal visual cortex and extending into the cortex in the ventral bank of the superior temporal sulcus, produce visual aspects of the syndrome, seen for example as a tendency to select non-food as well as food items (Weiskrantz and Saunders 1984). Anatomically, there are connections from the inferior temporal visual cortex to the amygdala (Herzog and Van Hoesen 1976), which in turn projects to the hypothalamus (Nauta 1961), thus providing a route for visual information to reach the hypothalamus (Amaral et al. 1992, Pitkanen 2000). This evidence, together with the evidence that damage to the hypothalamus can disrupt feeding (Winn et al. 1984, Dunnett et al. 1985, Winn et al. 1990, Clark et al. 1991), thus indicates that there is a system that includes visual cortex in the temporal lobe, projections to the amygdala, and further connections to structures such as the lateral hypothalamus, which is involved in behavioural responses made on the basis of learned associations between visual stimuli and primary (unlearned) reinforcers such as the taste of food (see Fig. 4.2). Given this evidence from lesion and anatomical studies, the contribution of each of these regions to the visual analysis and learning required for these functions in food selection will be considered using evidence from the activity of single neurons in these regions.

5.4.6.2   Inferior Temporal visual cortex

Recordings were made from single neurons in the inferior temporal visual cortex while rhesus monkeys performed visual discriminations, and while they were shown visual stimuli associated with positive reinforcement such as food, with negative reinforcement such as aversive hypertonic saline, and neutral visual stimuli (Rolls, Judge and Sanghera 1977). It was found that during visual discrimination inferior temporal neurons often had sustained visual responses with latencies of 100–140 ms to the discriminanda, but that these responses did not depend on whether the visual stimuli were associated with reward or punishment. This was shown in a visual discrimination learning paradigm in which one visual stimulus is associated with reward (for example glucose taste, or fruit-juice taste), and another visual stimulus is associated with an aversive taste, such as saline, and then the reinforcement contingency was reversed. (That is, the visual stimulus, for example a triangle, to which the monkey had to lick in order to obtain a taste of fruit juice, was after the reversal associated with saline: if the monkey licked to the triangle after the reversal, he obtained mildly aversive salt solution.) An example of such an experiment is shown in Fig. 4.6 on page 76. The neuron responded more to the triangle, both before reversal when it was associated with fruit juice, and after reversal, when the triangle was associated with saline. Thus the reinforcement association of the visual stimuli did not alter the response to the visual stimuli, which was based on the physical properties of the stimuli (for example their shape, colour, or texture). The same was true for the other neurons recorded in this study. This independence from reward association seems to be characteristic of neurons right through the temporal visual cortical areas, and must be true in earlier cortical areas too, in that they provide the inputs to the inferior temporal visual cortex.

This conclusion, that the responses of inferior temporal neurons during visual discriminations do not code for whether a visual stimulus is associated with reward or punishment, is also consistent with further findings (Ridley et al. 1977, Jarvis and Mishkin 1977, Gross et al. 1979, Sato et al. 1980), including an investigation in which macaques search for food-related stimuli in complex visual scenes (Rolls, Aggelopoulos and Zheng 2003a). Further it was found that inferior temporal neurons did not respond only to food-related visual stimuli, or only to aversive stimuli, and were not dependent on hunger, but rather that in many cases their responses depended on physical aspects of the stimuli such as shape, size, orientation, colour, or texture (Rolls, Judge and Sanghera 1977, Rolls and Deco 2002).

Nor are reward-related, including food reward-related representations found in the perirhinal cortex (which anatomically connects the inferior temporal visual cortex to the hippocampus), in that the neurons do not respond differently to the sight of food and non-food objects, and do not respond differently to the visual stimuli in a visual discrimination task (Hölscher and Rolls 2002, Hölscher, Rolls and Xiang 2003b). Instead, perirhinal cortex neurons have activity related to the active resetting of short-term memories required in delayed match to sample tasks (Hölscher and Rolls 2002), and to long-term familiarity memory (Hölscher, Rolls and Xiang 2003b, Rolls, Franco and Stringer 2005b).

A fundamental point about pattern association networks for stimulus–reinforcement association learning can be made from what we have considered (see also Section 4.4.4). It is that sensory processing in the primate brain proceeds as far as the invariant representation of objects independently of reward vs punishment associations. The reason for this systems-level brain design is, I propose, because the visual properties of the world about which reward associations must be learned are generally objects (for example the sight of a banana, or of an orange), and are not just raw pixels or edges, with no invariant properties, which is what is represented in the retina and V1.

The findings described thus indicate that the responses of neurons in the inferior temporal visual cortex do not reflect the association of visual stimuli with reinforcers such as food. Given these findings, and the lesion evidence described above, it is thus likely that the inferior temporal cortex is an input stage for this process. The next structure on the basis of anatomical connections (see Fig. 4.2) is the amygdala, and this is considered next.

5.4.6.3 Amygdala

In recordings made from 1754 amygdaloid neurons, it was found that 113 (6.4%), of which many were in a dorsolateral region of the amygdala known to receive directly from the inferior temporal visual cortex (Herzog and Van Hoesen 1976), had visual responses that in most cases were sustained while the monkey looked at effective visual stimuli (Sanghera, Rolls and Roper-Hall 1979). The latency of the responses was 100–140 ms or more. The majority (85%) of these visual neurons responded more strongly to some stimuli than to others, but physical factors that accounted for the responses such as orientation, colour, and texture could not usually be identified. It was found that 22 (19.5%) of these visual neurons responded primarily to foods and to objects associated with food (see e.g. Fig. 4.57). Further, although some neurons responded in a visual discrimination task to the visual stimulus that indicated food reward, but not to the visual stimulus associated with aversive saline, only minor modifications of the neuronal responses were obtained when the association of the stimuli with reinforcement was reversed in the reversal of the visual discrimination (see Section 4.6.4). Thus even the responses of these neurons were not invariably associated with whichever stimulus was associated with food reward (see further Rolls (1992b), Rolls (2000d) and Section 4.6.3). A comparable population of neurons with responses apparently partly but not uniquely related to aversive visual stimuli was also found (Sanghera, Rolls and Roper-Hall 1979).

Amygdala neurons with responses that are probably similar to these have also been described by Ono and colleagues (Ono et al. 1980, Ono, Tamura, Nishijo, Nakamura and Tabuchi 1989, Nishijo et al. 1988, Ono and Nishijo 1992). When Nishijo et al. (1988) tested four amygdala neurons in a simpler relearning situation than reversal in which salt was added to a piece of food such as a water melon, the neurons' responses to the sight of the water-melon appeared to diminish. However, in this task it was not clear whether the monkeys continued to look at the stimuli during extinction. It will be of interest in further studies to investigate whether in extinction evidence can be found for a rapid decrease in the neuronal responses to visual stimuli formerly associated with reward, even when fixation of the stimuli is adequate (see Rolls (1992b) and Rolls (2000d)).

Wilson and Rolls (2005) (see also Rolls (2000d)) extended the analysis of the responses of these amygdala neurons by showing that while they do respond to (some) stimuli associated with primary reinforcement such as food, they do not respond if the reinforcement must be determined on the basis of a rule (such as stimuli when novel are negatively reinforced, and when familiar are positively reinforced). This is consistent with the evidence that the amygdala is involved when reward must be determined, as normally occurs during feeding, by association of a stimulus with a primary reinforcer such as the taste of food, but is not involved when reinforcement must be determined in some other ways (see Rolls (2000d)). In the same study (Wilson and Rolls 2005), it was shown that these amygdala neurons that respond to food can also respond to some other stimuli while they are relatively novel. It is suggested that it is by this mechanism that when relatively novel stimuli are encountered, they are investigated, e.g. by being smelled and then placed in the mouth, to assess whether the new stimuli are foods (Rolls 2000d).

The failure of this population of amygdala neurons to respond only to reinforcing stimuli, and the difficulty in reversing their responses, are in contrast with the responses of certain populations of neurons in the caudal orbitofrontal cortex and in a region to which it projects, the basal forebrain, which do show very rapid (in one or two trials) reversals of their responses in visual discrimination reversal tasks (Thorpe, Rolls and Maddison 1983, Wilson and Rolls 1990b, Wilson and Rolls 1990a) (see Section 4.5). On the basis of these findings, it is suggested that the orbitofrontal cortex is more involved than the amygdala in the rapid readjustments of behavioural responses made to stimuli such as food when their reinforce-ment value is repeatedly changing, as in discrimination reversal tasks (Thorpe, Rolls and Maddison 1983, Rolls, Critchley, Mason and Wakeman 1996b, Deco and Rolls 2005d). The ability to flexibly alter responses to stimuli based on their changing reinforcement associations is important in motivated behaviour (such as feeding) and in emotional behaviour, and it is this flexibility that it is suggested the orbitofrontal cortex adds to a more basic capacity which the amygdala implements for stimulus–reinforcement learning (Rolls 1990d, Rolls 1999a, Deco and Rolls 2005d).

These findings thus suggest that the amygdala could be involved in a rather inflexible circuit by which visual stimuli are associated with reinforcement. Neuronal responses here do not code uniquely for whether a visual stimulus is associated with reinforcement, partly because the neurons do not reverse rapidly, and partly because the neurons can respond to relatively novel stimuli, which monkeys frequently pick up and place in their mouths for further exploration. Neurons with responses more closely related to reinforcement are found in areas to which the amygdala projects, such as the lateral hypothalamus, substantia innom-inata, and ventral striatum, and this may be because of the inputs these structures receive from the orbitofrontal cortex. The amygdala may thus be a somewhat slow and inflexible system, compared with the orbitofrontal cortex which has developed greatly in primates, in learning about which visual stimuli have the taste and smell of food. Consistent with the hypothesis that the amygdala can play some role in learning associations of visual stimuli to the taste, smell and texture of food (see Fig. 4.2), some neurons with taste, olfactory and oral texture and temperature responses are found in the primate amygdala (Sanghera, Rolls and Roper-Hall 1979, Ono, Nishino, Sasaki, Fukuda and Muramoto 1980, Ono, Tamura, Nishijo, Nakamura and Tabuchi 1989, Nishijo, Ono and Nishino 1988, Ono and Nishijo 1992, Scott, Karadi, Oomura, Nishino, Plata-Salaman, Lenard, Giza and Aou 1993, Kadohisa, Rolls and Verhagen 2005b) (see example in Fig. 4.53).

5.4.7 Functions of the orbitofrontal cortex in feeding

Damage to the orbitofrontal cortex alters food preferences, in that monkeys with damage to the orbitofrontal cortex select and eat foods that are normally rejected (Butter et al. 1969, Baylis and Gaffan 1991) (Fig. 5.19). Their food choice behaviour is very similar to that of monkeys with amygdala lesions (Baylis and Gaffan 1991). Lesions of the orbitofrontal cortex also lead to a failure to correct feeding responses when these become inappropriate. Examples of the situations in which these abnormalities in feeding responses are found include: (a) extinction, in that feeding responses continue to be made to the previously reinforced stimulus; (b) reversals of visual discriminations, in that the monkeys make responses to the previously reinforced stimulus or object; (c) Go/Nogo tasks, in that responses are made to the stimulus that is not associated with food reward; and (d) passive avoidance, in that feeding responses are made even when they are punished (Butter 1969, Iversen and Mishkin 1970, Jones and Mishkin 1972, Tanaka 1973, Rosenkilde 1979, Fuster 1996).

To investigate how the orbitofrontal cortex may be involved in feeding and in the correction of feeding responses when these become inappropriate, recordings were made of the activity of 494 orbitofrontal neurons during the performance of a Go/Nogo task, reversals of a visual discrimination task, extinction, and passive avoidance (Thorpe, Rolls and Maddison 1983). First, neurons were found that responded in relation to the preparatory auditory or visual signal used before each trial (15.1%), or non-discriminatively during the period in which the

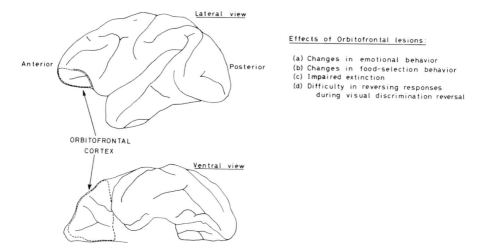

Fig. 5.19 The orbitofrontal cortex of the monkey. The effects of orbitofrontal lesions include: (a) changes in emotional behaviour; (b) changes in food-selection behaviour; (c) impaired extinction; (d) difficulty in reversing responses during visual discrimination reversal.

discriminative visual stimuli were shown (37.8%). These neurons are not considered further here. Second, 8.6% of neurons had responses that occurred discriminatively during the period in which the visual stimuli were shown. The majority of these neurons responded to whichever visual stimulus was associated with reward, in that the stimulus to which they responded changed during reversal (see examples in Figs. 4.30 and 4.31). However, six of these neurons required a combination of a particular visual stimulus in the discrimination and reward in order to respond (see example in Fig. 4.32). Further, none of this second group of conditional reward neurons responded to all the reward-related stimuli including different foods that were shown, so that in general this group of neurons coded for a combination of one or several visual stimuli and reward. Thus information that particular visual stimuli had previously been associated with reinforcement was represented in the responses of orbitofrontal neurons. Third, 9.7% of neurons had responses that occurred after the lick response was made in the task to obtain reward. Some of these responded independently of whether fruit juice reward was obtained, or aversive hypertonic saline was obtained on trials on which the monkey licked in error or was given saline in the first trials of a reversal. Through these neurons information that a lick had been made was represented in the orbitofrontal cortex. Other neurons in this third group responded only when fruit juice was obtained, and thus through these neurons information that food reward had been given on that trial was represented in the orbitofrontal cortex. Such neurons reflect the taste of the liquid received, and are in a part of the orbitofrontal cortex which is close to, and probably receives inputs from, the secondary taste cortex (Baylis, Rolls and Baylis 1994, Rolls, Yaxley and Sienkiewicz 1990). Other neurons in this group ('error neurons') responded when saline was obtained when a response was made in error, or when saline was obtained on the first few trials of a reversal (but not in either case when saline was simply placed in the mouth), or when reward was not given in extinction, or when food was taken away instead of being given to the monkey, but did not respond in all these situations in which reinforcement was omitted or punishment was given. Thus through these neurons task-selective information that reward had been omitted or punishment given was represented in the responses of these neurons (see Section 4.5.5).

These three groups of neurons found in the orbitofrontal cortex could together provide for computation of whether the reinforcement previously associated with a particular stimulus was still being obtained, and generation of a signal if a match was not obtained. This signal could be partly reflected in the responses of the last subset of ('error') neurons with task-selective responses to non-reward or to unexpected punishment. This signal could be used to alter the monkey's behaviour, leading for example to reversal to one particular stimulus but not to other stimuli, to extinction to one stimulus but not to others, etc. It could also lead to the altered responses of the orbitofrontal differential neurons found as a result of learning in reversal, so that their responses indicate appropriately whether a particular stimulus is now associated with food reinforcement (see Appendix 2).

Thus the orbitofrontal cortex contains neurons that appear to be involved in altering behavioural responses when these are no longer associated with reward or become associated with punishment. In the context of feeding it appears that without these neurons the primate is unable to suppress his behaviour correctly to non-food objects, in that altered food preferences are produced by orbitofrontal damage (Butter et al. 1969). It also appears that without these neurons the primate is unable to correct his behaviour when it becomes appropriate to break a learned association between a stimulus and a reward such as food (Jones and Mishkin 1972). The orbitofrontal neurons could be involved in the actual breaking of the association, or in the alteration of behaviour when other neurons signal that the connection is no longer appropriate. As shown here, the orbitofrontal cortex contains neurons with responses that could provide the information necessary for, and the basis for, the unlearning. This type of unlearning is important in enabling animals to alter the environmental stimuli to which motivational responses such as feeding have previously been made, when experience shows that such responses have become inappropriate. In this way they can ensure that their feeding and other motivational responses remain continually adapted to a changing environment.

This evidence on how the primate orbitofrontal cortex is involved in feeding has been greatly extended by the discoveries described in Sections 5.4.2–5.4.4 that the secondary and tertiary taste and olfactory cortices are present in the orbitofrontal regions, that it is the reward value of food that is represented here as shown by the finding that satiety reduces the responsiveness of these neurons, and that the representation of the flavour of food is formed here in the brain. These findings show that the primary reward value of food produced by its taste and smell is represented in the primate orbitofrontal cortex. Consistent with this, in humans a representation of the taste, smell and texture of food has been demonstrated in the orbitofrontal cortex (O'Doherty, Rolls, Francis, Bowtell, McGlone, Kobal, Renner and Ahne 2000, O'Doherty, Rolls, Francis, Bowtell and McGlone 2001b, De Araujo, Kringelbach, Rolls and Hobden 2003a, Rolls, Kringelbach and De Araujo 2003c, De Araujo, Kringelbach, Rolls and McGlone 2003b, De Araujo, Kringelbach, Rolls, McGlone and Phillips 2003c, De Araujo and Rolls 2004) (Fig. 4.22 and Fig. 5.15). The findings described in Section 5.4.5 also confirm the very rapid visual-to-taste learning and reversal that take place in the primate orbitofrontal cortex. The fact that the texture of food in the mouth, and the mouth feel of fat, an important factor in the palatability of food, are also represented in the primate orbitofrontal cortex (Rolls, Critchley, Browning, Hernadi and Lenard 1999a, Verhagen, Rolls and Kadohisa 2003, Rolls, Verhagen and Kadohisa 2003e, Kadohisa, Rolls and Verhagen 2004) also implicates this region as a crucial region for indicating the reward value of food, as well as for learning which stimuli are associated with food reward (Rolls 2004g, Rolls 2004h).

The more rapid reversal of neuronal responses in the orbitofrontal cortex, and in a region to which it projects, the basal forebrain (Thorpe, Rolls and Maddison 1983, Wilson and Rolls 1990b, Wilson and Rolls 1990a), than in the amygdala suggest that the orbitofrontal cortex is more involved than the amygdala in the rapid readjustments of behavioural responses made to stimuli when their reinforcement value is repeatedly changing, as in discrimination reversal tasks (Thorpe, Rolls and Maddison 1983, Rolls 1999a, Deco and Rolls 2005d). The ability to flexibly alter responses to stimuli based on their changing reinforcement associations is important in motivated behaviour (such as feeding) and in emotional behaviour, and it is this flexibility which it is suggested the orbitofrontal cortex adds to a more basic capacity that the amygdala implements for stimulus–reinforcement learning.

The great development of the orbitofrontal cortex in primates, yet the similarity of its connections to those of the amygdala (see Fig. 4.51), and its connections with the amygdala, lead to the suggestion that in evolution, and as part of continuing corticalization of functions, the orbitofrontal cortex has come to be placed hierarchically above the amygdala, and is especially important when rapid readjustment of stimulus–reinforcement associations is required (Rolls 1990d). This suggestion is also consistent with the indication that whereas in rodents subcortical structures such as the amygdala and hypothalamus have access to taste information from the precortical taste system, the same does not occur in primates; and that some precortical processing of taste in relation to the control of feeding occurs in rodents (see above and Scott and Giza (1992) and Rolls and Scott (2003)). In contrast, there is great development and importance of cortical processing of taste in primates, and it is very appropriate that the orbitofrontal cortex area just described is found just medial to the secondary taste cortex, which is in primates in the caudolateral orbitofrontal cortex. It appears that close to this orbitofrontal taste cortex the orbitofrontal cortical area just described develops, and receives inputs from the visual association cortex (inferior temporal cortex), the olfactory (pyriform) cortex, and probably from the somatosensory cortex, so that reward associations between these different modalities can be determined rapidly.

An interesting topic for the future is whether the satiety signals summarized in Sections 5.2 and 5.3 also gain access to the orbitofrontal cortex, and how they modulate there the taste, olfactory and visual neuronal responses to food. As shown in Fig. 4.22, the activation of a part of the human orbitofrontal cortex does correlate with the pleasantness of the flavour of food, and its activation decreases when food is eaten to satiety. The signals that produce this effect will include sensory-specific satiety, and also the other satiety signals such as gastric distension described in Section 5.3.

5.4.8   Functions of the striatum in feeding

Parts of the striatum receive inputs from many of the structures involved in the control of feeding, and have connections on through other parts of the basal ganglia which may influence behavioural output. Moreover, damage to different parts of the striatum can affect feeding in a number of ways. We therefore discuss here its role as one of the behavioural output systems for feeding which enable the structures such as the orbitofrontal cortex and amygdala which decode the reward value of sensory stimuli including food to connect to behaviour. Further aspects of basal ganglia function in terms of an output system for emotional stimuli to produce behavioural responses are described in Chapter 4, and a more complete description (with Figures), including its role in the pharmacology of reward, is provided in Chapter 8.

Figure 8.6 on page 322 shows where the striatum (which includes the caudate nucleus, the putamen, and the ventral striatum consisting of the nucleus accumbens and olfactory tubercle) is in the primate brain. Figure 8.7 shows some of the connections of the different parts of the striatum. Hypotheses on how the basal ganglia actually operate as neural networks are described in Chapter 8 (Section 8.4) and by Rolls and Treves (1998) (Chapter 9). In this Section, we focus on the role of the striatum in feeding.

5.4.8.1 Effects of lesions of the striatum on feeding, and connections of the striatum

Damage to the nigrostriatal bundle, which depletes the striatum of dopamine, produces aphagia (lack of eating) and adipsia (lack of drinking) associated with a sensori-motor disturbance in the rat (Ungerstedt 1971, Marshall et al. 1974, Stricker and Zigmond 1976, Stricker 1984). Many of the brain systems implicated in the control of feeding, such as the amygdala and orbitofrontal cortex, have projections to the striatum, which could provide a route for these brain systems to lead to feeding responses (Rolls 1979, Rolls 1984a, Rolls 1986b, Mogenson, Jones and Yim 1980, Rolls and Williams 1987b, Rolls and Williams 1987a, Rolls and Johnstone 1992, Williams, Rolls, Leonard and Stern 1993) (see Figs. 8.6 and 8.7 and Section 8.4). We now consider how each part of the striatum is involved in the control of feeding, using evidence from the connections of each part, the effects of lesions to each part, and especially the type of neuronal activity in each part of the primate striatum during feeding. A more general discussion of basal ganglia function is provided in Section 8.4, and only aspects especially relevant to feeding are considered here.

5.4.8.2 The ventral striatum

The ventral striatum, which includes the nucleus accumbens, the olfactory tubercle (or anterior perforated substance of primates), and the islands of Calleja, receives inputs from limbic structures such as the amygdala and hippocampus, and from the orbitofrontal cortex, and projects to the ventral pallidum (see further Groenewegen, Berendse, Meredith, Haber, Voorn, Wolters and Lohman (1991), Gurney, Prescott and Redgrave (2001a), Section 8.4.1; and Figs. 8.6 and 8.7). The ventral pallidum may then influence output regions by the subthalamic nucleus/globus pallidus/ventral thalamus/ premotor cortex route, or via the mediodorsal nucleus of the thalamus/prefrontal cortex route (Heimer et al. 1982). The ventral striatum may thus be for limbic structures what the neostriatum is for neocortical structures, that is a route for limbic structures to influence output regions. There is evidence linking the ventral striatum and its dopamine input to reward, for manipulations of this system alter the incentive effects that learned rewarding stimuli (e.g. a light associated with food) have on behaviour (Everitt and Robbins 1992, Robbins and Everitt 1992). For example, depletion of dopamine in the ventral striatum of rats using the neurotoxin 6-hydroxydopamine abolished the effect that a light previously associated with the delivery of food normally has in prolonging responding when food is no longer being delivered (Everitt and Robbins 1992, Robbins and Everitt 1992). Eating and body weight were not impaired. Thus it is the effects on feeding that result from stimulus–reinforcement association learning, in which the amygdala and orbitofrontal cortex are implicated, that the ventral striatum appears to influence behavioural output. In particular, the ventral striatum may allow the affective states retrieved by the basolateral amygdala to conditioned stimuli to influence instrumental behaviour by for example Pavlovian-instrumental transfer, and facilitating locomotor approach to food which appears to be in rats a Pavlovian process (Cardinal et al. 2002, Cardinal and Everitt 2004). However, opioid receptors in the nucleus accumbens influence the palatability of food (especially fat) in rats, mediating this effect via the lateral hypothalamus (Kelley 2004b). Further, in a human fMRI study, we found that activation in the nucleus accumbens was produced by the texture of fat in the mouth (De Araujo and Rolls 2004), providing further evidence that a sensory input that has strong effects on the palatability of food can influence this brain system.

Because of its possible role as an output structure for the amygdala and orbitofrontal cortex to enable learned associations between previously neutral stimuli and rewards such as food to influence behaviour, the activity of neurons in the ventral striatum has been analysed in macaques during feeding and during tasks that require stimulus–reinforcement association learning, such as visual discrimination tasks in which one visual stimulus predicts (is a discriminative stimulus for) the taste of food, and the other visual stimulus is a discriminative stimulus for the taste of saline (Rolls and Williams 1987b, Rolls and Williams 1987a, Williams, Rolls, Leonard and Stern 1993). A number of different types of neuronal response were found, as described in Section 8.4.3.1. One population of neurons was found to respond differently to visual stimuli which indicate that if a lick response is made, the taste of glucose will be obtained, and to other visual stimuli which indicate that if a lick response will be made, the taste of aversive saline will be obtained. Examples of the responses of a neuron of this type are shown in Fig. 8.8 on page 326. The neuron increased its firing rate to the visual stimulus which indicated that saline would be obtained if a lick was made (the S–), and decreased its firing rate to the visual stimulus which indicated that a response could be made to obtain a taste of glucose (the S+). The differential response latency of this neuron to the reward-related and to the saline-related visual stimulus was approximately 150 ms (see Fig. 8.8), and this value was typical.

Of the neurons that responded to visual stimuli that were rewarding, relatively few responded to all the rewarding stimuli used. That is, only few (1.8%) ventral striatal neurons responded both when food was shown and to the positive discriminative visual stimulus, the S+ (e.g. a triangle shown on a video monitor), in a visual discrimination task. Instead, the reward-related neuronal responses were typically more context- or stimulus-dependent, responding, for example, to the sight of food but not to the S+ which signified food (4.3%), differentially to the S+ or S– but not to food (4.0%), or to food if shown in one context but not in another context. Some neurons were classified as having taste or olfactory responses to food (see Table 8.1; Williams, Rolls, Leonard and Stern (1993)). Some other neurons (1.4%) responded to aversive stimuli. These neurons did not respond simply in relation to arousal, which was produced in control tests by inputs from different modalities, for example by touch of the leg.

These neurons with reinforcement-related responses represented 13.9% of the neurons recorded in the ventral striatum, and may receive their inputs from structures such as the amygdala and orbitofrontal cortex, in which some neurons with similar responses are found (see above).

In that the majority of the neurons recorded in the ventral striatum did not have unconditional sensory responses, but instead the response typically depended on memory, for whether the stimulus was recognized, or for whether it was associated with reinforcement, the function of this part of the striatum does not appear to be purely sensory. Rather, it may provide one route for such memory-related and emotional and motivational stimuli to influence motor output. This is consistent with the hypothesis that the ventral striatum is a link for learned incentive (e.g. rewarding) stimuli (Everitt and Robbins 1992, Cardinal et al. 2002, Cardinal and Everitt 2004), and also for other limbic-processed stimuli such as faces and novel stimuli, to influence behaviour (Mogenson, Jones and Yim 1980, Rolls 1984a, Rolls 1989b, Rolls 1990a, Rolls and Williams 1987b, Rolls and Williams 1987a, Williams, Rolls, Leonard and Stern 1993, Rolls and Treves 1998, Rolls 1999a). The role of the ventral striatum in feeding may thus be to provide a route for learned incentive stimuli such as the sight of food to influence behavioural responses such as approach to food.

In addition, the food reward system appears to be influenced by opiate systems (Levine and Billington 2004), and in rodents one area implicated in these effects is the nucleus accumbens (Zhang, Gosnell and Kelley 1998, Kelley 2004b) (see Section 8.5). The activation of the nucleus accumbens produced in humans by the texture of fat in the mouth (De Araujo and Rolls 2004) also shows that sensory inputs that have strong effects on the palatability of food can influence this brain system, so that the role of the ventral striatum in feeding may not be only in learned incentive effects.

5.4.8.3 The caudate nucleus

In the head of the caudate nucleus (Rolls, Thorpe and Maddison 1983c), which receives inputs particularly from the prefrontal cortex (see Figs. 8.6 and 8.7), many neurons responded to environmental stimuli which were cues to the monkey to prepare for the possible initiation of a feeding response. Thus, 22.4% of neurons recorded responded during a cue given by the experimenter that a food or non-food object was about to be shown, and fed if food, to the monkey (see Section 8.4.3.4). Comparably, in a visual discrimination task made to obtain food, 14.5% of the neurons (including some of the above) responded during a 0.5 s tone/light cue which preceded and signalled the start of each trial (see Figs. 8.11 and 8.12). It is suggested that these neurons are involved in the utilization of environmental cues for the preparation for movement, and that disruption of the function of these neurons contributes to the akinesia or failure to initiate movements (including those required for feeding) found after depletion of dopamine in the striatum (Rolls, Thorpe and Maddison 1983c).

Some other neurons (25.8%) responded if food was shown to the monkey immediately prior to feeding by the experimenter, but the responses of these neurons typically did not occur in other situations in which food-related visual stimuli were shown, such as during the visual discrimination task. Comparably, some other neurons (24.3%) responded differentially in the visual discrimination task, for example to the visual stimulus which indicated that the monkey could initiate a lick response to obtain food (see Fig. 8.13), yet typically did not respond when food was simply shown to the monkey prior to feeding (see Section 8.4.3.4). The responses of these neurons thus occur to particular stimuli that indicate that particular motor responses should be made, and are thus situation-specific, so that it is suggested that these neurons are involved in stimulus–motor response (habit) connections. In that their responses are situation-specific, they are different from the responses of the orbitofrontal cortex and hypothalamic neurons described above with visual responses to the sight of food (Rolls, Thorpe and Maddison 1983c). It is thus suggested that these neurons in the head of the caudate nucleus could be involved in relatively fixed feeding responses made in particular, probably well-learned, situations to food, but do not provide a signal that reflects whether a visual stimulus is associated with food, and on the basis of which any response required to obtain the food could be initiated. Rather, it is likely that the systems described above in the temporal lobe, hypothalamus and orbitofrontal cortex are involved in this more flexible decoding of the food value of visual stimuli.

In the tail of the caudate nucleus, which receives inputs from the inferior temporal visual cortex (see Figs. 8.6 and 8.7), neurons were found that responded to visual stimuli such as gratings and edges, but that showed habituation which was rapid and pattern-specific (Caan, Perrett and Rolls 1984). It was suggested that these neurons are involved in orientation to patterned visual stimuli, and in pattern-specific habituation to these stimuli (Caan, Perrett and Rolls 1984). These neurons would thus appear not to be involved directly in the control of feeding, although a disturbance in the ability to orient normally to a changed visual stimulus could indirectly have an effect on the ability to react normally to food.

5.4.8.4 The putamen

In the putamen, which receives from the sensori-motor cortex, neurons were found with activity that occurred just before mouth or arm movements made by the monkey (Rolls, Thorpe, Boytim, Szabo and Perrett 1984b). Disturbances in the normal function of these neurons might be expected to affect the ability to initiate and execute movements, and thus might indirectly affect the ability to feed normally.

5.4.8.5 Synthesis: the functions of the striatum in feeding and reward

These neurophysiological studies show that in different regions of the striatum neurons are found that may be involved in orientation to environmental stimuli, in the use of such stimuli in the preparation for and initiation of movements, in the execution of movements, in stimulus–response connections appropriate for particular responses made in particular situations to particular stimuli, and in allowing learned reinforcers, including food, to influence behaviour. Because of its many inputs from brain systems involved in feeding and from other brain systems involved in action, it may provide a crucial route for signals that have been decoded through sensory pathways and limbic structures, and that code for the current reward value of visual, olfactory, and taste stimuli, to be interfaced in an arbitration or selection mechanism, to produce behavioural output. The issue then arises of how the striatum, and more generally the basal ganglia, might operate to perform such functions.

We can start by commenting on what functions must be performed in order to link the signals that control feeding to action. It has been shown above that through sensory pathways representations of objects in the environment are produced. These are motivation-independent, and are in, for example, the primary taste cortex and the inferior temporal visual cortex in primates (see Fig. 4.2). After this stage, the sensory signals are interfaced to motivational state, so that the signals in, for example, the orbitofrontal cortex reflect not only the taste of the food, but also whether the monkey is hungry. The sensory signals are also passed in these structures (e.g. the orbitofrontal cortex and amygdala) through association memories, so that the outputs reflect whether a particular stimulus has been previously, and is still, associated with a primary reward. (This process will include conditioned effects from previous ingestion which reflect the energy obtained from the food, sickness produced by it, etc.) These neurons thus reflect the reward value of food, and neurons in this system can be driven by visual, olfactory, and/or taste stimuli. Now, it is of fundamental importance that these reward-related signals should not be interfaced directly to feeding movements, such as chewing. (Brainstem systems which perform such functions might, in a limited way, assist in the execution of feeding movements later in the feeding sequence.) Instead, what is required is that the food-related reward signals should enter an arbitration or selection mechanism, which takes into account not only the other rewards (with their magnitude) that are currently available, but also the cost of obtaining each reward (see further Sections 3.3 and 8.4). A proposal is developed at the conceptual level in Section 8.4 about how the basal ganglia are involved in these functions

(Rolls 1979, Rolls 1984a, Rolls 1994b, Rolls and Williams 1987b, Rolls and Johnstone 1992, Rolls and Treves 1998, Rolls 1999a). Other possible outputs from the orbitofrontal cortex to action selection mechanisms include the cingulate cortex (see Section 4.7) and the dorsolateral prefrontal cortex (Cardinal et al. 2002, Matsumoto et al. 2001, Rushworth et al. 2004, Hikosaka and Watanabe 2000, Watanabe, Hikosaka, Sakagami and Shirakawa 2002).

5.5   Obesity, bulimia, and anorexia

We conclude this Chapter on the brain mechanisms involved in affective responses to food, and appetite control, by considering some of the disturbances in these systems that may contribute to obesity and other eating disorders. This is an increasingly important issue, because the incidence of obesity is apparently rising[15], and because there are many diseases associated with a body weight that is much above normal. These diseases include hypertension, cardiovascular disease, hypercholesterolaemia, and gall bladder disease; and in addition obesity is associated with some deficits in reproductive function (e.g. ovulatory failure), and with an excess mortality from certain types of cancer (Garrow 1988, Barsh and Schwartz 2002, Cummings and Schwartz 2003).

There are many factors that can cause or contribute to obesity in humans (Brownell and Fairburn 1995, Rolls 2007f, Rolls 2007g).

Genetic factors may be of some importance, with for example 11% of the variance in resting metabolic rate in a population of humans attributable to inheritance (Garrow 1988, Barsh and Schwartz 2002). A small proportion of cases of obesity can be related to dysfunctions of the peptide systems in the hypothalamus, with for example 4% of obese people having deficient (MC4) receptors for melanocyte stimulating hormone (Barsh, Farooqi and O'Rahilly 2000, Cummings and Schwartz 2003, Horvath 2005). Cases of obesity that can be related to changes in the leptin system are very rare (Farooqi et al. 2001). Further, obese people generally have high levels of leptin, so leptin production is not the problem, and instead leptin resistance (i.e. insensitivity) may be somewhat related to obesity, with the resistance perhaps related in part to smaller effects of leptin on arcuate nucleus NPY/AGRP neurons (Munzberg and Myers 2005). However, although there are similarities in fatness within families, these are as strong between spouses as they are between parents and children, so that these similarities cannot be attributed to genetic influences, but presumably reflect the effect of family attitudes to food and weight.

Another factor is *food palatability*, which with modern methods of food production can now be greater than would have been the case during the evolution of our feeding control systems. These evolved so that internal signals from for example gastric distension and glucose utilization could act to decrease the pleasantness of the sensory sensations produced by feeding sufficiently by the end of a meal to stop further eating. However, the greater palatability of modern food may mean that this balance is altered, so that there is a tendency for the greater palatability of food to be insufficiently decreased by a standard amount of food eaten, so that extra food is eaten in a meal.

Similarly, given that it is now possible to make available a very wide range of food flavours, textures, and appearances, another factor that could contribute to a tendency towards obesity

---

[15]However, van den Pol (2003) argues that when corrected for changes in the age distribution in the population, the increase in obesity may be more modest, perhaps 7–8%.

is that food intake may be enhanced by the *variety* of food because *sensory-specific satiety* to one food may nevertheless leave other foods still somewhat pleasant to eat.

Another factor that could contribute to obesity is *fixed meal times*, in that the normal control of food intake by alterations in inter-meal interval is not available, and food may be eaten at a meal-time even if hunger is not present.

Making food *salient*, for example by placing it on display, may increase food selection particularly in the obese (Schachter 1971, Rodin 1976, Cornell, Rodin and Weingarten 1989), and portion size is a factor, with more being eaten if a large portion of food is presented (Kral and Rolls 2004), though whether this is a factor that can lead to obesity and not just alter meal size is not yet clear.

Gastric emptying rate may be quite an important factor, for although gastric emptying rate is slower for high energy density foods, this does not fully compensate for the energy density of the food (Hunt and Stubbs 1975, Hunt 1980).

Indeed, it is notable that obese people tend to eat high *energy density* foods and to visit restaurants with high energy density (e.g. high fat) foods. It is also a matter of clinical experience that gastric emptying is faster in obese than in thin individuals, so that gastric distension may play a less effective role in contributing to satiety in the obese.

A factor related to this is *eating rate*, which is typically fast in the obese, and may provide insufficient time for the full effect of satiety signals as food reaches the intestine to operate.

Another potential factor is *stress*, which can induce eating and could contribute to a tendency to obesity. (Placing a paper clip on the tail of a rat induces mild stress, and in the presence of food, overeating and obesity can be produced. The overeating is reduced by antianxiety drugs.)

On the *energy output* side, the lack of exercise, and the presence of good room heating, may tend to limit energy output, and thus contribute to obesity. It should be noted though that obese people do not generally suffer from a very low metabolic rate: in fact, as a population, in line with their elevated body weight, obese people have higher metabolic rates than normal weight humans (Garrow 1988) (at least at their obese body weights: it might be interesting to investigate this further).

Models of binge eating which draw a parallel to addiction are described in Section 8.3.3. In one rat model of binge eating, access to sucrose for several hours each day can lead to binge-like consumption of the sucrose over a period of days (Colantuoni, Rada, McCarthy, Patten, Avena, Chadeayne and Hoebel 2002, Avena and Hoebel 2003a, Avena and Hoebel 2003b, Spangler, Wittkowski, Goddard, Avena, Hoebel and Leibowitz 2004). The binge-eating is associated with the release of dopamine. Moreover, the model brings binge eating close to an addictive process, at least in this model, in that after the binge-eating has become a habit, sucrose withdrawal decreases dopamine release in the accumbens, altered binding of dopamine to its receptors in the ventral striatum is produced, and signs of withdrawal from an addiction occur including teeth chattering. In withdrawal, the animals are also hypersensitive to the effects of amphetamine. Another rat model investigates binge eating of fat, and is investigating whether the reinforcing cues associated with this can be reduced by the GABA-B receptor agonist baclofen (Corwin and Buda-Levin 2004).

Anorexia nervosa is a disturbance of food intake in which food intake is reduced severely (typically in girls in late adolescence), a paradoxical reduction in appetite occurs, and body weight may be so much reduced that the condition becomes life threatening (Beumont, Burrows and Caspar 1987, Barbarich, Kaye and Jimerson 2003). The factors that lead to anorexia are not well understood, but the alteration in body image (in which anorexics feel that their bodies are much less thin than they are) has been related to altered binding of 5-HT (5-hydroxy-tryptamine, a monoamine neurotransmitter, with cell bodies in the raphe nucleus in the brainstem, and receptors abundant on layer 5 cortical pyramidal cells) in the parietal cortex (Bailer and Kaye 2003). Further, depletion of the amino acid tryptophan in the diet, which can reduce brain levels of 5HT, decreases anxiety more in anorexics than in controls (Bailer and Kaye 2003). It is also notable that anorexics feel better when they starve, as this reduces their levels of anxiety (Barbarich et al. 2003), which are, it must be said, much focussed on their being fatter than they wish, so that cause and effect may not be entirely separate here. Much remains to be understood, in relation to both the causes of and the treatment of eating disorders, but some of the scientific bases for such understanding are now being advanced.

5.6 Conclusions on reward, affective responses to food, and the control of appetite

We have seen in this Chapter that the reward value of food, and its subjective complement, the rated affective pleasantness of food, is decoded in primates including humans only after several stages of analysis. First the representation of the taste of the food (its identity and intensity) is made explicit in the primary taste cortex. Only later, in the orbitofrontal cortex, is the reward value made explicit in the representation, for it is here that satiety signals modulate the responses of the taste and flavour neurons. Thus in the control of food intake, the reward value or pleasantness is crucial to the design of how food intake is controlled, and the reward value is represented only in specialized cortical areas. The orbitofrontal cortex is moreover where multimodal representations of food are built, which include taste, texture, olfactory, and visual components. The actual satiety signals are complex, and include sensory-specific satiety, computed in the orbitofrontal cortex, gastric distension, gut satiety signals, plasma glucose, and hormones such as leptin.

The primate orbitofrontal cortex is more closely related to the changing affective value of food than the amygdala, in that the orbitofrontal cortex shows responses that decrease to zero as the reward decreases to zero with satiety, and in that the orbitofrontal cortex tracks (and probably computes) the changing reward value of stimuli as they are altered by stimulus–reinforcer association learning and reversal.

The outputs of the orbitofrontal cortex reach brain regions such as the striatum, cingulate cortex, and dorsolateral prefrontal cortex where behavioural responses to food may be elicited because these structures produce behaviour which makes the orbitofrontal cortex reward neurons fire, as they represent a goal for behaviour. At the same time, outputs from the orbitofrontal cortex and amygdala, in part via the hypothalamus, may provide for appropriate autonomic and endocrine responses to food to be produced, including the release of hormones such as insulin.

6 Thirst

6.1 Introduction

In this Chapter, the systems that control thirst are described. These systems operate analogously to those involved in the control of feeding, although in the case of thirst the actual stimuli that initiate the thirst and drinking are relatively simple and prescribed, and so the way in which these signals control the motivated behaviour can be analysed quite precisely. For comparison, in Chapter 9 we consider the processing of rewards relevant to sexual behaviour, in which the conditions that initiate the drive are not simply homeostatic to maintain the internal milieu.

We focus on the rewards relevant to thirst and drinking. In the case of thirst there are internal signals that indicate that there is a need for water. The water is a reward, in that the organism will work to obtain the water. The signals that make the water rewarding originate internally. In the case of thirst, the internal signals reflect the volumes of the cellular and extracellular fluid. Thirst and drinking operate to maintain the constancy of the internal milieu. The internal signals operate to alter the reward value that water has for the thirsty organism. The reward signals are conveyed primarily by the taste and sight of water.

In this Chapter, we will consider where in information processing in these sensory systems the sensory stimulation produced by water is decoded not just as a physical stimulus, but is coded in terms of its reward value. An important aspect of brain organization is that these two aspects of information processing are kept separate, at least in primates including humans. Another important aspect of brain organization for this type of reward is that the learning of which visual stimuli are water, or are associated with water, takes place in specialized parts for the brain of this type of learning, and takes place after analysis of what the stimulus is.

Thirst is a sensation normally aroused by a lack of water and associated with a desire to drink water. The mechanisms involved in the control of drinking are useful to study, not only because of their medical relevance, but also because the stimuli that lead to drinking can be identified, measured and manipulated, so allowing the basis of a relatively complex, motivated behaviour to be analysed. The type of control of the reward value produced by the taste of water being modulated by internal thirst signals is analogous to the control of the reward value of the taste of food by internal hunger and satiety signals. However, thirst is a useful case to study because the internal signals that control thirst can be defined and precisely measured. A summary of the control signals for thirst is provided in Section 6.6 and Fig. 6.8 on page 286.

Body water is contained within two main compartments. The intracellular water accounts for approximately 40% of body weight, and the extracellular water is approximately 20% of body weight, divided between the blood plasma (the blood without the cells) (5% of body weight) and the interstitial fluid (the fluid between/outside the cells of the body and not in the blood vascular system) (15% of body weight) (see Fig. 6.1). After water deprivation, significant depletions of both the cellular and extracellular fluid compartments are found. To discover whether changes in either or both fluid compartments can act as stimuli for drinking,

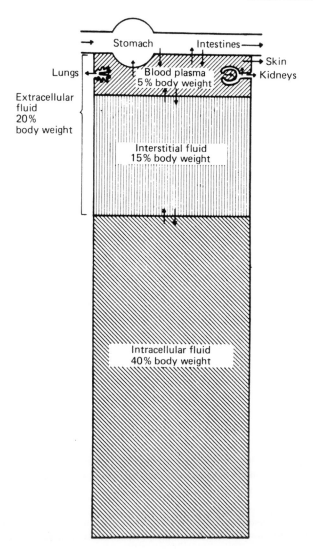

Fig. 6.1 Body water compartments. Arrows represent fluid movement. (After Rolls and Rolls 1982)

effects of selective depletion of one of the compartments on drinking, and the mechanisms activated, have been investigated as described below. References to original sources are contained in Rolls and Rolls (1982a), Rolls, Wood and Rolls (1980a), Grossman (1990), and Fitzsimons (1992).

6.2   Cellular stimuli for drinking

The drinking that occurs when the body fluids become concentrated due to net water loss or the ingestion of foods rich in salts such as meat appears to be initiated by cellular dehydration, leading to cell shrinkage. Evidence for this is that the administration of concentrated sodium chloride solution leads to withdrawal of water from the cells by osmosis and produces drinking. (Osmosis is the process by which water may be withdrawn through the semipermeable membrane of cells if the concentration of salts and other osmotically active substances outside the cells is increased.) The effective change appears to be cellular dehydration and not an increase in absolute osmotic pressure (i.e. osmolality, as measured by freezing-point depression), in that administration of hypertonic substances such as sodium chloride and sucrose, which remain outside the cells and therefore cause cellular dehydration by osmosis, stimulates drinking. In contrast, similar concentrations of substances such as glucose, urea, and methylglucose, which cross the cell membrane and therefore do not lead to cellular dehydration, stimulate little or no drinking.

Increases in sodium concentration rather than cellular dehydration might be thought to be the thirst stimulus, but this seems unlikely since drinking is stimulated by the application of sucrose (which withdraws water from cells but does not raise sodium concentration) either directly to brain tissue (Blass and Epstein 1971, Peck and Novin 1971) or into the cerebral ventricles.

The degree of cellular dehydration must be monitored accurately, because sufficient water is consumed to dilute administered hypertonic sodium chloride solutions to the same concentration as the body fluids, that is to the same effective osmotic pressure (isotonicity).

Cellular dehydration as a stimulus for drinking is sensed centrally, in the brain, rather than peripherally, in the body, in that low doses of hypertonic sodium chloride (or sucrose) infused into the carotid arteries, which supply the brain, produced drinking in the dog. Peripheral infusions of the same magnitude had no effect on drinking (Wood, Rolls and Ramsay 1977).

The brain regions in which cellular dehydration is sensed and leads to drinking appear to be near or lie in a region extending from the preoptic area through the hypothalamus, and including tissue surrounding the anteroventral part of the third ventricle, to the zona incerta posteriorly (Fig. 6.2). In these regions (but not in other brain regions) injections of small volumes of mildly hypertonic sodium chloride or sucrose lead to drinking, which at least at some sites is motivationally specific, as drinking, but not eating, is elicited (Blass and Epstein 1971, Peck and Novin 1971). Consistent with the hypothesis that these brain regions are involved in drinking in response to cellular dehydration, small lesions here can specifically impair drinking in response to cellular thirst stimuli yet leave drinking in response to other thirst stimuli intact, although more non-specific effects of the lesions are common (Rolls and Rolls 1982a).

6.3 Extracellular thirst stimuli

6.3.1 Extracellular stimuli for thirst

Thus far we have considered only the effect of loss of fluid from inside cells on thirst. Although the amount of fluid in the extracellular fluid (ECF) compartment is less than that in the cells, it is vital for the organism that the ECF be conserved to avoid debilitating changes in vascular fluid volume and pressure. The effects of loss of extracellular fluid include fainting, caused by insufficient blood reaching the brain. In addition to the physiological and hormonal mechanisms that contribute to the maintenance of the ECF volume [e.g. baroreceptor reflexes stimulated by a fall in blood pressure, antidiuretic hormone (ADH) (which reduces

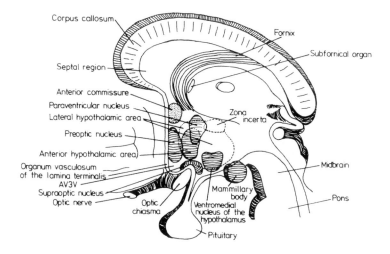

Fig. 6.2 Sagittal three-dimensional representation of the brain to illustrate some brain regions implicated in the control of drinking. AV3V: anteroventral region of the third ventricle. (After Rolls and Rolls 1982)

the excretion of water in the urine), and aldosterone (which reduces the excretion of sodium ion in the urine)], the behavioural response of drinking ensures that plasma volume does not fall to dangerously low levels.

The extracellular compartment has two components: the intravascular which contains the plasma, and the extravascular or interstitial fluid. These two components are in equilibrium and the receptors for controlling the ECF volume are located within the vasculature. ECF volume can become depleted in a variety of clinical conditions, which are accompanied by the loss of isotonic fluid as a result of vomiting, diarrhoea, or blood loss. (Isotonic fluid is fluid that is at the same 'strength' or effective osmotic pressure as the body fluids.) Significant ECF volume depletion will cause the release of antidiuretic hormone, which will reduce renal fluid loss. There might also be a need to replenish lost fluid, and it is advantageous that thirst often follows the ECF depletion in these clinical conditions.

There are several ways that ECF volume can be depleted experimentally in order to study the role of ECF volume in thirst. Obvious methods include haemorrhage, lowering the sodium content of the diet, and encouraging excessive sweating, urine production, or salivation, depending on the species being tested. However, ECF can be removed quickly and simply by injecting high concentrations of colloids (gum acacia or polyethylene glycol) either into the peritoneal cavity or subcutaneously. Isotonic fluid accumulates around the colloid, thereby depleting the ECF. Such depletion leads to a reduction in urine flow, and an increase in water intake that is related to the magnitude of the depletion. Some hours after the onset of thirst, a marked appetite for sodium develops and the ingestion of sodium restores the volume and composition of the ECF to normal.

The drinking that follows ECF depletion could be mediated by receptors in the vasculature. The role of such putative receptors in thirst can be studied by either constricting or expanding blood vessels in regions where such manipulations would be interpreted as under- or over-filling. Such studies have indicated that the receptors for extracellular thirst are located in two

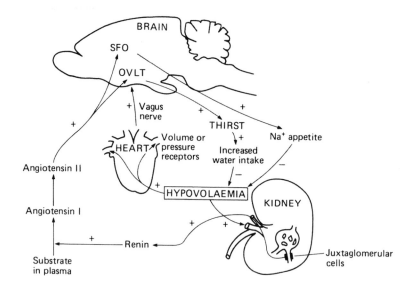

Fig. 6.3 A summary of the mechanisms involved in extracellular thirst. SFO, subfornical organ; OVLT, organum vasculosum of the lamina terminalis. (After Rolls and Rolls 1982)

main regions of the vasculature, in and around the kidneys and the heart (see Fig. 6.3), as shown by the following evidence.

6.3.2 Role of the kidney in extracellular thirst: the renin–angiotensin system

In the rat, ligation of the inferior vena cava, which reduces venous return to the heart and reduces arterial blood pressure, leads to a marked increase in water intake and a positive fluid balance due to decreased urine flow. If both kidneys are removed before ligation, water intake is significantly reduced, which suggests that an essential thirst stimulus following caval ligation could be a reduction in blood pressure to the kidneys. In order to test this hypothesis, Fitzsimons reduced the pressure to the kidneys by partially constricting the renal arteries, and found that water intake increased (see Fitzsimons (1992)).

When reductions in blood pressure or volume are sensed by the juxtaglomerular apparatus in the kidneys, the enzyme renin is released. Renin acts on substrate in the plasma to form angiotensin I, which is converted to angiotensin II, a vasoactive octapeptide (see Figs. 6.2 and 6.3). Angiotensin II is an active dipsogen in that intravenous infusions stimulate copious drinking (Fitzsimons and Simons 1969).

The receptors for angiotensin-induced drinking are located in the central nervous system, since injections into localized brain regions of doses of angiotensin at least 1000 times smaller than those required peripherally stimulate rats in fluid balance to drink large quantities of water (Epstein, Fitzsimons and Rolls 1970). Not only is angiotensin very potent, it is also very specific. Drinking is the only behavioural response that follows its administration and this drinking is highly motivated. A wide variety of species (including mammals, birds, and reptiles) have been shown to drink after administration of angiotensin (see Rolls and Rolls (1982a)).

Since the initial discovery that intracranial angiotensin stimulates drinking, much work has been aimed at locating precisely the receptive site(s) in the brain. Angiotensin does not cross the blood–brain barrier, but the circumventricular organs, which are located on the surface of the cerebral ventricles, are outside the blood–brain barrier. Several circumventricular organs have now been suggested as receptive sites for angiotensin, and one of these is the subfornical organ (SFO) (see Fig. 6.4). Local application of angiotensin to the SFO in very low doses (1.0 pg) can stimulate drinking, and lesions of the SFO or application to it of a competitive angiotensin receptor-blocking agent, at least in the rat, can abolish drinking in response to intravenous angiotensin without affecting drinking in response to cellular thirst stimuli (Simpson, Epstein and Camardo 1977). The SFO has been shown electrophysiologically to contain angiotensin-sensitive neurons (Phillips and Felix 1976), and anatomically to send projections to the medial preoptic area, the supraoptic nucleus, and the brain close to the anteroventral part of the third ventricle (AV3V) (Miselis, Shapiro and Hand 1979). Injections of low doses of angiotensin in the region of another circumventricular organ, the organum vasculosum of the lamina terminalis (OVLT) in the anteroventral part of the third ventricle (see Fig. 6.3), also elicit drinking (Phillips 1978). Relatively large lesions in this region, which included damage to fibres from the SFO, reduced drinking in response to angiotensin (and to hypertonic sodium chloride) (Buggy and Johnson 1977a, Buggy and Johnson 1977b, Thrasher, Brown, Keil and Ramsay 1980a, Thrasher, Jones, Keil, Brown and Ramsay 1980b). Thus there is reasonable evidence that there are specialized and localized regions of neural tissue in or near the SFO and the OVLT involved in drinking produced by angiotensin (see Rolls and Rolls (1982a)).

6.3.3 Cardiac receptors for thirst

Local changes in volume and pressure in and around the heart are involved in extracellular thirst. Reducing the blood flow to the heart by partially constricting the thoracic inferior vena cava in the dog (a method used to produce low-output experimental cardiac failure) markedly increased water intake, which led to excessive oedema (Ramsay, Rolls and Wood 1975). Inflation of a balloon in the abdominal inferior vena cava also led to drinking which was correlated with the maximal fall in central venous pressure, but some drinking still occurred after administration of an angiotensin receptor-blocking agent and presumably was mediated by cardiac receptors (Fitzsimons and Moore-Gillon 1980). It is still not clear precisely where such cardiac receptors are located, but it seems most likely that they are in the low-pressure (venous) circulation around the heart (see Fig. 6.3), since the compliance of these vessels is high, making them responsive to changes in blood volume. It is thought that the information from these receptors is carried to the central nervous system via the vagosympathetic nerves, which normally exert an inhibitory effect on thirst.

6.4 Control of normal drinking

It has been shown above that there are mechanisms by which depletion of the cellular or the extracellular fluid compartments can stimulate drinking. An important question is to what extent these mechanisms are normally activated during thirst and drinking, whether produced by water deprivation, or occurring when there is free access to water. Perhaps habit is one factor normally important in the initiation of drinking, but are deficits in the body fluid compartments normally involved in the initiation of drinking?

To gain evidence on this, it is first important to know whether deficits in the body fluid compartments are produced, for example, by water deprivation. There are deficits in both fluid compartments produced by water deprivation (Rolls, Wood and Rolls 1980a, Rolls and Rolls 1982a). This is the case not only in the rat, dog, and monkey, but also in humans (Rolls and Rolls 1982a, Rolls, Wood, Rolls, Lind, Lind and Ledingham 1980b). Next, it is found that the deficit in the cellular fluid compartment is large enough to lead to drinking, as shown by threshold measurements determined for the initiation of drinking in response to cellular dehydration. For example, following infusions of sodium chloride in the monkey, the threshold increase in plasma concentration necessary to evoke drinking was found to be 7 mOsmol kg^{-1} H$_2$O, which was less than the increase produced by water deprivation for 24 h (Wood, Maddison, Rolls, Rolls and Gibbs 1980). Other evidence comes from repletion experiments. When, after water deprivation, intravenous water preloads were given that effectively abolished the cellular fluid deficit, drinking was reduced by 65% in the rat and by 85% in the monkey (Wood, Maddison, Rolls, Rolls and Gibbs 1980, Wood, Rolls and Rolls 1982). If the ECF deficit is corrected by intravenous infusions of isotonic sodium chloride, then drinking is reduced by 20% and 5% in the rat and monkey, respectively (see Rolls, Wood and Rolls (1980a)). Thus depletion of the fluid compartments is an important determinant of drinking after water deprivation, with the depletion in the cellular compartment being more important, particularly in the primate (see further Rolls, Wood and Rolls (1980a) and Rolls and Rolls (1982a)).

In humans, it was found that with free access to water, the osmotic and extracellular thresholds for the elicitation of thirst were not normally reached before the humans had water to drink (Phillips, Rolls, Ledingham and Morton 1984). Thus in humans, at least when working in an air-conditioned temperature-controlled environment, drinking may anticipate needs. This anticipation is likely to be at least partly based on learning, so that after some time, actual body fluid deficits would be avoided. Humans would thus learn to initiate drinking based on any stimuli that are associated later with thirst signalled by cellular or extracellular body fluid deficits. In this way, drinking might become conditioned to stimuli such as large meals, salty food, or hot temperatures and dry conditions, or even to time of day. Of course, the primary thirst signals would be important for setting up this learning, but after the learning, the drinking would occur to the conditioned stimuli, and the primary thirst signals would not be activated. One would expect the primary thirst signals to become activated again if conditions changed, an example of which might be moving from sedentary work in an air-conditioned environment to physical work outdoors in a hot country. As a result of the activation of primary thirst signals, new learning would produce appropriate conditioned drinking for the new conditions.

Another factor in humans that may lead to primary body fluid deficit signals being unusual is that there is frequently available a large set of attractive drinks, including soft drinks, tea, and coffee.

Another interesting aspect of thirst is that in humans it was found that infusions of angiotensin did not always elicit drinking (Phillips, Rolls, Ledingham, Morton and Forsling 1985). Moreover, large variations of angiotensin concentrations are found when a human

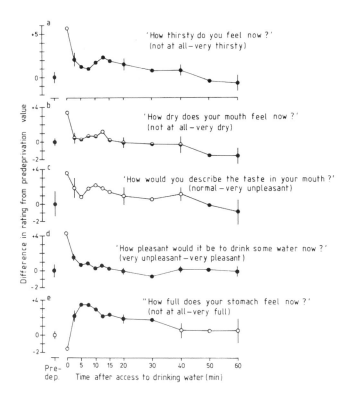

Fig. 6.4 The pleasantness of the taste of water is increased by water deprivation in humans, and decreases rapidly during drinking to satiety, before the water depletion of the body fluids has been completed. This is shown in the fourth graph from the top. In this diagram the effects of 24 h water deprivation on human subjective ratings of thirst and other sensations are shown by the difference between the predeprivation rating (pre-dep.) and the rating at time 0, taken 24 h later just before access to the water was given. The way in which the ratings changed after drinking started at time 0 is also shown. The significance of the changes relative to the value after 24 h water deprivation, at time 0, is indicated by closed circles (P < 0.01), half-filled circles (P < 0.05), or open circles (not significant). (After Rolls, Wood, Rolls, Lind, Lind and Ledingham, 1980; and Rolls and Rolls, 1982)

moves for example from lying down to standing up. The reason for this is that the change of posture in humans to standing upright on two legs produces a sudden drop in pressure in the renal arteries (as blood accumulates initially in the lower half of the standing body), and the release of angiotensin (stimulated by the reduced pressure in the renal arteries) produces vasoconstriction, which helps to compensate for the reduced blood pressure. Under these conditions (just standing up), thirst is not necessarily appropriate, and it may therefore be that the renin–angiotensin system is less important in humans than in other animals. It is nevertheless important to know about angiotensin in humans, for under some pathological conditions such as congestive heart failure, much angiotensin may be released as part of the body's attempt to compensate for some of the lack of fluid on the arterial side of the

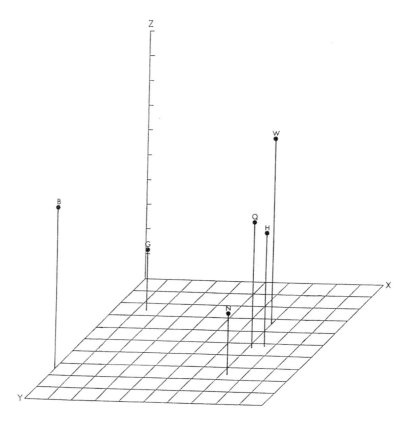

Fig. 6.5 The space produced by multidimensional scaling (MDS) of the responses of primate orbitofrontal cortex neurons to different tastes. The representation of water (W) is well separated from that of the prototypical tastes glucose (G), salt (N), bitter (Q, quinine) and sour (H, HCl). B, Blackcurrant juice. (After Rolls, Yaxley and Sienkiewicz 1990)

circulation (see Fitzsimons (1992)). However, to the extent that such pathologically high levels of angiotensin may produce thirst and lead to drinking, this drinking is inappropriate, for it may merely exacerbate the problem. Under these conditions, appropriate clinical care might include monitoring of water and fluid intake, to ensure that it is not excessive.

6.5 Reward and satiety signals for drinking

Drinking still occurs when ingested water is allowed to drain from a fistula in the oesophagus, stomach or duodenum. This is found in the rat, dog, and monkey (Rolls, Wood and Rolls 1980a, Rolls and Rolls 1982a, Gibbs, Rolls and Rolls 1986), and indicates that the reward for drinking is provided by oropharyngeal (and other pregastric) sensations such as the taste of water (at least in the first instance; compensatory learning may occur after prolonged experience). In fact, even a small quantity (e.g. 0.1 ml) of water delivered orally is sufficient to reinforce drinking, whereas much more water (e.g. 1–2 ml) must be delivered for the rat to learn a response in order to deliver water intragastrically (Epstein 1960) or intravenously

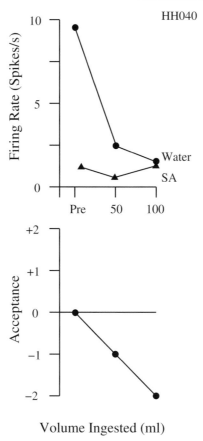

Fig. 6.6 An orbitofrontal cortex neuron in the monkey responding to the taste of water when thirsty, and gradually responding less to the taste of water during drinking to satiety. SA, spontaneous activity of the neuron; Pre, the firing rate before satiety was produced, by allowing the monkey to drink 100 ml water. The acceptability of the water is shown in the lower graph, on a scale from +2 indicating strong acceptance to −2 indicating strong rejection when satiety has been reached. (After Rolls, Sienkiewicz and Yaxley 1989.)

(Nicolaidis and Rowland 1974). This underlines the importance of exteroceptors in detecting and responding correctly to the presence of water, and shows that the presence of water in the gut or the dilution of plasma are not the primary rewards that normally control the animal's drinking.

A subjective analysis of the oropharyngeal control of drinking found that humans report (using a quantitative visual analogue rating scale) that the pleasantness of the taste of water is increased when they are thirsty as a result of water deprivation for 24 h, relative to the non-deprived condition (Rolls, Wood, Rolls, Lind, Lind and Ledingham 1980b) (see Fig. 6.4). It thus appears that oropharyngeal factors such as taste and swallowing maintain drinking and provide the incentive (or reward) for drinking.

There are neurons in the orbitofrontal cortex taste regions that respond to the 'taste' of water. Examples of this type of neuron are shown in Fig. 4.20 on page 98. The neuron responded much more to the taste of water than to other stimuli. There are many such neurons

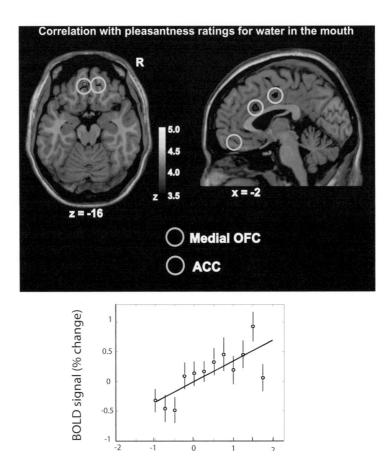

Fig. 6.7 Representation of the pleasantness of the taste of water in the human brain. Correlations with the pleasantness of the taste of water in a group random effects analysis. Top left: Regions of the medial caudal orbitofrontal where the activation was correlated with the subjective pleasantness ratings of water throughout the experiment. Bottom: A scatter plot showing the values of the BOLD signal in the medial orbitofrontal cortex (mean across subjects, ± s.e.m.), with the regression line shown. Top right: The regions of anterior cingulate cortex (ACC) where activation was correlated with the subjective pleasantness ratings of water given throughout the experiment. (After DeAraujo, Kringelbach, Rolls and McGlone, 2003.) (See colour plates section.)

in the orbitofrontal cortex (Rolls, Yaxley and Sienkiewicz 1990). Although there might not be water receptors per se on the tongue, the presence of water in the mouth may be signalled by the presence of non-viscous liquid in the mouth, and the absence of firing of sweet, salt, bitter, sour, and umami neurons. (The saliva in the mouth will be diluted when water is in the mouth.) In any case, the processing that has taken place by the time taste information reaches the orbitofrontal cortex results in a population of neurons that conveys information about the presence of water in the mouth, and that is approximately as large a population as that devoted to the other prototypical tastes sweet, salt, bitter, and sour (Rolls, Yaxley and

Sienkiewicz 1990).

The coding provided by these populations of taste-responsive neurons in the orbitofrontal cortex can be visualized using multidimensional scaling (MDS), as shown in Fig. 6.5. MDS is based on a distance measure of the representations provided by different neurons. It is based, for example, on the correlations between the response profiles of different neurons to a set of stimuli. If all the different neurons respond similarly to two stimuli, they will be close together in the MDS space. If the different neurons have differences in their responses to the two stimuli, the stimuli will be far apart in the space. The results of MDS on a population of taste neurons in the orbitofrontal cortex is shown in Fig. 6.5. It can be seen that the prototypical taste stimuli are well separated from each other, and that water is well separated from each of the other stimuli, in at least some dimensions of the space. Thus the 'taste' of water is clearly represented as being separate from that of other tastes in the primate orbitofrontal cortex.

The representation of taste in the primate orbitofrontal cortex is probably of the reward value of the taste of water, in that the responses of these neurons to the taste of water is reduced to zero by feeding the monkey to satiety (see Fig. 6.6; Rolls, Sienkiewicz and Yaxley (1989b)). After the reward value of the taste of water has been decoded in the orbitofrontal cortex, the output systems that link to action may be analogous to those described in Chapter 5 for hunger. For example, there are neurons in the lateral hypothalamus of the monkey that respond to the taste of water if the monkey is thirsty (Rolls, Burton and Mora 1976, Rolls and Rolls 1982a, Rolls, Murzi, Yaxley, Thorpe and Simpson 1986, Rolls, Rolls and Rowe 1983b). There are also neurons in the primate lateral hypothalamus that respond in a motivation-selective way to the sight of a visual stimulus associated with the sight of water but not of food when both thirst and hunger are present (see Fig. 5.12).

The human orbitofrontal cortex also has a corresponding representation of the pleasantness of the taste of water, in that as shown in Fig. 6.7, activations in the orbitofrontal cortex and parts of the anterior cingulate cortex were correlated with the subjective pleasantness (but not intensity) ratings for water in the mouth (De Araujo, Kringelbach, Rolls and McGlone 2003b). In this investigation, the brain activations were measured to the delivery of water in the mouth while the subjects were thirsty, and then again after the subjects had drunk water to satiety. The pleasantness of the taste of the water was decreased by drinking it to satiety, and the brain activations in the orbitofrontal cortex and cingulate cortex were correlated with the changes of the subjective pleasantness of water in the mouth. The control solution was a tasteless solution with the same ionic components as saliva.

In the termination of drinking, gastric and post-gastric factors such as gut stimulation by water, and the systemic effects of absorbed water are important, and oropharyngeal factors are of less importance. If, for example, drinking is measured with an oesophageal, gastric or duodenal fistula open, then much more water (e.g. 1.5–10 times) is consumed than normally or when the fistula is closed (Maddison, Wood, Rolls, Rolls and Gibbs 1980, Rolls, Wood and Rolls 1980a). Gastric distension appears to be one factor in satiety, for if drinking is allowed to terminate normally in the monkey, and then a gastric cannula is opened to allow water in the stomach to drain out, drinking starts again very promptly (Maddison, Wood, Rolls, Rolls and Gibbs 1980). Gastric distension can only operate normally if ingested water reaches the intestine to inhibit gastric emptying, because excessive drinking occurs with a duodenal fistula open (Maddison, Wood, Rolls, Rolls and Gibbs 1980). Gut stimulation by water, and possibly activation of immediately post-absorptive hepatic-portal mechanisms, may also contribute to satiety, because intraduodenal infusions of water are relatively more effective in terminating

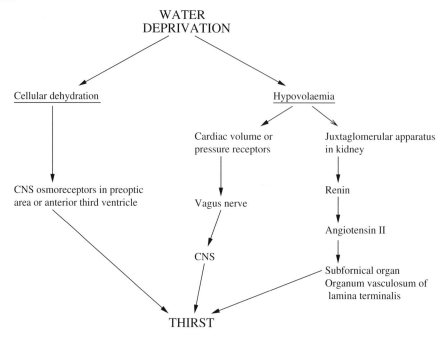

Fig. 6.8 A summary of the factors that can lead to drinking after water deprivation. (After Rolls and Rolls 1982)

drinking than intravenous infusions (Wood, Maddison, Rolls, Rolls and Gibbs 1980).

In the monkey and other relatively rapid drinkers such as the dog and human, systemic dilution produced by ingested water is not rapid enough to account for the termination of drinking, although, within 15–20 minutes after access to water, dilution of the body fluids is occurring (Rolls, Wood, Rolls, Lind, Lind and Ledingham 1980b, Rolls and Rolls 1982a). This dilution does at least contribute to satiety, since equivalent dilution produced by intravenous infusions of water reduces drinking (Wood, Maddison, Rolls, Rolls and Gibbs 1980).

The termination of drinking is best considered as the sequential activation of a number of contributing factors, starting with oropharyngeal stimulation by water (which appears to make a partial contribution to satiety as shown by observations that drinking with an oesophageal fistula open does usually stop in very rapid drinkers such as the dog (Towbin 1949); followed by gastric distension (which humans report subjectively to occur rapidly as satiety develops (Rolls, Wood, Rolls, Lind, Lind and Ledingham 1980b)); followed by gut and hepatic-portal stimulation by water; and finally systemic dilution and expansion (see Rolls, Wood, Rolls, Lind, Lind and Ledingham (1980b) and Rolls and Rolls (1982a)). Thus the reward value of the taste of water can be reduced by preabsorptive factors such as gastric distension, and later systemic dilution can contribute to satiety.

6.6 Summary

(see Fig. 6.8)

Drinking can be initiated by depletion of either the cellular or extracellular fluid compartments.

Both cellular and extracellular thirst stimuli (i.e. cellular dehydration and hypovolaemia) are produced by water deprivation in a variety of mammalian species, including man. Experiments in which the deficits in the fluid compartments are selectively repleted indicate that changes in both compartments contribute to drinking following water deprivation, but that changes in the cellular compartment are the more important.

Cellular dehydration as a thirst stimulus is indicated by the shrinkage of cells in or near the preoptic area of the brain.

Extracellular depletion as a thirst stimulus is indicated by activation of the renin–angiotensin system, and by signals from volume receptors in the low-pressure circulation on the venous side of the heart. Angiotensin is sensed by neurons in the subfornical organ, which have connections to a brain region close to the preoptic area.

Drinking is maintained or reinforced by oropharyngeal factors such as the taste of water, and it appears that the pleasantness of the taste of water in humans is influenced by the degree of thirst.

When water is consumed, the following changes occur in sequence and all contribute to the termination of drinking: oropharyngeal stimulation by water, gastric distension and gut stimulation by water, and finally systemic dilution.

7 Brain-stimulation reward

7.1 Introduction

Electrical stimulation at some sites in the brain is rewarding, in that animals including humans will work to obtain the stimulation. This phenomenon has been very useful in helping to understand the brain mechanisms that implement reward.

The discovery that rats would learn to stimulate electrically some regions of the brain was reported by Olds and Milner (1954). Olds noticed that rats would return to a corner of an open field apparatus where stimulation had just been given. He stimulated the rat whenever it went to the corner and found that the animals rapidly learned to go there to obtain the stimulation, by making delivery of it contingent on other types of behaviour, such as pressing a lever in a Skinner box or crossing a shock grid (Olds 1977) (see Fig. 7.1).

The electrical stimulation is usually delivered through electrodes insulated to within 0.1–0.5 mm of the tip and permanently implanted so that the tip is in a defined location in the brain. The stimulation usually consists of pulses at a frequency of 50–100 Hz delivered in a train 300–500 ms long. At self-stimulation sites the animal will repeatedly perform the operant response to obtain one train of stimulation for each press. The rate of lever pressing provides a measure of the self-stimulation behaviour. The phenomenon can be called brain-stimulation reward because the animal will work to obtain the stimulation of its brain. Brain-stimulation reward has been found in all vertebrates tested. For example, it occurs in the goldfish, pigeon, rat, cat, dog, monkey, and humans (Rolls 1975). Brain-stimulation reward can also refer to reward produced by injections of pharmacological agents into the brain. For example, animals will learn to inject small amounts of amphetamine to certain parts of the brain. Pharmacological aspects of reward are described in Chapter 8.

7.2 The nature of the reward produced

One way in which the nature of the reward produced by brain stimulation can be tested in animals is by altering the drive (e.g. the hunger) of the animal to determine how this influences the reward produced by the stimulation. At some brain sites, for example in the lateral hypothalamus, a reduction of hunger can reduce the self-stimulation rate (Hoebel 1969, Hoebel 1976). As a reduction of hunger reduces both food reward (in that the animal will no longer work for food), and brain-stimulation reward at some brain sites, it is suggested that the stimulation at these brain sites is rewarding because it mimics the effect of food reward for a hungry animal (Hoebel 1969, Rolls 1975). This modulation of brain-stimulation reward by hunger is found at lateral hypothalamic sites (Rolls, Burton and Mora 1980c) and of all sites I have tested, most profoundly in the orbitofrontal cortex (Mora, Avrith, Phillips and Rolls 1979).

It is important to note that this modulation by satiety is not just a general effect on performance of, for instance, drowsiness, because a reduction of hunger may reduce self-stimulation

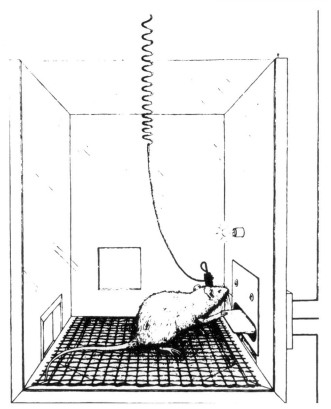

Fig. 7.1 A rat pressing a lever in order to obtain brain-stimulation reward. The reward is provided by a 0.5 s train of pulses of stimulation at typically 50–100 Hz delivered each time the rat presses the bar. (After Olds 1956.)

at some sites but not at others (Rolls 1975). Further, at some sites hunger may facilitate self-stimulation, while at other sites thirst may facilitate self-stimulation. For example, in an experiment by Gallistel and Beagley (1971) rats chose stimulation on one electrode if they were hungry and on a different electrode if they were thirsty (see Fig. 7.2). One interesting and useful feature of this experiment is that a choice rather than a rate measure of the reward value of the brain stimulation was used. The advantage of the choice measure is that any general effect such as arousal or drowsiness produced by the treatment which could affect response rate has a minimal effect on the outcome of the experiment. The experiment shows that at some sites brain-stimulation reward can be equivalent to a specific natural reward, such as food for a hungry animal or water for a thirsty animal.

Support for this view that brain-stimulation reward can mimic the effects of a natural reward such as food comes from neurophysiological experiments described below in which brain-stimulation reward and food reward have been shown to activate the same neurons in the hypothalamus.

At some other sites, the brain-stimulation reward produces effects that mimic those of sexual rewards. For example, at sites in the posterior hypothalamus but not in the lateral hypothalamus in male rats, castration decreases the self-stimulation, and subsequent androgen

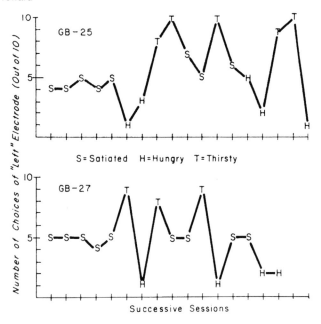

Fig. 7.2 Water and food reward effects produced by electrical stimulation of the brain in two rats. If the rats were thirsty (T) they chose to press a lever that delivered electrical stimulation to one brain site, and if they were hungry (H) they chose to press the other lever that delivered stimulation to another brain site. If the rats were satiated (S) for both food and water, then the preference for the two sites was approximately equal. (Reprinted with permission from Gallistel and Beagley 1971.)

replacement injections produced a differential facilitation of the posterior hypothalamic self-stimulation (Caggiula 1970, Olds 1958, Olds 1961).

At other sites natural drives such as hunger and thirst do not modulate self-stimulation, so that some other reward process, perhaps more related to emotion as described next, must underlie the reward produced (Rolls 1975).

A different type of evidence on the nature of the reward produced by electrical stimulation of the brain comes from direct reports of the sensations elicited by the stimulation in humans. During the investigation of, or treatment of, epilepsy, tumours or Parkinson's disease, electrical stimulation has been given to localized brain regions to evaluate the functioning of particular regions. Sem-Jacobsen (1968) and Sem-Jacobsen (1976) reported on the effects of stimulation at 2639 sites in 82 patients. Pleasant smells were evoked by the stimulation at nine sites, and unpleasant at six. Pleasant tastes were evoked at three sites, and unpleasant at one. Sexual responses were elicited at two sites. These types of finding are consistent with the food-related and other effects of the stimulation at some sites inferred from experiments with animals.

The relative paucity of reports of this type in humans may be because brain sites in the temporal and frontal lobes are usually investigated and the electrodes do not normally reach the basal regions such as the hypothalamus that are often investigated in animals.

More common in humans are reports that mood changes are elicited by stimulation at some sites. In Sem-Jacobsen's series, at 360 points the patients became relaxed, at ease, had a feeling of well-being and/or were a little sleepy (classed as Positive I). At 31 sites the patients in addition showed enjoyment, frequently smiled and might want more stimulation (Positive

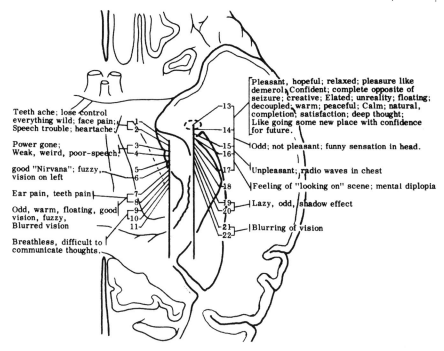

Pleasant, hopeful; relaxed; pleasure like demerol, Confident; complete opposite of seizure; creative; Elated; unreality; floating; decoupled; warm; peaceful; Calm; natural, completion; satisfaction; deep thought; Like going some new place with confidence for future.

Odd; not pleasant; funny sensation in head.

Unpleasant; radio waves in chest

Feeling of "looking on" scene; mental diplopia

Lazy, odd, shadow effect

Blurring of vision

Teeth ache; lose control everything wild; face pain; Speech trouble; heartache.

Power gone; Weak, weird, poor-speech.

good "Nirvana"; fuzzy, vision on left

Ear pain, teeth pain

Odd, warm, floating, good vision, fuzzy, Blurred vision

Breathless, difficult to communicate thoughts.

Fig. 7.3 Summary of subjective states evoked by electrical stimulation at different sites along two tracks in the human temporal lobe on a diagrammatic representation of the stimulating points. (Reprinted from Stevens, Mark, Ervin, Pacheco and Suematsu 1969)

II). At eight sites (in seven patients) the patients laughed out loud, enjoyed themselves, positively liked the stimulation and wanted more (Positive III). These and other reports of mood changes were produced by the stimulation. Thus at some brain sites in humans electrical stimulation can produce mood changes, stimulation may be desired, and this may be associated with self-stimulation (Heath 1954, Heath 1963, Heath 1972, Bishop, Elder and Heath 1963, Stevens, Mark, Ervin, Pacheco and Suematsu 1969, Delgado 1976, Sem-Jacobsen 1976, Valenstein 1974, Halgren 1992). Examples of some of the effects produced by electrical stimulation in tracks made into the temporal lobe during neurosurgery are illustrated in Fig. 7.3.

The evidence available from animals and humans thus suggests that the nature of the reward produced at different self-stimulation sites depends on the site: at some sites (e.g. the lateral hypothalamus and the secondary taste cortex in the orbitofrontal region) the stimulation may be equivalent to a specific natural reward such as food for a hungry animal. At other sites the stimulation may produce more general changes in mood and may thus be desired. At other sites (e.g. some parts of the orbitofrontal cortex and amygdala) it is possible that the stimulation taps into brain systems concerned with learning about stimulus–reinforcer associations, where of course primary reinforcers must be represented, and where the output pathways must be capable of signalling (secondary) reinforcement if they are to implement the effects that secondary reinforcers have. This analysis makes it clear that brain self-stimulation may occur for any one of a number of reasons and that a single basis for brain-stimulation reward should not be expected.

It is now to the neural bases of brain-stimulation reward that we turn. We will be concerned not only with the neural mechanisms of brain-stimulation reward at different sites, but also with what can be learned about reward processes in the brain from studies of brain-stimulation reward.

For example, one question before us will be how it happens that animals will only work for food (i.e. find it rewarding) when they are hungry. Another question is why brain-stimulation reward continues for hours on end with no appearance of satiety. Is the elicitation of a reward by a sensory stimulus something that normally can continue indefinitely, and if so, how does the system normally arrange for any one reward not to dominate behavioural choice for long periods? Another question, examined in Chapter 8, will be how studies of the pharmacology of brain-stimulation reward relate to our understanding of the control of mood, and what they tell us about the neural basis of addiction.

7.3 The location of brain-stimulation reward sites in the brain

To understand the neural mechanisms of brain-stimulation reward it is first necessary to know where brain self-stimulation sites are located. One group is located along the general course of the medial forebrain bundle, passing lateral to the midline from the ventral tegmental area of the midbrain posteriorly, through the lateral hypothalamus, preoptic area and nucleus accumbens, toward the prefrontal cortex (orbitofrontal cortex in the monkey) anteriorly (Fig. 7.4) (Olds and Olds 1965, Rolls 1971c, Rolls 1974, Rolls 1975, Rolls 1976a, Rolls and Cooper 1974, Mora, Avrith and Rolls 1980, Rolls, Burton and Mora 1980c). Many cell groups and neural pathways follow this path or much of this general course. For example, there is the medial forebrain bundle itself, interconnecting forebrain and brainstem regions with hypothalamic and other diencephalic systems. There are fibres connected to neurons in prefrontal self-stimulation sites, which pass many self-stimulation sites in their course through the brain (Routtenberg, Gardner and Huang 1971, Rolls and Cooper 1973, Rolls and Cooper 1974). In addition there are dopamine-containing fibres in the mesolimbic and mesocortical systems ascending from cell group A10 in the ventral tegmental region to the ventral striatum and orbitofrontal cortex, as well as in the substantia nigra (cell group A9) coursing to the striatum (see Sections 8.3 and 8.4). It is likely that many neural systems are activated by electrodes in this group of sites and it is possible that stimulation of any one of a number of systems in this region may support self-stimulation.

A second group of self-stimulation sites is in limbic and related areas such as the amygdala, nucleus accumbens, and prefrontal cortex (orbitofrontal cortex in the monkey) (Rolls 1974, Rolls 1975, Rolls 1976a, Rolls, Burton and Mora 1980c, Mora, Avrith and Rolls 1980). This group of sites is highly interconnected neurophysiologically with the first group lying along the general course of the medial forebrain bundle, in that stimulation in any one of these reward sites activates neurons in the others in primates (Rolls, Burton and Mora 1980c) (see below).

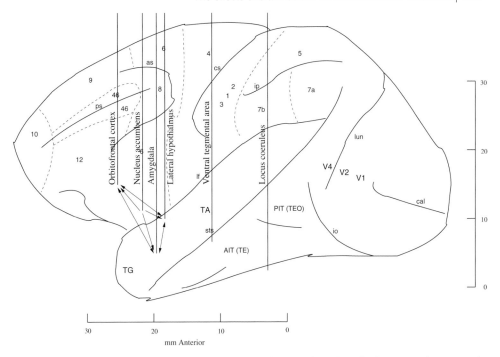

Fig. 7.4 Some brain sites in primates at which electrical stimulation of the brain can produce reward. The arrows indicate that stimulation at any one of these sites activates neurons in all of the other sites connected by arrows, as shown by Rolls, Burton and Mora (1980). The scales show the stereotaxic base planes. Abbreviations as in Fig. 4.1.

7.4 The effects of brain lesions on intracranial self-stimulation

Lateral or posterior hypothalamic self-stimulation rate is decreased (but not abolished) by small lesions in or near the medial forebrain bundle, particularly if the lesions are caudal to (i.e. behind) the self-stimulation electrode (Boyd and Gardner 1967, Olds and Olds 1969, Stellar and Stellar 1985). Ipsilateral, but not contralateral, lesions are effective. Thus a unilaterally organized system that can be disrupted particularly by posterior lesions at least modulates hypothalamic self-stimulation. Lesions that destroy most of the locus coeruleus do not abolish self-stimulation from regions anterior to it through which its fibres pass, so that it is unlikely that the cells of the locus coeruleus support self-stimulation even from these sites (Clavier 1976, Clavier and Routtenberg 1976). Cells in the dopamine A10 pathway are important for self-stimulation of some sites such as the ventral tegmentum, but not for self-stimulation of all sites, in that neurotoxic lesions of the dopamine inputs to the nucleus accumbens abolish self-stimulation of only some sites (Phillips and Fibiger 1989).

It is interesting to note that self-stimulation can occur after ablation of most of the forebrain in rats. Huston and Borbely (1973) were able to show this by requiring only a simple response of tail-raising (or lowering) which their forebrain-ablated rats were able to learn in order to obtain posterior hypothalamic stimulation (although extinction was impaired). This finding underlines the view that self-stimulation can occur because of the activation of one of a number of systems, and suggests that the basic mechanisms for rewarded behaviour must be represented at a low level in the brain. Forebrain areas may be related to reward, not because they are essential for all rewarded behaviour, but because they are concerned with decoding complex sensory inputs and determining whether these inputs are associated as a result of previous learning with reward; and with executing complex, instrumental, motor responses to obtain reward (see below).

Evidence that neurons with cell bodies in the lateral hypothalamus are involved in the reward effects produced by stimulation there comes from studies in which neurotoxic lesions of the lateral hypothalamus (which damage cell bodies there but not fibres of passage such as the dopaminergic fibres) attenuate self-stimulation of the lateral hypothalamus (and of sites anterior to it) (Lestang, Cardo, Roy and Velley 1985). It is possible that descending lateral hypothalamic neurons that mediate reward synapse on to dopamine neurons in the ventral tegmental area, and that the dopamine connection is important in the reward produced (Wise 1989, Shizgal and Murray 1989). However, the dopamine connection does not appear to be an essential part of the substrate of lateral hypothalamic brain-stimulation reward, for unilateral 6-OHDA lesions of the dopamine cell bodies in the ventral tegmentum did not attenuate lateral hypothalamic self-stimulation (Phillips and Fibiger 1976, Fibiger, LePiane, Jakubovic and Phillips 1987).

7.5 The neurophysiology of reward

By recording from single neurons while stimulation is delivered at the threshold current to self-stimulation electrodes[16], it is possible to determine which neural systems are actually activated by brain-stimulation reward. In the rat it is clear that during hypothalamic self-stimulation, neurons in the prefrontal cortex, amygdala and some areas of the brainstem, as well as in the hypothalamus itself, are activated (Rolls 1974, Rolls 1975, Rolls 1976a, Ito 1976). In the monkey it has been found that neurons in the lateral hypothalamus, orbitofrontal cortex, amygdala, nucleus accumbens, and ventral tegmental area are activated during self-stimulation of any one of these sites or of the nucleus accumbens (see Fig. 7.4) (Rolls 1974, Rolls 1975, Rolls 1976a, Rolls, Burton and Mora 1980c). Thus in the monkey, there is a highly interconnected set of structures, stimulation in any one of which will support self-stimulation and will activate neurons in the other structures.

7.5.1 Lateral hypothalamus and substantia innominata

Mainly in the monkey, it has been possible to record in the alert, behaving animal from neurons activated by brain-stimulation reward, and to determine whether these neurons are also activated by natural rewards such as food given to the hungry animal or during learning. When recording in the lateral hypothalamus and substantia innominata (which is lateral and rostral to the lateral hypothalamus) from neurons activated by brain-stimulation reward, it was found that some neurons (approximately 13% in one sample of 764 neurons) altered their activity in relation to feeding (Rolls 1974, Rolls 1975, Rolls 1976a, Rolls 1979, Rolls, Burton and Mora 1980c). This is the same population of hypothalamic neurons with feeding-related

---

[16]The threshold current for self-stimulation is the minimum amount of current for a given stimulation pulse-width required to produce self-stimulation at a given self-stimulation site.

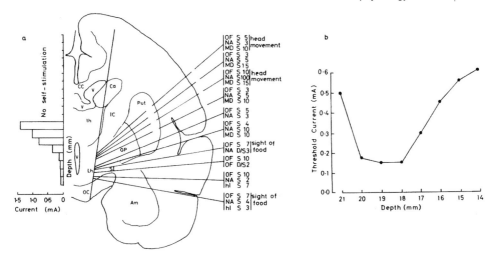

Fig. 7.5 a. Neurons activated by both brain-stimulation reward and the sight of food were found at the lower end of this microelectrode track in the macaque lateral hypothalamus. Neurons higher up the track in the globus pallidus were activated by brain-stimulation reward and also by head movements. The neurons were trans-synaptically (S) or possibly in some cases directly (D/S) activated with the latencies shown in ms from self-stimulation sites in the orbitofrontal cortex (OF), nucleus accumbens (NA), mediodorsal nucleus of the thalamus (MD), or lateral hypothalamus (hl). b. Self-stimulation through the recording microelectrode occurred with low currents if the microelectrode was in the hypothalamus close to the neurons activated by the sight of food. (From Rolls 1975; Rolls, Burton and Mora 1980.)

responses described in Chapter 5. Indeed, the neurons with feeding-related responses were discovered originally when we sought to determine what functions the hypothalamic neurons activated by brain-stimulation reward perform.

In the original sample of 764 neurons, some altered their activity only during the ingestion of some substances, so that their activity appeared to be associated with the taste of food. Many more of these neurons (approximately 11% of the total sample) altered their activity before ingestion started, while the animal was looking at the food (Rolls, Burton and Mora 1976, Rolls, Sanghera and Roper-Hall 1979a). The activity of this second set of neurons only occurred to the sight of food if the monkey was hungry (Burton, Rolls and Mora 1976), and becomes associated with the sight of food during learning (Mora, Rolls and Burton 1976b). Thus the activity of these neurons is associated with the sight and/or taste of food in the hungry animal, that is with the presentation of food reward.

To determine whether the activity of these neurons precedes, and could thus mediate, the responses of the hungry animal to food reward, their latency of activation was measured using a shutter that opened to reveal a food or a non-food-related visual stimulus (Rolls, Sanghera and Roper-Hall 1979a). The latency for different neurons was 150–200 ms, and compared with a latency of 250–300 ms for the earliest electrical activity recorded from the genioglossus muscle associated with the motor responses of a lick made to obtain food when the food-related visual stimulus was shown (see Fig. 5.10). (Upper motor neuron firing would occur in close temporal relation to the electromyogram recorded from this muscle.) Thus the motor response to the food could not result in the food-related activity of the hypothalamic neurons. This is consistent with the view that these neurons activated both by food reward and brain-stimulation reward are involved in mediating the reactions of the animal to food. These reactions to the food reward include the initiation of feeding behaviour, as well as endocrine and autonomic responses to the food (Fig. 4.2).

These hypothalamic neurons only respond to the sight or taste of food when the monkey is hungry (Burton, Rolls and Mora 1976, Rolls, Murzi, Yaxley, Thorpe and Simpson 1986). This is part of the evidence that implicates these neurons in the reward produced by the sight or taste of food if hunger is present. It is also thus very interesting that self-stimulation in the lateral hypothalamus is reduced by feeding the monkey to satiety (Rolls, Burton and Mora 1980c). As noted earlier, this indicates that the reward produced by the electrical stimulation of the lateral hypothalamus is like food for a hungry monkey, in that the reward value of each is reduced by feeding the monkey to satiety. In an additional experiment, it was shown that the current passed through the microelectrode that had recorded from food-related neurons in the lateral hypothalamus was lowest when the electrode was at the depth of the feeding-related neurons (see Fig. 7.5) (Rolls 1975, Rolls, Burton and Mora 1980c).

Taken together, these results show that brain-stimulation reward of the lateral hypothalamus occurs because it activates and thus mimics the effects that food reward has on these neurons. In a reciprocal way, the fact that self-stimulation of a number of brain sites, including the lateral hypothalamus, activates these neurons also activated by food when the food is rewarding provides useful evidence that the firing of these neurons actually produced reward. This is one of the valuable outcomes of research on brain-stimulation reward – it helps to show whether the firing of neurons activated by natural rewards is causally related to producing reward, and does not reflect some other process produced by food, such as salivation to food.

It is also worth noting that hypothalamic self-stimulation does not depend on direct activation of dopamine neurons, in that the refractory periods of directly activated neurons that mediate lateral hypothalamic reward are in the region of 0.6–1.2 ms, whereas the refractory periods of the dopamine neurons, which are small and unmyelinated, are in the range 1.2–2.5 ms (Rolls 1971c, Rolls 1971a, Yeomans 1990). Further, dopamine does not appear to be an essential part of the substrate of lateral hypothalamic brain-stimulation reward, for unilateral 6-OHDA lesions of the dopamine cell bodies in the ventral tegmentum did not attenuate lateral hypothalamic self-stimulation (Phillips and Fibiger 1976, Fibiger et al. 1987).

7.5.2   Orbitofrontal cortex

The orbitofrontal cortex is one of the brain regions in which excellent self-stimulation is produced in primates (Mora, Avrith, Phillips and Rolls 1979, Phillips, Mora and Rolls 1979, Phillips, Mora and Rolls 1981, Rolls, Burton and Mora 1980c, Mora, Avrith and Rolls 1980). The self-stimulation is like lateral hypothalamic self-stimulation in that it is learned rapidly, and occurs at a high rate. It has been shown that the self-stimulation of the orbitofrontal cortex is hunger-dependent, in that feeding a monkey to satiety produces great attenuation of orbitofrontal cortex self-stimulation (Mora, Avrith, Phillips and Rolls 1979). Of all the brain-stimulation reward sites studied in the monkey, it is the one at which feeding to satiety has the most profound effect in reducing self-stimulation (Rolls, Burton and Mora 1980). The orbitofrontal self-stimulation pulses have also been shown to drive neurons strongly in the lateral hypothalamus with latencies of only a few ms (Rolls 1975, Rolls 1976a, Rolls, Burton and Mora 1980c). On the basis of these findings, it was suggested that orbitofrontal cortex stimulation in primates is rewarding because it taps into food-reward mechanisms.

This proposal has been greatly elaborated by the discovery of the way in which the primate orbitofrontal cortex analyses the stimuli that implement food reward (and other types of reward too). The investigations of the neurophysiology of the orbitofrontal cortex that led to these discoveries were prompted by the fact that the orbitofrontal cortex is a good site for brain-stimulation reward, and that lateral hypothalamic food-related neurons are activated by rewarding stimulation of the lateral hypothalamus (Rolls 1974, Rolls 1975, Rolls 1976a, Rolls 1976b, Rolls, Burton and Mora 1980c). The discoveries included the following, considered in more detail in Chapters 4 and 5:

1. The secondary taste cortex is in the orbitofrontal cortex (Rolls, Yaxley and Sienkiewicz 1990, Baylis, Rolls and Baylis 1994).

2. The representation in the secondary taste cortex is of the reward value of taste, in that the responses of taste neurons here (but not in the primary taste cortex) are reduced to zero when the monkey feeds himself or herself to normal, physiological satiety (Rolls, Sienkiewicz and Yaxley 1989b, Rolls, Scott, Sienkiewicz and Yaxley 1988, Yaxley, Rolls and Sienkiewicz 1988). There is also a representation of the reward value of the 'taste' of water in the primate orbitofrontal cortex (Rolls, Sienkiewicz and Yaxley 1989b), and activations in the human orbitofrontal cortex are correlated with the pleasantness of the water in the mouth (De Araujo, Kringelbach, Rolls and McGlone 2003b).

3. The reward value of olfactory stimuli is represented in the secondary and tertiary cortical olfactory areas in the primate orbitofrontal cortex (Critchley and Rolls 1996b), representations which are themselves built for some orbitofrontal olfactory neurons by association with the primary reinforcer of taste (Rolls, Critchley, Mason and Wakeman 1996b, Critchley and Rolls 1996b). The subjective pleasantness of odour is correlated with activations in the human orbitofrontal cortex (Rolls, Kringelbach and De Araujo 2003c, O'Doherty, Rolls, Francis, Bowtell, McGlone, Kobal, Renner and Ahne 2000).

4. The reward value of visual stimuli such as the sight of food is represented in the primate orbitofrontal cortex (Critchley and Rolls 1996b), and the learning of the representation of which visual stimuli are rewarding is built in the orbitofrontal cortex by visual-to-taste reward learning (Rolls, Critchley, Mason and Wakeman 1996b), which can occur in one trial, and be reversed in one trial, by neurons in the orbitofrontal cortex (Thorpe, Rolls and Maddison 1983, Rolls, Critchley, Mason and Wakeman 1996b).

5. There is a representation of the mouth feel of food, including information about the presence of fat, in the orbitofrontal cortex, mediated through the somatosensory system (Rolls, Critchley, Browning, Hernadi and Lenard 1999a, Verhagen, Rolls and Kadohisa 2003, De Araujo and Rolls 2004) (see Chapter 5). These sensory inputs converge on to some orbitofrontal neurons that represent the pleasantness or reward value of taste, and are themselves likely to make a major contribution to the evaluation of the palatability (reward value) of food in the mouth (Rolls, Critchley, Browning, Hernadi and Lenard 1999a, Rolls, Verhagen and Kadohisa 2003e). Activations in the human orbitofrontal cortex are correlated with the subjective pleasantness of food during investigations with a whole food of sensory-specific satiety (Kringelbach, O'Doherty, Rolls and Andrews 2003).

6. The pleasantness of touch is represented in the human orbitofrontal cortex (Rolls, O'Doherty, Kringelbach, Francis, Bowtell and McGlone 2003d).

7. Activations in the human medial orbitofrontal cortex correlate with abstract rewards such as monetary gain in a probabilistic monetary reward task (O'Doherty, Kringelbach, Rolls, Hornak and Andrews 2001a).

These discoveries thus extend the explanation of why orbitofrontal cortex electrical stimulation can produce reward. It does so by activating representations concerned with the reward value of a whole spectrum of rewarding sensory stimuli, including the taste, smell, and texture of food, the reward value of water, the reward value of touch, and also abstract rewards such as monetary gain.

The fact that brain-stimulation reward of the orbitofrontal cortex occurs supports the evidence that this region implements the reward value of sensory stimuli related to food, as well as to other stimuli. The orbitofrontal cortex may be related to reward not only because it represents the reward value of a number of primary reinforcers (e.g. taste and touch), but also because it is involved in learning associations between primary reinforcers and the stimuli (such as the sight of food) with which they are associated. For this pattern-association learning (and reversal) process, the orbitofrontal cortex must contain a representation of both the primary reinforcer and the to-be-associated (e.g. visual) stimulus (see Appendix 1). Moreover, the firing of neurons that convey the fact that a secondary reinforcer is reinforcing must themselves if activated produce reward, and this, as well as the activation of representations of primary reinforcers such as taste and touch, implements the reward value of electrical stimulation of the orbitofrontal cortex.

It is noted that in rats the reward value of what may be a corresponding though less developed region, the sulcal prefrontal cortex, does not depend on the integrity of the dopamine inputs to this region (Phillips and Fibiger 1989). This suggests that activation of neurons in the orbitofrontal cortex is the fundamental component of reward produced by activation of this region, and not any possible activation of dopamine neurons or dopamine inputs to the prefrontal cortex.

Moreover, the findings considered above are consistent with the possibility that one way in which dopaminergic activation produced by the psychomotor stimulants such as amphetamine and cocaine produces reward is by activating the reward mechanisms just discussed in the orbitofrontal cortex (Phillips, Mora and Rolls 1981, Voellm, De Araujo, Cowen, Rolls, Kringelbach, Smith, Jezzard, Heal and Matthews 2004), and regions to which it projects such as the nucleus accumbens (Phillips, Blaha and Fibiger 1989, Phillips and Fibiger 1990).

7.5.3 Amygdala

Self-stimulation pulses applied to the monkey amygdala activate lateral hypothalamic and orbitofrontal cortex neurons also activated by the taste, sight or smell of food (Rolls 1976a, Rolls, Burton and Mora 1980c). This is one explanation of why electrical stimulation of the amygdala can produce reward.

Another, consistent, explanation is that neurons in the amygdala can be activated by the taste of food, or by the sight of food (Sanghera, Rolls and Roper-Hall 1979, Ono, Nishino,

Sasaki, Fukuda and Muramoto 1980, Rolls 2000d, Nishijo, Ono and Nishino 1988, Wilson and Rolls 1993, Scott, Karadi, Oomura, Nishino, Plata-Salaman, Lenard, Giza and Aou 1993, Kadohisa, Rolls and Verhagen 2005b, Wilson and Rolls 2005).

The underlying conceptual reason though for an involvement of activation of amygdala neurons in brain-stimulation reward is that the amygdala is a region, evolutionarily old, implicated in stimulus–reward association learning (see Chapter 4). For its output to be interpreted as a secondary reinforcer, some part of the output of the amygdala must be interpretable by the rest of the brain as being positively reinforcing; and for the amygdala to play a role in such pattern association learning, the primary reward (e.g. the taste of food) must be represented in the amygdala. Electrical stimulation of the amygdala could also tap into this representation of primary reward. In addition, electrical stimulation of the amygdala may produce reward because it taps into systems concerned more generally with rewards, including those produced by facial expression (see Chapter 4).

7.5.4 Nucleus accumbens

The nucleus accumbens is a self-stimulation site in primates and rats (Rolls 1971b, Rolls 1974, Rolls, Burton and Mora 1980c). The rewarding electrical stimulation here produces activation of neurons in the lateral hypothalamus and orbitofrontal cortex also activated by the sight and taste of food (Rolls, Burton and Mora 1980c). This may be a sufficient explanation for self-stimulation of the nucleus accumbens.

However, a more conceptual explanation is as follows. The accumbens may be a system through which conditioned incentives (secondary reinforcers) learned about in the orbito-frontal cortex and amygdala are connected to influence instrumental action. In particular, although the nucleus accumbens is not involved in action–outcome learning itself, it does allow the affective states retrieved by the basolateral amygdala (BLA) to conditioned stimuli to influence instrumental behaviour by for example Pavlovian-instrumental transfer, and facilitating locomotor approach to food which appears to be in rats a Pavlovian process (Cardinal et al. 2002). Such a role in for example processing a signal that facilitates approach would imply that the animal would work to obtain electrical stimulation of the output, which has to be interpretable as being rewarding if the secondary reinforcing properties of stimuli are to be interpreted by this route by the rest of the brain.

It may be that, because dopamine inputs to this region enhance the secondary reinforcing properties of incentive stimuli (Cador, Robbins and Everitt 1989, Everitt and Robbins 1992)[17], presumably by facilitating transmission through the nucleus accumbens, psychomotor stimulants such as amphetamine and cocaine come to produce their rewarding properties (see Section 8.3). Moreover, brain-stimulation reward of some sites such as the ventral tegmental area where dopamine cell bodies are located occurs because of activation of nucleus accumbens neurons through the dopaminergic ascending connections (see Section 8.3).

7.5.5 Central gray of the midbrain

Electrical stimulation of some regions of the brain can lead to analgesia in animals ranging from rats to humans and can be equivalent in its pain-reducing properties to large doses of morphine (Liebeskind and Paul 1977). These analgesic effects can last for hours after only

[17]They showed that amphetamine injections into the nucleus accumbens enhanced the reinforcing properties of conditioned incentive stimuli.

seconds of stimulation. The analgesia is often for only part of the body, so that a strong pinch to one side but not to the other might be ignored. This shows that the stimulation-produced analgesia is not simply some general interference with the animal's ability to respond to stimulation.

The effective stimulation sites are in the medial brainstem, and extend from the rostral medulla (nucleus raphe magnus), through the midbrain central grey matter, towards the hypothalamus. There is no clear relation with brain-stimulation reward mechanisms, because at some sites analgesia and self-stimulation are found and at others the stimulation is aversive but is followed by analgesia (Koob and Le Moal 1997).

It has been shown that naloxone, a specific morphine antagonist, reverses, at least partly, stimulation-produced analgesia in both the rat and humans (Akil, Mayer and Liebeskind 1976, Adams 1976). The endogenous morphine-like peptide enkephalin (Hughes 1975, Hughes, Smith, Kosterlitz, Fothergill, Morgan and Morris 1975, Cooper et al. 2003) injected intraventricularly yields analgesia (Beluzzi, Grant, Garsky, Sarantakis, Wise and Stein 1976), and central grey matter stimulation releases this substance or a peptide similar to it (Liebeskind, Giesler and Urca 1985). Further, there are stereospecific opiate-binding sites in the central grey matter, and elsewhere in the brain (Kuhar, Pert and Snyder 1973). These findings raise the possibility that stimulation-produced analgesia is effective because it causes the release of a naturally occurring morphine-like substance which acts on opiate receptors in the central grey matter and elsewhere to induce analgesia.

The stimulation at these brainstem sites may be rewarding because of activation of enkephalin-containing neurons which make synapses on to the dopamine neurons in the ventral tegmental area (Phillips and Fibiger 1989). The central gray stimulation may be rewarding because it is part of an endogenous opiate-containing system that controls the threshold for pain, which in emergency situations might be elevated, presumably to avoid being disabled by severe pain in situations that threaten survival.

7.6 Some of the properties of brain-stimulation reward

There are several properties of brain-stimulation reward that seemed surprising when they were discovered. However, by understanding these properties of brain-stimulation reward, we come to see that these are also properties of natural rewards, and we thus enhance our understanding of some of the properties of natural rewards.

7.6.1 Lack of satiety with brain-stimulation reward

One of the most striking properties of brain-stimulation reward is its persistence and lack of satiety. A record of a rat working for brain-stimulation reward for 24 h essentially without stopping is shown in Fig. 7.6. At the time that this was first discovered (see, e.g., Olds (1958)) it seemed quite extraordinary, because normally we do not work for a reward for that long. With eating, for example, we like the taste of food but during the course of a meal its reward value drops to zero, and we no longer work for it. The folk psychology was that reward somehow produced satiety, so we never worked for a reward for long. But the evidence from brain-stimulation reward showed that reward per se does not produce satiety.

This finding was useful, because it led to reconsideration of what happens with food reward (see Rolls (1975)), which does not, of course, itself produce satiety either, as the sham

48 Hours
Anterior Hypothalamic Electrode # 253

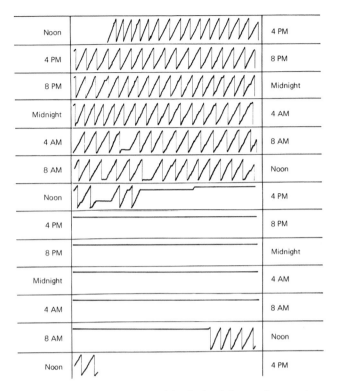

Fig. 7.6 This cumulative record shows that intracranial self-stimulation can be very vigorous and persistent. Each time the rat bar-pressed (for a 0.5-s train of electrical stimulation) the pen stepped once vertically. After 500 steps, it resets to 0. A four-hour time period is shown along the horizontal axis. (From J. Olds 1958.)

feeding experiments described in Section 5.2 show very clearly. The point with respect to feeding is that normally when food accumulates in the stomach and intestine it does produce peripheral satiety signals, and via these brain mechanisms reduces the reward value of sensory stimulation produced by the sight, smell, and taste of food, as shown in Chapter 5. But there is little about food reward per se that produces satiety. The only respect in which giving food reward does affect satiety is that there is some sensory-specific satiety, which, as described in Chapter 5, is sufficient to produce variety effects in food reward, but is not sufficient to reduce food reward to zero, and stop feeding (as shown by the continuing feeding in the sham feeding preparation). So the finding of little satiety produced by brain-stimulation reward is actually in line with other rewards, and the persistence of brain-stimulation reward helped to underline this. It is just that normally when we have a food or water reward, we ingest the food or water, and thereby close the loop and produce negative feedback to reduce the reward value of the food. As discussed in Chapter 9, there may be special mechanisms to turn off the rewards associated with sexual behaviour in males just after ejaculation.

The conclusion is that in general reward itself does not produce satiety, apart from some sensory-specific satiety to help behaviour to switch after some time to another reward, and there are special mechanisms usually associated with the rewarded behaviour (such as the ingestion of food) that act to neurally turn off the reward.

7.6.2 Rapid extinction

Extinction from self-stimulation can be very rapid (Seward, Uyeda and Olds 1959) even when the manipulandum is withdrawn, so that non-rewarded responses are prevented (Howarth and Deutsch 1962).

A factor that determines the number of responses in extinction is the time elapsed since the last reward (Howarth and Deutsch 1962), which was not found to apply for thirsty rats trained for water, that is where there is a string relevant drive (Quartermain and Webster 1968).

Perhaps the major factor that accounts for the rapid extinction of self-stimulation often reported is that no relevant drive is present. If rats are hungry, extinction from brain-stimulation reward is very prolonged (Deutsch and Di Cara 1967). Thus one conclusion that can be made from studies with brain-stimulation reward is that resistance to extinction depends on the presence of an appropriate drive.

The role of a relevant drive in the rapidity of extinction was demonstrated for conventional reinforcers by Panksepp and Trowill (1967b), who found a trend towards rapid extinction in satiated rats previously rewarded with chocolate milk.

Another factor that contributes to rapid extinction is the short time between pressing the manipulandum and receiving brain-stimulation reward, in contrast to the one or two seconds delay between pressing a manipulandum and then finding food or water reward available in a cup (Gibson, Reid, Sakai and Porter 1965, Panksepp and Trowill 1967a). Keesey (1964) also found that errors in learning a brightness discrimination are increased when the brain-stimulation reward is delayed.

This conclusion is relevant to interpreting investigations relevant to animal welfare. Although an animal may work for a reward, if it shows rapid extinction when the reward is no longer available, this could be because there is little motivation for that particular reward.

7.6.3 Priming

Rats will run along a runway to obtain electrical stimulation at the end of the runway. If some of the electrical stimulation is given in addition at the start of the runway, then the rats will run faster (Gallistel 1969). The stimulation given at the start of the runway is said to have a priming effect, which decays gradually (see Fig. 7.7 – the priming effect decayed over a particularly long time in this rat). Priming stimulation (given by the experimenter) can also cause a rat to return to a self-stimulation lever and start self-stimulating. This may be useful if the rat does not bar-press at once when it is put in a self-stimulation box, i.e. if it shows an 'overnight decrement effect'.

One factor that may contribute to the priming effect is arousal. It has been shown that arousal, measured by EEG (electroencephalogram) desynchronization and by increased locomotor activity, is produced by stimulation of reward sites along the medial forebrain bundle (MFB) (Rolls 1971c, Rolls 1971b, Rolls 1975, Rolls and Kelly 1972). This arousal decays in a very similar way to the priming effect, as shown, for example, in Fig. 7.7. The arousal must at least influence medial forebrain bundle (MFB) self-stimulation. Because of its similarities to the priming effect, it may well mediate the priming effect, at least in part. Similarities

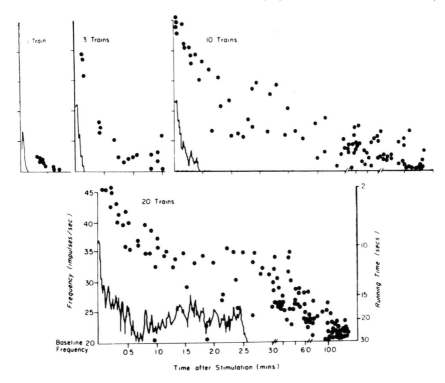

Fig. 7.7 The priming effect of brain-stimulation reward. Running speed (closed circles) for brain-stimulation reward as a function of time after different numbers of priming trains of stimulation given before the first trial (after Gallistel 1969). The firing rate (continuous line) of a neuron in the reticular activating system of the midbrain as a function of time after different numbers of trains of stimulation delivered at a lateral hypothalamic self-stimulation site is shown for comparison (after Rolls 1971a–c, 1975).

include the temporal nature of the decay, the greater magnitudes and durations of the effects produced by more stimulation trains (see Fig. 7.7), and the refractory periods of the neurons through which the effects are produced (Rolls 1971c, Rolls 1971a, Rolls 1974). Arousal may contribute not only to priming effects, but also to differences between some self-stimulation sites. For example, arousal is elicited by rewarding stimulation of MFB, but not nucleus accumbens, sites, and differences between these sites include hyperactivity and fast rates of self-stimulation at MFB self-stimulation sites (Rolls 1971b, Rolls 1974, Rolls 1975).

A second factor that may contribute to priming effects is incentive motivation, that is the motivation that can be produced by giving a reward. For example, if satiated animals are primed with an intraoral reward of chocolate milk, then they will resume bar-pressing to obtain more chocolate milk (Panksepp and Trowill 1967b). It is important that this effect is seen most markedly under zero-drive conditions, e.g. when an animal is neither hungry nor thirsty. These are the conditions under which self-stimulation experiments are often run. Incentive motivation is seen in other situations with natural reward, e.g. as the salted-nut phenomenon (Hebb 1949), and as the increase in the rate of ingestion seen at the start of a meal (LeMagnen 1971) (see Sections 3.3, 4.6.1.2 and 5.3.1).

This second factor may be relevant to investigations in animal welfare, in which it may be found that animals will work to obtain certain rewards if they have just been given or shown them, but do not appear to rank these rewards highly when they are pitted in long-term preference tests against more important rewards, such as those relevant to internal homeostatic states such as hunger and thirst (Dawkins 1990, Mason, Cooper and Clareborough 2001). Such rewards may be acting as low priority rewards, which are chosen temporarily after they have been presented due to incentive motivational effects. Care must thus be used in the design of preference tests in animals when these are used to provide evidence about the priority the animals give to different reinforcers, to ensure that such priming or incentive motivational effects are adequately controlled for. In addition, care must be taken that the animal is choosing a stimulus or condition as a goal, and is not just acting out of habit. As shown in Section 4.6.1.2, overtraining can lead to behaviour being controlled by stimulus–response associations or habits, and the value of the goal may not be taken into account in behavioural tests if they are run under habit as compared to instrumental goal value conditions, as shown for example by reward devaluation experiments.

A third factor that may contribute to priming effects is conflict. Kent and Grossman (1969) showed that only some rats needed priming after an interval in which self-stimulation was prevented by withdrawal of the lever. In the 'primer' rats the stimulation seemed to produce reward and aversion in that self-stimulation was accompanied by squeaking and defecation. It was suggested that during the time away from the bar the reward decayed more rapidly than the aversion, so that self-stimulation was not resumed without priming. It was also found that 'non-primer' rats could be converted into 'primers' by pairing painful tail shock with the brain-stimulation reward. Although Kent and Grossman (1969) labelled one group of their rats as 'non-primers', a priming effect can be demonstrated in this type of animal using, for example, a runway (Reid, Hunsicker, Kent, Lindsay and Gallistel 1973).

Thus there are several explanations of the priming effect which are not necessarily contradictory and which may all contribute to the priming effect.

7.7 Stimulus-bound motivational behaviour

Electrical stimulation at some brain sites can elicit feeding, drinking and other consummatory types of behaviour (Valenstein, Cox and Kakolewski 1970). The behaviour may be called 'stimulation-bound' because it occurs during the electrical stimulation, or 'stimulus-bound' because the behaviour is associated with a particular goal object, for example food pellets. If small-tipped stimulation electrodes are used relatively specific behaviours are elicited, such as drinking with electrodes near the zona incerta, and feeding with electrodes in the lateral hypothalamus (Olds, Allan and Briese 1971, Huang and Mogenson 1972).

A frequently observed feature of such behaviour is plasticity, that is stimulus-bound feeding can develop into stimulus-bound drinking if food is removed from the environment and replaced with water (Valenstein et al. 1970). It is as if the stimulation activates the animal and the behaviour that is elicited depends on which environmental stimuli are available for the animal to respond to, for example, food to chew or water to lap. This type of interpretation receives support from the observation that a mild continuous tail-pinch (with, for example, a paper clip) leads to 'stimulus-bound' types of behaviour such as eating in the rat (Antelman and Szechtman 1975). Because of such findings, it is difficult to interpret stimulus-bound behaviour produced by brain stimulation as a proof of activation of a hunger or thirst mechanism — rather it could be a more general type of behavioural activation.

It is worth noting that although stimulus-bound behaviour may not represent activation of a specific drive (e.g. hunger), there is evidence that reward elicited by electrical stimulation can be relatively specific. For example, it may be equivalent to food for a hungry animal or water for a thirsty animal (see Section 7.2).

7.8 Conclusions

Animals, including humans, will learn to stimulate electrically certain areas of the brain. At some sites the stimulation may be equivalent to a natural reward such as food for a hungry animal, in that hunger increases working for brain-stimulation reward at these (but not at other) sites.

It has been found in the monkey that one population of neurons activated by the brain-stimulation reward at these sites is in the region of the lateral hypothalamus and substantia innominata. Some of these neurons are also activated by the sight and/or taste of food if the monkey is hungry, that is when the food is rewarding. The latency of the responses of these neurons to the sight of food is 150–200 ms. This is longer than the responses of sensory neurons to visual stimuli in the inferotemporal cortex and dorsolateral amygdala, but shorter than the latency of the animal's behavioural responses to the sight of food, as shown by electrographic recording of the muscles that implement the motor responses. Thus it is possible that these hypothalamic neurons mediate some of the reactions of the hungry animal to food reward, such as the initiation of feeding and/or autonomic and endocrine responses.

In a comparable way, brain-stimulation reward of the primate orbitofrontal cortex occurs because it is activating systems normally concerned with decoding and representing taste, olfactory, tactile and visual rewards.

In this way reward-related processes can be identified and studied by analysing the operations (from sensory input through central control processes to motor output) that are involved in the responses of animals to rewarding stimuli.

Self-stimulation of some sites may occur because neurons whose activity is associated with food reward are activated by stimulation at these sites.

At other sites, brain-stimulation reward may be produced because the stimulation mimics other types of natural reward such as, in the nucleus accumbens, the effects of secondary reinforcers.

At other sites, as shown by verbal reports in humans, the electrical stimulation is rewarding because it is producing mood states such as a feeling of happiness normally produced by emotional stimuli.

The findings with brain-stimulation reward are helpful, because they provide additional evidence about whether a particular part of the brain is involved in reward processes. Consistent with this point, in general, brain-stimulation reward does not occur in brain areas involved in early sensory processing (e.g. in visual cortical areas up to and including the inferior temporal visual cortex), where on independent grounds it is believed that in primates the reward value of stimuli is not represented (see Chapter 4). Nor does brain-stimulation reward occur in general in motor structures such as the globus pallidus (see Fig. 7.5), nor in motor cortical areas (see Rolls (1974) and Rolls (1975)). Thus the evidence from brain-stimulation reward complements the other evidence described in this book that it is at special stages of the pathways that lead from sensory input to motor output that reward is represented, and that this is part of brain design (see further Chapters 2–11).

Brain-stimulation reward also historically helped to draw attention to important points, such as the fact that reward per se does not produce satiety (Section 7.6.1); that the time between the operant response and the delivery of the reward (or a stimulus associated with the reward) has important implications for what happens when the reward is no longer available (Section 7.6.2); and that effects such as rapid extinction, and priming, are found under low-drive conditions, that is, when the motivation for the reward is low (Sections 7.6.2 and 7.6.3).

7.9 Apostasis

[18] There was a great deal of research on electrical brain-stimulation reward in the years after its discovery (reported by Olds and Milner (1954)) until 1980. After that, research on brain-stimulation reward tailed off. Why was this? I think that one reason was that by the middle 1970s it was becoming possible to study reward mechanisms in the brain directly, by recording from single neurons, in order to provide a fundamental understanding of how natural rewards are being processed by the brain (see Rolls (1974), Rolls (1975), Rolls (1999a), and this book). This led to the analysis of the neural mechanisms involved in the sensory processing, and eventually to an understanding of the decoding of the reward value, in the taste, olfactory, visual, and touch systems of primates. In the case of visual processing, this involved investigating the learning mechanisms that enable visual stimuli to be decoded as rewarding based on pattern-association learning between visual stimuli and primary reinforcers such as taste (see Rolls and Treves (1998), Rolls and Deco (2002), and Appendix 1). By analysing such sensory information processing, an explanation for why electrical stimulation of some parts of the brain could produce reward became evident.

At the same time, the investigations of brain-stimulation reward were very helpful, because they provided additional evidence that neurons putatively involved in reward because of the nature of their responses (e.g. hypothalamic, orbitofrontal cortex, or amygdala neurons responding to the sight, smell, or taste of food) were actually involved in food reward, because electrical stimulation which activated these neurons could produce reward (see Rolls (1975), Rolls (1999a), and Chapters 4–6).

In a comparable way, electrical brain-stimulation reward was also of significance because it pointed the way towards brain regions such as the ventral tegmental area dopamine neurons, which, via their projections to the nucleus accumbens, can influence brain processing normally involved in decoding by the amygdala and orbitofrontal cortex environmental stimuli as being rewarding, and enabling these signals to influence behaviour (see Section 8.4.3.1). The relation of this brain dopamine system to reward led eventually to the discoveries that this dopamine neural system, and its projections to the orbitofrontal cortex, are involved in the rewarding and indeed addictive properties of drugs of abuse such as amphetamine and cocaine (Phillips, Mora and Rolls 1981, Phillips and Fibiger 1989, Koob and Le Moal 1997) (see Section 8.3).

A second reason why research on electrical brain-stimulation reward decreased after about 1980 is that it then became possible to study the pharmacological substrates of reward not only by investigating how pharmacological agents affect electrical brain-stimulation reward, which required very careful controls to show that the drugs did not affect rewarded behaviour

---

[18]Apostasis, from the Greek, meaning standing apart or away from; hence a meta-statement (literally an 'about' statement) or a comment. Different from the Latin p.s. (postscriptum translated as post script) which means written after.

just because of motor or arousal side effects (see Section 8.3), but also by investigating directly the self-administration of pharmacological agents, both systemically and even directly to the brain (e.g. Phillips, Mora and Rolls (1981)). The results of these investigations, described in Section 8.3, taken together with the increasing understanding of brain mechanisms involved in natural reward processing and learning (see Chapters 4–6), led directly to rapid advances in understanding the processing in the neural systems that provides the neural basis of the self-administration of drugs (see Section 8.3).

Brain-stimulation reward, though less investigated today, does nevertheless provide a way to present repeatedly for hours on end a reward that does not satiate. Indeed, the persistence of responding to obtain brain-stimulation reward was one of the startling facts that led to the clear exposition of how reward and satiety signals are very distinct in their sensory origin, and how motivational signals such as hunger and thirst actually modulate the reward value of sensory input produced, for example, by the taste of food (see Chapter 5). Studies with brain-stimulation reward emphasized the fact that (apart from some sensory-specific satiety), the delivery of reward per se does not produce satiety.

The discoveries with brain-stimulation reward also led to advances in understanding behaviour under low-drive conditions, including priming effects and rapid extinction, and this understanding is relevant to interpreting modern studies in animal welfare.

8 Pharmacology of emotion, reward, and addiction; the basal ganglia

8.1 Introduction

It is well established that pharmacological manipulations of the catecholamine transmitters in the brain (dopamine and noradrenaline) alter self-stimulation rate (see Rolls (1975) and Rolls (1974)). For example, amphetamine, which enhances the release of dopamine and noradrenaline from axon terminals at synapses, increases hypothalamic self-stimulation rate. Drugs that reduce catecholamine levels (e.g. α-methyl-p-tyrosine) or that block catecholamine receptors (e.g. the 'neuroleptic' or 'anti-psychotic' drugs chlorpromazine, haloperidol, and spiroperidol) reduce self-stimulation rates. These catecholamine systems have been teased apart, and it is now clear that noradrenaline is not involved in brain-stimulation reward (Section 8.2), but that dopamine is involved in brain-stimulation reward at some brain sites (Section 8.3.1).

This evidence is complemented by findings with self-administration of the psychomotor stimulant addictive drugs amphetamine and cocaine, which produce their reward by acting on the dopaminergic projection to the nucleus accumbens (see Section 8.4.6), itself implicated in the secondary reinforcing properties of stimuli.

Dopamine appears to modulate transmission that links reward systems in structures such as the amygdala and orbitofrontal cortex via their connections to the ventral striatum to behavioural response selection and execution systems. This leads to an examination in Section 8.4 of the functions of the basal ganglia in behavioural output.

Opiate reward systems are considered in Section 8.5, and after that the pharmacology of depression (Section 8.6) and anxiety (Section 8.7), and the implicated brain systems, are considered. Finally in this Chapter we give an overview of the different behavioural selection and output systems involved in reward, punishment, emotion, and motivation (Section 8.9).

In the remainder of Section 8.1, an introduction to some of the pharmacology of the dopamine systems in the brain is provided, because of its importance in understanding the pharmacology of reward.

The two catecholamines found in the brain with which we are concerned are dopamine (DA), and noradrenaline (NA) (which is also known by its Greek name norepinephrine). A schematic view of a dopaminergic synapse showing some of the ways in which pharmacological agents used to analyse self-stimulation affect its function is shown in Fig. 8.1 (see also Cooper, Bloom and Roth (2003)). Tyrosine is converted to dihydroxyphenylalanine (DOPA) in the presence of the enzyme tyrosine hydroxylase. The drug α-methyl-p-tyrosine blocks this step, and thus inhibits the synthesis of DA. DOPA is converted to DA. (In noradrenergic synapses, DA is converted to NA in the presence of the enzyme dopamine-β-hydroxylase. This latter step is inhibited by disulfiram, so that the administration of disulfiram prevents the synthesis of NA but not of DA.)

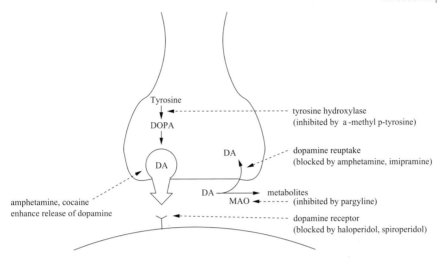

Fig. 8.1 Schematic diagram showing how pharmacological agents affect a dopaminergic synapse. The presynaptic terminal above is shown separated by the synaptic cleft from the postsynaptic cell below. DOPA, dihydroxyphenylalanine; DA, dopamine; MAO, monoamine oxidase.

Dopamine is normally released from the presynaptic membrane in vesicles when an action potential occurs. The released dopamine travels across the synaptic cleft to activate dopamine receptors (of which there are several types) in the postsynaptic membrane. The pharmacological agents haloperidol, spiroperidol, and pimozide block the DA receptors in the postsynaptic membrane. The drug amphetamine enhances the release of DA from the presynaptic membrane.

After dopamine is released into the synapse, and some of it activates the postsynaptic receptors, the remaining dopamine is removed from the synapse quickly by a number of mechanisms. One is reuptake into the presynaptic terminal. This process involves dopamine transporter (DAT), and is blocked by amphetamine and by cocaine, which both thus increase the concentration of dopamine in the synapse. Another mechanism for removing DA from the synapse is by monoamine oxidase (MAO), which destroys the DA. MAO is present in the synapse, and also in the presynaptic mechanism. MAO inhibitors (MAOI) thus also increase the concentration of DA in the synapse (and also of NA in noradrenergic synapses, and 5-hydroxytryptamine (5-HT, serotonin) in serotonergic synapses). Another mechanism is diffusion out of the synaptic cleft.

A number of comparisons between noradrenergic and dopaminergic mechanisms can usefully be remembered when interpreting the actions of pharmacological agents on self-stimulation. α-Methyl-p-tyrosine inhibits the synthesis of NA and DA, while disulfiram inhibits the synthesis of NA but not DA. Amphetamine releases both NA and DA. Phentolamine blocks NA-receptors but not DA-receptors. Spiroperidol and pimozide block DA-receptors and not NA-receptors. Chlorpromazine and haloperidol block both DA- and NA-receptors to some extent (as well as having other actions). The drug 6-hydroxydopamine can cause degeneration of both NA and DA nerve terminals. Some of the antidepressant drugs (such as the tricyclic reuptake inhibitors, and the MAOIs) facilitate both NA and DA mechanisms, but also considerably 5-HT mechanisms.

The catecholamines DA and NA (norepinephrine) are located in brain cells whose course

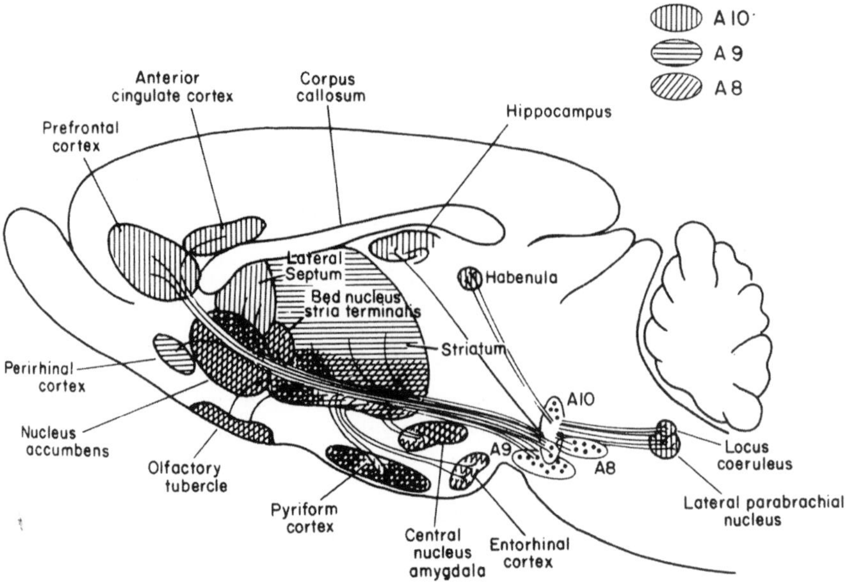

Fig. 8.2 Schematic diagram illustrating the distribution of the main central neuronal pathways containing dopamine. The stippled regions indicate the major nerve-terminal areas and their cell groups of origin. The cell groups in this figure are named according to the nomenclature of Dahlström and Fuxe (1965). The A9 cell group in the substantia nigra pars compacta is one of the main DA-containing cell groups, and gives rise mainly to the nigro-striatal dopamine pathway terminating in the striatum. The A10 cell group in the ventral tegmental area is the other main DA-containing cell groups, and gives rise mainly to the meso-limbic DA pathway which terminates in the nucleus accumbens and the olfactory tubercle (together known as the ventral striatum), and the meso-cortical DA pathway which terminates in prefrontal, anterior cingulate, and some other cortical areas. (After Cooper, Bloom and Roth 2002).

has been traced using histofluorescence techniques (Dahlström and Fuxe 1965, Ungerstedt 1971, Bjorklund and Lindvall 1986, Cooper, Bloom and Roth 2003). The mesostriatal dopamine projection (see Fig. 8.2) originates mainly (but not exclusively) from the A9 dopamine cell group in the substantia nigra, pars compacta, and projects to the (dorsal or neo-) striatum, in particular the caudate nucleus and putamen. The mesolimbic dopamine system originates mainly from the A10 cell group, and projects to the nucleus accumbens and olfactory tubercle, which together constitute the ventral striatum (see Fig. 8.2). In addition there is a mesocortical dopamine system projecting mainly from the A10 neurons to the frontal cortex, but especially in primates also to other cortical areas, including parts of the temporal cortex. However, these pathways are not completely separate from the mesostriatal projection system, in that the A10 neurons project into the ventromedial part of the striatum, and in that a dorsal and medial set of neurons in the A9 region with horizontally oriented dendrites project into the olfactory tubercle and amygdala (see Phillips and Fibiger (1989)).

The ascending noradrenergic pathways, at one time suggested to be involved in brain-stimulation reward, are as follows. Noradrenaline cell bodies in the locus coeruleus (cell group A6 according to the nomenclature of Dahlström and Fuxe (1965)) give rise to ascending pathways which form a dorsal bundle in the pons and midbrain, ascend through the medial forebrain bundle, and innervate the cortex and hippocampus (Fig. 8.3). The 'ventral NA

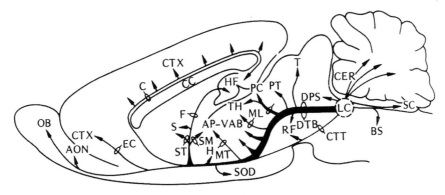

Fig. 8.3 Diagram of the projections of the locus coeruleus noradrenergic pathways viewed in the sagittal plane. Abbreviations: AON, anterior olfactory nucleus; AP-VAB, ansa peduncularis-ventral amygdaloid bundle system; BS, brainstem nuclei; C, cingulum; CC, corpus callosum; CER, cerebellum; CTT, central tegmental tract; CTX, cerebral neocortex; DPS, dorsal periventricular system; DTB, dorsal catecholamine bundle; EC, external capsule; F, fornix; H, hypothalamus; HF, hippocampal formation; LC, locus coeruleus; ML, medial lemniscus; MT, mammillothalamic tract; OB, olfactory bulb; PC, posterior commissure; PT, pretectal area; RF, reticular formation; S, septal area; SC, spinal cord; SM, stria medullaris; SOD, supraoptic decussations; ST, stria terminalis; T, tectum; TH, thalamus. (Reprinted with permission from Cooper, Bloom and Roth 2002).

pathway' arises from cell groups A1, A2, A5, and A7, and has terminals in the lower brain stem, midbrain, and hypothalamus and preoptic area.

8.2 The noradrenergic hypothesis

Stein (1967) and Stein (1969), noting the points made in the first paragraph of Section 8.1, and that many self-stimulation sites occurred along the course of the dorsal noradrenergic bundle from its origin in the locus coeruleus (cell group A6) through the hypothalamus towards its termination in the neocortex, formulated the noradrenergic theory of reward. According to this theory, activation of noradrenergic axons in this pathway by electrical stimulation at self-stimulation sites, and the consequent release of noradrenaline at its terminals, mediates brain-stimulation reward (Stein 1967, Stein 1969, Crow 1976).

Evidence against this theory comes from several sources. Rolls (1974) found that rats treated with disulfiram, which depletes the brain of noradrenaline, could self-stimulate if aroused, but were usually too drowsy to do so. Rolls, Kelly and Shaw (1974a) came to a similar conclusion when they found that the doses of disulfiram required to reduce hypothalamic self-stimulation rates produced a major attenuation of spontaneous locomotor activity. Interestingly, the dopamine receptor-blocking agents pimozide or spiroperidol (used following an earlier study by Wauquier and Niemegeers (1972)) produced a much greater attenuation of self-stimulation rate than of locomotor activity, suggesting that dopamine was more closely related to brain-stimulation reward at these sites than was noradrenaline. The finding of Clavier and Routtenberg (1976) and Clavier (1976) that lesions to the locus coeruleus did not attenuate self-stimulation along the course of the dorsal noradrenergic bundle also argues strongly against the noradrenergic theory of reward.

8.3 Dopamine and reward

8.3.1 Dopamine and electrical self-stimulation of the brain

There is better evidence that dopamine is involved in self-stimulation of some brain sites. Following the observation described above, that dopamine-receptor blockade with spiroperidol attenuated hypothalamic self-stimulation without producing an arousal deficit (Rolls, Kelly and Shaw 1974a), it was shown that spiroperidol attenuated self-stimulation at different sites in the rat (Rolls, Kelly and Shaw 1974a, Rolls, Rolls, Kelly, Shaw and Dale 1974b). It was also shown that spiroperidol attenuated self-stimulation even when the motor response required to obtain the stimulation was made simple in order to minimize the effect of motor impairment (Mora, Sanguinetti, Rolls and Shaw 1975). Spiroperidol also attenuates self-stimulation in the monkey (Mora, Rolls, Burton and Shaw 1976c). These findings were consistent with the observation that self-stimulation in the rat can be obtained in the ventral mesencephalon near the A10 dopamine-containing cell bodies (Crow, Spear and Arbuthnott 1972), and in the monkey from the nucleus accumbens (Rolls, Burton and Mora 1980c). However, strong supporting evidence is needed in view of the situation emphasized by Rolls and his colleagues that it is difficult to exclude the possibility that dopamine-receptor blockade interferes with self-stimulation by producing a motor impairment (see also Fibiger (1978)).

Evidence supporting a role for dopamine in brain-stimulation reward came from experiments with apomorphine, which directly stimulates dopamine receptors. It was found that apomorphine attenuates self-stimulation of the prefrontal cortex in the rat and of the comparable region in the monkey, the orbitofrontal cortex (Mora, Phillips, Koolhaas and Rolls 1976a). Both areas are rich in dopamine-containing terminals of the mesocortical (A10) dopamine system. An attenuation of self-stimulation by the dopamine-receptor stimulant apomorphine would be predicted in a system in which the release of dopamine influenced the reward produced by stimulation of the prefrontal cortex.

In these experiments, self-stimulation with electrodes in the caudate nucleus was not attenuated by the apomorphine, so that this self-stimulation could not depend on dopamine (even though dopamine is present in this region), and the attenuation of prefrontal self-stimulation produced by the apomorphine could not have been due to a general disruption of behaviour. In a further investigation of the role of dopamine in brain-stimulation reward in the prefrontal cortex, it was found that the administration of apomorphine intravenously decreases the firing rate of neurons in the medial prefrontal cortex of the rat (Mora, Sweeney, Rolls and Sanguinetti 1976d) (as does the local iontophoretic administration of dopamine (Bunney and Aghajanian 1976)), and that dopamine is released from this region during electrical stimulation of medial prefrontal reward sites (Mora and Myers 1977). This evidence thus suggests that the mesocortical dopamine system can influence brain-stimulation reward of the prefrontal cortex in the rat and the corresponding orbitofrontal cortex in the monkey, but dopamine may not be essential for self-stimulation of the prefrontal cortex, as lesions of the dopaminergic fibres which ascend to the prefrontal cortex may not abolish prefrontal cortex self-stimulation (Phillips and Fibiger 1978).

In studies with unilateral lesions of the dopamine pathways, it has been found that damage to the dopamine pathways attenuates brain-stimulation reward of the far lateral hypothalamus where the dopamine pathways project, but not in a more central part of the lateral hypothalamus, nor in the nucleus accumbens, and only partly in the medial prefrontal cortex (Fibiger et al. 1987, Phillips and Fibiger 1989). This again indicates that activation of dopamine pathways may be sufficient for brain-stimulation reward, but is not involved in brain-stimulation reward of all brain sites.

When electrodes are activating the dopaminergic A10 system, for example when the electrodes are in the ventral tegmental area, the system through which the reward is mediated appears to be via the dopamine terminals in the nucleus accumbens, in that injections of the dopamine receptor-blocking agent spiroperidol into the nucleus accumbens attenuated the tegmental self-stimulation (Mogenson, Takigawa, Robertson and Wu 1979). Thus, when dopamine is involved in brain-stimulation reward, the reward appears to be mediated by tapping into the nucleus accumbens system, a system which is involved in learned incentive effects on behaviour (see Sections 4.9.2, 7.5.4, and 8.4). The evidence described in Section 8.3.2 implicates this ventral striatal system also in the reward produced by systemic self-administration of the psychomotor stimulant drugs such as amphetamine and cocaine.

Thus there is reasonable evidence that dopamine is involved in brain-stimulation reward of some sites, for example of the ventral tegmental area where the A10 dopamine neuron cell bodies are located, but that dopamine is not involved in self-stimulation at all sites. Analyses of the pharmacology of brain-stimulation reward do need to show that reward, rather than performance, is affected by experimental variables. Effects on self-stimulation rate are difficult to interpret unless (as shown above) controls for side effects on performance are included. Also, as emphasized by Fibiger (1978), drug effects may depend on the initial rate of bar-pressing shown by the animal. But to equalize initial self-stimulation rates at different sites does not help, because although the self-stimulation rate at some sites may be low, stimulation at these sites may be preferred to stimulation at other sites (Valenstein 1964), and this could influence the effects of drugs. With rate measures, it is at least necessary to determine how the rate of bar-pressing is affected by the stimulation current intensity and to determine how this relation is affected by experimental variables. This led to the use in later studies (see Phillips and Fibiger (1989)) of graphs which show how the rate of self-stimulation is related to the current intensity (or the number of pulses of stimulation obtained with each response) (see example in Fig. 8.4). If this rate-intensity curve is moved to the left by a treatment, the implication is that the treatment has resulted in more reward for each lever press (because less current per press is needed). Conversely, if the curve moves to the right, this is interpreted as less reward per press, in that more current for each press is required to maintain responding at half its maximal rate. Other measures of reward are the time spent in the side of the box in which stimulation is given, and a runway in which reward can be measured independently of performance (Edmonds and Gallistel 1977, Phillips and Fibiger 1989, Stellar and Rice 1989).

Self-stimulation of sites in the ventral tegmental area (VTA, where there are cell bodies of the A10 dopamine neurons that project to the nucleus accumbens), increases the release of dopamine in the nucleus accumbens (Fiorino, Coury, Fibiger and Phillips 1993), and VTA self-stimulation (but not substantia nigra pars compacta self-stimulation) was abolished by dopamine depleting lesions at the hypothalamic level (Phillips, LePiane and Fibiger 1982). Consistently, blocking dopamine receptors in the nucleus accumbens with spiroperidol reduced self-stimulation of the ipsilateral (but not in an elegant control, of the contralateral) VTA (Mogenson et al. 1979). Moreover, dopamine-depleting lesions of the nucleus accumbens (with 6-hydroxydopamine) attenuate self-stimulation of the ventral tegmental area (Phillips and Fibiger 1989).

A conclusion from these studies is that dopamine neurons in the VTA can support self-stimulation behaviour, but that non-dopaminergic neurons can also support brain-stimulation

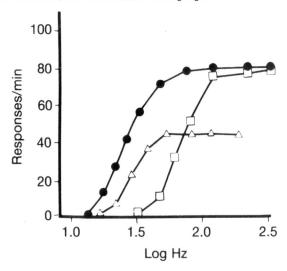

Fig. 8.4 Amphetamine can increase the reward value of brain-stimulation reward in regions such as the ventral tegmental area and posterior hypothalamus where the stimulation activates the dopamine system (see Koob 1992; A. Phillips and Fibiger 1989). Pimozide or spiroperidol, which block dopamine receptors, can reduce the reward value of brain-stimulation reward. This can be measured in graphs showing the rate of lever pressing (responses/min) vs the frequency (in Hz) of the brain stimulation pulses obtained for each lever press. Such a graph is shown with no drug as filled circles. After pimozide, the curve (open squares) moves to the right, interpreted as showing that more pulses of brain stimulation are needed with pimozide to produce the same amount of reward. If the curve is shifted down (open triangles), this indicates that the drug interferes with performance, e.g. the ability of the animal to work, and this can be produced by high doses of pimozide. Amphetamine has the effect of shifting the baseline curve to the left (not shown). This implies that each press produces more reward, because each train of electrical stimulation produced by a lever press releases more dopamine when amphetamine is present. After Stellar and Rice (1989).

reward even in forebrain areas such as the nucleus accumbens and medial prefrontal cortex to which the dopamine neurons project (Phillips and Fibiger 1989). The unsurprising implication of the latter conclusion is that in the regions in which dopamine fibres make synapses, electrical stimulation of the postsynaptic neurons can produce reward.

Amphetamine can increase the reward value of brain-stimulation reward in regions such as the ventral tegmental area and posterior hypothalamus where the stimulation activates the dopamine system (Phillips and Fibiger 1989, Koob 1992). The facilitation is measured in a rate of lever pressing vs current intensity curve, which shifts to the left when amphetamine or cocaine is present (see Fig. 8.4 which shows a rate of pressing vs current pulse frequency curve). This implies that each press produces more reward, because each train of electrical stimulation produced by a lever press releases more dopamine when amphetamine is present.

8.3.2 Self-administration of dopaminergic substances, and addiction

In this Section evidence is summarized that a major class of drug, the psychomotor stimulants such as amphetamine and cocaine, produce their reward by acting on a dopaminergic mechanism in the nucleus accumbens (Liebman and Cooper 1989, Phillips and Fibiger 1990, Koob 1992, Koob 1996, Koob and Le Moal 1997, Everitt 1997), which receives a dopaminergic input from the A10 cell group in the ventral tegmental area. These drugs are addictive, and under-standing their mode of action in the brain helps to clarify how these drugs produce their effects.

1. Amphetamine (which increases the release of dopamine and noradrenaline) is self-administered intravenously by humans, monkeys, rats, etc.

2. Amphetamine self-injection intravenously is blocked by dopamine receptor blockers such as pimozide and spiroperidol (Yokel and Wise 1975). The implication is that the psychomotor stimulants produce their reward by causing the release of dopamine which acts on dopamine receptors. The receptor blocker at first increases the rate at which the animal will work for the intravenous injection. The reason for this is that with each lever press for amphetamine, less reward is produced than without the receptor blockade, so the animal works more to obtain the same net amount of reward. This is typical of what happens with low rate operant response behaviour when the magnitude of the reward is reduced. The rate increase is a good control which shows that the dopamine receptor blockade at the doses used does not produce its reward-reducing effect by interfering with motor responses.

3. Apomorphine (which activates D2 dopamine receptors) is self-administered intravenously.

4. Intravenous self-administration of indirect DA agonists such as D-amphetamine and cocaine is much decreased by 6-OHDA lesions of the nucleus accumbens (see Lyness, Friedle and Moore (1980), Roberts, Koob, Klonoff and Fibiger (1980), Koob (1992), and Koob (1996)). In a complementary way, the self-administration of the psychomotor stimulants increases the release of dopamine in the nucleus accumbens (DiChiara, Acquas and Carboni 1992).

5. Rats will learn to self-administer very small quantities of amphetamine to the nucleus ac-cumbens. This effect is abolished by 6-OHDA lesions of the meso-limbic dopamine pathway.

6. It is however notable that the self-administration of opiates and alcohol occurs even when the meso-limbic dopamine system is lesioned (Koob 1992, Koob and Le Moal 1997).

All these points of evidence combine to show that the psychomotor stimulants (though not necessarily all other self-administered drugs) produce their effects by an action on the nucleus accumbens (Koob and Le Moal 1997, Weiss and Koob 2001). The neurons activated by cocaine in the nucleus accumbens are not in general the same as those activated by water reward (Deadwyler, Hayashizaki, Cheer and Hampson 2004), indicating that there is some continuing specificity of the type of reward encoded that is maintained from the input regions such as the orbitofrontal cortex and amygdala which project to the ventral striatum (see also Section 8.4.3.1). The addictive effects of the dopaminergic drugs implemented via the ventral striatum may be related to 'incentive salience' effects whereby 'wanting' or motivation for the drug-related stimuli is sensitized (Robinson and Berridge 2003, Berridge and Robinson 1998).

In work to understand the factors that influence addiction, Brebner, Childress and Roberts (2002) have found that baclofen, a $GABA_B$ receptor agonist, decreases the reinforcing value of cocaine in rats. (The reinforcement value of the drug is measured by the use of an exponentially increasing ratio schedule of lever presses for each self-injection of cocaine, with rats typically working for as many as approximately 200 lever presses for a single injection of cocaine, but not working beyond this in the ratio. With baclofen, the reinforcing value of the injection is less, in that the animals will work for perhaps only 25 lever presses for each injection. Lever pressing itself can still occur, and some other reinforcers are still effective, in that the baclofen-treated rats will still lever press for food.) The effective site of action of the baclofen appears to be to influence the dopamine-containing neurons, for injections of baclofen into the ventral tegmental area, where the dopamine-containing cell bodies of the A10 group that project to the nucleus accumbens and other areas are located, also disrupt the intravenous self-administration of dopamine, but nucleus accumbens injections of baclofen are much less effective. The possible relevance to binge eating and its possible similarity to addiction is being investigated in a rodent model of binge eating in which rats eat large amounts of fat, and baclofen can influence this (Corwin and Buda-Levin 2004).

8.3.3   Behaviours associated with the release of dopamine

The functional role of dopamine can be investigated by determining what factors influence its release. The release can be assayed by push–pull techniques in which a slow stream of fluid is transfused through a small cannula in the ventral striatum, and fluid is at the same time sucked out through another tube, allowing chemical assay of substances in the trans-fusate. Another method is to use in vivo chronoamperometry using stearate modified graphite paste electrodes to monitor changes in dopamine release (Phillips, Pfaus and Blaha 1991). Preparatory behaviours for feeding, including foraging for food, food hoarding, and perform-ing instrumental responses to obtain food, are more associated with dopamine release than is the consummatory behaviour of feeding itself (Phillips et al. 1991). Also, stimuli condi-tioned to cocaine delivery may release small amounts of dopamine in the nucleus accumbens (Phillips, Stuber, Heian, Wightman and Carelli 2003b).

In a complementary way, dopamine-depleting lesions of the nucleus accumbens disrupt appetitive behaviour produced by food-related stimuli at doses that do not affect eating itself. Similarly, Everitt, Cador and Robbins (1989) showed in rats that neurotoxic lesions of the basolateral amygdala reduced the rate of operant responding for a secondary sexual reward but not copulatory behaviour itself, and that infusions of amphetamine to the nucleus accumbens restored rates of working for the secondary sexual reward.

In another study, Pfaus, Damsma, Nomikos, Wenkstern, Blaha, Phillips and Fibiger (1990) showed that dopamine release in the nucleus accumbens increased in male rats during a 10 min period in which a male and female rat were placed in the same enclosure but were separated by a wire mesh screen, and increased further when the rats were allowed to copulate (see also Phillips et al. (1991)). The dopamine release decreased after the first ejaculation. If a new female was placed behind the mesh screen, the dopamine release increased again, and sexual behaviour was reinstated (Fiorino, Coury and Phillips 1997). (The reinstatement is known as the Coolidge effect.) In a whole series of studies, Robbins, Cador, Taylor and Everitt (1989) showed that conditioned reinforcers (for food) increase the release of dopamine in the nucleus accumbens, and that dopamine-depleting lesions of the nucleus accumbens attenuate the effect of conditioned (learned) incentives on behaviour.

Dopamine release in the nucleus accumbens shell is also increased in rats by the adminis-tration of most drugs of abuse, and conditioned stimuli associated with the delivery of drugs of abuse such as morphine also increase the release of dopamine in the nucleus accumbens shell (DiChiara 2002). In addition, foods can also increase the release of dopamine in the shell part of the nucleus accumbens, though this effect tends to habituate over repeated days of presentation (DiChiara 2002).

In an interesting rat model of binge eating, Colantuoni et al. (2002) have shown that access to sucrose for several hours each day can lead to binge-like consumption of the sucrose over a period of days. The binge-eating is associated with the release of dopamine. Moreover, the model brings binge eating close to an addictive process, at least in this model, in that after the binge-eating has become a habit, sucrose withdrawal decreases dopamine release in the accumbens, altered binding of dopamine to its receptors in the ventral striatum is produced, and signs of withdrawal from an addiction occur including teeth chattering. In withdrawal, the animals are also hypersensitive to the effects of amphetamine (Avena and Hoebel 2003a, Avena and Hoebel 2003b). An interesting question about this model is whether stressors that increase the release of dopamine such as placing the rats' feet into cold water, if repeated daily, would also cause similar effects. These effects might be similar not only at the pharmacological level, but also at the behavioural level. For example, would animals given such daily repeated stressors show a 'cross-addiction' to sucrose; or to amphetamine? Could this provide a model of the effects of repeated stress on binge eating? In any case, there are interesting implications for the understanding and treatment of binge-eating disorder and bulimia in humans.

The neural substrates for these reward effects of dopamine release in the nucleus accumbens and their relation to addiction will be considered later in the light of the evidence described in the next few Sections (see also Section 8.4.6).

The nucleus accumbens however may not be the only place in the primate brain where dopamine release can produce reward, for Phillips, Mora and Rolls (1981) showed that monkeys will learn to self-administer very small quantities of amphetamine to the orbitofrontal cortex, which receives a strong projection from the dopamine pathways. Further, Voellm, De Araujo, Cowen, Rolls, Kringelbach, Smith, Jezzard, Heal and Matthews (2004) showed that the administration of amphetamine to drug-naive (non-addicted) human subjects activates the medial prefrontal cortex. The (Pavlovian) conditioned cues that support addiction and may lead to relapse to addiction by Pavlovian-instrumental transfer (see Section 4.6.1.2 and Cardinal et al. (2002)) may operate in part via the orbitofrontal cortex, for Childress et al. (1999) have shown that cocaine-related cues shown visually in a video to addicts activate the orbitofrontal cortex, and also parts of the anterior cingulate and medial prefrontal cortex. Moreover, the orbitofrontal cortex activation in humans to these drug-conditioned cues can be decreased by baclofen, the GABA-B agonist described above (Childress et al. 1999). In rodents, cues associated by Pavlovian learning with drug administration also influence the prefrontal and cingulate cortices and related areas (Kelley and Berridge 2002, Kelley 2004b). Presumably dopaminergic substances produce reward in the orbitofrontal cortex by influencing the reward systems known to be present in this region. The reward signals processed in the orbitofrontal cortex include the sight, smell, and taste of food, pleasure produced by touch, the reward value of face expression, social reinforcers, and monetary reinforcers (see Chapters 4 and 5). The orbitofrontal cortex, and also the amygdala, are likely to be the main sources via which these reinforcers gain access to the nucleus accumbens, and may influence dopamine neuron firing.

Although the majority of the studies have focused on rewarded behaviour, there is also evidence that dopamine can be released by stimuli that are aversive. For example, Rada, Mark and Hoebel (1998) showed that dopamine was released in the nucleus accumbens when rats worked to escape from aversive hypothalamic stimulation (see also Hoebel (1997), and Leibowitz and Hoebel (1998)). Also, Gray, Young and Joseph (1997) describe evidence that

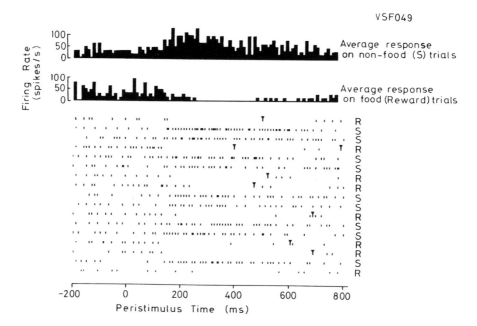

Fig. 8.8 Responses of a ventral striatal neuron in a visual discrimination task. The neuron reduced its firing rate to the S+ on food reward trials (R), and increased its firing rate to the S− on non-food trials (S) on which aversive saline was obtained if a lick was made. Rastergrams and peristimulus time histograms are shown. The inverted triangles show where lick responses were made on the food reward (R) trials. (After Rolls and Williams 1987a; and Williams, Rolls, Leonard and Stern 1993.)

is made, the taste of aversive saline will be obtained. Responses of an example of a neuron of this type are shown in Fig. 8.8. The neuron increased its firing rate to the visual stimulus that indicated that saline would be obtained if a lick was made (the S−), and decreased its firing rate to the visual stimulus that indicated that a response could be made to obtain a taste of glucose (the S+). The differential response latency of this neuron to the reward-related and to the saline-related visual stimulus was approximately 150 ms (see Fig. 8.8), and this value was typical. This neuron thus coded for the valence of the visual stimuli (i.e. whether the visual stimulus was associated with a reward vs a punisher).

Of the neurons that responded to visual stimuli that were rewarding, relatively few responded to all the rewarding stimuli used. That is, only few (1.8%) ventral striatal neurons responded both when food was shown and to the positive discriminative visual stimulus, the S+ (e.g. a triangle shown on a video monitor), in a visual discrimination task. Instead, the reward-related neuronal responses were typically more context or stimulus-dependent, responding for example to the sight of food but not to the S+ which signified food (4.3%), differentially to the S+ or S− but not to food (4.0%), or to food if shown in one context but not in another context. Some neurons were classified as having taste or olfactory responses to food (see Table 8.1; Williams, Rolls, Leonard and Stern (1993); Rolls and Williams (1987a)). Some other neurons (1.4%) responded to aversive stimuli. These neurons did not respond simply in relation to arousal, which was produced in control tests by inputs from different modalities, for example by touch of the leg. Thus, as shown in Table 8.1, 13.9% of primate ventral striatal neurons encoded the valence of visual stimuli (Rolls and Williams 1987a, Williams, Rolls, Leonard and Stern 1993). Neurons in the ventral striatum with activity related to the expectation of reward were also found by Schultz, Apicella, Scarnati and Ljungberg (1992).

Table 8.1 Types of neuronal response found in the macaque ventral striatum (after Williams, Rolls, Leonard and Stern 1993)

		No./1013	%
1	Visual, recognition-related		
	-novel	39	3.5
	-familiar	11	1.1
2	Visual, association with reinforcement		
	-aversive	14	1.4
	-food	44	4.3
	-food and S+	18/1004	1.8
	-food, context dependent	13	1.3
	-opposite to food/aversive	11	1.1
	-differential to S+ or S− only	44/1112	4.0
3	Visual		
	-general interest	51	5.0
	-non-specific	78/1112	7.0
	-face	17	1.7
4	Movement-related, conditional	50/1112	4.5
5	Somatosensory	76/1112	6.8
6	Cue related	177/1112	15.9
7	Responses to all arousing stimuli	9/1112	0.8
8	Task-related (non-discriminating)	17/1112	1.5
9	During feeding	52/1112	4.7
10	Peripheral visual and auditory stimuli	72/538	13.4
11	Unresponsive	608/1112	54.7

Another population of ventral striatal neurons responded to novel visual stimuli. An example is shown in Fig. 8.9.

Other ventral striatal neurons responded to faces; to other visual stimuli than discriminative stimuli and faces; in relation to somatosensory stimulation and movement; or to cues that signalled the start of a task (see Table 8.1) (Rolls and Williams 1987a, Williams, Rolls, Leonard and Stern 1993). The cue-related neurons in the ventral striatum were similar to those found in the head of the caudate nucleus (see Section 8.4.3.4), in that they responded to warning cues that signalled the start of a trial, and stopped responding to the cue if it no longer signalled the start of a trial (see example in Fig. 8.11). As shown in Table 8.1, 15.9% of ventral striatal neurons had cue-related responses. These (and other neurons shown in Table 8.1) can thus be described as encoding the salience of stimuli, and respond independently of the valence of the stimuli. Thus valence and salience are represented independently by different populations of neurons in the primate ventral striatum (see Table 8.1).

The neurons with responses to reinforcing or novel visual stimuli may reflect the inputs to the ventral striatum from the amygdala, orbitofrontal cortex, and hippocampus, and are consistent with the hypothesis that the ventral striatum provides a route for learned reinforcing and novel visual stimuli to influence behaviour. It was notable that although some neurons responded to visual stimuli associated with reward (see Table 8.1), 1.4% responded to visual stimuli associated with punishment, and 12% responded to arousing visual stimuli or non-specifically to visual stimuli (see Table 8.1). It was also notable that these neurons were

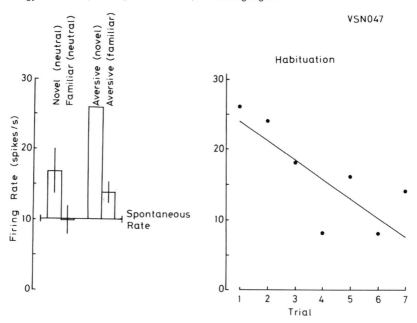

Fig. 8.9 Responses of a ventral striatal neuron to novel visual stimuli. On the right it is shown that the response to novel stimuli, an increase in firing rate to 25 spikes/s from the spontaneous rate of 10 spikes/s, habituated over repeated presentations of the stimulus. The lack of response shown in the left panel to the familiar stimulus was thus only achieved after habituation produced by 4–7 presentations of the stimulus. It is also shown that the neuron responded to aversive stimuli when they had not been seen for more than one day (Aversive (novel)), but did not respond to aversive visual stimuli (such as the sight of a syringe from which the monkey was fed saline, Aversive (familiar)), even though the latter produced arousal. (From Williams, Rolls, Leonard and Stern 1993.)

not restricted to the nucleus accumbens, but were found also in the adjacent ventral part of the head of the caudate nucleus (Rolls and Williams 1987a, Williams, Rolls, Leonard and Stern 1993, Rolls, Thorpe and Maddison 1983c), which also receives projections from both the amygdala (Amaral and Price 1984) and orbitofrontal cortex (Seleman and Goldman-Rakic 1985).

In human fMRI studies, activations have been described in the ventral striatum that reflect whether monetary rewards can be obtained, and indeed more activation is found for the larger rewards (Knutson, Adams, Fong and Hommer 2001). Interestingly, one of the strongest activations that is found in the ventral striatum is produced by temporal difference reward/punishment prediction errors in Pavlovian (i.e. classical conditioning) tasks (O'Doherty, Dayan, Friston, Critchley and Dolan 2003a, McClure, Berns and Montague 2003, Seymour, O'Doherty, Dayan, Koltzenburg, Jones, Dolan, Friston and Frackowiak 2004). For example, in a classical conditioning task, a first visual stimulus probabilistically predicted high vs low pain, and a second visual stimulus perfectly predicted whether the pain would be high or low on that trial. Activation of the ventral striatum and a part of the insula was related to the temporal difference error, which arose for example at the transition between the first and second visual stimulus if the first visual stimulus had predicted low pain, but the second informed the subject that the pain would be high (Seymour et al. 2004).

The ventral striatum activations may reflect the operation of a 'critic' in reinforcement learning, in that activations in it are related to temporal difference errors in Pavlovian conditions in which actions are not made (O'Doherty, Dayan, Schultz, Deichmann, Friston and Dolan 2004). In contrast, activation in the dorsal striatum may be closely related to temporal difference prediction errors used to correct an actor, as these activations occurred during an instrumental version of the task in which the subjects had to choose between two stimuli associated with a high probability or low probability of obtaining juice reward (O'Doherty et al. 2004). (The distinction between a 'critic' and an 'actor' in reinforcement learning is described in Appendix 1, Section A.5.3.)

Activations in the ventral striatum related to temporal difference reward/punishment prediction errors in a monetary reward *decision* task are exemplified in a study by Rolls, McCabe and Redoute (2007b). In this probabilistic monetary reward decision task, the subjects could choose either on the right to obtain a large reward with a value of 30 pence, or on the left to obtain a smaller reward with a value of 10 pence with a probability of 0.9. On the right, in different trial blocks, the probability of the large reward was 0.9 (making the expected value which approximates probability × reward value = 27 pence); or the probability was 0.33 making the expected value 10 pence; or the probability was 0.16 making the expected value 5 pence. (On the trials on which a reward was not obtained, 0 pence was the reward value.) (Expected utility approximates expected value = probability × reward value as described in Section 11.2.6). The participants learned in the blocks of 30 trials with the different expected values on the right whether to press on the right or the left to maximize their winnings. They took typically less than 10 trials to adjust to the unsignalled change in expected value every 30 trials, and analysis was performed for the last 20 trials of each block when the expected value had been learned.

The design of the task meant that sometimes the participants were expecting a low probability of a high reward of 30 pence, and unexpectedly obtained a high reward value of 30 pence. On these trials, the temporal difference prediction error from the expected value part of the trial to the reward value part of the trial when subjects were informed whether they would obtain the large reward was positive. On other trials when the expected value was high but probabilistically no reward was obtained, the temporal difference prediction error from the expected value part of the trial to the reward value part of the trial was negative. (Temporal difference (TD) errors are described in Appendix 1, Section A.5.3). It was found that the fMRI BOLD signal in the nucleus accumbens reflected this temporal difference error signal, calculated at the part of the trial when the reward prediction changed from the expected value for that trial block to the actual reward available on that trial, as shown in Fig. 8.10.

Further analyses showed that the activation in the ventral striatum was positively correlated with the reward actually obtained on that trial but not with the expected value. Thus the TD error correlation arose in the nucleus accumbens because at the time that the expected value period ended and the subject was informed about how much reward had been obtained on that trial, the BOLD signal changed to a higher value for large rewards, and to a lower value for low or no reward, from a value that was not a function of the expected value on that trial. A TD error correlation was also found in left cortical area 44 (Broca's area) (as shown in Fig. 8.10), but here the TD correlation arose because the activation became low when the subject was informed that no reward was obtained on a trial, and it appeared that the area was activated especially when the decision was difficult, between two approximately equal values of the expected value. In a part of the midbrain near the dopamine neurons at [14 −20 −16], there

TD error signal in the ventral striatum in a probabilistic monetary decision-making task

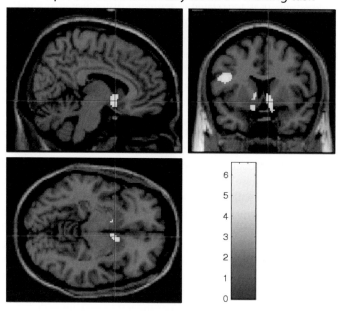

Fig. 8.10 Temporal Difference (TD) error signal in the ventral striatum in a probabilistic monetary decision-making task. The correlation between the TD error and the activation in the nucleus accumbens was significant in a group random effects analysis fully corrected at the cluster level with p<0.048 (voxel z=3.84) at MNI coordinates [8 8 –8]. (From Rolls, McCabe and Redoute, 2007.) (See colour plates section.)

was also a correlation with the TD error, but here this was related to a negative correlation between the BOLD signal in the expected value period of each trial and the expected value. (The TD error was thus positive for example whatever reward became available if it was a low expected value trial block, and the TD error was negative if it was a high expected value trial block.) This shows that TD error regressions with functional neuroimaging can arise for a number of different reasons. In this investigation, the reward value on a trial was correlated with the activation in parts of the orbitofrontal cortex, and the expected value was negatively correlated with activations in the anterior insula [–38 24 16], and these cortical areas may be the origins of some of the signals found on other brain areas.

These findings do exemplify the fact that activation of the ventral striatum does reflect the changing expectations of reward (see Appendix 1, Section A.5.3) during the trials of a task, and indeed this is what is illustrated at the neuronal level in Fig. 8.8, where the neuron altered its firing rate within 170 ms of the monkey being shown a visual stimulus that indicated whether reward or saline was available on that trial. Given that ventral striatal neurons of the type illustrated in Fig. 8.8 alter their activity when the visual stimulus is shown informing the macaque about whether reward is available on that trial, it is in fact not surprising that the fMRI correlation analyses do pick up signals during trials that can be interpreted as temporal difference error signals. Whether these fMRI correlations with a temporal difference error reflect more than the activity of neurons that respond as shown in Fig. 8.8 to the predicted reward value ($\hat{v}$ of Appendix 1, Section A.5.3) rather that the phasic temporal difference error (Δ) will be interesting to examine in the future.

8.4.3.2 Tail of the caudate nucleus, and posteroventral putamen

The projections from the inferior temporal cortex and the prestriate cortex to the striatum arrive mainly, although not exclusively, in the tail (and genu) of the caudate nucleus and in the posteroventral portions of the putamen (Kemp and Powell 1970, Saint-Cyr, Ungerleider and Desimone 1990b). The activity of single neurons was analysed in the tail of the caudate nucleus and adjoining part of the ventral putamen by Caan, Perrett and Rolls (1984). Of 195 neurons analysed in two macaque monkeys, 109 (56%) responded to visual stimuli, with latencies of 90–150 ms for the majority of the neurons. The neurons responded to a limited range of complex visual stimuli, and in some cases responded to simpler stimuli such as bars and edges. Typically (for 75% of neurons tested) the neurons habituated rapidly, within 1–8 exposures, to each visual stimulus, but remained responsive to other visual stimuli with a different pattern. This habituation was orientation-specific, in that the neurons responded to the same pattern shown at an orthogonal orientation. The habituation was also relatively short term, in that at least partial dishabituation to one stimulus could be produced by a single intervening presentation of a different visual stimulus. These neurons were relatively unresponsive in a visual discrimination task, having habituated to the discriminative stimuli that had been presented in the task on many previous trials. Consistent findings were obtained by Brown, Desimone and Mishkin (1995).

Given these responses, it may be suggested that these neurons are involved in short-term pattern-specific habituation to visual stimuli. This system would be distinguishable from other habituation systems (involved, for example, in habituation to spots of light) in that it is specialized for patterned visual stimuli that have been highly processed through visual cortical analysis mechanisms, as shown not only by the nature of the neuronal responses, but also by the fact that this system receives inputs from the inferior temporal visual cortex. It may also be suggested that this sensitivity to visual pattern change may have a role in alerting the monkey's attention to new stimuli. This suggestion is consistent with the changes in attention and orientation to stimuli produced by damage to the striatum.

In view of these neurophysiological findings, and the finding that in a visual discrimination task neurons that reflected the reinforcement contingencies of the stimuli were not found, Caan, Perrett and Rolls (1984) suggested that the tail of the caudate nucleus is not directly involved in the development and maintenance of reward or punishment associations to stimuli (and therefore is not closely involved in emotion-related processing), but may aid visual discrimination performance by its sensitivity to change in visual stimuli. Neurons in some other parts of the striatum may, however, be involved in connecting visual stimuli to appropriate motor responses. For example, in the putamen some neurons have early movement-related firing during the performance of a visual discrimination task (Rolls, Thorpe, Boytim, Szabo and Perrett 1984b); and some neurons in the head of the caudate nucleus respond to environmental cues that signal that reward may be obtained (Rolls, Thorpe and Maddison 1983c).

8.4.3.3 Postero-ventral putamen

Following these investigations on the caudal striatum which implicated it in visual functions related to a short-term habituation or memory process, a further study was performed to investigate the role of the posterior putamen in visual short-term memory tasks (Johnstone and Rolls 1990, Rolls and Johnstone 1992). Both the inferior temporal visual cortex and the prefrontal cortex project to the posterior ventral parts of the putamen (Goldman and Nauta 1977, Van Hoesen, Yeterian and Lavizzo-Mourey 1981) and these cortical areas are known to subserve a variety of complex functions, including functions related to memory. For example, cells in both areas respond in a variety of short-term memory tasks (Fuster 1973, Fuster 1996, Fuster and Jervey 1982, Baylis and Rolls 1987, Miyashita and Chang 1988).

Two main groups of neurons with memory-related activity were found in the postero-ventral putamen in a delayed match-to-sample (DMS) task. In the task, the monkey was shown a sample stimulus, and had to remember it during a 2–5 s delay period, after which if a matching stimulus was shown he could make one response, but if a non-matching stimulus was shown he had to make no response (Johnstone and Rolls 1990, Rolls and Johnstone 1992).

First, 11% of the 621 neurons studied responded to the test stimulus which followed the sample stimulus, but did not respond to the sample stimulus. Of these neurons, 43% responded only on non-match trials (test different from sample), 16% only on match trials (test same as the sample), and 41% to the test stimulus irrespective of whether it was the same or different from the sample. These neuronal responses were not related to the licking motor responses since (i) the neurons did not respond in other tasks in which a lick response was required (for example, in an auditory delayed match-to-sample task which was identical to the visual delayed match-to-sample task except that auditory short-term memory rather than visual short-term memory was required; in a serial recognition memory task; or in a visual discrimination task), and (ii) a periresponse time spike-density function indicated that the stimulus onset better predicted neuronal activity.

Second, 9.5% of the neurons responded in the delay period after the sample stimulus, during which the sample was being remembered. These neurons did not respond in the auditory version of the task, indicating that the responses were visual modality-specific (as were the responses of all other neurons in this part of the putamen with activity related to the delayed match-to-sample task). Given that the visual and auditory tasks were very similar apart from the modality of the input stimuli, this suggests that the activity of the neurons was not related to movements, or to rewards or punishers obtained in the tasks (and is thus not closely linked to emotion-related processing), but instead to modality-specific short-term memory-related processing.

In recordings made from pallidal neurons it was found that some responded in both visual and auditory versions of the task (Johnstone and Rolls 1990, Rolls and Johnstone 1992). Of 37 neurons responsive in the visual DMS task that were also tested in the auditory version, seven (19%) responded also in the auditory DMS task. The finding that some of the pallidal neurons active in the DMS task were not modality-specific, whereas only visual modality-specific DMS units were located in the postero-ventral part of the striatum, provides evidence that the pallidum may represent a further stage in information processing in which information from different parts of the striatum can converge.

8.4.3.4 Head of the caudate nucleus

The activity of 394 neurons in the head of the caudate nucleus and most anterior part of the putamen was analysed in three behaving rhesus monkeys (Rolls, Thorpe and Maddison 1983c). Of these neurons, 64.2% had responses related to environmental stimuli, movements, the performance of a visual discrimination task, or eating. However, only relatively small proportions of these neurons had responses that were unconditionally related to visual (9.6%), auditory (3.5%), or gustatory (0.5%) stimuli, or to movements (4.1%). Instead, the majority of the neurons had responses that occurred conditionally in relation to stimuli or movements, in that the responses occurred in only some test situations, *and were often dependent on the performance of a task by the monkeys.* Thus, it was found that in a visual discrimination task 14.5% of the neurons responded during a 0.5 s tone/light cue that signalled the start of each trial (cue-related neurons); 31.1% responded in the period in which the discriminative visual stimuli were shown, with 24.3% of these responding more either to the visual stimulus that predicted food reward or to that that predicted punishment (by a taste of saline) (reward prediction neurons); and 6.2% responded in relation to lick responses.

An example of a *cue-related* neuron in the head of the caudate nucleus that started re-sponding as soon as a tone/light-emitting diode (LED) cue was presented indicating that a trial was about to start is shown in Fig. 8.11. At time 0 a discriminative visual stimulus was shown, which indicated if for example it was a triangle that reward could be obtained, or if it was a square that saline would be obtained if a lick was made. The reward trials (R) on which a lick could be made to obtain fruit juice, and saline (S) trials on which a lick should not be made otherwise a drop of aversive saline was obtained, each occurred with probability 0.5. This cue-related neuron stopped responding soon after the visual stimulus appeared, and did not discriminate between reward (R) and punishment (S) trials. It was thus a cue neuron and not a reward-predicting neuron. It could be described as encoding *salience* but not valence. Further evidence that the neuron was not reward or punishment related is that it did not respond on trials on which a food reward was shown (F), or an aversive visual stimulus was shown (A).

If the lick tube was moved away from the lips by a few mm so that juice reward could not be obtained (but the tone/LED still sounded, and was followed by a discriminative visual stimulus), the neuron stopped responding to the tone/LED cue, providing evidence that it was only when the tone/LED cue predicted the start of a trial in the visual discrimination task that the head of caudate neuron responded to the cue. This is shown by the middle set of trials in Fig. 8.11. Approximately half of the cue-related neurons tested showed this learning whereby they only responded to a warning cue normally used to start a trial if it actually did signal the start a trial. It typically took just a few trials for this trial predicting effect of a tone/LED cue to be learned and unlearned by these neurons.

Most of these cue-related neurons learned to respond to whichever cue, either a 500 Hz tone, or a light-emitting diode, signalled the start of a trial (see example in Fig. 8.12).

An example of a *reward-predicting* neuron in the head of the caudate nucleus that started responding as soon as a cue was available that a trial was about to start, and which contin-ued firing after a visual stimulus was shown which indicated that a lick response could be made to obtain juice reward (R), but which stopped firing after a visual stimulus was shown that indicated that if a lick response was made, aversive saline (S) would be obtained, is shown in Fig. 8.13. The reward (R) and saline (S) trials each occurred with probability 0.5. This type of neuron, common in the head of the primate caudate nucleus, thus increased its firing as soon as the probability of reward increased at the start of a trial to 0.5, learned to respond to the first cue that signalled the start of a trial, and stopped responding as soon as the probability of reward decreased to 0 on punishment (S) trials. These neurons typi-cally did not respond in relation to the cue stimuli, to the visual stimuli, or to movements, when these occurred independently of the task or performance of the task was prevented, for example by withdrawing the lick tube from which fruit juice could be obtained (Rolls, Thorpe and Maddison 1983c) (as illustrated for a cue-related neuron in Fig. 8.11). That is, the responses of these neurons reflected whether reward would be obtained, and more generally, reflect how much reward will be obtained (Cromwell and Schultz 2003). Similar

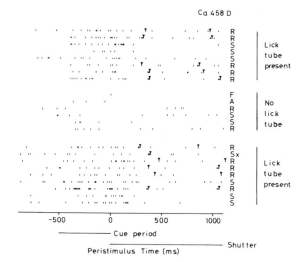

Fig. 8.11 Responses of a cue-related neuron in the head of the caudate nucleus in a Go/NoGo visual discrimination task in which the visual stimulus was presented at time 0. Each trial is a single row of the rastergram, each action potential is represented by a single dot, and a lick made to obtain fruit juice is represented by an inverted triangle. R, Reward trials on which fruit juice was obtained. S, Salt trials on which if a lick was made, a small drop of saline was obtained. Tone and light emitting diode cues were provided starting 500 ms before the visual stimulus was shown. Top set of trials: normal performance of the task with the lick tube close to the mouth. Middle set of trials: the lick tube was removed out of reach, but the tone/LED cue, and discriminative visual stimuli, were still provided. Bottom set of trials: normal performance of the task with the lick tube close to the mouth. F, food reward was shown. A, an aversive visual stimulus was shown. (After Rolls, Thorpe and Maddison, 1983.)

neurons in the head of the caudate nucleus responded to punishment-predicting stimuli, and indeed approximately as many neurons responded to the saline punishment-associated visual stimulus in the Go/NoGo visual discrimination task as to the juice reward-predicting stimulus (Rolls, Thorpe and Maddison 1983c, Rolls, Thorpe, Maddison, Roper-Hall, Puerto and Perrett 1979b, Rolls 1984b). Thus some neurons in the head of the caudate nucleus encode the *valence* of visual stimuli. Consistently, Watanabe, Lauwereyns and Hikosaka (2003) have found that one population of neurons in the primate caudate nucleus responds to rewarded eye movements, and a separate population to unrewarded eye movements.

Similar types of response were found when the neurons were tested outside the visual discrimination task, during feeding. Of the neurons tested during feeding, 25.8% responded when the food was seen by the monkey, 6.2% when he tasted it, and 22.4% during a cue given by the experimenter that a food or non-food object was about to be presented. Further evidence on the nature of these neuronal responses was that many of the neurons with cue-related responses only responded to the tone/light cue stimuli when they were cues for the performance of the task or the presentation of food as described above, and some responded to the different cues used in the task (tone/LED) and feeding test (an arm movement made by the experimenter to reach behind a screen to obtain a food or non-food object) situations (Rolls, Thorpe and Maddison 1983c).

The finding that such neurons may respond to environmental stimuli only when they are significant in predicting for example the onset of a trial (a cue neuron), or the delivery of

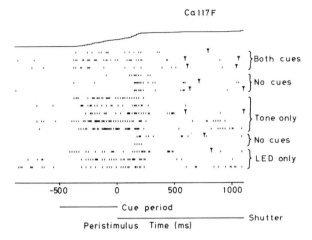

Ca 117F

Both cues

No cues

Tone only

No cues

LED only

-500 0 500 1000

Cue period

Shutter

Peristimulus   Time (ms)

Fig. 8.12 Responses of a cue-related neuron in the head of the caudate nucleus in a Go/NoGo visual discrimination task in which the visual stimulus was presented at time 0, when a mechanical shutter opened to reveal the discriminative stimulus. Each trial is a single row of the rastergram, each action potential is represented by a single dot, and a lick made to obtain fruit juice on Reward trials only is represented by an inverted triangle. Tone and/or light emitting diode (LED) cues were provided starting 500 ms before the visual stimulus was shown. If no 500 ms warning cue was given for the start of a trial, the neuron responded to the first indication that a trial was beginning, the sound of the shutter opening at time 0. The neuron did not predict whether reward would or would not be obtained, in that there was no differential neuronal response on Reward trials (on which licks were made), compared to non-reward trials (on which licks were correctly not made). The line at the top shows the cusum (cumulative sum) statistic. (After Rolls, Thorpe and Maddison, 1983.)

reward (a reward-predicting neuron) (Rolls, Thorpe, Maddison, Roper-Hall, Puerto and Perrett 1979b, Rolls, Thorpe and Maddison 1983c), was confirmed by Evarts and his colleagues. They showed that some neurons in the putamen only responded to the click of a solenoid when it indicated that a fruit juice reward could be obtained (Evarts and Wise 1984). The findings have also been confirmed by Tremblay and Schultz (1998) (see also Schultz, Tremblay and Hollerman (2003)), who reported that macaque caudate neurons come to respond during learning to cues related to the preparation of movement or expectation of reward, and do not respond to cues that do not predict such events.

We have found that this decoding of the significance of environmental events that are signals for the preparation for or initiation of a behavioural response is represented in the firing of a population of neurons in the dorsolateral prefrontal cortex, which projects into the head of the caudate nucleus (E. T. Rolls and G. C. Baylis, unpublished observations 1984). These neurons only respond to the tone cue if it signals the start of a trial of the visual discrimination task, just as do the corresponding population of neurons in the head of the caudate nucleus. The indication that the decoding of significance is performed by the prefrontal cortex, and that the striatum receives only the results of the cortical computation, is considered below and elsewhere (Rolls and Williams 1987b).

These findings indicate that the head of the caudate nucleus and most anterior part of the putamen contain populations of neurons that respond to predictive sensory cues that enable preparation for the performance of tasks such as feeding and tasks in which movements must be initiated, and others that respond during the performance of such tasks in relation

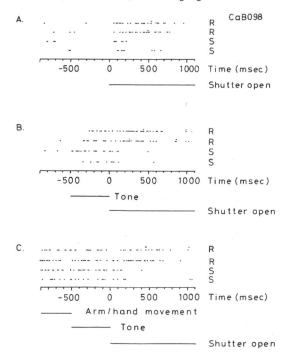

Fig. 8.13 Responses of a reward-predicting neuron in the head of the caudate nucleus in a Go/NoGo visual discrimination task in which the visual stimulus was presented at time 0. Each trial is a single row of the rastergram, each action potential is represented by a single dot, and a lick made to obtain fruit juice is represented by a vertical pair of dots. R, Reward trials on which fruit juice was obtained. S, Salt trials on which if a lick was made, a small drop of saline was obtained. A. The neuron started to respond approximately 80 ms after the start of the trial when a shutter opened to reveal the discriminative stimulus, continued to respond on reward trials until after the fruit juice was obtained, and stopped responding at approximately 160 ms on trials on which the punisher-related stimulus (S) was shown. B. The neuron started responding soon after a cue tone sounded indicating the start of a trial. C. The neuron started responding at the earliest indication that the trial would start, an arm movement made by the macaque to press a button to start the trial. (After Rolls, Thorpe and Maddison, 1983.)

to sensory cue that predict reward, and that the majority of these neurons have no uncondi-tional sensory or motor responses. It has therefore been suggested (Rolls, Thorpe, Maddison, Roper-Hall, Puerto and Perrett 1979b, Rolls, Thorpe and Maddison 1983c) that the anterior neostriatum contains neurons that are important for the utilization of environmental cues for the preparation for behavioural responses, and for particular behavioural responses made in particular situations to particular environmental stimuli, that is in stimulus–motor response habit formation. Different neurons in the cue-related group often respond to different sub-sets of environmentally significant events, and thus convey some information that would be useful in switching behaviour, in preparing to make responses, and in connecting inputs to particular responses (Rolls, Thorpe, Maddison, Roper-Hall, Puerto and Perrett 1979b, Rolls, Thorpe and Maddison 1983c, Rolls 1984b). Striatal neurons with similar types of response have also been recorded by Wolfram Schultz and colleagues (Schultz, Apicella, Romo and Scarnati 1995a, Tremblay and Schultz 1998, Cromwell and Schultz 2003, Schultz et al. 2003).

Striatal tonically active interneurons (TANs) which have high spontaneous firing rates and respond by decreasing their firing rates may respond to similar cue-predicting and reward-predicting events (Graybiel and Kimura 1995), presumably by receiving inhibitory inputs from the principal striatal neurons described above, the medium spiny neurons.

In human fMRI studies, activations have been described in the striatum that reflect whether monetary rewards can be obtained (Delgado, Nystrom, Fissell, Noll and Fiez 2000, Knutson et al. 2001). They presumably reflect the activity of the reward-predicting neurons (Rolls, Thorpe, Maddison, Roper-Hall, Puerto and Perrett 1979b, Rolls, Thorpe and Maddison 1983c, Rolls 1984b). Activations to monetary reward only if it is being worked for instrumentally (Zink et al. 2004) may reflect the type of task dependence illustrated for a cue-related neuron in Fig. 8.11. Human striatal fMRI activations to non-rewarding but salient stimuli (Zink et al. 2003) may reflect the types of trial-predicting (i.e. cue-related) neurons shown in Figs. 8.11 and 8.12 but not reward-predicting neurons of the type shown in Fig. 8.13.

One would expect human striatal activations also to be demonstrable to punishment-predicting stimuli, given that approximately half of the reward/punishment-predicting neurons respond to punishment-predicting stimuli (Rolls, Thorpe, Maddison, Roper-Hall, Puerto and Perrett 1979b, Rolls, Thorpe and Maddison 1983c, Rolls 1984b), and there is some human fMRI evidence for this (Seymour et al. 2004). It is a difficulty for the dopamine reward prediction error hypothesis (Schultz et al. 1995b, Schultz, Dayan and Montague 1997, Waelti et al. 2001, Schultz 2004) that it cannot account for the formation of striatal neurons that fire to predict punishment. [In particular, if dopamine neurons decrease their firing rate if an expected reward is not received or a punishment is received (Mirenowicz and Schultz 1996, Waelti, Dickinson and Schultz 2001, Tobler, Dickinson and Schultz 2003), then this would not promote learning in the striatum whereby striatal neurons might respond more to the stimulus (e.g. a discriminative stimulus in a visual discrimination task) that predicted punishment.] However, such reward and punisher predicting information is reflected in the firing of orbitofrontal cortex neurons, some of which predict reward, and others of which predict punishment (see Section 4.5), and it is presumably by this orbitofrontal cortex route that punishment-predicting neurons in the head of the caudate nucleus receive this information (rather than being reinforced into this type of firing by a dopamine reward error prediction signal).

It is very interesting that the type of neuron shown in Fig. 8.13 has certain similarities to the midbrain dopamine neurons described by Schultz and colleagues (Schultz et al. 1995b, Mirenowicz and Schultz 1996, Waelti et al. 2001), except that the dopamine neurons respond to the transitions in reward probabilities, rather than the reward probabilities themselves which is what appears to be encoded by the type of head of caudate neuron shown in Fig. 8.13. Thus an alternative to the hypothesis that the dopamine neurons provide a reward-prediction error teaching signal (see Section 8.3.4) is that the firing of the dopamine neurons may reflect feedback connections from these striatal regions as well as from the hypothalamus in which similar neurons are found (see Sections 4.9.4, 4.9.5, and 5.4.1.2) to the dopamine neurons in the substantia nigra, pars compacta, and ventral tegmental area. These feedback connections would then influence the dopamine neurons for short periods primarily when the firing of the striatal neurons changed, implemented by a high-pass filtering effect. This would leave much more open what the functions of the dopamine neurons are (see Sections 8.3.4 and 8.4.7), in that a simple feedback effect might be being implemented (from striatum to the dopamine neurons and back), perhaps to dynamically reset thresholds or gains in the striatum.

8.4.3.5 Anterior putamen

It is clear that the activity of many neurons in the putamen is related to movements (Anderson 1978, Crutcher and DeLong 1984a, Crutcher and DeLong 1984b, DeLong et al. 1984). There is a somatotopic organization of neurons in the putamen, with separate areas containing neurons responding to arm, leg, or orofacial movements. Some of these neurons respond only to active movements, and others to active and to passive movements. Some of these neurons respond to somatosensory stimulation, with multiple clusters of neurons responding, for example, to the movement of each joint. Some neurons in the putamen have been shown in experiments in which the arm has been given assisting and opposing loads to respond in relation to the direction of an intended movement, rather than in relation to the muscle forces required to execute the movement (Crutcher and DeLong 1984b). Also, the firing rate of neurons in the putamen tends to be linearly related to the amplitude of movements (Crutcher and DeLong 1984b), and this is of potential clinical relevance, since patients with basal ganglia disease frequently have difficulty in controlling the amplitude of their limb movements.

In order to obtain further evidence on specialization of function within the striatum, the activity of neurons in the putamen has been compared with the activity of neurons recorded in different parts of the striatum in the same tasks (Rolls, Thorpe, Boytim, Szabo and Perrett 1984b). Of 234 neurons recorded in the putamen of two macaque monkeys during the performance of a visual discrimination task and the other tests in which other striatal neurons have been shown to respond (Rolls, Thorpe and Maddison 1983c, Caan, Perrett and Rolls 1984), 68 (29%) had activity that was phasically related to movements (Rolls, Thorpe, Boytim, Szabo and Perrett 1984b). Many of these responded in relation to mouth movements such as licking. Similar neurons were found in the substantia nigra, pars reticulata, to which the putamen projects (Mora, Mogenson and Rolls 1977). The neurons did not have activity related to taste, in that they responded, for example, during tongue protrusion made to a food or non-food object. Some of these neurons responded in relation to the licking mouth movements made in the visual discrimination task, and always also responded when mouth movements were made during clinical testing when a food or non-food object was brought close to the mouth. Their responses were thus unconditionally related to movements, in that they responded in whichever testing situation was used, and were therefore different from the responses of neurons in the head of the caudate nucleus (Rolls, Thorpe and Maddison 1983c).

Of the 68 neurons in the putamen with movement-related activity in these tests, 61 had activity related to mouth movements, and seven had activity related to movements of the body. Of the remaining neurons, 24 (10%) had activity that was task-related in that some change of firing rate associated with the presentation of the tone cue or the opening of the shutter occurred on each trial (Rolls, Thorpe, Boytim, Szabo and Perrett 1984b), four had auditory responses, one responded to environmental stimuli (Rolls, Thorpe and Maddison 1983c), and 137 were not responsive in these test situations.

These findings (Rolls, Thorpe, Boytim, Szabo and Perrett 1984b) provide further evidence that differences between neuronal activity in different regions of the striatum are found even in the same testing situations, and also that the inputs that activate these neurons are derived functionally from the cortex which projects into a particular region of the striatum (in this case sensori-motor cortex, areas 3, 1, 2, 4, and 6).

8.4.4   What computations are performed by the basal ganglia?

The neurophysiological investigations described in Section 8.4.3 indicate that reinforcement-related signals do affect neuronal activity in some parts of the striatum, particularly in the ventral striatum. This finding suggests that pharmacological agents such as dopaminergic drugs that produce reward by acting on the ventral striatum may do so because they are tapping into a system normally involved in providing a route to behavioural output for signals carrying information about learned incentives. Some questions arise. Does the ventral striatum process the inputs in any way before passing them on? Can the ventral striatum be considered as one part of a larger computational system that includes all parts of the basal ganglia, and that operates as a single system with inputs from all parts of the cerebral cortex, allowing selection by competition between all the inputs as well as convergence between them to produce a single behavioural output stream? How do the outputs of the basal ganglia lead to or influence action?

One way to obtain evidence on the information processing being performed by the striatum is to compare neuronal activity in the striatum with that in its corresponding input and output structures. For example, the taste and visual information necessary for the computation that a visual stimulus is no longer associated with taste reward is represented by the activity of different neurons in the orbitofrontal cortex, and the putative result of such a computation, namely neurons that respond in this non-reward situation, are also found in the orbitofrontal cortex (Thorpe, Rolls and Maddison 1983, Rolls 1999a, Rolls 2000e, Rolls 2004b). However, such neurons that represent the necessary sensory information for this computation, and neurons that respond to the non-reward, were not found in the head of the caudate nucleus or the ventral striatum (Rolls, Thorpe and Maddison 1983c, Williams, Rolls, Leonard and Stern 1993). Instead, in the head of the caudate nucleus, neurons in the same test situation responded in relation to whether the monkey had to make a response on a particular trial, that is many of them responded more on Go than on No-Go trials. This could reflect the output of a cognitive computation performed by the orbitofrontal cortex, indicating whether on the basis of the available sensory information, the current trial should be a Go trial, or a No-Go trial because a visual stimulus previously associated with punishment had been shown.

Similarly, neurons were not found in the ventral striatum that are tuned to all the visual reward, taste reward, olfactory reward, and visual non-reward functions about which macaque orbitofrontal cortex neurons carry information (see Chapter 4). Instead the ventral striatal neurons were usually less easy to classify in these sensory ways, and were especially engaged when tasks were being performed. For example, many of the ventral striatal neurons that respond to visual inputs do so preferentially on the basis of whether the stimuli are recognized, or are associated with reinforcement (Williams, Rolls, Leonard and Stern 1993). Much of the sensory and memory-related processing required to determine whether a stimulus is a face, is recognized, or is associated with reinforcement has been performed in and is evident in neuronal responses in structures such as the amygdala (Leonard, Rolls, Wilson and Baylis 1985, Rolls 2000d), orbitofrontal cortex (Thorpe, Rolls and Maddison 1983, Rolls 2000e, Rolls 2004b) and hippocampal system (Rolls and Treves 1998, Rolls 1999c, Rolls and Stringer 2005, Rolls, Franco and Stringer 2005b, Rolls, Xiang and Franco 2005c, Rolls and Xiang 2006).

Similar comparisons can be made for the head and tail of the caudate nucleus, and the posterior putamen (Rolls and Johnstone 1992, Rolls and Treves 1998).

In these four parts of the striatum in which a comparison can be made of processing in the striatum with that in the cortical area that projects to that part of the striatum, it thus appears that the full information represented in the cortex does not reach the striatum, but that rather the striatum receives the output of the computation being performed by a cortical area, and could use this to initiate, switch, or alter behaviour.

The hypothesis arises from these findings that some parts of the striatum, particularly the caudate nucleus, ventral striatum, and posterior putamen, receive the output of these memory-related and cognitive computations, but do not themselves perform them. Instead, on receiving the cortical and limbic outputs, the striatum may be involved in switching behaviour as appropriate as determined by the different, sometimes conflicting, information received from these cortical and limbic areas. On this view, the striatum would be particularly involved in the selection of behavioural responses, and in producing one coherent stream of behavioural output, with the possibility to switch if a higher priority input was received. This process may be achieved by a laterally spreading competitive interaction between striatal or pallidal neurons, which might be implemented by the direct inhibitory connections between nearby neurons in the striatum and globus pallidus. In addition, the inhibitory interneurons within the striatum, the dendrites of which in the striatum may cross the boundary between the matrix and striosomes, may play a part in this interaction between striatal processing streams (Groves 1983, Graybiel and Kimura 1995, Groves, Garcia-Munoz, Linder, Manley, Martone and Young 1995).

Dopamine could play an important role in setting the sensitivity of this response selection function, as suggested by direct iontophoresis of dopamine on to single striatal neurons, which produces a similar decrease in the response of the neuron and in its spontaneous activity in the behaving macaque (Rolls, Thorpe, Boytim, Szabo and Perrett 1984b, Rolls and Williams 1987b).

In addition to this response selection function by competition, the basal ganglia may, by the convergence discussed, enable signals originating from non-motor parts of the cerebral cortex to be mapped into motor signals to produce behavioural output. The ways in which these computations might be performed are considered next.

8.4.5 How do the basal ganglia perform their computations?

On the hypothesis just raised, different regions of the striatum, or at least the outputs of such regions, would need to interact. Is there within the striatum the possibility for different regions to interact, and is the partial functional segregation seen within the striatum maintained in processing beyond the striatum? For example, is the segregation maintained throughout the globus pallidus and thalamus with projections to different premotor and even prefrontal regions reached by different regions of the striatum, or is there convergence or the possibility for interaction at some stage during this post-striatal processing?

Given the anatomy of the basal ganglia, interactions between signals reaching the basal ganglia could happen in a number of different ways. One would be for each part of the striatum to receive at least some input from a number of different cortical regions. As discussed above, there is evidence for patches of input from different sources to be brought adjacent to each other in the striatum (Van Hoesen et al. 1981, Seleman and Goldman-Rakic 1985, Graybiel and Kimura 1995). For example, in the caudate nucleus, different regions of association cortex project to adjacent longitudinal strips (Seleman and Goldman-Rakic 1985). Now, the dendrites of striatal neurons have the shape of large plates which lie at right angles to the incoming cortico-striatal fibres (Percheron, Yelnik and François 1984, Percheron, Yelnik and

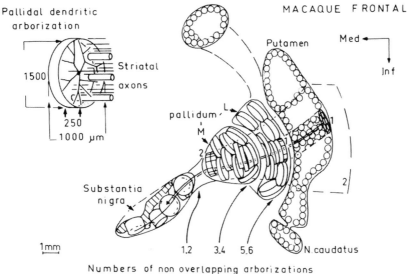

Pallidal dendritic arborization

1500

250

1000 μm

Striatal axons

MACAQUE FRONTAL

Putamen

Med

Inf

pallidum

L

M

2

2

Substantia nigra

1mm

1.2 3.4 5.6

N.caudatus

Numbers of non overlapping arborizations

Fig. 8.14 Semi-schematic spatial diagram of the striato-pallido-nigral system (see text). The numbers represent the numbers of non-overlapping arborizations of dendrites in the plane shown. L, lateral or external segment of the globus pallidus; M, medial or internal segment of the globus pallidus. The inserted diagram in the upper left shows the geometry of the dendrites of a typical pallidal neuron, and how the flat dendritic arborization is pierced at right angles by the striatal axons, which make occasional synapses en passage. (Reprinted with permission from Percheron, Yelnik and François 1984b.)

François 1984b, Percheron, Yelnik, François, Fenelon and Talbi 1994) (see Figs. 8.14 and 8.15). Thus one way in which interaction may start in the basal ganglia is by virtue of the same striatal neuron receiving inputs on its dendrites from more than just a limited area of the cerebral cortex. This convergence may provide a first level of integration over limited sets of cortico-striatal fibres. The large number of cortical inputs received by each striatal neuron, in the order of 10,000 (Wilson 1995), is consistent with the hypothesis that convergence of inputs carrying different signals is an important aspect of the function of the basal ganglia. The computation that could be performed by this architecture is discussed below for the inputs to the globus pallidus, where the connectivity pattern is comparable.

8.4.5.1 Interaction between neurons and selection of output

The regional segregation of neuronal response types in the striatum described above is consistent with mainly local integration over limited, adjacent sets of cortico-striatal inputs, as suggested by this anatomy. Short-range integration or interactions within the striatum may also be produced by the short length (for example 0.5 mm) of the intra-striatal axons of striatal neurons. These could produce a more widespread influence if the effect of a strong input to one part of the striatum spread like a lateral competition signal (cf. Groves (1983); Groves et al. (1995)). Such a mechanism could contribute to behavioural response selection in the face of different competing input signals to the striatum. The lateral inhibition could operate, for example, between the striatal principal (that is medium spiny) neurons by direct connections (they receive excitatory connections from the cortex, respond by increasing their firing rates,

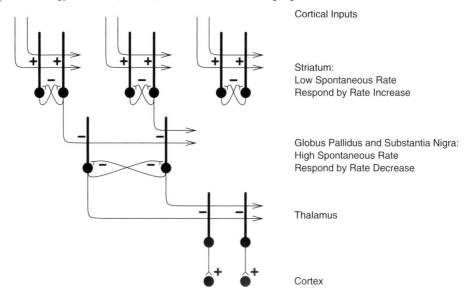

Fig. 8.15 Simple hypothesis of basal ganglia network architecture. A key aspect is that in both the striatum, and in the globus pallidus and substantia nigra pars reticulata, there are direct inhibitory connections (−) between the principal neurons, as shown. These synapses use GABA as a transmitter. Excitatory inputs to the striatum are shown as +. (From Rolls and Treves 1998, and Rolls 1999a.)

and could inhibit each other by their local axonal arborizations, which spread in an area as large as their dendritic trees, and which utilize GABA as their inhibitory transmitter). Further lateral inhibition could operate in the pallidum and substantia nigra (see Fig. 8.15). Here again there are local axon collaterals, as widespread as the very large pallidal and nigral dendritic fields. The lateral competition could again operate by direct connections between the neurons.

[Note that pallidal and nigral cells have high spontaneous firing rates (often 25–50 spikes/s), and respond (to their inhibitory striatal inputs) by reducing their firing rates below this high spontaneous rate. Such a decrease in the firing rate of one neuron would release inhibition on nearby neurons, causing them to increase their firing rates, equivalent to responding less. It is very interesting that direct inhibitory connections between the neurons can implement selection, even though at the striatal level the neurons have low spontaneous firing rates and respond by increasing their firing rates, whereas in the globus pallidus and substantia nigra pars reticulata the neurons have a high spontaneous firing rate, and respond by decreasing their firing rate.]

A selection function of this type between processing streams in the basal ganglia, even without any convergence anatomically between the processing streams implemented by feed-forward inputs, might provide an important computational raison d'être for the basal ganglia. The direct inhibitory local connectivity between the principal neurons within the striatum and globus pallidus would seem to provide a simple, and perhaps evolutionarily old, way in which to implement competition between neurons and processing streams. This might even be a primitive design principle that characterizes the basal ganglia. A system such as the basal ganglia with direct inhibitory recurrent collaterals may have evolved easily because it is easier to make stable than architectures such as the cerebral cortex with recurrent excitatory connections. The basal ganglia architecture may have been especially appropriate in motor systems in which instability could produce movement and co-ordination difficulties (Rolls and Treves 1998, Rolls 1999a). Equations that describe the way in which this mutual inhibition between the principal neurons can result in contrast enhancement of neuronal activity in the different competing neurons, and thus selection, are provided by Grossberg (1988), Gurney et al. (2001a), and Gurney, Prescott and Redgrave (2001b).

This hypothesis of lateral competition between the neurons of the basal ganglia can be sketched simply (see also Fig. 8.15 and Rolls and Treves (1998) Chapter 9, where a more detailed neuronal network theory of the operation of the basal ganglia is presented). The inputs from the cortex to the striatum are excitatory, and competition between striatal neurons is implemented by the use of an inhibitory transmitter (GABA), and direct connections between striatal neurons, within an area which is approximately co-extensive with the dendritic arborization. Given that the lateral connections between the striatal neurons are collaterals of the output axons, the output must be inhibitory on to pallidal and nigral neurons. This means that to transmit signals usefully, and in contrast with striatal neurons, the neurons in the globus pallidus and substantia nigra (pars reticulata) must have high spontaneous firing rates, and respond by reducing their firing rates. These pallidal and nigral neurons then repeat the simple scheme for lateral competition between output neurons by having direct lateral inhibitory connections to the other pallidal and nigral neurons. When nigral and pallidal neurons respond by reducing their firing rates, the reduced inhibition through the recurrent collaterals allows the connected pallidal and nigral neurons to fire faster, and also at the same time the main output of the pallidal and nigral neurons allows the thalamic neurons to fire faster. The thalamic neurons then have the standard excitatory influence on their cortical targets.

The simple, and perhaps evolutionarily early, aspect of this basal ganglia architecture is that the striatal, pallidal, and nigral neurons implement competition (for selection) by direct inhibitory recurrent lateral connections of the main output neurons on to other output neurons, with the inputs to each stage of processing (e.g. striatum, globus pallidus) synapsing directly on to the output neurons that inhibit each other (see Fig. 8.15).

Another possible mechanism for interaction within the striatum is provided by the dopaminergic pathway, through which a signal that has descended from, for example, the ventral striatum to the dopamine neurons in the midbrain might thereby influence other parts of the striatum (see Section 8.3.4). Because of the slow conduction speed of the dopaminergic neurons, this latter system would probably not be suitable for rapid switching of behaviour, but only for more tonic, long-term adjustments of sensitivity.

Further levels for integration within the basal ganglia are provided by the striato-pallidal and striato-nigral projections (Percheron, Yelnik and François 1984, Percheron, Yelnik and François 1984b, Percheron, Yelnik, François, Fenelon and Talbi 1994). The afferent fibres from the striatum again cross at right angles a flat plate or disc formed by the dendrites of the pallidal or nigral neurons (see Fig. 8.14). The discs are approximately 1.5 mm in diameter, and are stacked up one upon the next at right angles to the incoming striatal fibres. The dendritic discs are so large that in the monkey there is room for only perhaps 50 such discs not to overlap in the external pallidal segment, for 10 non-overlapping discs in the medial pallidal segment, and for one overlapping disc in the most medial part of the medial segment of the globus pallidus and in the substantia nigra.

One result of this convergence achieved by this stage of the medial pallidum/substantia

ventral striatum in this may be to enable Pavlovian conditioned stimuli to influence the level of instrumental responding by Pavlovian-instrumental transfer (see Sections 4.6.1.2, 4.6.3, 8.4.2 and 7.5.4).

8.5 Opiate reward systems, analgesia, and food reward

Electrical stimulation of some regions of the brain can lead to analgesia in animals ranging from rats to humans and can be equivalent in its pain-reducing properties to large doses of morphine (Liebeskind and Paul 1977). These analgesic effects can last for hours after only seconds of stimulation. The analgesia is often for only part of the body, so that a strong pinch to one side but not to the other might be ignored. This shows that the stimulation-produced analgesia is not simply some general interference with the animal's ability to respond to stimulation. The effective stimulation sites are in the medial brainstem, and extend from the rostral medulla (nucleus raphe magnus), through the midbrain central grey matter, towards the hypothalamus. As described in Section 7.5.5, at some sites both analgesia and self-stimulation are found, and at other sites the stimulation is aversive but is followed by analgesia. It has been shown that naloxone, a specific morphine antagonist, reverses, at least partly, stimulation-produced analgesia in both the rat and in humans (Adams 1976, Akil et al. 1976). The endogenous morphine-like peptide enkephalin (Hughes 1975, Hughes et al. 1975) injected intraventricularly yields analgesia (Beluzzi et al. 1976), and central grey matter stimulation releases this substance or a peptide similar to it (Liebeskind et al. 1985). Further, there are stereospecific opiate-binding sites in the central grey matter, and elsewhere in the brain (Kuhar et al. 1973). These findings raise the possibility that stimulation-produced analgesia is effective because it causes the release of a naturally occurring morphine-like substance which acts on opiate receptors in the central grey matter and elsewhere to provide analgesia. The function of this pain-reduction may be, after injury and the initial behavioural reaction to it to prevent further injury, to reduce the on-going effects of continuing severe pain, which could otherwise impair the animal's ability to cope well behaviourally with other needs.

At some of these analgesia-producing sites the electrical stimulation can produce reward (see Koob and Le Moal (1997)). The reward at these sites might be related to the pain-reducing effect of the release of opiates, which can itself be pleasurable and positively reinforcing. However, it is also known that endogenous opiates can be released by behaviours such as grooming (Dunbar 1996), and this may be part of the mechanism by which grooming produces pleasure and relaxation, for blockade of opiate receptors with naloxone greatly reduces grooming interactions.

The food reward system appears to be influenced by opiate systems (Levine and Billington 2004). For example, peripheral morphine injections increase the intake of a high fat palatable diet more than a high carbohydrate diet in rats, whereas injections of naloxone decreased intake of a preferred diet relative to a nonpreferred diet (see Levine and Billington (2004)). Ann Kelley and her group have shown that injections of a μ-opioid receptor agonist into the nucleus accumbens increase the intake of a high fat diet much more than of a high carbohydrate diet (Zhang et al. 1998), and in addition, naltrexone injected into the amygdala decreased the intake of a preferred diet more than of a non-preferred diet (Levine and Billington 2004). Interestingly, humans report a reduction in the pleasantness of sucrose solution following administration of naltrexone, but can still discriminate between sucrose solutions (Bertino et al. 1991, Levine and Billington 2004). Thus there is evidence that brain opioid systems are involved in influencing the palatability of and hedonic reactions to foods, and that in rodents some of these effects are related to actions on the nucleus accumbens and amygdala (see also Berridge and Robinson (2003)). In this context, it is of interest that in humans brain areas influenced by the texture of oral fat include the orbitofrontal cortex, the perigenual cingulate cortex, and also a ventral part of the striatum (De Araujo and Rolls 2004).

8.6 Pharmacology of depression in relation to brain systems involved in emotion

One class of antidepressant drug, the tricyclic antidepressants, of which imipramine is an example, blocks the reuptake of 5-HT (5-hydroxy-tryptamine, serotonin), NA (noradrenaline), and DA (dopamine), in that order of potency. (They inhibit the presynaptic transporters with that order of efficacy.) Another class of drug that has antidepressant properties, the monoamine oxidase inhibitors, blocks the oxidative breakdown of all three of these monoamines. Both types of drug increase the concentration of the catecholamines NA and DA in the synaptic cleft of catecholaminergic neurons, and the catecholamine hypothesis of affective disorders was based on this type of evidence, and also on the concentrations of these monoamines and their metabolites in the brains of depressed patients. The catecholamine hypothesis was that low concentrations of the catecholamines produced depression, and that the antidepressant drugs worked by increasing the concentrations again. However, the catecholamine hypothesis is too simple as it stands, for at least two reasons (Cooper, Bloom and Roth 2003). First, most of the antidepressant treatments affect 5-HT (which is an indoleamine rather than a catecholamine like DA and NA), and indeed some newer drugs such as fluoxetine (Prozac) are relatively selective 5-HT reuptake inhibitors (SSRIs). Second, when antidepressant drugs are given, the pharmacological effects described take place within hours, whereas the antidepressant effects may take up to 6 weeks to become apparent.

One reason that the rapid increase of concentration of 5-HT produced by most of the antide-pressant drugs does not work rapidly appears to be that there are 5-HT_{1A} autoreceptors on the 5-HT cell bodies in the raphe nucleus (and also on the post-synaptic neurons), and when these are activated by the elevated 5-HT, the potassium conductance is increased, producing hyper-polarization of the 5-HT neurons, which decreases their firing, counteracting any influence of the potentially elevated 5-HT concentrations produced by most antidepressant drugs. It may be that this autoreceptor-mediated negative feedback becomes attenuated with a time course of weeks, and then the antidepressant drugs start to influence depression (see e.g. Celada, Puig, Armagos-Bosch, Adell and Artigas (2004)). Also, the blockade of 5-HT_{2A} receptors by some atypical antipsychotic drugs may improve the clinical effects of SSRIs, perhaps by an action on the prefrontal cortex (Celada et al. 2004). Selective noradrenaline reuptake inhibitors (NRIs) such as reboxetine may also be useful in treating depression (Brunello, Mendlewicz, Kasper, Leonard, Montgomery, Craig Nelson, Paykel, Versiani and Racagni 2002).

Overall, the evidence tends to support the hypothesis that central 5-HT is involved in depression, with probably some involvement of NA but much less evidence that DA is involved (Cooper, Bloom and Roth 2003). The traditional way forward for pharmacological research in this area involves screening a large number of new drugs for potential antidepressant effects. This research has not been closely linked to understanding of the brain systems involved in

In terms of sensory analysis, we have seen in Chapters 4 and 5 how sensory systems set up representations of objects in the world that are without reward/punishment valence, but are suitable as inputs to succeeding stages of processing such as the orbitofrontal cortex and amygdala where the valence can be learned by pattern association with primary reinforcers such as taste and touch. We have seen how the representations are highly appropriate as inputs to pattern-association mechanisms, in that they can be read with a dot product type of decoding that is very neurophysiologically plausible, implemented in the brain by adding in the post-synaptic neuron the contributions of many thousands of inputs each weighted by its synaptic connection strength (see Rolls and Treves (1998) and Rolls and Deco (2002)), and in that each input carries information that is essentially independent (within the limits enforced by the number of stimuli being processed). After this pattern association, we have a representation that is coded in terms of its reward/punishment valence. We also have other sensory stimuli that are decoded by the brain as being primary, that is unlearned, reinforcers, such as the taste of food (Chapter 5), or pleasant touch or pain (Chapter 4), or many others (Table 2.1). We should think of these representations coded in terms of reward and punishment as potential goals for action. Although Milner and Goodale (1995) have characterized the dorsal visual system as being appropriate for the control of action, and the ventral visual system projecting to the primate temporal lobe as being appropriate for perception, the view taken here is that the ventral visual system is also involved in action, indeed is at the heart of action, by providing the representations that are the goals for action. It is precisely because the goals for action are typically objects in the world that the ventral visual system, which is involved in the representation of objects, is an important component of the action system (see further Rolls and Deco (2002) and Rolls and Treves (1998)).

We have seen then that reward and punishment decoding systems require certain types of sensory system, so that an important way of understanding much sensory information processing is to realize that it is involved in producing representations suitable as goals for action. The reasons for brain design that have resulted in it using rewards and punishers (including expected rewards and punishers) as goals for actions are considered in Chapter 3. The issue considered here is how, in the brain, reward and punishment systems, which encode goals, are connected to output systems. One feature of the output systems is that they must be built to try to obtain activation of the reward representations in the brain, and to avoid or escape from activation of punishment-related representations in the brain. A second feature is that of response selection, and a third is that of cost–benefit 'analysis' (see Chapter 3).

In Section 8.4, we considered the operation of the basal ganglia in terms of receiving inputs from many reward systems. We showed how they could implement a selection based on competition between inputs, the strongest current reward or punishment (in the common currency, see Chapter 3) winning. Some of the mechanisms for ensuring that one reward does not dominate behaviour for too long include satiety mechanisms, sensory-specific satiety, etc. (see Chapter 5). We showed how the basal ganglia could perhaps also map (by association) the selected reward on to the other systems that also project into the basal ganglia. These other inputs, from the cerebral cortex, include motor and somatosensory systems so that the rewards could produce responses with which they had been associated in the past. This would implement response–reinforcer (i.e. action–outcome) or stimulus–response habit learning. The other cortical inputs though come from all areas of cerebral cortex, so effectively the reinforcers could be associated to much more complex actions than just 'responses' of the type represented in primary motor and somatosensory areas (see Rolls and Treves (1998)). The basal ganglia could thus in principle provide one way in which the rewards and punishment representations in the brain could be interfaced to response and action systems. This is an implicit route to action (see Chapter 10), and in line with this, the basal ganglia do not have backprojections to the cortical areas that project into them. This is in contrast with memory systems such as the hippocampus, orbitofrontal cortex, and amygdala, which do have backprojections to the cortical areas from which they receive, potentially allowing retrieval of information from those systems about memories and emotional states (see Rolls and Treves (1998)). In contrast, the basal ganglia, with no such backprojections, may not allow such explicit retrieval, and indeed we are not aware of how our motor system solves and is processing well-learned problems.

In addition to the basal ganglia route, and the route for explicit reasoning about courses of action to take concerning rewards and punishments (see Section 10.3), there are some other possible routes for stimuli that are reinforcers to influence behaviour. There may for example be many brainstem connections between aversive sensory inputs such as the pain-related inputs coming from the C and Aδ fibres, and brainstem response systems. Such systems operate at the reflex level, enabling for example a limb to be pulled away from a noxious stimulus. However, in terms of the definition given in Chapter 1 for reinforcers, which require operant, that is arbitrary, acts to be learnable to the stimuli, such brainstem reflexes would not qualify as being involved in (instrumental) behavioural responses to reinforcers. There may be other sensory-motor routes that also operate at a relatively low level, and that may correspondingly not qualify as reward or punishment systems. To qualify, the systems have to provide a representation of the goals for actions, and allow arbitrary (operant) responses to be learned to obtain such rewards or avoid or escape from such punishers.

Although the basal ganglia are key brain systems involved in this function in terms of habit (stimulus–response) learning, other brain systems, such as the cingulate cortex, may be especially important in action–outcome learning (see Section 4.7). Now that we have clear hypotheses about how and where rewards and punishers are decoded and represented by the brain, it must be an aim of future research to clarify and better understand how the selection is made between the different goals, how the costs of actions are taken into account (perhaps because they are encoded into the common currency as punishers and expected punishers), and how responses for obtaining the selected goals are made.

9 Sexual behaviour, reward, and brain function; sexual selection of behaviour

9.1 Introduction

One of the themes of this Chapter is the brain control of sexual behaviour, and especially how the brain has evolved to respond to different types of reward to produce sexual behaviour that is adaptive, that is, increases fitness. Part of the Chapter is therefore concerned with what is known of the brain mechanisms that underlie sexual behaviour. Understanding the actual neural mechanisms is important not only because this helps to clarify the behaviour itself, but also because this is a foundation for understanding medical and other disorders of these systems, and treatments for them.

However, because there have been many advances recently in understanding and theorizing about the different patterns of sexual behaviour and why they have evolved, part of the aim of this Chapter is to suggest what reward systems could account for this behaviour, and what the properties are of these reward systems. Specific hypotheses are presented about the operation of the neural systems that could implement these reward-related processes. This is intended to be an approach to how the different types of behaviour observed could be produced by particular reward systems designed by natural selection during evolution, and to provide a basis for investigations of the actual neural mechanisms that implement these processes. The aim thus is to link much recent research on sociobiology, evolutionary psychology and the Darwinian adaptive approaches to different types of sexual behaviour, to new ideas introduced here about how these behaviours could be produced by the sculpting during evolution of systems that are sensitive to different types of reward. The aim is to provide a better understanding of how natural selection may operate in the course of evolution to produce different types of behavioural adaptation by selecting for different types of reward system. The possibility that during evolution a variety of different reward systems could have their sensitivity set differently in different individuals, leading to tendencies towards different types of behaviour in different individuals, each with its own way of being adaptive, is introduced. These new ideas are intended to provide a foundation for future studies of the actual reward systems in the brain that implement these different aspects of sexual behaviour each with its underlying evolutionary 'strategy'[19].

---

[19] We should note at the outset that there may be two types of evolutionary 'strategy'. A first is to have genetically specified polymorphism, with the two types of individual existing in a mixed evolutionarily stable state (ESS). An example is that some individuals might be 'hawks', and others 'doves', in social situations. The behaviours might be set to occur probabilistically by the genes, and do not necessarily imply a polymorphism (Dawkins 1986a). A second is to have a conditional strategy, in which an individual might change strategy, based on an assessment of the situation. For example, if one's opponent is large, one might not play a hawk. Conditional strategies can also lead to evolutionarily stable states (Maynard Smith 1984). Of the examples that are included in this Chapter, some might be polymorphic (mixed) ESSs, e.g. attractiveness (though this can in humans be conditionally modified too!). Probably the majority are conditional ESSs, e.g. the tendency for flirtation, as these are likely to be more effective

The selection processes that lead to the development of some aspects of sexual behaviour are related to the adaptive value of the function being performed. For example, being healthy and strong enables a male to survive long enough to reproduce, and to fight off competitors for females. Reward systems built by genes that favour these characteristics evolve by what we can call natural selection, in a use of the term that is close to that of Darwin (Darwin 1859, Darwin 1871). A distinguishing concept here is that the body survives long enough and is healthy enough to reproduce, and when natural selection is used in its narrow sense here it implies 'survival selection'.

However, Darwin (1871) also recognized that evolution can occur by sexual selection, when what is being selected for has no inherent adaptive or survival value for the individual, but is attractive to potential mates (intersexual selection), or helps individuals of the same sex to compete better with each other (intra-sexual selection, for e.g. male–male competition). The most cited example is the peacock's large tail, which does not have survival value for the peacock (and indeed it is somewhat of a handicap to have a very long tail), but, because it is attractive to the peahen, becomes prevalent in the population. It turns out that sexual selection may lead to all sorts of behaviours being selected, which have in common that they make the bearer attractive to the opposite sex of the species, and are thus useful in courtship, but which would normally be considered as non-sexual types of behaviour, such as kindness and humour (Miller 2000). Thus in this Chapter we also consider the reward and punishment systems that may be built by sexual selection (see Section 9.6).

There will be primary reinforcers to consider specified by genes, and then in addition the possibility of learning associations between previously neutral stimuli and these primary reinforcers. A major emphasis in this book is that reward and punishment systems are built to guide behaviour efficiently and appropriately for the specifying genes, and in this Chapter I show how sexual selection as well as natural ('survival') selection is involved in this process. Insofar as the states elicited by rewards and punishers are emotional states (see Chapters 2 and 3), this Chapter thus extends the understanding of emotion to systems shaped by sexual selection.

The intentional stance is adopted in much writing about sociobiology and evolutionary psychology, and is sometimes used here, but should not be taken literally. It is used just as a shorthand. An example is that it might be said that genes are selfish. But this does not mean at all that genes think about whether to be selfish, and then take the decision. Instead it is just shorthand for a statement along the lines 'genes produce behaviour that operates in the context of natural selection to maximize the number of copies of the gene in the next generations'. Much of the behaviour produced is implicit or unconscious, and when the intentional stance is used as a descriptive tool, it should not be taken to mean that there is usually any explicit or conscious processing involved in the behavioural outcome.

Some of the points may seem 'obvious' once they have been made, if the reader is a neo-Darwinian used to the approach taken in evolutionary biology. However, a potential problem of sociobiology is that its stories do seem plausible, given Darwinism – but many stories are plausible. So we must be careful to seek evidence too, not just plausibility; and we need to know how much of the variance of behaviour is accounted for by each sociobiological account of a type of behaviour. In the long term, once sociobiological hypotheses have been presented, they must be tested.

when information is available on which to base the conditional choice (Maynard Smith 1984, Dawkins 1986a). In many of the cases, the type of strategy that is in operation strictly remains to be determined.

One of the themes of this Chapter is how the underlying physiology of reward is related to the sexual behaviour shown by different types of women, and different types of men. One of the key ideas is that reward systems become tuned to biological functions that they serve. For this reason, there will be discussion of the biological functions that could be implemented by different aspects of sexual behaviour.

Sexual behaviour is an interesting type of motivated behaviour to compare with feeding and drinking. For both feeding and drinking, there are internal signals such as plasma glucose or cellular dehydration related to homeostatic control that set the levels of food or water reward in order to produce the appropriate behaviour. In the case of sexual behaviour, there are no similar short-term homeostatic controls. However, the reward value of sexual behaviour has to be set so that it does perhaps occur sufficiently often to lead to successful reproductive behaviour, in terms of passing an individual's genes into the next generation, and helping them to thrive in the offspring. There are several factors that contribute to this, including internal (steroid) hormonal signals that on a seasonal basis, or in relation to the stage of an oestrus cycle, set the relative reward value of sexual behaviour. For example, in rats at the stage of the oestrus cycle when oestrogen is high the appetite for food is suppressed and sexual behaviour is rewarding. The hormonal status can even be set by the environmental stimuli. For example, Lehrman and colleagues (see Lehrman (1965)) described a series of events in ring doves in which seasonal factors lead to bow-cooing in the male, the sight of which stimulates the female to become receptive as a result of hormonal changes. External signals can also adjust the reward value of sexual behaviour. For example, it has been claimed that female macaques release a pheromone (actually produced by bacteria in the vagina under the influence of androgenic hormones in the female) that acts to promote sexual behaviour in males (Baum, Everitt, Herbert and Keverne 1977). (In this example, a 'male' hormone produced in females 'controls' male sexual behaviour through the effect of the pheromone!) Thus both internal and external stimuli can act to influence the reward value of sexual behaviour. In addition, some of the rewards and punishers related to courtship may have no survival or adaptive value for the individual, but have evolved instead by the process of sexual selection (see Section 9.6).

9.2   Mate selection, attractiveness, and love

What factors are decoded by our brains to influence mate attractiveness (reward value) and selection? Many factors are involved in mate selection, and they are not necessarily the same for selection of a short term vs a long-term partner. The selection of a long-term partner in species with long-term relatively monogamous relationships is influenced for example by parental investment, which is a major evolutionary adaptive factor in promoting long-term relationships. Thus in humans, males choose females because human males do make a parental investment; and females compete for males. Indeed, the selection of a long-term partner in humans is mutual, and this tends to reduce sex differences in partner choice. Consistent with this, David Buss has shown that in contrast, human sex differences in mate selection are more evident in short-term mating (Buss 1989, Buss 1994, Buss 1999).

Species with shared parental investment are primarily those where two parents can help the offspring to survive better than one, and this includes many birds (where one bird must sit on the eggs to incubate them, while the other finds food), and humans (where the human infant is born so immature[20] that care of the offspring for a number of years could, when humans were evolving, make it more likely that the offspring, containing the father's genes, would survive, and then reproduce). Most other mammals are not good models of human pair mate selection and pair bonding, because there is generally less advantage to joint care of the young, and the female, who has made the major investment of the gestation period for the baby, and breast feeding it post-partum (for the whole of which period she will remain relatively infertile), generally assumes most of the responsibility for bringing up her young. In most mammals, females will maximize their reproductive success, given the cost of gestation and lactation, by focussing on the successful rearing of offspring. In contrast, male mammals do not invest by gestation and lactation in their offspring, and the most effective way for males to influence their reproductive success is to maximize the number of fertilizations they achieve, and this is a major factor in mammalian mate selection. This tendency is tempered in humans by the advantage of male investment in the offspring, as ensuring that the immature offspring survive sufficiently long that the chances of their reproductive success is high is an adaptive investment.

9.2.1 Female preferences

Factors that across a range of species influence female selection of male mates include the following.

1. Athleticism. The ability to compete well in mate selection (including being healthy and strong), as this will be useful for her genes when present in her male offspring. Athleticism may be attractive (rewarding) also as an indicator of protection from male marauding (single females are at risk in some species of abuse, and forced copulation, which circumvents female mate choice), from predators, and as an indicator of hunting competency (meat was important in human evolution (Aiello and Wheeler 1995), although the hunt may also have been co-opted by sexual selection as a mating ritual giving the males a chance to show off). Consistent with these points, Buss and Schmitt (1993) showed that women show a strong preference for tall, strong, athletic men.

2. Resources, power and wealth. In species with shared parental investment (which include many birds and humans), having power and wealth may be attractive to the female, because they are indicators of resources that may be provided for her young. Women should desire men who show willingness to invest resources (which should be defensible, accruable and controllable) in his partner. Women place a greater premium on income or financial prospects than men (Buss 1989). Further, in a cross-cultural study of 37 cultures with 10,047 participants, it was found that irrespective of cultural/political/social background, women consistently placed more value on financial resources (100% more) than men (see Buss (1989), Buss et al. (1990) and Buss (1994)). Women value a man's love as an indicator of resource commitment.

3. Status. Both now and historically, status hierarchies are found in many cultures (and species, for example monkeys' dominance hierarchies, and chickens' pecking order). Status correlates with the control of resources (e.g. alpha male chimpanzees take precedence in feeding), and therefore acts as a good cue for women. Women should therefore find men of high status attractive (e.g. rock stars, politicians, and tribal rulers), and these men should be able to attract the most attractive partners (Betzig 1986). Consistent with this, Buss (1989)

---

[20] Humans are born secondarily altricial (where altricial is the opposite of precocial) because of the narrow female pelvis of humans associated with bipedality, which results in gestation being shortened from an estimated 21 to 9 months (Gould 1985).

showed cross-culturally that women regard high social status as more valuable than do men; and Udry and Eckland (1984) showed that attractive women marry men of high status.

4. Age. Status and higher income are generally only achieved with age, and therefore women should generally find older men attractive. Buss (1989) showed cross-culturally that women prefer older men (3.42 years older on average; and marriage records from 27 countries showed that the average age difference was 2.99 years).

5. Ambition and industriousness, which may be good predictors of future occupational status and income, are attractive. Valued characteristics include those that show a male will work to improve their lot in terms of resources or in terms of rising up in social status (Kyl-Heku and Buss 1996). Cross-culturally, women rated ambition/industriousness as highly desirable (Buss 1989).

6. Testosterone-dependent features may also be attractive. These features include a strong (longer and broader) jaw, a broad chin, strong cheekbones, defined eyebrow ridges, a forward central face, and a lengthened lower face (secondary sexual characteristics which are a result of pubertal hormone levels). High testosterone levels are immuno-suppressing, so these features may be indicators of immuno-competence (and thus honest indicators of fitness). The attractiveness of these masculinized features increases with increased risk of conception across the menstrual cycle (Penton-Voak, Perrett, Castles, Kobayashi, Burt, Murray and Minamisawa 1999, Johnston, Hagel, Franklin, Fink and Grammer 2001). The implication is that the neural mechanism controlling perception of attractiveness must be sensitive to oestrogen/progesterone levels in women.

Another feature thought to depend on prenatal testosterone levels is the 2nd/4th digit ratio. A low ratio reflects a testosterone-rich uterine environment. It has been found that low ratios correlate with female ratings of male dominance and masculinity, although the relationship to attractiveness ratings was less clear (Swaddle and Reierson 2002).

7. Symmetry (in both males and females) may be attractive, in that it may reflect good development in utero, a non-harmful birth, adequate nutrition, and lack of disease and parasitic infections. Fluctuating asymmetry (FA) reflects the degree to which individuals deviate from perfect symmetry on bilateral features (e.g. in humans, both ears, both feet, both hands and arms; in other species, bilateral fins, bilateral tail feathers). Greater asymmetry may reflect deviations in developmental design resulting from the disruptive effects of environmental or genetic abnormalities, and in some species is associated with lower fecundity, slower growth, and poorer survival. A low fluctuating asymmetry may thus be a sign of reproductive fitness (Gangestad and Simpson 2000). In a number of bird species, attractive (symmetric) males employ a strategy of investing more in extra-pair mating than in paternal care, and maximize their reproductive success in this way (Moller and Thornhill 1998). In humans, more symmetrical men reported more lifetime partners (r=0.38), and more extra-pair partners; and women's choice of extra-pair partners was predicted by male symmetry (see Gangestad and Simpson (2000)). Moreover, women rate men as more attractive if they have high symmetry (low FA). Intellectual ability (which may be attractive to women) is also correlated with symmetry (Gangestad and Thornhill 1999). A further type of evidence here is that the frequency of human female orgasm (which probably results in high sperm retention) correlates with low fluctuating asymmetry (FA) (i.e. being symmetrical) in male partners (Thornhill, Gangestad and Comer 1995).

8. Dependability and faithfulness may be attractive, particularly where there is paternal investment in bringing up the young, as these characteristics may indicate stability of resources

(Buss et al. 1990). Emotionally unstable men may also inflict costs on women, and thus women rate emotional stability and maturity as important. For example, jealousy might lead to abuse.

9. Risk-taking by men may be attractive to women, perhaps because it is a form of competitive advertising: surviving the risk may be an honest indicator of high quality genes (Barrett et al. 2002).

10. Characteristics that may not be adaptive in terms of the survival of the male, but that may be attractive because of inter-sexual sexual selection, are common in birds, perhaps less common in most mammals, though present in some primates (Kappeler and van Schaik 2004), and may be present in humans (see Section 9.6). An example of a sexually selected characteristic that may not increase the survival of the individual, but that may be attractive to females and thus increase the fitness of the male in terms of whether his genes are passed on to the next generation by reproduction, is the peacock's tail. These characteristics may in some cases be an honest indicator of health, in the sense that having a large gaudy tail may be a handicap.

11. Odour. The preference by women for the odour of symmetrical men is correlated with the probability of fertility of women as influenced by their cycle (Thornhill and Gangstad 1999). Another way in which odour can influence preference is by pheromones which are related to major histocompatibility complex (MHC) genes, which may provide a molecular mechanism for producing genetic diversity by influencing those who are considered attractive as mates, as described in Section 9.8.

It is important to note that physical factors such as high symmetry and that are indicators of genetic fitness may be especially attractive when women choose short term partners, and that factors such as resources and faithfulness may be especially important when women choose long-term partners, in what may be termed a conditional mating strategy (Gangstad and Simpson 2000, Buss 1999). This conditionality means that the particular factors that influence preferences alter dynamically, and preferences will often depend on the prevailing circumstances, including the current opportunities and costs.

9.2.2 Male preferences

Males are not always indiscriminate[21]. When a male chooses to invest (for example to produce offspring), there are preferences for the partner with whom they will make the investment. Accurate evaluation of female quality (reproductive value) is therefore important, and a male will need to look out for cues to this, and find these cues attractive (rewarding). The factors that influence attractiveness include the following (see also Barrett et al. (2002)).

1. Youth. As fertility and reproductive value in females is linked to age (reproductive value is higher when younger, and actual fertility in humans peaks in the twenties), males (unlike females) place a special premium on youth. It is not youth per se that men find attractive, but indicators of youth, for example neotenous traits such as blonde hair and wide eyes. An example of this preference is that Buss (1989) showed that male college students preferred an age difference on average of 2.5 years younger. Another indicator of youth might be a small body frame, and it is interesting that this might contribute to the small body frame of some women in this example of sexual dimorphism.

---

[21] In fact, males are probably rarely indiscriminate, in that producing sperm and performing sexual behaviour do have costs, including for example the risk of catching disease.

2. Beauty. Features that are most commonly described as the most attractive tend to be those that are oestrogen-dependent, e.g. full lips and cheeks, and short lower facial features. (Oestrogen caps the growth of certain facial bones.) Like testosterone, oestrogen also affects the immune system, and its effects might be seen as 'honest indicators' of genetic fitness.

For example, in one study, Johnston and Franklin (1993) found that when subjects were able to evolve a computer generated image into their ideal standard of female beauty, the beautiful composite had a relatively short lower face, small mouth, and full lips.

In a cross-cultural study, people of different races agreed in their ratings of the attractiveness of faces of Asian, Hispanic, black, and white women (Cunningham, Roberts, Barbee and Druen 1995). In meta-analyses of 11 studies, Langlois, Kalakanis, Rubenstein, Larson, Hallam and Smoot (2000) demonstrated that (a) raters agree about who is and is not attractive, both within and across cultures; (b) attractive children and adults are judged and treated more positively than unattractive children and adults, even by those who know them; and (c) attractive children and adults exhibit more positive behaviours and traits than unattractive children and adults. In an fMRI study, it was found that attractive faces produce more activation of the human medial orbitofrontal cortex than unattractive faces (O'Doherty et al. 2003b).

Further, small babies were even shown to gaze for longer at slides of the more attractive woman when shown pairs of pictures of women that differed in attractiveness (Langlois, Roggman, Casey and Ritter 1987, Langlois, Ritter, Roggman and Vaughn 1991). In another study, 12-month-olds interacted with a stranger. The infants showed more positive affective tone, less withdrawal, and more play involvement with a stranger who wore a professionally constructed attractive than unattractive mask; and played longer with an attractive than an unattractive doll (Langlois, Roggman and Reiser-Danner 1990). These results extend and amplify earlier findings showing that young infants exhibit visual preferences for attractive over unattractive faces. Both visual and behavioural preferences for attractiveness are evidently exhibited much earlier in life than was previously supposed.

Women appear to spend more time on fashion and enhancing beauty than men. Why should this be, when in most mammals it is men who may be gaudy to help in their competition for females, given that females make the larger investment in offspring? In humans, there is of course value to investment by males in their offspring, so women may benefit by attracting a male who will invest time and resources in bring up children together. But nevertheless, women do seem to invest more in bearing and then raising children, so why is the imbalance so marked, with women apparently competing by paying attention to their own beauty and fashion? Perhaps the answer is that males who are willing to make major investments of time and resources in raising the children of a partner are a somewhat limiting resource (as other factors may make it advantageous genetically for men not to invest all their resources in one partner), and because women are competing to obtain and maintain this scarce resource, being beautiful and fashionable is important to women. Faithful men may be a limited resource because there are alternative strategies that may have a low cost, whereas women are essentially committed to a considerable investment in their offspring. These factors lead to greater variability in men's strategies, and thus contribute to making men who invest in their offspring a more limited resource than women who invest in their offspring.

3. Body fat. The face is not the only cue to a woman's reproductive capacity. Although the ideal body weight varies significantly with culture (in cultures with scarcity, obesity is attractive, and relates to status), the ideal distribution of body fat seems to be a universal standard, as measured by the waist-to-hip ratio (which cancels out effects of actual body

weight). Consistently, across cultures, men preferred an average ratio of 0.7 (small waist/bigger hips) when rating female figures (line drawings and photographic images) for attractiveness (Singh 1993, Singh 1995, Singh and Young 1995, Singh and Luis 1995). Thornhill and Grammer (1999) also found high correlations between rating of attractiveness of nude females by men of different ethnicity. Long term health risks (diabetes, hypertension, coronary disease, and stroke) are also associated with a high waist-to-hip ratio, which may therefore be an 'honest indicator' of fitness.

4. Fidelity. The desire for fidelity in females is most obviously related to her concealed ovulation (see next paragraph and Section 9.5), and therefore the degree of paternity certainty males may suffer. Males therefore place a premium on a woman's sexual history. Virginity was a requisite for marriage both historically (before the arrival of contraceptives) and cross-culturally (in non-Westernised societies where virginity is still highly valued) (Buss 1989). Nowadays, female monogamy in previous relationships is a sought after characteristic in future long term partners (Buss and Schmitt 1993). (Presumably with simple genetic methods now available for identifying the father of a child, the rational thought system (see Chapter 10) might place less value on fidelity with respect to paternity issues as paternity can be established genetically, yet the implicit emotional system may still place high value on fidelity, as during evolution, fidelity was valued as an indicator of paternity probability.) The modern rational emphasis might be especially placed on valuing fidelity because this may indicate less risk of sexually transmitted disease, and perhaps the emotional value of fidelity will be a help in this respect.

5. Attractiveness and the time of ovulation. Although ovulation in some primates and in humans is concealed[22], it would be a premium for men to pick up other cues to ovulation, and find women highly desirable at these times. Possible cues include an increased body temperature reflected in the warm glow of vascularized skin (van der Berge and Frost 1986), and pheromonal cues. Indeed, male raters judged the odours of T-shirts worn during the follicular phase as more pleasant and sexy than odours from T-shirts worn during the luteal phase (Singh and Bronstad 2001). In macaques, male interest in females increases during the fertile period, and alpha males more often mate guard females during the fertile phase of the cycle, with possible cues related to the high levels of oestrogen at the time of ovulation (Engelhardt, Pfeifer, Heistermann, Niemitz, Van Hoof and Jodges 2004). Women generally do not know when they are ovulating (and in this sense ovulation may be double blind), but there is a possibility that ovulation could unconsciously affect female behaviour. In fact, Event-Related Potentials (ERPs) were found to be greater to sexual stimuli in ovulating women, and these could reflect increased affective processing of the stimuli (Krug, Plihal, Fehm and Born 2000). This in turn might affect outward behaviour of the female, helping her to attract a mate at this time.

In most species, females invest heavily in the offspring in terms of providing the eggs and providing the care (from gestation until weaning, and far beyond weaning in the case of humans). Females are therefore a 'limited resource' for males allowing the females to be the choosier sex during mate choice. This leads therefore to strong levels of male intra-sexual selection, resulting in males typically being the larger and/or more flamboyant sex (an example is the male mandrill's brightly coloured face in comparison to the dull one of

---

[22]Perhaps so that males may be uncertain who the father is of a baby, and thus not threaten infanticide–see Section 9.3

the female's). If the sex roles become somewhat reversed, however, this can alter. Dramatic female ornamentation can be seen in the pipefish (a relative of the seahorse). Male pipefish overwhelmingly find the larger, most ornamented females the most attractive (Berglund and Rosenqvist 2001). This stems from the fact that the males of these species have evolved a brood pouch (which, in some species, is vascularised) into which the female can oviposit her eggs. Moreover, the size of the (male) brood pouch (which determines how many embryos a male can store) is also another limiting factor that females compete over. This accounts for why the males are the choosier sex and why females compete in pipefish. Female competition is also found in the spotted sandpiper – a bird with an unusual polyandrous breeding system (i.e. a breeding system with one female with multiple males) (Oring 1986). Here, females arrive on the breeding ground first and must attract males to it. The females must defend from other females the territory that contains the individual territories of their male consorts. The males then provide the important resource of incubating the clutch on their own, and therefore become unavailable as mates. This often leads to a chronic shortage of available males, and thus, female competition is intense, and displays are extremely vigorous and occasionally lead to physical combat. Similar polyandrous tactics are also seen in the jacana (Jenni and Collier 1972).

In humans, male investment in caring for the offspring means that male choice has a strong effect on intrasexual selection in women. Female cosmetic use and designer clothing could be seen as weapons in this competition, and perhaps are reflected in extreme female self-grooming behaviour such as cosmetic surgery, or pathological disorders such as anorexia, bulimia and body dysmorphic disorder. The modern media, by bombarding people with images of beautiful women, may heighten intrasexual selection even further, pushing women's competitive mating mechanisms to a major scale.

Finally in this section, we should note that in addition to the benefits of particular mate choices, the costs also need to be assessed (Kokko, Brooks, McNamara and Houston 2002, Kokko, Brooks, Jennions and Morley 2003), and both the benefits and costs may vary across time.

9.2.3   Pair-bonding, and Love

Attachment to a particular partner by pair bonding in a monogamous relationship, which in humans becomes manifest in love between pair-bonded parents, and which occurs in humans because of the advantage to the man of investing in his offspring, may have special mechanisms to facilitate it. Species in which attachment has been investigated include the prairie vole. In monogamous species of prairie voles, mating can increase pair-bonding (as measured by partner preference). Oxytocin, a hormone released from the posterior pituitary, whose other actions include the milk let-down response, is released during mating. Exogenous administration of oxytocin facilitates pair bonding in both female and male prairie voles (Carter 1998). In female prairie voles, antagonists of oxytocin interfere with partner preference formation. In female prairie voles, the endogenous release of oxytocin is thus important in partner preference and attachment. Thus oxytocin has been thought of as the 'hormone of love'. Oxytocin gene knock-out mice fail to recognize familiar conspecifics after repeated social exposures, and injection of oxytocin in the medial amygdala restores social recognition (Ferguson, Aldag, Insel and Young 2001, Winslow and Insel 2004). In males, the effects of oxytocin are facilitated by vasopressin, another posterior pituitary hormone whose other effects include promoting the retention of water by the kidney. In the case of vasopressin, it has been possible to show that the vasopressin V1a receptor (V1aR) is expressed in higher concentration in the ventral forebrain of monogamous prairie voles than in promiscuous (i.e. polygamous) meadow voles, and that viral vector V1aR transfer into the forebrain of the meadow mouse increases its partner preference (i.e. makes it more like a monogamous prairie vole) (Lim, Wang, Olazabal, Ren, Terwilliger and Young 2004, Young and Wang 2004). Thus a single gene may be important in influencing monogamy vs promiscuity in voles. Stress, or the administration of the hormone corticosterone which is released during stress, can facilitate the onset of new pair bonds (DeVries, DeVries, Taymans and Carter 1996).

Are similar mechanisms at work in humans to promote pair-bonding and love? There is as yet no definitive evidence, but in humans, oxytocin is released by intercourse, and especially at the time of orgasm, in both women and men (Meston and Frohlich 2000, Kruger, Haake, Chereath, Knapp, Janssen, Exton, Schedlowski and Hartmann 2003). Moreover, although orgasm is thought not to occur in females in most non-human species, it does occur in some female non-human primates (e.g. the Japanese macaque, Macaca fuscata), where it is more likely to occur if the female is mating with a high-ranking male (Troisi and Carosi 1998), and it is possible that this serves as a reward for mating with high-ranking males, and at the same time promotes cryptic choice. (Cryptic female choice is the postcopulatory ability of females to favour one male of the same species over another (Thornhill 1983, Ben-Ari 2000, Birkhead and Pizzari 2002, Birkhead 2000).) It has also been reported that women desiring to become pregnant are more likely to have an orgasm after their partner ejaculates (Singh, Meyer, Zambarano and Hurlbert 1998) (see further Section 9.4).

9.3   Parental attachment, care, and parent–offspring conflict

Many mammal females make strong attachments to their own offspring, and this is also facilitated in many species by oxytocin. One model is the sheep, in which vaginal-cervical stimulation and suckling, which release both oxytocin and endogenous opioids, facilitate maternal bonding (Keverne 1995, Keverne, Nevison and Martel 1997). Oxytocin injections can cause ewes to become attached to an unfamiliar lamb presented at the time oxytocin is released or injected, and oxytocin antagonists can block filial bonding in sheep. Perhaps oxytocin had an initial role in evolution in the milk let-down reflex, and then became appropriate as a hormone that might facilitate mother–infant attachment.

In humans the evidence is much more correlative, but oxytocin release during natural childbirth, and rapid placing of the baby to breast feed and release more oxytocin (Carter 1998, Nissen, Uvnas-Moberg, Svennson, Stock, Widstrom and Winberg 1996, Uvnas-Moberg 1997, Uvnas-Moberg 1998), might facilitate maternal attachment to her baby. This provides an argument in favour (other things being equal) of natural childbirth (Odent 1999). Prolactin, the female hormone that promotes milk production, may also influence maternal attachment. It is certainly a major factor in humans that bonding can change quite suddenly at the time that a child is born, with women having a strong tendency to shift their interests markedly towards the baby as soon as it is born (probably in part under hormonal influences), and this can result in relatively less attachment behaviour to the husband. Understanding the scientific basis for this, and stimulated by this understanding, counselling couples about how their affections and attachments may alter at the time of the birth of a child, may be and should be

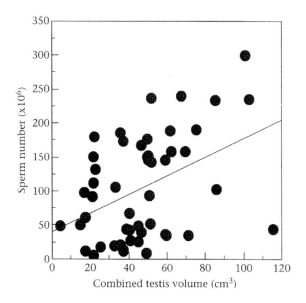

Fig. 9.1 Relation between number of sperm contained in human ejaculate volume and the size of the testes. The relation was significant at P=0.002 in the sample of 50 men. (From Simmons, Firman, Rhodes and Peters 2004.)

see Section 9.6.)

In such a social system, such as that of the swallow, the wife needs a reliable husband with whom she mates (so that he thinks the offspring are his, which for the system to be stable they must be sometimes) to help provide resources for 'their' offspring. (Remember that a nest must be built, the eggs must be incubated, and the hungry young must be well fed to help them become fit offspring. Here fit means successfully passing on genes into the next generation – see Dawkins (1986b)). But the wife (or at least her genes) also benefits by obtaining as fit genes as possible, by sometimes cheating on her husband. To ensure that her husband does not find out and therefore leave her and stop caring for the young, she deceives the husband by committing her adultery as much as possible secretly, perhaps hiding behind a bush to mate with her lover. So the (swallow) wife maximizes care for her children using her husband, and maximizes her genetic potential by finding a lover with fit genes that are likely to be attractive in her sons to other females (see Ridley (1993b)).

Could anything like the situation just described for birds such as swallows also apply to humans? It appears that it might apply, at least in part, and that similar evolutionary factors might influence human sexual behaviour, and hence make obtaining particular stimuli in the environment rewarding to humans. We need to understand whether this is the case, in order to understand the rewards that drive sexual behaviour in humans. One line of evidence already described is the large testis and penis size of men. In humans, it has been shown that the number of sperm ejaculated is related to testis size (Simmons, Firman, Rhodes and Peters 2004). Fig. 9.1 shows this relation, and also indicates the large variation in both testis size and number of sperm contained in an ejaculate in humans, indicating that there is the potential for variation between humans to play a role in sperm competition. This potential may not be fully realised in modern humans perhaps because of contraceptive practices, in that extrapair paternity rates are estimated at around 4% in modern times (see below), though double paternity in some dizygotic twins does show that conditions for sperm competition in humans can occur (Simmons et al. 2004). (We will get on to the reason for the large penis size soon.) A second line is that some studies in humans of paternity using modern DNA tests suggest that in fact the woman's partner (e.g. husband) is not the father of about 14% of their children. Although surprising, this has been claimed in a study in Liverpool, and in another in the south of England (Baker and Bellis 1995) (see Ridley (1993b)). In other studies, the extrapair paternity rate has been estimated at closer to 2%, although 28% of men and 22% of women did report extrapair copulations (Simmons et al. 2004). Further, an approximate estimate across 53,619 humans in 5 studies yields 24% of men and 20% of women reporting extrapair copulations (estimate made from data in Simmons et al. (2004)). In the data reviewed by Simmons et al. (2004), an approximate estimate of the extra-pair paternity rate is 4%, but there were great variations, with estimates in some traditional cultures of 10–11.8%. The latter estimates are particularly interesting, because estimates of extrapair paternity rates from North American and European cultures, practised in birth control and taught by particular mores, may not reflect the behaviour of our ancestors, selection between whom has shaped the behaviour of modern humans. On balance, these data suggest that while sperm competition may not be a major factor in modern humans, it may be to some extent, and might have been much more important in our ancestors, and have shaped our behaviour to at least some extent. So the possible effects of sperm competition in influencing modern human behaviour are worth exploring further.

So might men produce large amounts of sperm, and have intercourse quite regularly, in order to increase the likelihood that the children produced are theirs, whether by their wife or by their mistress? When women choose men as their lovers, do they choose men who are likely to produce children who are fit, that is children good at passing on their genes, half of which originate from the woman? It appears that women might choose like this, as described below, and that this behaviour may even select genetically for certain characteristics in men, because the woman finds these characteristics rewarding during mate selection. Of course, if such a strategy were employed (presumably mainly unconsciously) all the time in women the system would break down (be unstable), because men would not trust their wives, and the men would not invest in making a home and bringing up their children[25]. So we would not expect this to be the only selective pressure on what women find attractive and rewarding as qualities in men. Pursuing this matter further, we might expect women to find reliability, stability, provision of a home, and help with bringing up her children to be rewarding when selecting a husband; and the likelihood of producing genetically fit children, especially sons who can themselves potentially have many children by a number of women, to be rewarding when selecting a lover (i.e. short-term mate).

What is even more extraordinary is that women may even have evolved ways of influencing whether it is the woman's lover, as opposed to her husband, who fathers her children. Apparently she may be able to do this even while deceiving her husband, even to the extent of having regular intercourse with him. The ways in which this might work have been inves-

---

[25] In some tribes, brothers help to bring up their sisters' children, because these children share some of the mother's brother's genes. The brother and sister of course will share some of the same genes, so the behaviour of the brother is appropriate in terms of increasing the fitness of his genes in a promiscuous society.

tigated in research described next (Baker and Bellis 1995, Baker 1996). Although much of the research on the sociobiological background of human sexual behaviour, including sperm warfare in humans, is quite new, and many of the hypotheses remain to be fully established and some can now be rejected (Birkhead 2000, Moore, Martin and Birkhead 1999), this research does have interesting potential implications for understanding the rewards that control human behaviour, and for this reason the research, and its potential implications, are considered here.

In the research by Baker and Bellis (1995) and others (see also Ridley (1993b)), it was claimed that if a woman has no orgasm, or if she has an orgasm more than a minute before the male ejaculates, relatively little sperm is retained in the woman. This is a low-retention orgasm. The claim was that if she has an orgasm less that a minute before him or up to 45 min after him, then much more of the sperm stays in the woman, and some of it is essentially sucked up by the cervix during and just following the later stages of her perceived orgasm. This is a high-retention orgasm. [This effect, known as upsuck, does not literally mean that seminal fluid is sucked up physically into the womb, with a resulting low volume of fluid lost during the outflow from the woman 30–45 min later. Instead, the mechanism of sperm retention claimed was that in a high-retention orgasm, more sperm enter the channels in the cervical mucus, and either swim right through them into the womb, or stay in the cervical mucus. In both high- and low-retention orgasms, the volume of the outflow, which includes more than sperm, was claimed to be similar (see Baker and Bellis (1995), p. 237).] After a high-retention orgasm, it was claimed (Baker and Bellis 1995) that the woman is more likely to conceive (by that intercourse) even if she already has sperm in her reproductive tract left from intercourse in the previous 4 or so days. Baker and Bellis (1995) then (using a questionnaire) found that in women who were faithful (having intercourse only with their husbands) about 55% of the orgasms were of the high-retention (i.e. most fertile) type. By contrast, in unfaithful women having intercourse with their husbands, only 45% of the copulations were high-retention, but 70% of the copulations with the lover were of the high-retention type. Moreover, the unfaithful women were having sex with their lovers at times of the month when they were most fertile, that is when they were just about to ovulate. The result in the research sample was that an unfaithful woman could have sex twice as often with her husband as with her lover, but was still slightly more likely to conceive a child by the lover than by the husband. Put another way, the women in this sample would be more than twice as likely to conceive during sex with their lover than with their partner[26]. Thus women appear to be able to influence to some extent who is the father of their children, not only by having intercourse with lovers, but also by influencing whether they will become pregnant by their lover. The ways in which reward mechanisms might help this process are described later in this Chapter. Some evidence for such selection is that domestic fowls (hens) appear to select which sperm fertilize their eggs, in that when inseminated with sperm of different cocks, the fertilization was non-random (Birkhead, Chaline, Biggins, Burke and Pizzari 2004).

These data are at present quite controversial, although there is evidence that women have orgasms more frequently after their partner has ejaculated when they desire to become pregnant (Singh et al. 1998), and this might be a mechanism for cryptic choice (Birkhead and Pizzari 2002) when mating with an attractive lover, in that a woman is more likely to have

---

[26]Given that 14% of children are not the children of the male partner according to Baker and Bellis, this suggests (and not taking into account fertility factors such as the time of month, whether the woman is more likely to synchronize ovulation with a lover, and possible differences in contraceptives used) that the average across the whole population of the number of copulations women have with lovers rather than their partners could be in the order of 7.5%. When effects of fertility etc. are taken into account, it will be less than 7.5%.

an orgasm with an attractive (symmetric) partner (Thornhill et al. 1995). If female orgasm is involved in influencing who the father is of a baby, then it might be expected that female orgasm might be somewhat variable in whether it occurs, as part of a putative selection process. Another possible contributory factor in the evolution of female orgasm is that it provides motivation to solicit multiple partners, for example if she does not have an orgasm with one partner, or if she has an orgasm with one partner who then enters a refractory state after ejaculation (cf. Hrdy (1999) and Hrdy (1996)). Indeed, polyandrous mating situations make it adaptive (in order to conceal paternity) for a female to be able to have orgasms without a long refractory period between each, that is to be able to have multiple orgasms. Although a similar argument might be applied to men, a refractory period might nevertheless be adaptive in men in part because of limited sperm resources, and the utility of competing with adequate sperm numbers when insemination does occur. Indeed, dominant males may release limited sperm because of their multiple matings, and this indeed is a factor cited as accounting for females competing for the first mating (Wedell, Gage and Parker 2002).

Another finding by Baker and Bellis (1995) indicates that men have evolved strategies to optimize the chances of their genes in this sperm selection process. One is that men were reported to ejaculate more sperm if they have not been for some time with the woman with whom they are having intercourse. An effect consistent with this is that a man who spends a greater (relative to a man who spends a lesser) proportion of time apart from the partner since the couple's last copulation report (a) that his partner is more attractive, (b) that other men find his partner more attractive, (c) greater interest in copulating with the partner, and (d) that his partner is more sexually interested in him (Shackelford, Le Blanc, Weekes-Shackelford, Bleske-Rechek, Euler and Hoier 2002). (This effect is not just dependent on the time since he has last inseminated his partner, but is related to the time the couple have been apart, so the effects may be interpreted as being related to possible insemination of the partner while away, and not just to sexual frustration (Shackelford et al. 2002)). The (evolutionary, adaptive) function of this may be for the man to increase the chances of his sperm in what could be a sperm war with the sperm of another man. The aim would be to outnumber the other sperm. Moreover, the man should do this as quickly as possible after returning from an absence, as time could be of the essence in determining which sperm get to the egg first if the woman has had intercourse with another man recently. The implication of this for reward mechanisms in men is that after an absence, having intercourse quite soon with the woman from whom the man has been absent should be very rewarding (and this is what is reported (Shackelford et al. 2002)). Possible neural mechanisms for this are considered later. There is good evidence that processes of this type do occur in some species. For example, Pizzari, Cornwallis, Lovlie, Jakobsson and Birkhead (2003) found in domestic fowl that males show status-dependent investment in female according to the level of female promiscuity: they progressively reduce sperm investment in a particular female but, on encountering a new female, instantaneously increase their sperm investment; and they preferentially allocate sperm to females with large sexual ornaments signalling superior maternal investment. These results indicate that female promiscuity leads to the evolution of sophisticated male sexual behaviour.

It even appears that there should be some reward value in having intercourse very soon with the woman after an absence, because the action of the glans penis, with its groove behind the head, may be to pull sperm already in the vagina out of it using repeated thrusting and pulling back (Baker and Bellis 1995) (at least in some ancestors, Birkhead (2000)). The potential advantage to this in the sperm warfare may be the biological function that, as a result of evolution, leads to thrusting and withdrawal of the penis during intercourse being rewarding (perhaps to both men and women). Such thrusting and withdrawal of the penis during intercourse should occur especially vigorously (and should therefore have evolved to become especially rewarding) after an absence by the man. The possible advantage in the sperm warfare that shaped our evolution could also result in its being rewarding for a man to have intercourse with a woman if he has just seen her having intercourse with another man. (This could be part of the biological background of why some men find videos showing sex involving women rewarding.) However, large numbers of sperm from a previous man usually remain in the vagina for only up to 45 min after intercourse, after which a flowback of sperm and other fluids (the discharge of semen and other secretions) from the vagina usually occurs. Thus the evolutionary shaping of the glans penis, and the rewards produced by thrusting and withdrawing it and the shaft of the penis in the vagina, are likely to have adaptive value more in our ancestors than in us.

Baker and Bellis (1995) proposed that a second human male strategy might be to ejaculate not only sperm that can potentially fertilize an egg, but also killer (or kamikaze) sperm that kill the sperm of another male, and blocker sperm that remain in the mucus at the entrance to the cervix blocking access through the channels in the mucus to other sperm. However, this hypothesis of different sperm types in humans is now strongly criticised, and there is little evidence for different sperm types in humans, and for kamikaze-like effects (Moore et al. 1999, Birkhead 2000, Short 1998). (Nevertheless, there are many interesting sperm adaptations for competition in other species. For example, in the wood mouse the sperm from one individual form 'trains' that increase the motility of the sperm twofold, thus facilitating fertilization by that individual's sperm (Moore, Dvorakova, Jenkins and Breed 2002).) Independently of this argument, given that (the majority of) sperm remain viable once out of the vagina and in the uterus or Fallopian tubes for up to about four days, it becomes important (read adaptive) for a man to have intercourse with his partner at least as often as say twice per week. This would ensure that at least some of the male partner's sperm were present to compete with any other sperm that might arrive as a result of an extra-pair copulation. So because of this function of sperm warfare, the brain should be built to make male intercourse with his partner rewarding at least approximately twice per week.

A third argument of Baker and Bellis (1995) (see also Smith (1984) and Baker and Bellis (1993)) is that it is important (in the fitness sense) that a male should help his lover to have an orgasm, which should occur only just before or for 45 min after he has ejaculated for the upsuck effect to operate. [The orgasm was proposed to cause the upsuck effect of sperm into the uterus. This might give the woman some control over whether she will accept new sperm, even when she has had intercourse and has blocking sperm in her. The operation of this female 'strategy' is facilitated by the facts that sperm remain in the vagina only for a short time because of the flowback, and because the acidity of the vagina makes sperm viable in the vagina for less than 12 h. The result is that the upsuck effect with a lover can operate preferentially on his (recently ejaculated) sperm, because many of the sperm from previous intercourse will be ejected within 45 min in the flowback, and the majority in the vagina will be dead within 12 h. Whether female orgasm does facilitate sperm retention and the likelihood of fertilization is not yet clear (Levin 2002).] For this reason, men should find intercourse with a lover very exciting and rewarding if this tends to increase the likelihood that their lover will have an orgasm. This biological function of an orgasm in women provides a general reason why men should find it rewarding when a woman has an orgasm (and should therefore try to produce orgasms in women, and be disappointed when they do not occur). This process might be helped if one factor that tended to produce ejaculation in men was knowledge that the woman was having an orgasm. Of course, the reverse may occur – a woman may be triggered to orgasm especially just after she receives an ejaculation, especially if it is from a male with whom (presumably mainly subconsciously) she wishes to conceive. (Indeed, there is evidence that women have orgasms more frequently when they desire to become pregnant (Singh et al. 1998), and with men with an index of healthy genes, low asymmetry (Thornhill et al. 1995, Thornhill and Gangestad 1996).) If she does not have an orgasm, she may fake an orgasm (as this is rewarding to the male), and this may be part of her deception mechanism.

Having now outlined some of the functions at play in sexual behaviour we are in a better position later in this Chapter to consider the brain processes that implement rewards to produce these different types of behaviour.

9.5　Concealed ovulation and its consequences for sexual behaviour

Women, and a few non-human primate species, have concealed ovulation. It is not clear to males, or to themselves, when they are fertile. Why do women conceal their ovulation? Diamond (1997) considers evidence that a first process that occurs in evolution is that promiscuity or harems in the mating system give rise to concealed ovulation. This is the 'many fathers' theory. The concealed ovulation (concealed even from the woman, so that she can deceive better – what might be termed 'deceiving conceiving') – makes sure that men do not know who the father is (because they do not know when ovulation has occurred), and thus will not attack the young. (It frequently occurs in the animal kingdom that males kill their female's children if they have been born of other males, a process that enables genes to maximize their own reproductive potential. This occurs because the female will stop lactating and will come back into a reproductive state so that the new male can reproduce. Moreover, it will minimize potential use of his resources in helping to bring up children without his genes.)

A second process can then occur in evolution: monogamy evolves. Monogamy, Diamond (1997) argues, has never evolved in species that have bold advertisement of ovulation. It usually evolved in species with (i.e. that already have) concealed ovulation – the 'daddy-at-home' theory. The concealed ovulation means that fathers stay at home all the time (and help), because they want to be assured of their paternity; and because they think that they are the father, because they have been at home (Simmen-Tulberg and Moller 1993). Thus the consequences of concealed ovulation may be that fathers find it rewarding (and have emotions about) staying at home with their partner to guard a primarily monogamous relationship. Indeed, monogamy can be thought of as a form of mate guarding.

Consistent with these hypotheses, it has been found that free-living Hanuman langur females do have long periods of receptivity during which the time of ovulation is variable, that there is the opportunity for paternity confusion in that ovulation is concealed from the males, that there is a dominant male who tries to monopolize the females, and that nevertheless non-dominant males father a substantial proportion of the offspring (Heistermann, Ziegler, van Schaik, Launhardt, Winkler and Hodges 2001). This is direct evidence that extended periods of sexual receptivity in catarrhine primates may have evolved as a female strategy to confuse paternity.

Concealed ovulation could also play a role in combination with female orgasm to enable female cryptic choice, which would it has been suggested (see Section 9.4) occur if a woman has an orgasm with a man who she wants to be the father of her children. The contribution of the concealed ovulation would be to promote male-male competition.

Thus the interests of females and males may not be consistent, and this leads to the development of measures and countermeasures. Concealed ovulation can be seen as a protection against infanticide. Concealed ovulation promotes polyandry, and this results in multiple matings, and sperm competition and sperm allocation as a response to this. Females may then counter with mechanisms for cryptic choice, such as for example selective orgasms.

9.6   Sexual selection of sexual and non-sexual behaviour

9.6.1   Sexual selection and natural selection

Darwin (1871) distinguished natural selection from sexual selection, and this distinction has been consolidated and developed (Fisher 1930, Fisher 1958, Zahavi 1975, Hamilton 1964, Hamilton 1996, Dawkins 1986b, Grafen 1990a, Grafen 1990b, Dawkins 1995, Miller 2000). Natural selection can be used in a narrow sense to refer to selection processes that lead to the development of characteristics that have a function of providing adaptive or survival value to an individual so that the individual can reproduce, and pass on its genes. In its narrow sense, natural selection can be thought of as 'survival or adaptation selection'. An example might be a gene or genes that specify that the sensory properties of food should be rewarding (and should taste pleasant) when we are in a physiological need state for food. Many of the reward and punishment systems described in this book deal with this type of reward and punishment decoding that has evolved to enable genes to influence behaviour in directions in a high-dimensional space of rewards and punishments that are adaptive for survival and health of the individual, and thus promote reproductive success or fitness of the genes that build such adaptive functionality. We can include kin-related altruistic behaviours (see Chapter 3) because the behaviour is adaptive in promoting the survival of kin, and thus promoting the likelihood that the kin (who contain one's genes) survive and reproduce. Resources and wealth are also understood as making males attractive and being selected by natural selection, in that the wealth and resources may be useful to the female in bringing up her children.

Darwin (1871) also recognized that evolution can occur by sexual selection, when what is being selected for has no inherent adaptive or survival value, but is attractive to potential mates (inter-sexual selection), or helps in competing with others of the same sex (intra-sexual selection). The most cited example is the peacock's large tail, which does not have survival value for the peacock (and indeed it is somewhat of a handicap to have a very long tail), but, because it is attractive to the peahen, becomes prevalent in the population. Indeed, part of the reason for the long tail being attractive may be that it is an honest signal of phenotypic fitness (or 'fitness indicator'), in that having a very long tail is a handicap to survival (Zahavi 1975), though the signalling system that reveals this only operates correctly if certain conditions apply (Grafen 1990a, Grafen 1990b, Maynard Smith and Harper 2003)[27]. The inherited genes for a long tail may be expressed in the female's sons, and they will accordingly be attractive to

---

[27]The conditions under which a handicap signalling system can lead to sexual selection are i: the female can correctly infer a male's quality from his advertisement (honesty); ii: signals are costly; and iii: a given signal is more costly for a male of low quality.

females in the next generation. Although the female offspring of the mating will not express the male father's attractive long-tail genes, these genes are likely to be expressed in her sons. The female has to evolve to find the characteristic being selected for in males attractive for this situation to lead to a runaway explosion of the characteristic being selected for by the choosiness of females. Indeed, the fact that the female who chose a long-tailed male has children following her mating with genes for liking long-tailed males, and for generating long tails, is part of what leads to the runaway process that can occur with sexual selection. The fact that the long tail is actually a handicap for the peacock, and so is a signal of general physical fitness in the male, may be one way in which sexual selection can occur stably (Zahavi 1975, Grafen 1990a, Grafen 1990b). The peacock tail example is categorized as sexual selection because the long tail is not adaptive to the individual with the long tail, though of course it is adaptive to have a long tail if females are choosing it because it indicates general physical fitness. However, sexual selection can occur when a revealing or index signal or fitness indicator is not associated with a handicap, but is hard to fake, so that it is necessarily an honest fitness indicator (Maynard Smith and Harper 2003). An example occurs in birds that may show bare skin as part of their courtship, providing a sign that they are parasite resistant (Hamilton and Zuk 1982). Handicaps are costly to produce, and should reduce fitness in contexts other than mating. If the signal is an index signal, it is relatively cost-free, cannot be easily faked, and should correlate with some trait that contributes to fitness in contexts other than mating (Maynard Smith and Harper 2003).

Some characteristics of sexual selection that help to separate it from natural or survival selection are as follows:

First, the sexually selected characteristic is sexually dimorphic, with the male typically showing the characteristic. (For example the peacock but not the peahen has the long tail.) This occurs because it is the female who is being choosy, and is selecting males. The female is the choosy one because she has a considerable investment in her offspring, whom she may need to nurture until birth, and then rear until independent, and for this reason has a much more limited reproductive potential than the male, who could in principle father large numbers of offspring to optimize his genetic potential. This is an example of a sexual dimorphism selected by inter-sexual selection. An example of a sexual dimorphism selected by intra-sexual selection is the deer's antlers.

Second, sexually selected characteristics are typically species-specific (consistent with choice by the female of the species of a relatively arbitrary feature in males that may not itself have survival value), whereas naturally selected characteristics may, because they have survival value for individuals, be found in many species within a genus, and even across genera.

Third, and accordingly, the competition is within a species for sexual selection, whereas competition may be across as well as within species for natural (survival) selection.

Fourth, sexual selection operates most efficiently in polygynous species, that is species where some (attractive) males must mate with two or more females, and unattractive males must be more likely to be childless. Polygyny does seem to have been present to at least some extent in our ancestors, as shown for example by body size differences, with males larger than females. This situation is selected because males compete hard with each other in polygynous species compared to monogamous, where there is less competition. In humans, the male is 10% taller, 20% heavier, 50% stronger in the upper body muscles, and 100% stronger in the hand grip strength than the average female (Miller 2000).

Fifth, the sexually selected characteristics are likely to be apparent after but not before puberty. In humans, one possible example is the deep male voice.

Sixth, there may be marked differences between individuals, as it is these differences that are being used for mate choice. In contrast, when natural or survival selection is operating efficiently, there may be little variation between individuals.

Seventh, the fitness indicator should be costly or difficult to produce, as in this way it can reflect real fitness, and be kept honest.

Overall, Darwinian natural or survival selection increases health, strength, and potentially resources, and survival of the individual, and thus ability to mate and reproduce. Inter-sexual sexual selection does not make the individual healthier, but does make the individual more attractive as a mate, as in female choice, an example of intersexual selection. Intrasexual sexual selection does not necessarily help survival of the individual, but does help in competition for a mate, for example in intimidation of one male by another (Darwin 1871, Kappeler and van Schaik 2004). The behaviours and characteristics involved in sperm competition described in this Chapter are produced by intrasexual sexual selection.

It turns out that many of the best examples of inter-sexual sexual selection are in birds (for example the peacock's tail, and the male lyre bird's tail). Some of the examples in birds may be related to the visual system of birds, which is good at identifying sign stimuli and innate releasing stimuli, and this may facilitate the evolution of elaborate displays. (Is the rhesus macaque's red posterior an exception?) In contrast, mammals have a more general-purpose visual system that can recognize objects invariantly, and does not therefore need to specialize in analysing particular low-level sensory features of stimuli (Rolls and Deco 2002). In mammals, including primates, the selection is often by size, strength, physical prowess, and aggressiveness, which provide for direct physical competition, and are examples of intra-sexual selection (Kappeler and van Schaik 2004).

It has been suggested that sexual selection is important for further types of characteristic in humans. For example, it has been suggested that human mental abilities that may be important in courtship such as kindness, humour, and telling stories, are the type of characteristic that may be sexually selected in humans (Miller 2000). Before assessing this (in Section 9.6.2), and illuminating thus some of what may be sexually selected rewards and punishers that therefore contribute to human affective states, we should note a twist in how sexual selection may operate in humans.

In humans, because babies are born relatively immature and may take years of demanding care before they can look after themselves, there is some advantage to male genes of providing at least some parental care for the children. That is, the father may invest in his offspring. In this situation, where there is a male investment, the male may optimize the chance of his genes faring well by being choosy about his wife. The implication is that in humans, sexual selection may be of female characteristics (by males), as well as of male characteristics (by females). This may mean that the differences between the sexes may not be as large as can often be the case with inter-sexual sexual selection, where the female is the main chooser. One example of how sexual selection may affect female characteristics is in the selection for large breasts. These may be selected to be larger in humans than is really necessary for milk production, by the incorporation of additional fat. This characteristic may be attractive to males (and hence produce affective responses in males) because it is a symbol relating to fertility and child rearing potential, and not because large breasts have any particular adaptive value. It has even been suggested that the large breast size makes them useful to males as a sign of reproductive potential, for their pertness is maximal when a (young) woman's fertility and reproductive potential is at its highest. Although large breasts may be less pert with age, and it might thus be thought to be an advantage for women not to have large breasts, it may be possible that this is offset by the advantageous signal of a pert but large breast when fertility and reproductive potential is at its maximal when young, as this may attract high status males (even though there may be disadvantages later) (Miller 2000). Thus it is possible that inter-sexual selection contributes to the large breast size of some women. The fact that the variation is quite large is consistent with this being a sexually selected, not survival-selected, characteristic. Thus sexual selection of characteristics may occur in women as well as in men.

We may also note that the term 'natural selection' encompasses in its broad sense both 'survival or adaptation selection', and sexual selection. Both are processes now understood to be driven by the selection of genes, and it is gene competition and replication into the next generation that is the driving force of biological evolution (Dawkins 1989, Dawkins 1986b). The distinction can be made that with 'survival or adaptation selection', the genes being selected for make the individual animal stronger, healthier, and more likely to survive and reproduce, whereas sexual selection operates by sexual choice selecting for genes that may have little survival value to the individual, but enable the individual to be selected as a mate or to compete for a mate in intra-sexual selection, and thus pass on the genes selected by intra-sexual or inter-sexual selection.

Insofar as the states elicited by rewards and punishers are emotional states (see Chapters 2 and 3), this Chapter thus extends the understanding of emotion to systems shaped by sexual selection. For example, sexual selection may select symmetric and thus attractive faces which may produce emotional states.

9.6.2 Non-sexual characteristics may be sexually selected for courtship

Miller (2000) has developed the hypothesis that courtship provides an opportunity for sexual selection to select non-sexual mental characteristics such as kindness, humour, the ability to tell stories, creativity, art, and even language. He postulates that these are "courtship tools, evolved to attract and entertain sexual partners". Sexual selection views organisms as advertisers of their phenotypic fitness, and Miller sees these characteristics as such signals. From this perspective, hunting is seen as a costly and inefficient exercise (in comparison with food gathering) undertaken by men to obtain small gifts of meat for women, but at the same time to show how competitive and fit the successful hunter is in relation to other men. Conspicuous waste, and conspicuous consumption, are often signs in nature that sexual selection is at work, with high costs for behaviours that seem maladaptive in terms of survival and natural selection in the narrow sense. The mental characteristics described above are not only costly in terms of time, but may rely on many genes operating efficiently for these characteristics to be expressed well, and so, Miller suggests, may be 'fitness indicators'. Consistent with sexual selection, there is also great individual variability in these characteristics, providing a basis for choice.

One mental characteristic that Miller suggests could have evolved in this way is kindness, which is very highly valued by both sexes (Buss 1999, Buss 1994). In human evolution, being kind to the mother's children may have been seen as an attractive characteristic in men during courtship, especially when relationships may not have lasted for many years, and the children might not be those of the courting male. Kindness may also be used as an indicator of future cooperation. In a sense kindness thus may indicate potential useful benefits, consistent with the fact that across cultures human females tend to prefer males who have high social status, good income, ambition, intelligence, and energy (Buss 1999, Buss 1994). Kindness may also be related to kin altruism (Hamilton 1964) or to reciprocal altruism (Trivers 1971), both of which are genetically adaptive strategies (see Chapter 2)[28]. Although the simple interpretation of all these characteristics is that they indicate a good provider and potential material and genetic benefits (and thus would be subject to natural or survival selection), Miller (2000) argues that at least kindness is being used in addition as a fitness indicator and is being sexually selected. Although morality can be related in part to kin and reciprocal altruism (Ridley 1996) (see Section 11.3), moral behaviour may bring reproductive benefits through the social status that it inspires (Zahavi and Zahavi 1997) or by direct mate choice for moralistic displays during courtship (Tessman 1995, Miller 2000). The suggestion made by Miller (2000) is that the status of moral behaviour helps to attract mates, because it may reflect fitness as the moral behaviour may have costs. He suggests that *"Morality is a system of sexually selected handicaps"*.

Miller (2000) (page 258 ff) also suggests that art, language and creativity can be explained by sexual selection, and that they are difficult to account for by survival selection. He suggests that art develops from courtship ornamentation, and uses bowerbirds as an evolutionary example. Male bowerbirds ornament their often enormous and structurally elaborate nests or bowers with mosses, ferns, shells, berries and bark to attract female bowerbirds. The nests are used just to attract females, and after insemination the females go off and build their own cup-shaped nests, lay their eggs, and raise their offspring by themselves with no male support. Darwin himself viewed human ornamentation and clothing as outcomes of sexual selection. Sexual selection for artistic ability does not mean of course that the art itself needs to be about sex. This example helps to show that sexual selection can lead to changes in what is valued and found attractive, in areas that might be precursors to art in humans. Miller (2000) suggests that language evolved as a courtship device in males to attract females. Miller (2000) also suggests that creativity may be related to systems that can explore random new ideas, and also is a courtship device in males to attract females.

One potential problem with this approach is that sexual selection favours fast runaway evolution, because sexual preferences are genetically correlated with the ornaments they favour (as described in section 9.6). Why does mental capacity not develop more rapidly, and with larger sex differences, in humans, if Miller (2000) is right? Why is there not a faster runaway? Miller suggests a number of possible reasons.

1. There is a high genetic correlation between human males and females, with 22/23 chromosomes the same.
2. The female's brain must evolve to be able to appreciate the male's mental adornment – and might even be one step ahead to judge effectively. Further, similar or partly overlapping brain mechanisms may be used to produce (in males) and perceive (in females). In addition, male self-monitoring (and female practice) may help appraisal. Males may even internalize female's appreciation systems, to predict their responses.
3. There is mutual choice in humans: males choose females because human males do make a parental investment; and females compete for males. Indeed, the selection of a long-term partner is mutual, and this tends to reduce sex differences. Consistent with this, David Buss has shown that, in contrast, human sex differences are more evident in short-term mating

[28] Interestingly, the etymology of kindness is Old English cynd, kin, hence looking after kin, relations.

(Buss 1989, Buss 1994, Buss 1999). It is likely in fact that sexual selection works mainly through long-term relationships, because of concealed ovulation in women. This means that only in a relatively long-term relationship is it likely that a man will become the father of a woman's child, because only if he mates with her regularly is there a reasonable probability that he will hit her fertile time.

Another criticism of the approach of Miller (2000) is that many of these characteristics may have survival value, and are not purely sexually selected. For example, language has many uses in problem solving, planning ahead, and correcting multiple step plans which are likely to be very important to enable immediate rewards to be deferred, and longer term goals to be achieved (see Chapter 10, and Pinker (1997)).

9.7 Individual differences in sexual rewards

Before considering how biological reward systems might have evolved in order to implement the types of behaviours just described, we first consider possible individual differences in these types of sexual behaviour, because these have implications for how the reward systems may differ in different individuals to produce these differences in sexual behaviour. We remind ourselves that genetic specification of different reward mechanisms could produce a polymorphic, fixed, evolutionarily stable strategy, as described in the first footnote of this Chapter on page 358. An alternative mechanism is a conditional strategy (see the same footnote), which can also be evolutionarily stable (Maynard Smith 1984). In many of the examples discussed here, it is not clear which is the more likely. We should also note that many factors are likely to produce differences between the emotional behaviour of males and females. For example, in many species, females are attracted to dominant males, thus further favouring male competitiveness. Further, females may be attracted to males favoured by other women. Both might be accounted for by their predictive relation to producing genetically successful male offspring.

In addition, when considering individual differences in sexual behaviour, it is important to remember that conditional mating strategies may be employed (Gangestad and Simpson 2000, Buss 1999). For example, physical factors such as high symmetry that are indicators of genetic fitness may be especially attractive when women choose short-term partners, and factors such as resources and faithfulness may be especially important when women choose long-term partners. Indeed, because of conditional strategies, the choices made in different situations or contexts may be quite dynamical. To a considerable extent differences between individuals may reflect different weightings given to different rewards (benefits) and punishers (costs) by different individuals, so that the behaviour on any one occasion (e.g. promiscuous vs faithful) may reflect how each of these rewards and punishers operate in a given context. Thus different individuals might tend to act in the different ways described below based on the values of a number of reward and punishment factors in a multidimensional (partly gene-specified) space, but should not be thought of as being simply of one type or another.

9.7.1 Overview

Is the range of stimuli and situations related to sexual behaviour that different people find rewarding different, and can any differences be related to a biological function such as sperm warfare? It is plausible that there are such differences, and that they could be related to sperm warfare. Although experimental data on this issue in relation to an underlying function such as sperm competition are not yet available, the possibilities are sufficiently plausible that they are worth elaborating, in part as a guide to stimulating further concepts and experimental research in this area.

A hypothesis that seems plausible is that some individuals might be of the type that would specialize in sperm warfare. Such individuals might find especially rewarding the types of stimuli that would make them especially successful in sperm warfare, and their resulting behaviour might reflect the stimuli they find most rewarding. If men, they might be built to find variety in sexual partners especially rewarding, and to be ambitious and competitive. This could increase their fitness, by enabling them potentially to have many children with different women. A risk of this 'unfaithful' strategy, which would tend to keep it in check, is that the man might make insufficient investment in helping any of his lovers and her children by him to ensure that the children flourish and themselves reproduce successfully. Women might avoid such men if they were not already in receipt of sufficient resources to provide for their children, and the partners of such women might require that they be faithful, even to the extent of guarding them. Such 'unfaithful' individuals, who would be likely to specialize in sperm warfare, if women, might be unfaithful and as a result be fit if they had a tendency to choose genetically fit men to be the father of their children, while at the same time having as a partner to help bring up the children another man who was not necessarily as genetically fit as their lover, but would help to bring up the children. For this to be an evolutionarily stable strategy, it might be expected that at least some of the children would be children of the partner, otherwise the deception might be too obvious. Part of the risk of this strategy, which keeps it in balance with others in the population, is that if her deception is discovered, the woman risks losing the resources being provided for her and her children by her partner. Too great a tendency to unfaithfulness would also be unstable because of the associated risks of sexually transmitted disease.

Other individuals in the population might be genetically predisposed to use a different strategy, of being faithful to their partner. This could benefit a faithful woman's genes, because her children would have a partner who could be relied on to help bring up the children, and put all his resources into this (because he would be sure that his genes were in the children, and because he would not be tempted by other women). (In addition, he might not be very attractive or successful in life, and might not have the opportunity to be tempted away.) Her fitness would be increased by the fact that her children would be likely to survive, but reduced by the fact that the genes with which she has mated would not be as advantageous, and nor would she benefit from the effect of pure variety of genes with which to combine her own, which is part of the advantage of sexual reproduction. There could also be an advantage to a man's genes for him to be faithful, because in being faithful he would be less likely to catch a disease, and would be more likely to put sufficient resources into his children to ensure that they have a good start in life; and would be more likely to attract a faithful woman as his partner, so that the children in whom he invested would be more likely to be his. The cost of this strategy would be that he might have fewer children than if he were unfaithful, and his children might, if the behaviour is controlled genetically, be less likely themselves to have large numbers of children, because they would not be likely to be the unfaithful type.

It is suggested that these different strategies, because each has associated advantages and costs, could be retained in a stable balance in populations in which genetic factors at least partly predisposed the individual to be of the unfaithful or faithful type[29]. Of course, in a real human population it might be expected that there would be continuous variation between individuals in the tendency to be faithful or unfaithful, and for the actual range of differences found in a population to be being constantly adjusted depending on the fitness of the different types of strategy, and on the environment too, such as the availability of resources (see the first footnote of this Chapter on page 358). (The availability of resources could affect the balance. For example, if food and other resources were readily available, so that the advantage of care by both parents was less than in more harsh environments in which perhaps the man might be specialized for hunting, then the relative advantages of unfaithfulness in the population would be higher.)

The two contrasted phenotypes might be kept in stable balance by the advantages of extra-pair copulations such as more reproductive success for males and more fit genes for females, and the advantages of not having extra-pair copulations such as being less likely to be cheated on oneself while one is away not mateguarding (if a male) and of losing resources if detected (if a female) (Simmons et al. 2004).

Evidence that genetic factors do actually influence the likelihood of infidelity comes from the finding of what might be called a 'promiscuity gene' (Hamer and Copeland 1998). The research (conducted at the National Institutes of Cancer in Washington) has so far been conducted in men, but there could be a parallel in women. Very interestingly in relation to the points made about dopamine and reward in this book, the gene affects the D4 dopamine receptor (DRD4), and in particular it comes in a long form or a short form. Approximately 30% of men in the study carried the long form of the gene, and they were likely to have 20% more sexual partners than those with the short form. Men with the long form were likely to have an average of 10 sexual partners in their lifetime, whereas those with the short form were less likely to have sought such variety. In a more recent study, it was found that two aspects of novelty seeking, exploratory excitability and impulsiveness, were higher in humans with the long form of the DRD4 gene (Keltikangas-Jarvinen, Elovainio, Kivimaki, Lichtermann, Ekelund and Peltonen 2003), though it must be noted that this effect was not substantiated in a meta-analysis (Kluger, Siegfried and Ebstein 2002), and in any case is infrequent and would not account for much of the variation found overall in the population. Hamer and colleagues also described a gene that influences sex drive that is different to that for promiscuity. This is a serotonin (i.e. 5-hydroxytryptamine)-related gene which influences anxiety (Greenberg, Li, Lucas, Hu, Sirota, Benjamin, Lesch, Hamer and Murphy 2000). Men with the high anxiety form of this gene had more frequent sex, and those with the calm, happy and optimistic form had less sex. These findings are starting to show that genetic approaches may provide an important type of support for the suggestion made in this Chapter that different strategies for sexual behaviour, and in particular a strategy to be faithful vs a strategy to be unfaithful, could be influenced at least in part by genes.

Next we will consider how natural selection (in the broad sense, including sexual selection) might make different types of stimuli differently rewarding to different people in order to produce these different types of behaviour. This will just be a possible scenario, because I know of little actual evidence on this. Then we will consider what such evidence might look like when it does become available.

---

[29]Richard Dawkins (1976) described a stable situation of this type with faithful and philanderer males, and coy and fast females.

9.7.2 How might different types of behaviour be produced by natural selection altering the relative reward value of different stimuli in different individuals?

We will consider what could occur hypothetically in different types of women, predisposed to be unfaithful and faithful, and in different types of men, predisposed to be unfaithful and faithful, for clarity. We remember that in practice there would be likely to be a continuous distribution of these differences in a human population. (We note that in addition to the two types of evolutionarily stable strategy outlined in first footnote of this Chapter on page 358, the different behaviours do not have to be equally successful. One type of behaviour might just be 'making the best of a bad job'.)

First we consider women who might be genetically predisposed to be unfaithful and promote sperm warfare. (Sometimes the shorthand used for this is 'unfaithful woman', but this should always be taken to mean 'genetically predisposed to be an unfaithful woman'.) We might suppose that they should be especially attractive to men, and may therefore tend to be youthful-looking and thin, to indicate that they are at a fertile period of their lives, and are not already pregnant. They should not be shy, might be extravert, and might be flirtatious in order to attract men. They should like (sexually) aggressive men (because this is an indicator that her sons with him would pass on her genes to women that they were able to take as lovers). They might even like a man aggressive to other men as in war, because in war his genes (potentially in his children with her) will tend to survive and to be passed on, and he will be a potential protection in war. Women with genes predisposing them to be unfaithful might be attracted to men with a 'reputation' – because this also indicates that they will produce sons who are good at passing on (her) genes; should be good at finding a partner for stability, to bring up her children, but also good at deceiving him; should like men with large testes (which could correlate with testosterone levels, and thus perhaps be indicated by secondary sexual characteristics such as body hair); should like men with a large penis (because this would be good at sperm warfare by sucking out other men's sperm, and thus is an indicator of genetic fitness in sperm warfare); should be able to assess men for sexual fitness, not necessarily fast but by evaluating his position in society, power, wealth, and bodily fitness (one index of which is the shape of the buttocks which may reflect running ability). She might herself be sexually aggressive, because it is important (in terms of fitness) that when she takes risks and is unfaithful, she chooses the right man, with genes that will make her children fit, and does not choose just any man. She might also be likely to control sexual behaviour, rather than be passive – she wants to control whether and when (in relation to whether she is fertile) a man impregnates her, and if and when in relation to his ejaculation she has an orgasm. (She might, for example, choose to have intercourse with a fit lover especially when she is most fertile, and to orgasm soon after him. She might choose to have intercourse with her partner at other times, and either not to have an orgasm, or to orgasm before he does, to prevent upsuck. For this reason, and partly to please her partner, she might fake her orgasms.) She might be especially attracted to novel men, and indeed might need some element of novelty to make her have an orgasm and thus be likely to conceive. In this respect, she should be built to be continually searching for something better. She might also for this reason, because it is advantageous to her to control when and with whom she has orgasms, appear to need more stimulation to have an orgasm, and be especially likely to have orgasms with novel men or in novel situations. She may also tend to reproduce young, because of the risk of disease. Such an unfaithful woman, because of the risk that her deception might be discovered, might use her attractiveness to make relationships with a number of men, and have backup policies with several men, as insurance and support for her young.

Second, we consider women whose genes might have built them to be faithful. She might be less attractive, and once with a partner might take fewer steps to be attractive (she might not be thin, and might be less worried about her weight; she might be less concerned with cosmetics and might dress sensibly rather than provocatively). She might be reliable, looking for domestic security (to provide reliable resources for her and her children, as she has chosen to put her resources into bringing up her children well, rather than taking risks and possibly having genetically more fit children with a lover but risking the support for all her children). She might be relatively passive during intercourse, and not try to control sex (because with only one male, she does not need to control whether/when a male ejaculates in her, and if/when she orgasms). Partly for this reason, she might find it relatively easy to have orgasms, because she does not need to control who fertilizes her, and because orgasms (associated with oxytocin release, see Section 9.2) might promote attachment to the (same) partner. Multiple orgasms in this situation could help, though they might be especially useful if the woman was 'trying' to conceive. The main prediction here is that orgasms would be much more consistent (either present or not) than in women genetically predisposed to be unfaithful. The woman genetically predisposed to be faithful might tend to reproduce older, because she has less risk of disease. She might be shy, could be introvert, and might be expected not to be a flirtatious type. She should make very stable relationships with friends in a supporting society (to ensure care of her young, a high priority to her, and to listen to gossip, to learn of potentially threatening males or females). She should disapprove of women with a reputation, as they are a threat to her security, e.g. by attracting her partner and thus threatening her resources.

Some evidence consistent with these hypotheses is that promiscuity is correlated with personality, in particular with extraversion, and with low conscientiousness and agreeableness (Schmitt 2004). These findings were made in a study involving 16,362 participants from 52 nations whose personality was measured by questionnaire on the Big Five personality dimensions, and on Relationship Exclusivity, which has two sub-components, Relationship Infidelity (identified by the items 'adulterous', 'not devoted', 'not faithful', 'not monogamous', 'polygamous', and 'unfaithful'), and Sexual Promiscuity (identified by the items 'loose' and 'promiscuous'). Impulsiveness may be an underlying characteristic, as impulsive sensation seeking is most closely related within the Big Five to low conscientiousness and agreeableness, and the strongest correlate of risky sexual behaviour is impulsive sensation-seeking (Zuckerman 1994, Hoyle, Fejfar and Miller 2000, Zuckerman and Kuhlman 2000). In a link to brain mechanisms, it has been found that humans with orbitofrontal cortex damage are impulsive (Berlin, Rolls and Kischka 2004, Berlin and Rolls 2004, Berlin, Rolls and Iversen 2005). Relationship infidelity was associated with low conscientiousness and agreeableness, that is, again with impulsive sensation seeking.

Men genetically predisposed to be unfaithful and to participate in sperm warfare might be built by their genes as follows. First, at the simple physical level, they might have large testes and a large penis, both good in sperm warfare (see above). Second, they should be successful with other women, as this indicates how well a woman's sons with them would pass her genes on to future generations. (This could be 'why' some women are interested in a man's reputation, and why this could help to make a man attractive.) These men could be competitive and aggressive (both sexually and in war, see above); have high testosterone (possibly indicated by bodily hair and other secondary sexual characteristics); be ambitious, wealthy, successful and powerful (because these indicate potential to provide resources); possibly creative, intellectual, musical, etc. because these may be ways to keep women interested, and may be used in courtship. (There is the suggestion that women are selecting men's brains to be good at courtship, so that a man's brain would parallel a peacock's 'tail', see Ridley (1993b) and Miller (2000); and if so, this selection might be particularly evident in unfaithful men.) Such men might also be good at deceit, as this would be an advantage in deception of their partner and their lover's partner.

Men genetically predisposed to be faithful might have smaller testes and penes on average; and have lower concentrations of testosterone and be less aggressive, and even possibly less ambitious. They should be less interested in and attracted by women other than their partner, that is they should be built less to keep searching for novelty; they should be stable, reliable, good at providing a home, and truthful, all of which would appeal to a woman genetically predisposed to be faithful. He should denounce men (or women) with a reputation, because they, and that type of behaviour, are a threat to him, given that he is inclined to make his major investment in one woman, and it is to his genes' advantage that the children he helps to bring up are his.

9.7.3   How being tuned to different types of reward could help to produce individual differences in sexual behaviour

Given the hypotheses discussed in Section 9.7.2 [and they are of course only hypotheses, although personality differences related to promiscuity are now being identified (Schmitt 2004)], it is now possible to ask how differences in sexual behaviour might be produced by genes influencing the different types of stimulation and situation that different individuals find rewarding. (We remember that an alternative to a polymorphic fixed ESS is a conditional strategy, see first footnote of this Chapter on page 358. A conditional strategy might not alter what would be found inherently rewarding, but might alter how different types of reward were perceived.) As above, when the term 'unfaithful man or woman' is used, it is simply shorthand for the description 'man or woman predisposed to be unfaithful'.

1. Unfaithful women could be built to find external (relative to internal) stimulation of the genitals particularly necessary for reward, because this helps them to control impregnation.

2. Unfaithful women could be built to need much (external and sometimes adventurous and novel) stimulation to produce enough reward/pleasure for them to orgasm. (This would be part of the control of the impregnation process, making it particularly likely that they would have an orgasm and facilitate fertilization with a lover, who would probably be more novel than a regular partner. It would also be part of the mechanism that would encourage them to keep searching for something better, because some novelty would tend to be arousing.)

3. It is possible that sensory-specific satiety, a reduction in sexual desire for a particular person with whom intercourse has just taken place, relative to other men, would be more pronounced in unfaithful women, as a mechanism to facilitate searching for new genes, and sperm competition.

4. Unfaithful women could be built to like control, both of whether and when sex occurs with a particular man, and during sex, partly by requiring particular types of stimulation (novel and external), and perhaps partly by making control per se rewarding and important to them.

5. Unfaithful women could be built to find social interactions, sometimes flirtatious and provocative, including clothes, cosmetics etc., with men (and with novel men perhaps especially), particularly rewarding, as a mechanism to attract and obtain potential lovers.

6. Unfaithful women could tend to be smaller, with oestrogen-dependent features such as wide eyes and a small lower face, to keep their bodies in trim, and to age less than faithful women, in order to attract males with fit genes. In fact, sexual dimorphism should be especially pronounced in those predisposed to be unfaithful.

7. In a complementary way, women predisposed to be faithful could be tuned to internal vs external stimulation during intercourse, to need less stimulation and particularly less novel stimulation to have an orgasm, to show less sensory-specific satiety for the partner, to be more passive rather than controlling before and during sex, and to be less socially provocative.

8. In a corresponding way, men predisposed to be unfaithful might be tuned to find it rewarding to produce an orgasm in women (because this is a way to facilitate the chances of their sperm in a sperm war), and therefore be willing to work hard for this; to find vigorous thrusting during intercourse particularly rewarding (to serve the biological function of increasing their chances in sperm competition); to be especially attracted to attractive, novel, and interactive women (to serve the biological function of finding genes able to produce fit daughters who will themselves attract males); and to not be satisfied for long with the same situation, but continually be searching for new relationships and lovers.

9. Partial reinforcement (i.e. only sometimes giving a reinforcer or reward) by an unfaithful woman should be greatly reinforcing to an unfaithful man (beyond the normal partial reinforcement effect, which itself increases the amount a person will work for a reward), because this is a test of how motivated and successful the man is to pass on his genes, a quality that the unfaithful woman will value for her sons. The unfaithful woman may even titrate the partial reinforcement level to see just how persistent, and thus potentially fit, the man is.

It may be emphasized that the reward processes that have just been described might be those to which different people are predisposed, and probably operate primarily through an implicit or unconscious system for rewards. In addition to this implicit system with its predispositions, humans have an explicit processing system which can of course influence the actual choice that is made (see Chapter 10).

9.8 The neural reward mechanisms that might mediate some aspects of sexual behaviour

In Section 9.4 sociobiological research on sexual behaviour was described. In Section 9.7 we speculated about possible individual differences in such sexual behaviour. In both these sections we produced hypotheses about how genes might influence sexual behaviour by building particular reward systems and mechanisms into animals. We now consider how the brain might implement these different reward processes. Might there be a few principles of operation of the brain reward systems that could help to account for the quite complex sexual behaviour that is apparent in humans? How are these mechanisms implemented neurophysiologically in the brain? We consider what is known on these issues in this Section. Although the actual brain mechanisms are not fully worked out, the intention of the approach being taken here is to suggest what could be implemented in the brain mechanisms that provide the rewards for sexual behaviour, to guide future research and thinking.

Examples of quite simple neurophysiological rules and processes that could govern the operation of reward mechanisms for sexual behaviour and that could account for many of the effects discussed above are given next.

1. Olfactory rewards and pheromones. Pheromones, which are typically olfactory stimuli, can trigger a number of different types of sexual behaviour, and thus either affect what is rewarding, or in some cases can act as rewards (Dulac and Torello 2003, Beauchamp and Yamazaki 2003).

First, pheromones can produce slow and long-lasting effects by influencing hormones, affecting for example reproductive cycles. They produce the Lee-Boot effect, in which the oestrous cycles of female mice housed together without a male slow down and eventually stop. They act in the Whitten effect, in which the mice start cycling again if they are exposed to the odour of a male or his urine. They act in the Vandenbergh effect, the acceleration in the onset of puberty in a female rodent caused by the odour of a male. They act in the Bruce effect, in which if a recently impregnated female mouse encounters a male mouse other than the one with which she mated, the pregnancy is very likely to fail. The new male can then mate with her. This form of genetic warfare happening after the sperm-warfare stage is clearly to the advantage of the new male's genes, and presumably to the advantage of the female's genes, because it means that her pregnancies will tend to be with males who are not only able to oust other males, but are with males who are with her, so that her offspring will not be harmed by the new male, and may even be protected. The pheromones that produce these effects are produced in males under the influence of testosterone (see Carlson (2004)). These effects depend on an accessory olfactory system, the vomeronasal organ and its projections to the accessory olfactory bulb. The accessory olfactory bulb in turn projects to the medial nucleus of the amygdala, which in turn projects to the preoptic area, anterior hypothalamus, and ventromedial hypothalamus, and these pheromonal effects are produced by influences on hormones such as luteinizing hormone (LH) and prolactin (PRL) (Dulac and Torello 2003). Pheromones can cause groups of women housed together to start cycling together. The evolutionary significance of the synchronized cycling might be to increase male–male competition and selection. In addition, shared care may be facilitated by synchronized breeding, and this could increase the survival of the offspring.

Second, pheromones can act as attracting or rewarding signals, and rapidly influence behaviour. For example, pheromones present in the vaginal secretions of hamsters attract males. In some monkeys, bacteria in the vagina produce more of a pheromone under the influence of an androgen (male sex hormone) produced in small quantities in the adrenal glands, and this pheromone increases the attractiveness of the female to the male (Baum et al. 1977). (In this case, male sexual behaviour is induced by a male hormone produced in females.) Male rats also produce pheromones, which are attractive to females. In humans, body odours are not generally described as attractive, but there is a whole industry based on perfume, the odour of a mate may become attractive by conditioning, and there is some evidence that androstenol, a substance found in the underarm sweat of males especially, may increase the number of social interactions that women have with men (Cowley and Brooksbank 1991). In humans, it has been reported that a putative female pheromone oestra-1,3,5,(10),16-tetraen-3ol-acetate (EST) activates the male anterior medial thalamus and right inferior frontal gyrus at concentrations that cannot be detected consciously (Sobel, Prabhakaran, Hartley, Desmond, Glover, Sullivan and Gabrieli 1999). It has also been reported that androstadien-3-one, a putative male pheromone, activates the preoptic area in women. Conversely, EST activates the hypothalamus in men. Both activate cortical olfactory areas in both men and women (Savic 2002, Savic 2001, Savic, Berglund, Gulyas and Roland 2001).

There is interesting recent research showing that pheromones act through the vomeronasal system, though this system appears to be vestigial and disconnected in humans and Old World monkeys (such as macaques) (Dulac and Torello 2003, Meredith 2001). The vomeronasal system in rodents includes receptors in a specialized organ in the nose that connect to the accessory olfactory bulb, and utilize a set of genes that specify approximately 293 types of V1R and 100 types of V2R olfactory pheromone receptor (Dulac and Torello 2003). Pheromones that activate these receptors are involved in behaviours in rodents such as (with the pheromone 2-sec-butyl-4,5-dihydrothiazole produced by male mice) inducing oestrus in females, inter-male aggression, and attracting females (Dulac and Torello 2003). Monti-Bloch and colleagues (Monti-Bloch, Jennings-White, Dolberg and Berliner 1994, Monti-Bloch, Jennings-White and Berliner 1998, Berliner, Monti-Bloch, Jennings-White and Diaz-Sanchez 1996) applied what they termed 'vomeropherins' to the vomeronasal system while they recorded negative potentials from the (probably vestigial) human vomeronasal organ. They found vomeropherins that activated the vomeronasal organ but not the olfactory epithelium. Conversely, conventional odourants activated the olfactory epithelium but not the vomeronasal organ. Interestingly, males and females were sensitive to different vomeropherins. In men, the vomeropherin pregna-4,20-diene-3,6-dione (PDD) in concentrations of 5×10^{-9} M activated the vomeronasal organ and reduced luteinizing-hormone pulsatility and levels, and follicle-stimulating hormone (FSH) pulsatility. The pheromone also reduced respiratory frequency, increased cardiac frequency, and produced changes in electrodermal activity and the EEG (electroencephalogram). No significant effects of this pheromone were produced in women. In women (but not in men) the vomeropherins PH56 and PH94B activated the vomeronasal organ, and increased electrodermal activity, skin temperature, and alpha-cortical (EEG) activity. These findings raise interesting possibilities requiring much further exploration about the function of the human vomeronasal organ and accessory olfactory system, including potential roles in acting as a reward, or in influencing reward systems. One factor though is that in humans the vomeronasal organ may be vestigial and not connected to the brain (Dulac and Torello 2003). Another is that most of the genes in humans that should produce accessory olfactory system pheromone receptors are pseudogenes[30], so that no receptors can be produced, with only 5 of the V1R pheromone genes believed not to be inactivated in humans (Dulac and Torello 2003). It appears that pheromonal effects in humans may be produced through the main olfactory system.

In a different line of research, it has been suggested that another way in which animals including humans respond to some pheromones as rewards or as aversive stimuli could be a molecular mechanism for producing genetic diversity by influencing those who are considered attractive as mates (Dulac and Torello 2003, Jacob, McClintock, Zelano and Ober 2002, Potts 2002, Beauchamp and Yamazaki 2003). In particular, major histocompatibility complex (MHC)-dependent abortion and mate choice, based on olfaction, can maintain MHC diversity, and probably functions both to avoid genome-wide inbreeding and produce

---

[30]A pseudogene is a DNA sequence that is related to a functional gene but cannot be transcribed owing to mutational changes or the lack of regulatory sequences.

MHC-heterozygous offspring with increased immune responsiveness (Eggert, Holler, Luszyk, Muller-Ruchholtz and Ferstl 1996, Apanius, Penn, Slev, Ruff and Potts 1997, Potts 2002, Penn and Potts 1998, Potts, Manning and Wakeland 1991, Beauchamp and Yamazaki 2003, Jacob et al. 2002). Each individual has approximately 50 MHC genes, each with 500 alleles (different possible types, one instance of which is provided by each parent). These genes are involved in the process by which a cell infected with an antigen (from a virus or bacterium) displays short peptide sequences of it at the cell surface, and the T lymphocytes of the immune system then recognize the fragment, and build an antibody to it. This MHC gene system must maintain great diversity to help detect uncommon antigens, with an advantage arising from mating with an individual with different MHC genes. At least some of the MHC genes are very closely associated with gene-specified pheromone receptors, with individual pheromone receptor cells often expressing one or a few MHC genes in a complex with specific V2R-specified receptors (Dulac and Torello 2003). In addition, for this system to work, the MHC-linked pheromone receptor must be linked to a genetically coded pathway that passes through the brain as far as the stage at which behavioural preferences are generated; and the MHC genes must specify the odours being produced. The system is very sensitive, in that if a mutation occurs in one of the MHC genes, this produces a discriminably different odour to a mouse (Schaefer, Yamazaki, Osada, Restrepo and Beauchamp 2002). In another example, the MHC type of a foetus is evident in the smell emanating from the (mouse) mother by half term (Beauchamp and Yamazaki 2003). It has been speculated that this may help a male to know whether he is the father of the baby, which can be useful to the male in a mixed mating situation. In an example from humans, odour1 'pheromones' from T shirts are rated as pleasant by Hutterite women if one or more (compared to the more typical zero) of the MHC genes of the stranger who produced the odour on the T shirt matches a paternal MHC gene of the woman making the rating (Jacob et al. 2002). This is in contrast to most studies in rodents, in which diversity was preferred. However, in the rodent studies, what was being preferred was some diversity against a background of many similar MHC genes. Putting the different studies together, the rule may be to have a preference to avoid mating with individuals with very similar MHC profiles (to help produce diverse MHC immune systems), but to prefer some similarity compared to none (to help minimize outbreeding costs (Bateson 1983, Ochoa and Jaffe 1999) and to preserve immunocompetence (Penn and Potts 1998)). It may be that these pheromone-like effects in humans are produced by receptors in the main olfactory system (Schaefer, Young and Restrepo 2001).

2. The attractiveness, reward value, and beauty of women to men is determined by a number of factors to which the brain must be sensitive (Buss 1989, Buss 1999, Barrett et al. 2002, Thornhill and Gangestad 1996, Betzig 1997). One factor is a low waist-to-hip ratio. Waist-to-hip ratio in women correlates negatively with oestrogen, age, fertility, and health, and positively with age. Low waist-to-hip ratios (0.6–0.7) in women are maximally attractive to men. One of the obvious ways in which a low ratio indicates fertility is that it will reflect whether the woman is pregnant. It may be partly because of the biologically relevant signals given by a low waist-to-hip ratio that thinness and dieting are rewarding, and this may even be selecting for a small body build in women. Other indicators with similar biological signalling functions that are therefore rewarding to men and make women attractive include a youthful face (sometimes almost a baby face, with a small nose); slow ageing; symmetry (because symmetry is reduced by environmental insults, e.g. parasites and toxins, and genetic disruptions such as mutations and inbreeding, and so reflects fitness); smooth unblemished

skin; etc. All these signals of attractiveness and beauty might be selected for particularly in women predisposed to be unfaithful (because they must attract genetically fit men as lovers, even if they cannot have them as partners). Sexual restraint in women could make them attractive to men because this implies chastity and thus protection of the potential investment of a man in bringing up putatively his children with that woman. In addition, the relative reward value of different signals may vary as a function of the environment. Women who perceive that they are in an environment where men are not likely to invest, act and dress in a more sexually provocative manner, and use copulation to attract desirable men. That is, women may be designed to show sexual restraint (thus giving cues of paternity reliability) when investing males may be accessible, and less sexual restraint (to access material benefits) when each male can or will invest little.

An implication for brain mechanisms is that all these factors that reflect attractiveness, which include information from face analysis, must be used in the brain to determine reward value. Part of this process is reflected in the greater activation found to attractive than unattractive faces in the medial orbitofrontal cortex (O'Doherty et al. 2003b).

3. The attractiveness of men is influenced by their power, status in society, wealth, and ambition as a predictor of these (Buss 1999). These factors are rewarding and attractive to women because they are an indication of the resources that can be provided by the man for the woman, to help bring up her children to maturity and reproduction. Aggressiveness and competitiveness with other men, and domination and success with other women, may be attractive because they indicate fitness (in terms of genetic potential) of the man's genes, and thus of hers in their children. (Aggression and competitiveness in men can thus be ascribed to women's choice.) Physical factors such as symmetry, firm buttocks and a muscular build also make men attractive to women because they serve as biological signals of health and fertility, and also possibly because they indicate that such men can cope well despite the 'handicap' of a high level of testosterone, which suppresses the immune system. These factors are reviewed by Buss (1999); Buss (1989); Barrett et al. (2002); Thornhill and Gangestad (1996); and in the articles in Betzig (1997). To a woman predisposed to be faithful, indicators of a man's potential parental investment in her children as indicated by caring, stability, and lack of reputation should make a man attractive.

The operation of some of these factors can be understood in terms of a parental investment model. The parental investment model implies that the sex investing more (most commonly the female) will be most choosy; whereas the sex investing least (most commonly the male) should be most competitive (Kenrick, DaSadalla, Groth and Trost 1990). High male parental investment in humans contrasts with most other mammalian species. So the above may be less true of humans. The result is that when one measures patterns for what makes a stranger attractive, they are like those of other mammals; whereas when one measures what makes a long-term partner attractive, more similar selectivity should be found between males and females – that is, the requirements for marriage (high investment) are much more stringent than for dating (low investment), and the balance may shift under these conditions from males selecting females mainly on attractiveness to males selecting females as partners who will be faithful and protect their investment (Kenrick et al. 1990).

4. Repeated thrusting and withdrawal of the penis during intercourse should be rewarding to the man (and possibly also to the woman), because it serves the biological function (in sperm warfare) of helping to remove from the vagina sperm that could remain from previous

intercourse, possibly with another male, for up to 12 h. If the only aim was to deposit semen in the vagina, then there would be little point in this repeated thrusting and withdrawal, which typically occurs in males 100–500 times during intercourse in humans (see Baker and Bellis (1995)). An implication for brain reward systems is that stimulation of the glans and of the shaft of the penis should be rewarding, but should only bring the man to ejaculate after a reasonable number of thrust and withdrawal cycles have been completed. Humans may emphasize this design feature, in that many more cycles are completed before ejaculation than in many other species such as macaques (and rats, an example of a species in which the male will ejaculate as soon as the hard cervical plug from previous copulation is removed).

5. Correspondingly, if the woman is to take advantage of the sperm retention effect she can use with a new lover, she should not be brought to orgasm by the first thrust or two, but only after the greater part of the thrusting has been completed should she be likely to be brought to orgasm. The woman may actually facilitate this process, by tightening her vagina during most of the thrusting (which would help the potential sperm-removal effect of the thrusting and withdrawal), and relaxing it later on during intercourse, soon before she has an orgasm. If she does have this relaxation later on, this would make it less likely that when the male ejaculates he would remove his own sperm if he keeps moving for a short time, or that she would expel his sperm by muscular contractions.

6. After ejaculation in a woman, a man's thrusting movements should no longer be rewarding (or he would tend to suck out his own sperm), and the penis should shrink quite soon and withdraw slowly so as not to suck out sperm. Moreover, he should not feel like intercourse with that woman for 30–45 min (as that is the time period within which significant amounts of his sperm remain in the vagina, before the flowback). Thus when it occurs after ejaculation, satiety should be rapid, strong, and last for at least the next 30–45 min in men. The reward that rubbing the penis has before ejaculation is described as turning rapidly to being unpleasant or even painful after ejaculation, and this switch from pleasure to pain is what would be predicted by the biological function being performed. That this switch may not be a simple switch controlled only by whether the neural circuitry has recently produced ejaculation is that introduction of a new female (in many animals and in humans) may enable the whole circuitry to be reset, resulting in rapid re-erection, re-initiation of thrusting movements, and the reward or pleasure associated with rubbing the penis, and eventually in ejaculation again in the new female. The adaptive value of this novelty effect (sometimes known as the Coolidge effect after a remark made by President Coolidge of the United States[31]) in potentially enhancing fitness is clear. The sperm competition hypothesis might predict that intercourse with the man's partner would only need to become very rewarding again within about four days, as by this time the woman would need 'topping up' with his sperm (Baker and Bellis 1995).

7. The rapid speed of a first ejaculation by a man into a woman, and the slow last one (which could be useful in conditions such as promiscuous mating, see Baker (1996)) could be due to the satiety mechanism having a longer time-course each time it is successively activated, perhaps as a result of some neural adaptation of the reward relative to the aversive aspects of

[31] The story is that Calvin Coolidge and his wife were touring a farm when Mrs Coolidge asked the farmer whether the continuous and vigorous sexual activity among the flock of hens was the work of only one rooster. The reply was yes. "You might point that out to Mr Coolidge", she said. The President then asked the farmer whether a different hen was involved each time. The answer, again, was yes. "You might point that out to Mrs Coolidge", he said.

the stimulation. This could be related to a sensory-specific satiety effect, which would need to be specific to the mate, and to the mating opportunities available.

8. We would predict that it should be rewarding to a man to induce an orgasm in a woman, because of its (probably not consciously realized or intended) biological function of increasing the likelihood, at least under conditions of sperm warfare, that conception of his child would occur. (Such an unconscious function could be a factor that might contribute to the reward value in both men and women of sex without a condom.)

9. In women, orgasm should be particularly likely to occur under conditions when they 'want' (perhaps subconsciously) to conceive, and this does appear to be the case (Singh et al. 1998). For this biological function, particularly in women predisposed to be unfaithful and therefore possibly trying to manipulate using sperm warfare which person they are impregnated by, orgasm might generally be difficult; might not always be stimulated to occur with the regular partner; might be more likely to occur with the lover; and with the lover might be especially stimulated by his ejaculation so that the upsuck effect for his sperm occurs optimally. Neurophysiological predictions are that the reward systems in unfaithful women might (relative to those in faithful women) be less easily activated, but particularly stimulated by novelty, especially by a novel man with genes perceived to be fit. Indeed, women predisposed to be unfaithful may find variety in sex, and sexual adventurousness, especially rewarding. They may always need something new, because they are built to always be looking for better sexual and related stimulation – because this predicts how fit their sons will be. This may extend to the courtship battle, which some believe may have played a role in the rapid evolution of the human brain (see Ridley (1993b)). The argument is that the most creative brains intellectually, musically, and artistically will be successful in having many children with women, because they can provide the variety that unfaithful women are predisposed to want — the variety of all sorts of stimulation is needed to keep an unfaithful woman interested in continuing her relationship with him, and thus in passing his genes into the next generation. The suggestion by G. F. Miller (Miller 1992, Miller 2000, Ridley 1993b) that brain size has evolved for courtship might be extended to be important also beyond initial courtship, to keeping a partner interested while children are raised.

10. In women, we might expect that refractoriness after orgasm might be stronger for unfaithful women, and to be at least partly sensory-specific (for the male with whom she has just had intercourse), because there may (at least in the past) have been an advantage to females to allow sperm competition to occur, implying intercourse with another male in the not too distant future. This would be less important for women predisposed to be faithful, in whom even multiple orgasms might occur, helping to reward her and her partner (see above) in the mutual relationship.

11. A neurophysiological mechanism operating in a man that made sex with a woman more rewarding if she was relatively novel could contribute to a number of phenomena. It could contribute to make the reward value of a particular woman for a man higher if he has not seen her for some time. The biological function of this is that then the chance is greater that she has had intercourse with another man, and a sperm competition situation, in which speed is of the essence, could be necessary. Evidence that men do have appropriate behaviour for this situation is that the volume a man ejaculates into a particular woman increases with the length of the time since he has last seen her (Baker and Bellis 1995). The same

neurophysiological mechanism could contribute to a form of sensory-specific satiety in which even after intercourse and ejaculation with one woman, a man may be quickly aroused again by another woman. (Possibly it is partly because of this arousing effect of a novel potential lover that the sight of others having intercourse, e.g. in a video, might be arousing. Also possibly related is that the sperm warfare hypothesis might predict that if a man saw someone else having intercourse with his partner, a fit response might be to have intercourse with her too, to promote sperm warfare. However, this would not be an adaptive response if the woman had not yet had an orgasm, and did subsequently have one as a result of the second intercourse.) A similar neurophysiological mechanism could also contribute to making a man wish to have intercourse perhaps every four days, or sooner if he suspects infidelity.

12. There should be at least a small tendency to become attached to (find more rewarding) a person with whom intercourse has occurred (especially if it leads to orgasm in the woman, as described in Section 9.2 on oxytocin). For the woman this is one way of seeking resources for her potential child, by becoming attached to a person who may now be disposed to provide resources to help his genes. For the man such an attachment mechanism is one way of increasing the probability that he will provide for his potential offspring with her, and thus for the success of his genes.

13. The rewards produced by tactile stimulation are such that touch can be rewarding and feel pleasant, and this can occur in situations that are not explicitly sexual as well as in more sexual episodes. One example is grooming in monkeys, which may be rewarding because it serves a number of functions, including removing skin parasites, indicating commitment to another by the investment of time, or by trusting another to touch one, as a preliminary to more sexual touch, etc. Where in the brain is the pleasantness of touch made explicit? Is it in or before the somatosensory cortex of primates, or primarily after this in some of the connected areas such as the insula, orbitofrontal cortex, or amygdala (see Figs. 4.1 and 4.2)? As shown in Chapter 4, one area of the brain in which the pleasantness of touch is made explicit is in a part of the orbitofrontal cortex. The area of the orbitofrontal cortex in which pleasant touch is represented was different from the area in which taste and odour are represented (see Chapter 4). This is an early indication that there may be brain mechanisms specialized for processing the affective or rewarding aspects of touch in humans. Doubtless there will be a number of brain regions in addition to the orbitofrontal cortex where such information is represented. Perhaps one function of the representation in the orbitofrontal cortex is to act as a representation of touch as a primary reinforcer or unconditioned stimulus in stimulus–reinforcement association learning (see Chapter 4). The orbitofrontal representation of pleasant touch may also be involved in the subjective affective feeling produced by the touch, for orbitofrontal cortex damage in humans does blunt the affective component of other affective stimuli such as pain (Melzack and Wall 1996). Aspects of touch that may make it particularly pleasant include slight unpredictability, and a psychological component that reflects what it is one believes is providing the touch, and who is performing the touching. It will be of interest to determine where in the somatosensory system such cognitive influences converge with inputs originating from touch receptors to alter the affective component of the touch.

With regard to tactile stimulation that women may find rewarding in the early stages of a relationship or sexual episode, gentle touch, hugging, and kissing on any part of the body may be rewarding, perhaps as an indicator of caring, protection, and investment of time offered by a man. Because of the importance to a woman of indicators of investment by a man, women also have fantasies and prefer literature that emphasizes romance, commitment, and attachment rather than explicit details of sexual encounters and the physical stimulation being exchanged (Ellis and Symons 1990). Stimulation of the nipples may be rewarding partly to promote the biological function of breast-feeding and attachment. Its sexually arousing effects might be related to the fact that such stimulation may cause the release of the hormone oxytocin, which stimulates movements or contractions of the uterus. The movements might have a biological function in relation to later orgasm and the upsuck effect.

With regard to more explicitly sexual genital stimulation in women, both external (clitoral and vulval) and internal (vaginal, including the G spot on the anterior wall of the vagina) stimulation can be rewarding and pleasant. The possibility that women predisposed to be unfaithful might require more such stimulation to produce an orgasm, might be especially stimulated by a novel lover with fit genes and by novelty in the situation, and might be biased towards finding external as compared with internal stimulation more rewarding has been introduced above, together with the biological functions that might be served by being made differentially sensitive to these different types of reward.

The active control of a sexual episode may be rewarding not only to men (because being in control of sex is likely to make his genes fit), but also particularly to women predisposed to be unfaithful, because they can then determine whether they proceed to intercourse with that particular man, and also whether they receive the right stimulation to have an orgasm with that particular man, with its biological function of controlling the likelihood of conception with that particular man. It is also possible that a lack of control could act as a reward sometimes in some women, because the feeling of being dominated by a particular man could indicate potential fitness in her sons with him (who might be likely to dominate other women).

The reward value that oral sex can have (in both males and females) could be related to the biological function of determining whether the other person is disease-free (using sight, smell, and taste), and, if performed randomly, of detecting infidelity in a partner (by smell, possibly reduced volume of ejaculate from a male, etc.) (Ridley 1993b).

9.9 Brain regions involved in the control of sexual behaviour, and especially in the rewards produced by sexual behaviour

In males, the preoptic area (see Fig. 9.2) is involved in the control of sexual behaviour (Hull, Meisel and Sachs 2002). Lesions of this region permanently abolish male sexual behaviour; electrical stimulation can elicit copulatory activity; metabolic activity is induced (as shown by c-fos) in the preoptic area during copulation; and small implants of testosterone into the preoptic area restore sexual behaviour in castrated rats (Hull et al. 2002, Carlson 2004, Everitt et al. 1989, Everitt 1990, Everitt and Robbins 1992). This region appears to have neurons in it that respond to sex-related rewards in primates, in that Aou et al. (1984) described some preoptic neurons in the male macaque that increased their firing rates when he could see a female macaque seated on a chair that he could pull towards him. The same neurons did not respond to the sight of food (personal communication), and so reflected information about the type of reward available. They also described neuronal activity changes in the medial preoptic area of the male monkey that were related to the commencement of sexual behaviour, penile erection, and the refractory period following ejaculation. Similarly, neuronal activity changes

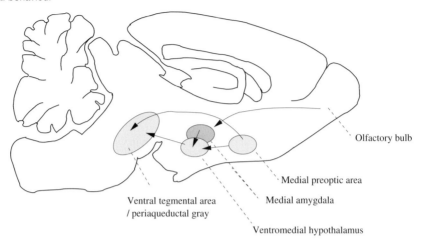

Olfactory bulb

Medial preoptic area

Ventral tegmental area / periaqueductal gray

Medial amygdala

Ventromedial hypothalamus

Fig. 9.2 Some of the brain regions implicated in sexual behaviour, shown on a midline view of a rat brain.

in the female medial preoptic area were related to the commencement of sexual behaviour and presentation. Increased neuronal activity in the dorsomedial hypothalamic nucleus in the male monkey and in the ventromedial hypothalamic nucleus in the female monkey were synchronized to each mating act. These findings, and studies using local electrical stimulation, suggested the involvement of medial preoptic area neurons in sexual arousal, and of male dorsomedial hypothalamic and female ventromedial hypothalamic neurons in copulation (Aou et al. 1984). Further evidence that these brain areas are involved in sex-related rewards is that the hormone testosterone affects brain-stimulation reward at some sites in this general region (e.g. in the posterior hypothalamus), but not at sites in, for example, the lateral hypothalamus (Caggiula 1970), where hunger modulates brain-stimulation reward (see Chapter 5).

In females, the medial preoptic area is involved in the control of reproductive cycles. It is probably also involved in controlling sexual behaviour directly (Blaustein and Erskine 2002). Neurons in it and connected areas respond to vagino-cervical stimulation in a hormone-dependent way (Blaustein and Erskine 2002). The ventromedial nucleus of the hypothalamus (VMH) is involved in some aspects of sexual behaviour, including lordosis (standing still in a receptive position) in rodents, and this behaviour can be reinstated in ovariectomized female rats by injections of oestradiol and progesterone into the ventromedial nucleus (Blaustein and Erskine 2002). Outputs from the VMH project to the periaqueductal gray of the midbrain, which is also necessary for female sexual behaviour such as lordosis in rodents (see Carlson (2004)), via descending influences on spinal cord reflexes implemented via the reticular formation neurons and the reticulospinal tracts (Pfaff 1980, Pfaff 1982, Priest and Pfaff 1995) (see Fig. 9.3). The VMH receives inputs from regions such as the medial amygdala.

The preoptic area receives inputs from the amygdala and orbitofrontal cortex, and thus receives information from the inferior temporal visual cortex (including information about face identity and expression), from the superior temporal auditory association cortex, from the olfactory system, and from the somatosensory system. The operation of these circuits has been described in Chapters 4 and 5. In one example described in Section 4.6.3, Everitt et al. (1989) showed that excitotoxic lesions of the basolateral amygdala disrupted appetitive sexual responses maintained by a visual conditioned reinforcer, but not the behaviour to

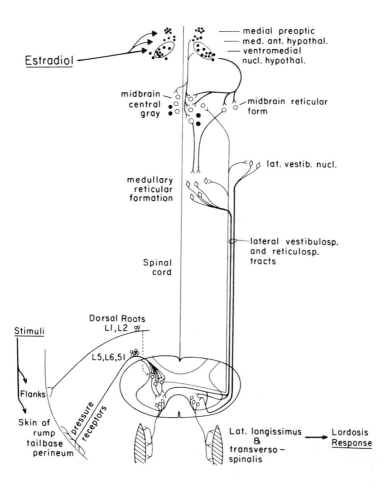

Fig. 9.3 Neural circuitry involved in the lordosis response of the female rat to flank, rump, and perineal stimulation by male rats after she is made sexually receptive by oestrogen (estradiol) in the hypothalamus. (Reproduced from Pfaff 1980 with permission.)

the primary reinforcer for the male rats, copulation with a female rat in heat (see further Everitt (1990) and Everitt and Robbins (1992)). (The details of the study were that the learned reinforcer or conditioned stimulus was a light for which the male rats worked on a FR10 schedule (i.e. 10 responses made to obtain a presentation of the light), with access to the female being allowed for the first FR10 completed after a fixed period of 15 min. This is a second order schedule of reinforcement.) For comparison, medial preoptic area lesions eliminated the copulatory behaviour of mounting, intromission and ejaculation to the primary reinforcer, the female rat, but did not affect the learned appetitive responding for the conditioned or secondary reinforcing stimulus, the light. The conclusion from such studies is that the amygdala is involved in stimulus–reinforcement association learning when the primary reinforcer is a sexual reward. On the other hand, the preoptic area is not involved in such stimulus–reinforcement association learning, but is involved in the rewarding effects of primary sexual rewards. Olfactory inputs reach the medial preoptic area via the medial amygdala and bed nucleus of the stria terminalis, and this pathway provides a route for olfactory stimuli to influence sexual behaviour (Hull et al. 2002). Somatosensory inputs from the genitals also reach the medial preoptic area, via the central tegmental field of the midbrain (Hull et al. 2002).

In an example illustrating part of the importance of the orbitofrontal cortex and of somatosensory reinforcers, evidence from fMRI indicates that the pleasantness of touch is represented especially in the orbitofrontal cortex (see Fig. 4.4). Presumably the pleasant effects of sexual touch are also represented in this and connected brain areas (see, e.g., Tiihonen, Kuikka, Kupila, Partanen, Vainio, Airaksinen, Eronen, Hallikainen, Paanila, Kinnunen and Huttunen (1994)). It is presumably by these neural circuits in the orbitofrontal cortex and amygdala that the effects related to the control of sexual behaviour described above are implemented, and much of the decoding of the relevant stimuli, and then their interpretation as primary reinforcers, or learning about their reinforcing properties by stimulus–reinforcement association learning, occurs. A number of the effects described in Section 9.8 are related to a diminution over time of the reward value produced by the same stimulus or individual, and the enhancement of behaviour produced by novel stimuli or individuals. It is also presumably in regions such as the orbitofrontal cortex and amygdala that such effects, which require a representation of individuals, and systems that can show a form of learning with stimulus repetition to implement sensory-specific satiety and novelty effects, are implemented.

The outputs of the preoptic area include connections to the lateral tegmental field in the midbrain, and in this region neurons are found that respond in relation to different aspects of male sexual behaviour (Shimura and Shimokochi 1990). However, it is likely that only some outputs of the orbitofrontal cortex and amygdala that control sexual behaviour act through the preoptic area. The preoptic area route may be necessary for computationally simple aspects of sexual behaviour such as copulation in males, but the attractive effect of sexual stimuli may survive damage to the medial preoptic area (see Carlson (2004)), suggesting that, as for feeding, outputs of the amygdala and orbitofrontal cortex can influence behaviour through the striatum (see Chapters 4 and 5).

During early development in males, the steroid hormone testosterone masculinizes the brain, and the effects produced include sexual dimorphism in a part of the preoptic area, which is larger in males than females (Morris, Jordan and Breedlove 2004). During puberty there are many changes in sexual behaviour, and associated with these some changes in brain connectivity and function occur, in for example the amygdala, prefrontal cortex, and striatum, but much remains to be understood, including to what extent these changes are steroid-dependent (Sisk and Foster 2004).

Much research remains to be performed to understand the details of the implementation of the rewards underlying sexual behaviour described earlier in this Chapter in brain regions such as the amygdala, orbitofrontal cortex, preoptic area, and hypothalamus.

9.10   Conclusion

We can conclude this Chapter by remembering that there is some evidence on how the brain produces sexual behaviour by being sensitive to certain rewards, and that reward systems for rewards of the type described in section 9.8 may have been built in the brain by genes as their way of increasing their fitness. It will be interesting to know how these different reward systems actually operate in the brain. In any case, the overall conclusion is that genes do appear to build reward systems that will lead to behaviour that will enhance their own survival in future generations. The issue of the role of reward (and punishment) systems in brain design by genetic variation and natural selection is described in Chapter 3.

10 Emotional feelings and consciousness: a theory of consciousness

10.1 Introduction

It might be possible to build a computer that would perform the functions of emotions described in Chapter 3, and yet we might not want to ascribe emotional feelings to the computer. We might even build the computer with some of the main processing stages present in the brain, and implemented using neural networks that simulate the operation of the real neural networks in the brain (see Chapter 4, Rolls and Treves (1998), Rolls and Deco (2002), and Appendices 1 and 2), yet we might not still wish to ascribe emotional feelings to this computer. This point often arises in discussions with undergraduates, who may say that they follow the types of point made about emotion in Chapters 4 and 5, yet believe that almost the most important aspect of emotions, the feelings, have not been accounted for, nor their neural basis described. In a sense, the functions of reward and punishment in emotional behaviour are described in Chapter 2 and 3, but what about the subjective aspects of emotion, what about the pleasure?

A similar point arises in Chapter 5, where parts of the taste, olfactory, and visual systems in which the reward value of the taste, smell, and sight of food is represented are described. Although the neuronal representation in the orbitofrontal cortex is clearly related to the reward value of food, and in humans the activations found with functional neuroimaging are directly correlated with the reported subjective pleasantness of the stimuli (see Chapters 4 and 5), is this where the pleasantness (the subjective hedonic aspect) of the taste, smell, and sight of food is represented and produced? Again, we could (in principle at least) build a computer with neural networks to simulate each of the processing stages for the taste, smell, and sight of food which are described in Chapter 5, and yet would probably not wish to ascribe feelings of pleasantness to the system we have simulated on the computer.

What is it about neural processing that makes it feel like something when some types of information processing are taking place? It is clearly not a general property of processing in neural networks, for there is much processing, for example that in the autonomic nervous system concerned with the control of our blood pressure and heart rate, of which we are not aware. Is it then that awareness arises when a certain type of information processing is being performed? If so, what type of information processing? And how do emotional feelings, and sensory events, come to feel like anything? These 'feels' are called qualia. These are great mysteries that have puzzled philosophers for centuries. They are at the heart of the problem of consciousness, for why it should feel like something at all is the great mystery.

Other aspects of consciousness may be easier to analyse, such as the fact that often when we 'pay attention' to events in the world, we can process those events in some better way. These are referred to as 'process' or 'access' aspects of consciousness, as opposed to the 'phenomenal' or 'feeling' aspects of consciousness referred to in the preceding paragraph (Block 1995a, Chalmers 1996, Allport 1988, Koch 2004, Block 1995b).

The puzzle of qualia, that is of the phenomenal aspect of consciousness, seems to be rather different from normal investigations in science, in that there is no agreement on criteria by which to assess whether we have made progress. So, although the aim of this Chapter is to address the issue of consciousness, especially of qualia, what is written cannot be regarded as being as firmly scientific as the other Chapters in this book. For most of the work in those, there is good evidence for most of the points made, and there would be no hesitation or difficulty in adjusting the view of how things work as new evidence is obtained. However, in the work on qualia, the criteria are much less clear. Nevertheless, the reader may well find these issues interesting, because although not easily solvable, they are very important issues to consider if we wish to really say that we understand some of the very complex and interesting issues about brain function, and ourselves.

With these caveats in mind, I consider in this Chapter the general issue of consciousness and its functions, and how feelings, and pleasure, come to occur as a result of the operation of our brains. A view on consciousness, influenced by contemporary cognitive neuroscience, is outlined next. I outline a theory of what the processing is that is involved in consciousness, of its adaptive value in an evolutionary perspective, and of how processing in our visual and other sensory systems can result in subjective or phenomenal states, the 'raw feels' of conscious awareness. However, this view on consciousness that I describe is only preliminary, and theories of consciousness are likely to develop considerably. Partly for these reasons, this theory of consciousness, at least, should not be taken to have practical implications.

10.2 A theory of consciousness

A starting point is that many actions can be performed relatively automatically, without apparent conscious intervention. An example sometimes given is driving a car. Such actions could involve control of behaviour by brain systems that are old in evolutionary terms such as the basal ganglia. It is of interest that the basal ganglia (and cerebellum) do not have backprojection systems to most of the parts of the cerebral cortex from which they receive inputs (see Section 8.4 and Rolls and Treves (1998)). In contrast, parts of the brain such as the hippocampus and amygdala, involved in functions such as episodic memory and emotion respectively, about which we can make (verbal) declarations (hence declarative memory, Squire (1992)) do have major backprojection systems to the high parts of the cerebral cortex from which they receive forward projections (see Figs. 10.1, 4.63 and 4.65). It may be that evolutionarily newer parts of the brain, such as the language areas and parts of the prefrontal cortex, are involved in an alternative type of control of behaviour, in which actions can be planned with the use of a (language) system that allows relatively arbitrary (syntactic) manipulation of semantic entities (symbols).

The general view that there are many routes to behavioural output is supported by the evidence that there are many input systems to the basal ganglia (from almost all areas of the cerebral cortex), and that neuronal activity in each part of the striatum reflects the activity in the overlying cortical area (see Section 8.4). The evidence is consistent with the possibility that different cortical areas, each specialized for a different type of computation, have their outputs directed to the basal ganglia, which then select the strongest input, and map this into action (via outputs directed, for example, to the premotor cortex). Within this scheme, the language areas would offer one of many routes to action, but a route particularly suited to

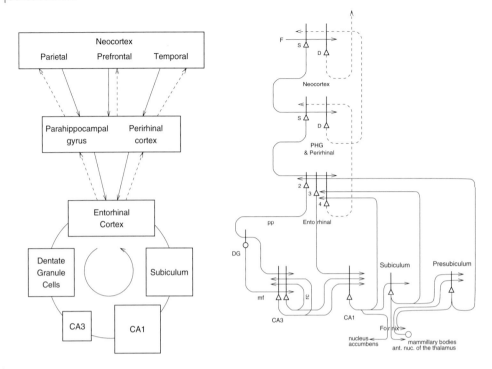

Fig. 10.1 Forward connections (solid lines) from areas of cerebral association neocortex via the parahippocampal gyrus and perirhinal cortex, and entorhinal cortex, to the hippocampus; and backprojections (dashed lines) via the hippocampal CA1 pyramidal cells, subiculum, and parahippocampal gyrus back to the neocortex. There is great convergence in the forward connections down to the single network implemented in the CA3 pyramidal cells; and great divergence again in the backprojections. Left: block diagram. Right: more detailed representation of some of the principal excitatory neurons in the pathways. Abbreviations: D, Deep pyramidal cells; DG, dentate granule cells; F, forward inputs to areas of the association cortex from preceding cortical areas in the hierarchy. mf: mossy fibres; PHG, parahippocampal gyrus and perirhinal cortex; pp, perforant path; rc, recurrent collaterals of the CA3 hippocampal pyramidal cells; S, superficial pyramidal cells; 2, pyramidal cells in layer 2 of the entorhinal cortex; 3, pyramidal cells in layer 3 of the entorhinal cortex; 5, 6, pyramidal cells in the deep layers of the entorhinal cortex. The thick lines above the cell bodies represent the dendrites.

planning actions, because of the syntactic manipulation of semantic entities which may make long-term planning possible. A schematic diagram of this suggestion is provided in Fig. 10.2.

Consistent with the hypothesis of multiple routes to action, only some of which utilize language, is the evidence that split-brain patients may not be aware of actions being performed by the 'non-dominant' hemisphere (Gazzaniga and LeDoux 1978, Gazzaniga 1988, Gazzaniga 1995). Also consistent with multiple, including non-verbal, routes to action, patients with focal brain damage, for example to the prefrontal cortex, may emit actions, yet comment verbally that they should not be performing those actions (Rolls, Hornak, Wade and McGrath 1994a, Hornak, Bramham, Rolls, Morris, O'Doherty, Bullock and Polkey 2003). In both these types of patient, confabulation may occur, in that a verbal account of why the action was performed may be given, and this may not be related at all to the environmental event that actually triggered the action (Gazzaniga and LeDoux 1978, Gazzaniga 1988, Gazzaniga 1995).

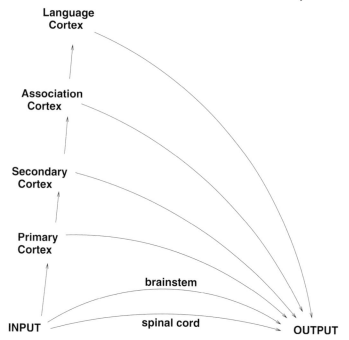

Fig. 10.2 Schematic illustration indicating many possible routes from input systems to action (output) systems. Cortical information-processing systems are organized hierarchically, and there are routes to output systems from most levels of the hierarchy.

It is accordingly possible that sometimes in normal humans when actions are initiated as a result of processing in a specialized brain region such as those involved in some types of rewarded behaviour, the language system may subsequently elaborate a coherent account of why that action was performed (i.e. confabulate). This would be consistent with a general view of brain evolution in which, as areas of the cortex evolve, they are laid on top of existing circuitry connecting inputs to outputs, and in which each level in this hierarchy of separate input–output pathways may control behaviour according to the specialized function it can perform (see schematic in Fig. 10.2). (It is of interest that mathematicians may get a hunch that something is correct, yet not be able to verbalize why. They may then resort to formal, more serial and language-like, theorems to prove the case, and these seem to require conscious processing. This is a further indication of a close association between linguistic processing, and consciousness. The linguistic processing need not, as in reading, involve an inner articulatory loop.)

We may next examine some of the advantages and behavioural functions that language, present as the most recently added layer to the above system, would confer.

One major advantage would be the ability to plan actions through many potential stages and to evaluate the consequences of those actions without having to perform the actions. For this, the ability to form propositional statements, and to perform syntactic operations on the semantic representations of states in the world, would be important.

Also important in this system would be the ability to have second-order thoughts about the type of thought that I have just described (e.g. I think that he thinks that ..., involving 'theory of mind'), as this would allow much better modelling and prediction of others' behaviour, and therefore of planning, particularly planning when it involves others[32]. This capability for higher-order thoughts would also enable reflection on past events, which would also be useful in planning. In contrast, non-linguistic behaviour would be driven by learned reinforcement associations, learned rules etc., but not by flexible planning for many steps ahead involving a model of the world including others' behaviour. (For an earlier view that is close to this part of the argument see Humphrey (1980).) [The examples of behaviour from non-humans that may reflect planning may reflect much more limited and inflexible planning. For example, the dance of the honey-bee to signal to other bees the location of food may be said to reflect planning, but the symbol manipulation is not arbitrary. There are likely to be interesting examples of non-human primate behaviour that reflect the evolution of an arbitrary symbol-manipulation system that could be useful for flexible planning, cf. Cheney and Seyfarth (1990), Byrne and Whiten (1988), and Whiten and Byrne (1997).]

It is important to state that the language ability referred to here is not necessarily human verbal language (though this would be an example). What it is suggested is important to planning is the syntactic manipulation of symbols, and it is this syntactic manipulation of symbols that is the sense in which language is defined and used here. The type of syntactic processing need not be at the natural language level (which implies a universal grammar), but could be at the level of mentalese (Rolls 1999a, Rolls 2004c, Fodor 1994).

It is next suggested that this arbitrary symbol-manipulation using important aspects of language processing and used for planning but not in initiating all types of behaviour is close to what consciousness is about. In particular, consciousness may be the state that arises in a system that can think about (or reflect on) its own (or other peoples') thoughts, that is in a system capable of second- or higher-order thoughts (Rosenthal 1986, Rosenthal 1990, Rosenthal 1993, Dennett 1991). On this account, a mental state is non-introspectively (i.e. non-reflectively) conscious if one has a roughly simultaneous thought that one is in that mental state. Following from this, introspective consciousness (or reflexive consciousness, or self consciousness) is the attentive, deliberately focused consciousness of one's mental states. It is noted that not all of the higher-order thoughts need themselves be conscious (many mental states are not). However, according to the analysis, having a higher-order thought about a lower-order thought is necessary for the lower-order thought to be conscious.

A slightly weaker position than Rosenthal's on this is that a conscious state corresponds to a first-order thought that has the capacity to cause a second-order thought or judgement about it (Carruthers 1996). Another position that is close in some respects to that of Carruthers and the present position is that of Chalmers (1996), that awareness is something that has direct availability for behavioural control, which amounts effectively for him in humans to saying that consciousness is what we can report (verbally) about[33]. This analysis is consistent with

---

[32] Second-order thoughts are thoughts about thoughts. Higher-order thoughts refer to second-order, third-order, etc., thoughts about thoughts...

[33] Chalmers (1996) is not entirely consistent about this. Later in the same book he advocates a view that experiences are associated with information-processing systems, e.g. experiences are associated with a thermostat (p. 297). He does not believe that the brain has experiences, but that he has experiences. This leads him to suggest that experiences are associated with information processing systems such as the thermostat in the same way as they are associated with him. "If there is experience associated with thermostats, there is probably experience everywhere: wherever there is a causal interaction, there is information, and wherever there is information, there is experience." (p. 297). He goes on to exclude rocks from having experiences, in that "a rock, unlike a thermostat, is not picked out as an information-processing system". My response to this is that of course there is mutual information between the physical world (e.g. the world of tastants, the chemical stimuli that can produce tastes) and the conscious world

the points made above that the brain systems that are required for consciousness and language are similar. In particular, a system that can have second- or higher-order thoughts about its own operation, including its planning and linguistic operation, must itself be a language processor, in that it must be able to bind correctly to the symbols and syntax in the first-order system. According to this explanation, the feeling of anything is the state that is present when linguistic processing that involves second- or higher-order thoughts is being performed.

It might be objected that this hypothesis captures some of the process aspects of consciousness, that is, what is useful in an information processing system, but does not capture the phenomenal aspect of consciousness. (Chalmers, following points made in his 1996 book, might make this point.) I agree that there is an element of 'mystery' that is invoked at this step of the argument, when I say that it feels like something for a machine with higher-order thoughts to be thinking about its own first- or lower-order thoughts. But the return point is the following: if a human with second-order thoughts is thinking about its own first-order thoughts, surely it is very difficult for us to conceive that this would not feel like something? (Perhaps the higher-order thoughts in thinking about the first-order thoughts would need to have in doing this some sense of continuity or self, so that the first-order thoughts would be related to the same system that had thought of something else a few minutes ago. But even this continuity aspect may not be a requirement for consciousness. Humans with anterograde amnesia cannot remember what they felt a few minutes ago, yet their current state does feel like something.)

It is suggested that part of the evolutionary adaptive significance of this type of higher-order thought is that it enables correction of errors made in first-order linguistic or in non-linguistic processing. Indeed, the ability to reflect on previous events is extremely important for learning from them, including setting up new long-term semantic structures. It was shown above that the hippocampus may be a system for such 'declarative' recall of recent memories (see also Squire, Stark and Clark (2004)). Its close relation to 'conscious' processing in humans (Squire has classified it as a declarative memory system) may be simply that it enables the recall of recent memories, which can then be reflected upon in conscious, higher-order, processing. Another part of the adaptive value of a higher-order thought system may be that by thinking about its own thoughts in a given situation, it may be able to understand better the thoughts of another individual in a similar situation, and therefore predict that individual's behaviour better (Humphrey (1980), Humphrey (1986); cf. Barlow (1997)).

As a point of clarification, I note that according to this theory, a language processing system is not sufficient for consciousness. What defines a conscious system according to this analysis is the ability to have higher-order thoughts, and a first-order language processor (which might be perfectly competent at language) would not be conscious, in that it could not think about its own or others' thoughts. One can perfectly well conceive of a system that obeyed the rules of language (which is the aim of much connectionist modelling), and implemented a first-order linguistic system, that would not be conscious. [Possible examples

(e.g. of taste) – if there were not, the information represented in the conscious processing system would not be useful for any thoughts or operations on or about the world. And according to the view I present here, the conscious processing system is good at some specialized types of processing (e.g. planning ahead using syntactic processing with semantics grounded in the real world, and reflecting on and correcting such plans), for which it would need reliable information about the world. Clearly Chalmers' view on consciousness is very much weaker than mine, in that he allows thermostats to be associated with consciousness, and in contrast to the theory presented here, does not suggest any special criteria for the types of information processing to be performed in order for the system to be aware of its thoughts, and of what it is doing.

of language processing that might be performed non-consciously include computer programs implementing aspects of language, or ritualized human conversations, e.g. about the weather. These might require syntax and correctly grounded semantics, and yet be performed non-consciously. A more complex example, illustrating that syntax could be used, might be 'If A does X, then B will probably do Y, and then C would be able to do Z.' A first-order language system could process this statement. Moreover, the first-order language system could apply the rule usefully in the world, provided that the symbols in the language system (A, B, X, Y etc.) are grounded (have meaning) in the world.]

In line with the argument on the adaptive value of higher-order thoughts and thus consciousness given above, that they are useful for correcting lower-order thoughts, I now suggest that correction using higher-order thoughts of lower-order thoughts would have adaptive value primarily if the lower-order thoughts are sufficiently complex to benefit from correction in this way. The nature of the complexity is specific – that it should involve syntactic manipulation of symbols, probably with several steps in the chain, and that the chain of steps should be a one-off (or in American usage, 'one-time', meaning used once) set of steps, as in a sentence or in a particular plan used just once, rather than a set of well learned rules. The first or lower-order thoughts might involve a linked chain of 'if ... then' statements that would be involved in planning, an example of which has been given above, and this type of cognitive processing is thought to be a primary basis for human skilled performance (Anderson 1996). It is partly because complex lower-order thoughts such as these that involve syntax and language would benefit from correction by higher-order thoughts that I suggest that there is a close link between this reflective consciousness and language.

The hypothesis is that by thinking about lower-order thoughts, the higher-order thoughts can discover what may be weak links in the chain of reasoning at the lower-order level, and having detected the weak link, might alter the plan, to see if this gives better success. In our example above, if it transpired that C could not do Z, how might the plan have failed? Instead of having to go through endless random changes to the plan to see if by trial and error some combination does happen to produce results, what I am suggesting is that by thinking about the previous plan, one might, for example, using knowledge of the situation and the probabilities that operate in it, guess that the step where the plan failed was that B did not in fact do Y. So by thinking about the plan (the first- or lower-order thought), one might correct the original plan in such a way that the weak link in that chain, that 'B will probably do Y', is circumvented.

To draw a parallel with neural networks: there is a **'credit assignment'** problem in such multistep syntactic plans, in that if the whole plan fails, how does the system assign credit or blame to particular steps of the plan? [In multilayer neural networks, the credit assignment problem is that if errors are being specified at the output layer, the problem arises about how to propagate back the error to earlier, hidden, layers of the network to assign credit or blame to individual synaptic connection; see Rumelhart, Hinton and Williams (1986) and Rolls and Deco (2002).] **My suggestion is that this solution to the credit assignment problem for a one-off syntactic plan is the function of higher-order thoughts, and is why systems with higher-order thoughts evolved. The suggestion I then make is that if a system were doing this type of processing (thinking about its own thoughts), it would then be very plausible that it should feel like something to be doing this.** I even suggest to the reader that it is not plausible to suggest that it would not feel like anything to a system if it were doing this.

Two other points in the argument should be emphasized for clarity. One is that the system that is having syntactic thoughts about its own syntactic thoughts would have to have its symbols grounded in the real world for it to feel like something to be having higher-order thoughts. The intention of this clarification is to exclude systems such as a computer running a program when there is in addition some sort of control or even overseeing program checking the operation of the first program. We would want to say that in such a situation it would feel like something to be running the higher level control program only if the first-order program was symbolically performing operations on the world and receiving input about the results of those operations, and if the higher-order system understood what the first-order system was trying to do in the world. The issue of symbol grounding is considered further in Section 10.4.

The second clarification is that the plan would have to be a unique string of steps, in much the same way as a sentence can be a unique and one-off string of words. The point here is that it is helpful to be able to think about particular one-off plans, and to correct them; and that this type of operation is very different from the slow learning of fixed rules by trial and error, or the application of fixed rules by a supervisory part of a computer program.

This analysis does not yet give an account for sensory qualia ('raw sensory feels', for example why 'red' feels red), for emotional qualia (e.g. why a rewarding touch produces an emotional feeling of pleasure), or for motivational qualia (e.g. why food deprivation makes us feel hungry). The view I suggest on such **qualia** is as follows. Information processing in and from our sensory systems (e.g. the sight of the colour red) may be relevant to planning actions using language and the conscious processing thereby implied. Given that these inputs must be represented in the system that plans, we may ask whether it is more likely that we would be conscious of them or that we would not. I suggest that it would be a very special-purpose system that would allow such sensory inputs, and emotional and motivational states, to be part of (linguistically based) planning, and yet remain unconscious (given that the processing being performed by this system is inherently conscious, as suggested above). It seems to be much more parsimonious to hold that we would be conscious of such sensory, emotional, and motivational qualia because they would be being used (or are available to be used) in this type of (linguistically based) higher-order thought processing system, and this is what I propose.

The explanation of emotional and motivational subjective feelings or qualia that this discussion has led towards is thus that they should be felt as conscious because they enter into a specialized linguistic symbol-manipulation system, which is part of a higher-order thought system that is capable of reflecting on and correcting its lower-order thoughts involved for example in the flexible planning of actions. It would require a very special machine to enable this higher-order linguistically-based thought processing, which is conscious by its nature, to occur without the sensory, emotional and motivational states (which must be taken into account by the higher-order thought system) becoming felt qualia. The sensory, emotional, and motivational qualia are thus accounted for by the evolution of a linguistic (i.e. syntactic) system that can reflect on and correct its own lower-order processes, and thus has adaptive value.

This account implies that it may be especially animals with a higher-order belief and thought system and with linguistic (i.e. syntactic, not necessarily verbal) symbol manipulation that have qualia. It may be that much non-human animal behaviour, provided that it does not require flexible linguistic planning and correction by reflection, could take place according to reinforcement-guidance (using, e.g., stimulus–reinforcer association learning in the amygdala and orbitofrontal cortex as described in Chapter 4, and rule-following [implemented, e.g., using habit or stimulus–response learning in the basal ganglia, see Section 8.4]). Such

involves conscious, verbally represented processing that can later be recalled (see Fig. 10.2 and Section 10.3).

It is of interest to comment on how the evolution of a system for flexible planning might affect emotions. Consider grief which may occur when a reward is terminated and no immediate action is possible (Rolls 1990d, Rolls 1995b, Rolls 1999a). It may be adaptive by leading to a cessation of the formerly rewarded behaviour, and thus facilitating the possible identification of other positive reinforcers in the environment. In humans, grief may be particularly potent because it becomes represented in a system that can plan ahead, and understand the enduring implications of the loss. (Thinking about or verbally discussing emotional states may also in these circumstances help, because this can lead towards the identification of new or alternative reinforcers, and of the realization that, for example, negative consequences may not be as bad as feared.)

This account of consciousness also leads to a suggestion about the processing that underlies the feeling of free will. Free will would in this scheme involve the use of language to check many moves ahead on a number of possible series of actions and their outcomes, and then with this information to make a choice from the likely outcomes of different possible series of actions. (If in contrast choices were made only on the basis of the reinforcement value of immediately available stimuli, without the arbitrary syntactic symbol manipulation made possible by language, then the choice strategy would be much more limited, and we might not want to use the term free will, as all the consequences of those actions would not have been computed.) It is suggested that when this type of reflective, conscious, information processing is occurring and leading to action, the system performing this processing and producing the action would have to believe that it could cause the action, for otherwise inconsistencies would arise, and the system might no longer try to initiate action. This belief held by the system may partly underlie the feeling of free will. At other times, when other brain modules are initiating actions (in the implicit systems), the conscious processor (the explicit system) may confabulate and believe that it caused the action, or at least give an account (possibly wrong) of why the action was initiated. The fact that the conscious processor may have the belief even in these circumstances that it initiated the action may arise as a property of its being inconsistent for a system that can take overall control using conscious verbal processing to believe that it was over-ridden by another system. This may be the reason why confabulation occurs.

In the operation of such a free-will system, the uncertainties introduced by the limited information possible about the likely outcomes of series of actions, and the inability to use optimal algorithms when combining conditional probabilities, would be much more important factors than whether the brain operates deterministically or not. (The operation of brain machinery must be relatively deterministic, for it has evolved to provide reliable outputs for given inputs.) The issue of whether the brain operates deterministically is not therefore I suggest the central or most interesting question about free will. Instead, analysis of which brain processing systems are engaged when we are taking decisions (see further Section 11.2), and which processing systems are inextricably linked to feelings as suggested above, may be more revealing.

Before leaving these thoughts, it may be worth commenting on the feeling of continuing self-identity that is characteristic of humans. Why might this arise? One suggestion is that if one is an organism that can think about its own long-term multistep plans, then for those plans to be consistently and thus adaptively executed, the goals of the plans would need to remain stable, as would memories of how far one had proceeded along the execution path of each plan. If one felt each time one came to execute, perhaps on another day, the next step of a plan, that the goals were different, or if one did not remember which steps had already been taken in a multistep plan, the plan would never be usefully executed. So, given that it does feel like something to be doing this type of planning using higher-order thoughts, it would have to feel as if one were the same agent, acting towards the same goals, from day to day, for which autobiographical memory would be important. Thus it is suggested that the feeling of continuing self-identity falls out of a situation in which there is an actor with consistent long-term goals, and long-term recall. If it feels like anything to be the actor, according to the suggestions of the higher-order thought theory, then it should feel like the same thing from occasion to occasion to be the actor, and no special further construct is needed to account for self-identity. Humans without such a feeling of being the same person from day to day might be expected to have, for example, inconsistent goals from day to day, or a poor recall memory. It may be noted that the ability to recall previous steps in a plan, and bring them into the conscious, higher-order thought system, is an important prerequisite for long-term planning which involves checking each step in a multistep process.

These are my initial thoughts on why we have consciousness, and are conscious of sensory, emotional and motivational qualia, as well as qualia associated with first-order linguistic thoughts. However, as stated above, one does not feel that there are straightforward criteria in this philosophical field of enquiry for knowing whether the suggested theory is correct; so it is likely that theories of consciousness will continue to undergo rapid development; and current theories should not be taken to have practical implications.

10.3   Dual routes to action

According to the present formulation, there are two major types of route to action performed in relation to reward or punishment in humans. Examples of such actions include those associated with emotion and motivation.

The first ('implicit') route is via the brain systems that have been present in non-human primates such as monkeys, and to some extent in other mammals, for millions of years. These systems include the amygdala and, particularly well-developed in primates, the orbitofrontal cortex. These systems control behaviour in relation to previous associations of stimuli with reinforcement. The computation which controls the action thus involves assessment of the reinforcement-related value of a stimulus. This assessment may be based on a number of different factors:

One is the previous reinforcement history, which involves stimulus–reinforcer association learning using the amygdala, and its rapid updating especially in primates using the orbitofrontal cortex. This stimulus–reinforcer association learning may involve quite specific information about a stimulus, for example of the energy associated with each type of food, by the process of conditioned appetite and satiety (Booth 1985).

A second is the current motivational state, for example whether hunger is present, whether other needs are satisfied, etc.

A third factor that affects the computed reward value of the stimulus is whether that reward has been received recently. If it has been received recently but in small quantity, this may increase the reward value of the stimulus. This is known as incentive motivation or the 'salted nut' phenomenon. The adaptive value of such a process is that this positive feedback of reward value in the early stages of working for a particular reward tends to lock the organism on to behaviour being performed for that reward. This means that animals that are for example almost equally hungry and thirsty will show hysteresis in their choice of action, rather than continually switching from eating to drinking and back with each mouthful of water or food. This introduction of hysteresis into the reward evaluation system makes action selection a much more efficient process in a natural environment, for constantly switching between different types of behaviour would be very costly if all the different rewards were not available in the same place at the same time. (For example, walking half a mile between a site where water was available and a site where food was available after every mouthful would be very inefficient.) The amygdala is one structure that may be involved in this increase in the reward value of stimuli early on in a series of presentations, in that lesions of the amygdala (in rats) abolish the expression of this reward-incrementing process which is normally evident in the increasing rate of working for a food reward early on in a meal (Rolls and Rolls 1973b, Rolls 1999a).

A fourth factor is the computed absolute value of the reward or punishment expected or being obtained from a stimulus, e.g. the sweetness of the stimulus (set by evolution so that sweet stimuli will tend to be rewarding, because they are generally associated with energy sources), or the pleasantness of touch (set by evolution to be pleasant according to the extent to which it brings animals of the opposite sex together, and depending on the investment in time that the partner is willing to put into making the touch pleasurable, a sign that indicates the commitment and value for the partner of the relationship, as in social grooming).

After the reward value of the stimulus has been assessed in these ways, behaviour is then initiated based on approach towards or withdrawal from the stimulus. A critical aspect of the behaviour produced by this type of 'implicit' system is that it is aimed directly towards obtaining a sensed or expected reward, by virtue of connections to brain systems such as the basal ganglia which are concerned with the initiation of actions (see Fig. 10.4). The expectation may of course involve behaviour to obtain stimuli associated with reward, which might even be present in a fixed chain or sequence.

Now part of the way in which the behaviour is controlled with this first ('implicit') route is according to the reward value of the outcome. At the same time, the animal may only work for the reward if the cost is not too high. Indeed, in the field of behavioural ecology animals are often thought of as performing optimally on some cost–benefit curve (see, e.g., Krebs and Kacelnik (1991)). This does not at all mean that the animal thinks about the long-term rewards, and performs a cost–benefit analysis using a lot of thoughts about the costs, other rewards (short and long term) available and their costs, etc (see Section 11.2.6.2). Instead, it should be taken to mean that in evolution the system has evolved in such a way that the way in which the reward varies with the different energy densities or amounts of food and the delay before it is received can be used as part of the input to a mechanism which has also been built to track the costs of obtaining the food (e.g. energy loss in obtaining it, risk of predation, etc.), and to then select given many such types of reward and the associated cost, the current behaviour that provides the most 'net reward'. Part of the value of having the computation expressed in this reward-minus-cost form is that there is then a suitable 'currency', or net reward value, to enable the animal to select the behaviour with currently the most net reward gain (or minimal aversive outcome).

Part of the evidence that this implicit route often controls emotional behaviour in humans is that humans with orbitofrontal cortex damage have impairments in selecting the correct

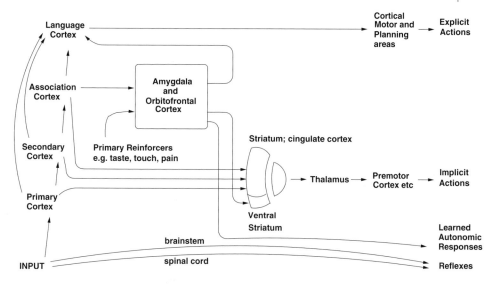

Fig. 10.4 Dual routes to the initiation of actions in response to rewarding and punishing stimuli. The inputs from different sensory systems to brain structures such as the orbitofrontal cortex and amygdala allow these brain structures to evaluate the reward- or punishment-related value of incoming stimuli, or of remembered stimuli. The different sensory inputs enable evaluations within the orbitofrontal cortex and amygdala based mainly on the primary (unlearned) reinforcement value for taste, touch, and olfactory stimuli, and on the secondary (learned) reinforcement value for visual and auditory stimuli. In the case of vision, the 'association cortex' that outputs representations of objects to the amygdala and orbitofrontal cortex is the inferior temporal visual cortex. One route for the outputs from these evaluative brain structures is via projections directly to structures such as the basal ganglia (including the striatum and ventral striatum) and cingulate cortex to enable implicit, direct behavioural responses based on the reward- or punishment-related evaluation of the stimuli to be made. The second route is via the language systems of the brain, which allow explicit (verbalizable) decisions involving multistep syntactic planning to be implemented.

action during visual discrimination reversal, yet can state explicitly what the correct action should be (Rolls, Hornak, Wade and McGrath 1994a, Rolls 1999b). The implication is that the intact orbitofrontal cortex is normally involved in making rapid emotion-related decisions, and that this emotion-related decision system is a separate system from the explicit system, which by serial reasoning can provide an alternative route to action. The explicit system may simply comment on the success or failure of actions that are initiated by the implicit system, and the explicit system may then be able to switch in to control mode to correct failures of the implicit system. Consistent evidence that an implicit system can control human behaviour is that in psychophysical and neurophysiological studies, it has been found that face stimuli presented for 16 ms and followed immediately by a mask are not consciously perceived, yet produce above chance identification (Rolls and Tovee 1994, Rolls, Tovee, Purcell, Stewart and Azzopardi 1994b, Rolls, Tovee and Panzeri 1999b, Rolls 2003, Rolls 2006c). In a similar backward masking paradigm, it was found that happy vs angry face expressions could influence how much beverage was wanted and consumed even when the faces were not consciously perceived (Winkielman and Berridge 2005, Winkielman and Berridge 2003). Thus unconscious emotion-related stimuli (in this case face expressions) can influence actions, and there is no need for processing to be conscious for actions to be initiated. Further, in blindsight, humans with damage to the primary visual cortex may not be subjectively aware of stimuli, yet may be able to guess what the stimulus was, or to perform reaching movements towards it (Weiskrantz 1998). Further, humans with striate cortex lesions may be influenced by emotional stimuli which are not perceived consciously (De Gelder, Vroomen, Pourtois and Weiskrantz 1999). Thus actions and emotions can be initiated without the necessity for the conscious route to be in control, and we should not infer that all actions require conscious processing.

The second ('explicit') route in (at least) humans involves a computation with many 'if ... then' statements, to implement a plan to obtain a reward. In this case, the reward may actually be deferred as part of the plan, which might involve working first to obtain one reward, and only then to work for a second more highly valued reward, if this was thought to be overall an optimal strategy in terms of resource usage (e.g. time). In this case, syntax is required, because the many symbols (e.g. names of people) that are part of the plan must be correctly linked or bound. Such linking might be of the form: 'if A does this, then B is likely to do this, and this will cause C to do this ...'. The requirement of syntax for this type of planning implies that an output to language systems in the brain is required for this type of planning (see Fig. 10.4). **Thus the explicit language system in humans may allow working for deferred rewards by enabling use of a one-off, individual, plan appropriate for each situation.** This explicit system may allow immediate rewards to be deferred, as part of a long-term plan. This ability to defer immediate rewards and plan syntactically in this way for the long term may be an important way in which the explicit system extends the capabilities of the implicit emotion systems that respond more directly to rewards and punishers, or to rewards and punishers with fixed expectancies such as can be learned by reinforcement learning (see Appendix 1, Section A.5).

Consistent with the point being made about evolutionarily old emotion-based decision systems vs a recent rational system present in humans (and perhaps other animals with syntactic processing) is that humans trade off immediate costs/benefits against cost/benefits that are delayed by as much as decades, whereas non-human primates have not been observed to engage in unpreprogrammed delay of gratification involving more than a few minutes (Rachlin 1989, Kagel, Battalio and Green 1995, McClure, Laibson, Loewenstein and Cohen 2004) (though this is a potentially interesting area for further investigation, see Section 11.2.6.2).

Another building block for such planning operations in the brain may be the type of short-term memory in which the prefrontal cortex is involved. This short-term memory may be, for example in non-human primates, of where in space a response has just been made. A development of this type of short-term response memory system in humans to enable multiple short-term memories to be held in place correctly, preferably with the temporal order of the different items in the short-term memory coded correctly, may be another building block for the multiple step 'if .... then' type of computation in order to form a multiple step plan. Such short-term memories are implemented in the (dorsolateral and inferior convexity) prefrontal cortex of non-human primates and humans (Goldman-Rakic 1996, Petrides 1996, Rolls and Deco 2002, Deco and Rolls 2003), and may be part of the reason why prefrontal cortex damage impairs planning and executive function (see Shallice and Burgess (1996)).

Of these two routes (see Fig. 10.4), it is the second that I have suggested above is related to consciousness. The hypothesis is that consciousness is the state that arises by virtue of having the ability to think about one's own thoughts, which has the adaptive value of enabling one to correct long multistep syntactic plans. This latter system is thus the one in which explicit, declarative, processing occurs. Processing in this system is frequently associated with reason and rationality, in that many of the consequences of possible actions can be taken into account. The actual computation of how rewarding a particular stimulus or situation is, or will be, probably still depends on activity in the orbitofrontal and amygdala, as the reward value of stimuli is computed and represented in these regions, and in that it is found that verbalized expressions of the reward (or punishment) value of stimuli are dampened by damage to these systems. (For example, damage to the orbitofrontal cortex renders painful input still identifiable as pain, but without the strong affective, 'unpleasant', reaction to it.)

This language system that enables long-term planning may be contrasted with the first system in which behaviour is directed at obtaining the stimulus (including the remembered stimulus) which is currently most rewarding, as computed by brain structures that include the orbitofrontal cortex and amygdala. There are outputs from this system, perhaps those directed at the basal ganglia and cingulate cortex, which do not pass through the language system, and behaviour produced in this way is described as implicit, and verbal declarations cannot be made directly about the reasons for the choice made. When verbal declarations are made about decisions made in this first ('implicit') system, those verbal declarations may be confabulations, reasonable explanations or fabrications, of reasons why the choice was made. These reasonable explanations would be generated to be consistent with the sense of continuity and self that is a characteristic of reasoning in the language system.

The question then arises of how decisions are made in animals such as humans that have both the implicit, direct reward-based, and the explicit, rational, planning systems (see Fig. 10.4). One particular situation in which the first, implicit, system may be especially important is when rapid reactions to stimuli with reward or punishment value must be made, for then the direct connections from structures such as the orbitofrontal cortex to the basal ganglia may allow rapid actions. Another is when there may be too many factors to be taken into account easily by the explicit, rational, planning, system, then the implicit system may be used to guide action.

In contrast, when the implicit system continually makes errors, it would then be beneficial for the organism to switch from automatic, direct, action based on obtaining what the orbitofrontal cortex system decodes as being the most positively reinforcing choice currently available, to the explicit conscious control system which can evaluate with its long-term planning algorithms what action should be performed next. Indeed, it would be adaptive for the explicit system to be regularly assessing performance by the more automatic system, and to switch itself in to control behaviour quite frequently, as otherwise the adaptive value of having the explicit system would be less than optimal.

Another factor that may influence the balance between control by the implicit and explicit systems is the presence of pharmacological agents such as alcohol, which may alter the balance towards control by the implicit system, may allow the implicit system to influence more the explanations made by the explicit system, and may within the explicit system alter the relative value it places on caution and restraint vs commitment to a risky action or plan.

There may also be a flow of influence from the explicit, verbal system to the implicit system, in that the explicit system may decide on a plan of action or strategy, and exert an influence on the implicit system that will alter the reinforcement evaluations made by and the signals produced by the implicit system. An example of this might be that if a pregnant woman feels that she would like to escape a cruel mate, but is aware that she may not survive in the jungle, then it would be adaptive if the explicit system could suppress some aspects of her implicit behaviour towards her mate, so that she does not give signals that she is displeased with her situation[34]. Another example might be that the explicit system might, because of its long-term plans, influence the implicit system to increase its response to for example a positive reinforcer. One way in which the explicit system might influence the implicit system is by setting up the conditions in which, for example, when a given stimulus (e.g. person) is present, positive reinforcers are given, to facilitate stimulus–reinforcement association learning by the implicit system of the person receiving the positive reinforcers. Conversely, the implicit system may influence the explicit system, for example by highlighting certain stimuli in the environment that are currently associated with reward, to guide the attention of the explicit system to such stimuli.

However, it may be expected that there is often a conflict between these systems, in that the first, implicit, system is able to guide behaviour particularly to obtain the greatest immediate reinforcement, whereas the explicit system can potentially enable immediate rewards to be deferred, and longer-term, multistep, plans to be formed. This type of conflict will occur in animals with a syntactic planning ability, that is in humans and any other animals that have the ability to process a series of 'if ... then' stages of planning. This is a property of the human language system, and the extent to which it is a property of non-human primates is not yet fully clear. In any case, such conflict may be an important aspect of the operation of at least the human mind, because it is so essential for humans to decide correctly, at every moment, whether to invest in a relationship or a group that may offer long-term benefits, or whether to pursue immediate benefits directly (Nesse and Lloyd 1992)[35].

Some investigations on deception in non-human primates have been interpreted as showing that animals can plan to deceive others (see, e.g., Griffin (1992), Byrne and Whiten (1988), and Whiten and Byrne (1997)), that is to utilize 'Machiavellian intelligence'. For example, a baboon might 'deliberately' mislead another animal in order to obtain a resource such as food (e.g. by screaming to summon assistance in order to have a competing animal chased from a food patch) or sex (e.g. a female baboon who very gradually moved into a position from which the dominant male could not see her grooming a subadult baboon) (see Dawkins (1993)). The attraction of the Machiavellian argument is that the behaviour for which it accounts seems to imply that there is a concept of another animal's mind, and that one animal is trying occasionally to mislead another, which implies some planning. However, such observations tend by their nature to be field-based, and may have an anecdotal character, in that the previous experience of the animals in this type of behaviour, and the reinforcements obtained, are not known (Dawkins 1993). It is possible, for example, that some behavioural responses that appear to be Machiavellian may have been the result of previous

---

[34]In the literature on self-deception, it has been suggested that unconscious desires may not be made explicit in consciousness (or actually repressed), so as not to compromise the explicit system in what it produces; see, e.g., Alexander (1975), Alexander (1979), Trivers (1976), Trivers (1985); and the review by Nesse and Lloyd (1992).

[35]As Nesse and Lloyd (1992) describe, some psychoanalysts ascribe to a somewhat similar position, for they hold that intrapsychic conflicts usually seem to have two sides, with impulses on one side and inhibitions on the other. Analysts describe the source of the impulses as the id, and the modules that inhibit the expression of impulses, because of external and internal constraints, the ego and superego respectively (Leak and Christopher 1982, Trivers 1985, Nesse and Lloyd 1992). The superego can be thought of as the conscience, while the ego is the locus of executive functions that balance satisfaction of impulses with anticipated internal and external costs. A difference of the present position is that it is based on identification of dual routes to action implemented by different systems in the brain, each with its own selective advantage.

instrumental learning in which reinforcement was obtained for particular types of response, or of observational learning, with again learning from the outcome observed. However, in any case, most examples of Machiavellian intelligence in non-human primates do not involve multiple stages of 'if ... then' planning requiring syntax to keep the symbols apart (but may involve associative learning which might lead to a description of the type 'if the dominant male sees me grooming a subadult male, I will be punished') (see Dawkins (1993)). Nevertheless, the possible advantage of such Machiavellian planning could be one of the adaptive guiding factors in evolution that provided advantage to a multistep, syntactic system that enables long-term planning, the best example of such a system being human language.

Another, not necessarily exclusive, advantage of the evolution of a linguistic multistep planning system could well be not Machiavellian planning, but planning for social co-operation and advantage. Perhaps in general an 'if ... then' multistep syntactic planning ability is useful primarily in evolution in social situations of the type: 'if X does this, then Y does that; then I would/should do that, and the outcome would be ... '. It is not yet at all clear whether such planning is required in order to explain the social behaviour of social animals such as hunting dogs, or socializing monkeys (Dawkins 1993).

However, in humans, members of 'primitive' hunting tribes spend hours recounting tales of recent events (perhaps who did what, when; who then did what, etc.), perhaps to help learn from experience about good strategies, necessary for example when physically weak men take on large animals (see Pinker and Bloom (1992)).

Thus, social co-operation may be as powerful a driving force in the evolution of syntactical planning systems as Machiavellian intelligence. What is common to both is that they involve social situations. However, such a syntactic planning system would have advantages not only in social systems, for such planning may be useful in obtaining resources purely in a physical (non-social) world. An example might be planning how to cross terrain given current environmental constraints in order to reach a particular place[36].

The thrust of this argument thus is that much complex animal, including human, behaviour can take place using the implicit, non-conscious, route to action. We should be very careful not to postulate intentional states (i.e. states with intentions, beliefs, and desires) unless the evidence for them is strong, and it seems to me that a flexible, one-off, linguistic processing system that can handle propositions is needed for intentional states. What the explicit, linguistic, system does allow is exactly this flexible, one-off, multistep planning-ahead type of computation, which allows us to defer immediate rewards based on such a plan.

Emotions as actions, and emotions as affects, are sometimes contrasted. My view on this is that sometimes emotions can lead to actions implicitly, without the need for conscious processing. However, when emotions involve longer term planning, then representation and processing in the explicit system is required, and affective feelings will then be inextricably linked to the processing.

---

[36]Tests of whether such multistep planning might be possible in even non-human primates are quite difficult to devise. One example might be to design a multistep maze. On a first part of the trial, the animal might be allowed to choose for itself, given constraints set on that trial to ensure trial unique performance, a set of choices through a maze. On the second part of that trial, the animal would be required to run through the maze again, remembering and repeating every choice just made in the first part of that trial. This part of the design is intended to allow recall of a multistep plan. To test on probe occasions whether the plan is being recalled, and whether the plan can be corrected by a higher-order thought process, the animal might be shown after the first part of a trial, that one of its previous free choices was not now available. The test would be to determine whether the animal can make a set of choices that indicate corrections to the multistep plan, in which the trajectory has to be altered before the now unavailable choice point is reached.

This discussion of dual routes to action has been with respect to the behaviour produced. There is of course in addition a third output of brain regions such as the orbitofrontal cortex and amygdala involved in emotion, which is directed to producing autonomic and endocrine responses. Although it has been argued in Chapter 2 that the autonomic system is not normally in a circuit through which behavioural responses are produced (i.e. against the James–Lange and related theories), there may be some influence from effects produced through the endocrine system (and possibly the autonomic system, through which some endocrine responses are controlled) on behaviour, or on the dual systems just discussed that control behaviour. For example, during female orgasm the hormone oxytocin may be released, and this may influence the implicit system to help develop positive reinforcement associations and thus attachment to her lover.

10.4 Content and meaning in representations: How are representations grounded in the world?

In Section 10.2 I suggested that representations need to be grounded in the world for a system with higher order thoughts to be conscious. I therefore now develop somewhat what I understand by representations being grounded in the world.

It is possible to analyse how the firing of populations of neurons encodes information about stimuli in the world (Rolls and Treves 1998, Rolls and Deco 2002). For example, from the firing rates of small numbers of neurons in the primate inferior temporal visual cortex, it is possible to know which of 20 faces has been shown to the monkey (Abbott, Rolls and Tovee 1996a, Rolls, Treves and Tovee 1997b). Similarly, a population of neurons in the anterior part of the macaque temporal lobe visual cortex has been discovered that has a view-invariant representation of objects (Booth and Rolls 1998). From the firing of a small ensemble of neurons in the olfactory part of the orbitofrontal cortex, it is possible to know which of eight odours was presented (Rolls, Critchley and Treves 1996a). From the firing of small ensembles of neurons in the hippocampus, it is possible to know where in allocentric space a monkey is looking (Rolls, Treves, Robertson, Georges-François and Panzeri 1998b). In each of these cases, the number of stimuli that is encoded increases exponentially with the number of neurons in the ensemble, so this is a very powerful representation (Abbott, Rolls and Tovee 1996a, Rolls, Treves and Tovee 1997b, Rolls and Treves 1998, Rolls and Deco 2002, Rolls, Aggelopoulos, Franco and Treves 2004, Franco, Rolls, Aggelopoulos and Treves 2004, Aggelopoulos, Franco and Rolls 2005). What is being measured in each example is the mutual information between the firing of an ensemble of neurons and which stimuli are present in the world. In this sense, one can read off the code that is being used at the end of each of these sensory systems.

However, what sense does the representation make to the animal? What does the firing of each ensemble of neurons 'mean'? What is the content of the representation? In the visual system, for example, it is suggested that the representation is built by a series of appropriately connected competitive networks, operating with a modified Hebb-learning rule (Rolls 1992a, Rolls 1994a, Wallis and Rolls 1997, Rolls 2000a, Rolls and Milward 2000, Stringer and Rolls 2000, Rolls and Stringer 2001a, Rolls and Deco 2002, Elliffe, Rolls and Stringer 2002, Stringer and Rolls 2002, Deco and Rolls 2004). Now competitive networks categorize their inputs without the use of a teacher (Kohonen 1989, Hertz et al. 1991, Rolls and Deco 2002). So which particular neurons fire as a result of the self-organization to represent a particular object or stimulus is arbitrary. What meaning, therefore, does the particular ensemble that fires to an object have? How is the representation grounded in the real world? The fact that there is mutual information (see Rolls and Treves (1998) and Rolls and Deco (2002)) between the firing of the ensemble of cells in the brain and a stimulus or event in the world does not fully answer this question.

One answer to this question is that there may be meaning in the case of objects and faces that it is an object or face, and not just a particular view. This is the case in that the representation may be activated by any view of the object or face. This is a step, suggested to be made possible by a short-term memory in the learning rule that enables different views of objects to be associated together (see Wallis and Rolls (1997), Rolls and Treves (1998), Rolls and Deco (2002), Rolls and Milward (2000) and Rolls and Stringer (2001a)). But it still does not provide the representation with any meaning in terms of the real world. What actions might one make, or what emotions might one feel, if that arbitrary set of temporal cortex visual cells was activated?

This leads to one of the answers I propose. I suggest that one type of meaning of representations in the brain is provided by their reward (or punishment) value: activation of these representations is the goal for actions. In the case of primary reinforcers such as the taste of food or pain, the activation of these representations would have meaning in the sense that the animal would work to obtain the activation of the taste of food neurons when hungry, and to escape from stimuli that cause the neurons representing pain to be activated. Evolution has built the brain so that genes specify these primary reinforcing stimuli, and so that their representations in the brain should be the targets for actions (see Chapter 3). In the case of other ensembles of neurons in, for example, the visual cortex that respond to objects with the colour and shape of a banana, and which 'represent' the sight of a banana in that their activation is always and uniquely produced by the sight of a banana, such representations come to have meaning only by association with a primary reinforcer, involving the process of stimulus–reinforcer association learning.

The second sense in which a representation may be said to have meaning is by virtue of sensory–motor correspondences in the world. For example, the touch of a solid object such as a table might become associated with evidence from the motor system that attempts to walk through the table result in cessation of movement. The representation of the table in the inferior temporal visual cortex might have 'meaning' only in the sense that there is mutual information between the representation and the sight of the table until the table is seen just before and while it is touched, when sensory–sensory association between inputs from different sensory modalities will be set up that will enable the visual representation to become associated with its correspondences in the touch and movement worlds. In this second sense, meaning will be conferred on the visual sensory representation because of its associations in the sensory–motor world. Thus it is suggested that there are two ways by which sensory representations can be said to be grounded, that is to have meaning, in the real world.

It is suggested that the symbols used in language become grounded in the real world by the same two processes.

In the first, a symbol such as the word 'banana' has meaning because it is associated with primary reinforcers such as the flavour of the banana, and with secondary reinforcers such as the sight of the banana. These reinforcers have 'meaning' to the animal in that evolution has built animals as machines designed to do everything that they can to obtain these reinforcers, so that they can eventually reproduce successfully and pass their genes onto the next generation[37]. In this sense, obtaining reinforcers may have life-threatening 'meaning' for animals, though of course the use of the word 'meaning' here does not imply any subjective state, just that the animal is built as a survival for reproduction machine[38].

In the second process, the word 'table' may have meaning because it is associated with sensory stimuli produced by tables such as their touch, shape, and sight, as well as other functional properties, such as, for example, being load-bearing, and obstructing movement if they are in the way (see Section 10.2).

10.5 Discussion

Some ways in which the current theory may be different from other related theories (Rosenthal 2004, Gennaro 2004, Carruthers 2000) follow.

The current theory holds that it is higher-order linguistic thoughts (HOLTs) (or higher order syntactic thoughts, HOSTs (Rolls 2004c, Rolls 2006a)) that are closely associated with consciousness, and this might differ from Rosenthal's higher-order thoughts (HOTs) theory (Rosenthal 1986, Rosenthal 1990, Rosenthal 1993, Rosenthal 2004) in the emphasis in the current theory on language. Language in the current theory is defined by syntactic manipulation of symbols, and does not necessarily imply verbal (or natural) language. The reason that strong emphasis is placed on language is that it is as a result of having a multistep, flexible, 'one-off', reasoning procedure that errors can be corrected by using 'thoughts about thoughts'. This enables correction of errors that cannot be easily corrected by reward or punishment received at the end of the reasoning, due to the credit assignment problem. That is, there is a need for some type of supervisory and monitoring process, to detect where errors in the reasoning have occurred.

This suggestion on the adaptive value in evolution of such a higher-order linguistic thought process for multistep planning ahead, and correcting such plans, may also be different from earlier work. Put another way, this point is that *credit assignment* when reward or punishment is received is straightforward in a one-layer network (in which the reinforcement can be used directly to correct nodes in error, or responses), but is very difficult in a multistep linguistic process executed once. Very complex mappings in a multilayer network can be learned if hundreds of learning trials are provided. But once these complex mappings are learned, their success or failure in a new situation on a given trial cannot be evaluated and corrected by the network. Indeed, the complex mappings achieved by such networks (e.g. networks trained by backpropagation of errors or by reinforcement learning) mean that after training they operate according to fixed rules, and are often quite impenetrable and inflexible (Rumelhart, Hinton and Williams 1986, Rolls and Deco 2002) (see also Appendix 1, Section A.5). In contrast, to correct a multistep, single occasion, linguistically based plan or procedure, recall of the steps just made in the reasoning or planning, and perhaps related episodic material, needs to occur, so that the link in the chain that is most likely to be in error can be identified. This may be part of the reason why there is a close relationship between declarative memory systems, which can explicitly recall memories, and consciousness.

---

[37]The fact that some stimuli are reinforcers but may not be adaptive as goals for action is no objection. Genes are limited in number, and can not allow for every eventuality, such as the availability to humans of (non-nutritive) saccharin as a sweetener. The genes can just build reinforcement systems the activation of which is generally likely to increase the fitness of the genes specifying the reinforcer (or may have increased their fitness in the recent past).

[38]This is a novel, Darwinian, approach to the issue of symbol grounding.

Some computer programs may have supervisory processes. Should these count as higher-order linguistic thought processes? My current response to this is that they should not, to the extent that they operate with fixed rules to correct the operation of a system that does not itself involve linguistic thoughts about symbols grounded semantically in the external world. If on the other hand it were possible to implement on a computer such a high-order linguistic thought–supervisory correction process to correct first-order one-off linguistic thoughts with symbols grounded in the real world (as described at the end of Section 10.4), then prima facie this process would be conscious. If it were possible in a thought experiment to reproduce the neural connectivity and operation of a human brain on a computer, then prima facie it would also have the attributes of consciousness[39]. It might continue to have those attributes for as long as power was applied to the system.

Another possible difference from earlier theories is that raw sensory feels are suggested to arise as a consequence of having a system that can think about its own thoughts. Raw sensory feels, and subjective states associated with emotional and motivational states, may not necessarily arise first in evolution.

A property often attributed to consciousness is that it is *unitary*. The current theory would account for this by the limited syntactic capability of neuronal networks in the brain, which render it difficult to implement more than a few syntactic bindings of symbols simultaneously (see Rolls and Treves (1998), McLeod, Plunkett and Rolls (1998), and Rolls and Deco (2002)). This limitation makes it difficult to run several 'streams of consciousness' simultaneously. In addition, given that a linguistic system can control behavioural output, several parallel streams might produce maladaptive behaviour (apparent as, e.g., indecision), and might be selected against. The close relationship between, and the limited capacity of, both the stream of consciousness, and auditory–verbal short-term working memory, may be that both implement the capacity for syntax in neural networks.

Whether syntax in real neuronal networks is implemented by temporal binding (see Malsburg (1990) and Singer (1999)) is still very much an unresolved issue (Rolls and Treves 1998, Rolls and Deco 2002)[40].

However, the hypothesis that syntactic binding is necessary for consciousness is one of the postulates of the theory I am describing (for the system I describe must be capable of correcting its own syntactic thoughts). The fact that the binding must be implemented in neuronal networks may well place limitations on consciousness that lead to some of its properties, such as its unitary nature. The postulate of Crick and Koch (1990) that oscillations and synchronization are necessary bases of consciousness could thus be related to the present

---

[39]This is a functionalist position. Apparently Damasio (2003) does not subscribe to this view, for he suggests that there is something in the 'stuff' (the 'natural medium') that the brain is made of that is also important. It is difficult for a person with this view to make telling points about consciousness from neuroscience, for it may always be the 'stuff' that is actually important.

[40]For example, the code about which visual stimulus has been shown can be read off from the end of the visual system without taking the temporal aspects of the neuronal firing into account; much of the information about which stimulus is shown is available in short times of 30–50 ms, and cortical neurons need fire for only this long during the identification of objects (Tovee, Rolls, Treves and Bellis 1993, Rolls and Tovee 1994, Tovee and Rolls 1995, Rolls and Treves 1998, Rolls and Deco 2002, Rolls 2003, Rolls 2006c) (these are rather short time-windows for the expression of multiple separate populations of synchronized neurons); and stimulus-dependent synchronization of firing between neurons is not a quantitatively important way of encoding information in the primate temporal cortical visual areas involved in the representation of objects and faces (Tovee and Rolls 1992, Rolls and Treves 1998, Rolls and Deco 2002, Rolls, Franco, Aggelopoulos and Reece 2003b, Rolls, Aggelopoulos, Franco and Treves 2004, Franco, Rolls, Aggelopoulos and Treves 2004, Aggelopoulos, Franco and Rolls 2005).

theory if it turns out that oscillations or neuronal synchronization are the way the brain implements syntactic binding. However, the fact that oscillations and neuronal synchronization are especially evident in anaesthetized cats does not impress as strong evidence that oscillations and synchronization are critical features of consciousness, for most people would hold that anaesthetized cats are not conscious. The fact that oscillations and stimulus-dependent neuronal synchronization are much more difficult to demonstrate in the temporal cortical visual areas of awake behaving monkeys (Tovee and Rolls 1992, Rolls and Treves 1998, Rolls and Deco 2002, Franco, Rolls, Aggelopoulos and Treves 2004, Aggelopoulos, Franco and Rolls 2005) might just mean that during the evolution of primates the cortex has become better able to avoid parasitic oscillations, as a result of developing better feedforward and feedback inhibitory circuits (Rolls and Treves 1998, Rolls and Deco 2002).

The current theory (see also Rolls (1995b), Rolls (1997a), Rolls (1999a), Rolls (2003), Rolls (2004c), and Rolls (2006a)) holds that consciousness arises by virtue of a system that can think linguistically about its own linguistic thoughts. The advantages for a system of being able to do this have been described, and this has been suggested as the reason why consciousness evolved. The evidence that consciousness arises by virtue of having a system that can perform higher-order linguistic processing is however, and I think might remain, circumstantial. [Why must it feel like something when we are performing a certain type of information processing? The evidence described here suggests that it does feel like something when we are performing a certain type of information processing, but does not produce a strong reason for why it has to feel like something. It just does, when we are using this linguistic processing system capable of higher-order thoughts.] The evidence, summarized above, includes the points that we think of ourselves as conscious when, for example, we recall earlier events, compare them with current events, and plan many steps ahead. Evidence also comes from neurological cases, from, for example, split-brain patients (who may confabulate conscious stories about what is happening in their other, non-language, hemisphere); and from cases such as frontal lobe patients who can tell one consciously what they should be doing, but nevertheless may be doing the opposite. (The force of this type of case is that much of our behaviour may normally be produced by routes about which we cannot verbalize, and are not conscious about.)

This raises the issue of the *causal role of consciousness*. Does consciousness cause our behaviour?[41] The view that I currently hold is that the information processing that is related to consciousness (activity in a linguistic system capable of higher-order thoughts, and used for planning and correcting the operation of lower-order linguistic systems) can play a causal role in producing our behaviour (see Fig. 10.4). It is, I postulate, a property of processing in this system (capable of higher-order thoughts) that it feels like something to be performing that type of processing. It is in this sense that I suggest that consciousness can act causally to influence our behaviour – consciousness is the property that occurs when a linguistic system is thinking about its lower-order thoughts, which may be useful in correcting plans.

---

[41]This raises the issue of the causal relation between mental events and neurophysiological events, part of the mind–body problem. My view is that the relationship between mental events and neurophysiological events is similar (apart from the problem of consciousness) to the relationship between the program running in a computer and the hardware on the computer. In a sense, the program causes the logic gates to move to the next state. This move causes the program to move to its next state. Effectively, we are looking at different levels of what is overall the operation of a system, and causality can usefully be understood as operating both within levels (causing one step of the program to move to the next), as well as between levels (e.g. software to hardware and vice versa). This is the solution I propose to this aspect of the mind–body (or mind–brain) problem.

The hypothesis that it does feel like something when this processing is taking place is at least to some extent testable: humans performing this type of higher-order linguistic processing, for example recalling episodic memories and comparing them with current circumstances, who denied being conscious, would prima facie constitute evidence against the theory. Most humans would find it very implausible though to posit that they could be thinking about their own thoughts, and reflecting on their own thoughts, without being conscious. This type of processing does appear, for most humans, to be necessarily conscious.

Finally, I provide a short specification of what might have to be implemented in a neural network to implement conscious processing. First, a linguistic system, not necessarily verbal, but implementing syntax between symbols implemented in the environment would be needed. This system would be necessary for a multi-step one-off planning system. Then a higher-order thought system also implementing syntax and able to think about the representations in the first-order linguistic system, and able to correct the reasoning in the first-order linguistic system in a flexible manner, would be needed. The system would also need to have its representations grounded in the world, as discussed in Section 10.4. So my view is that consciousness can be implemented in neural networks, (and that this is a topic worth discussing), but that the neural networks would have to implement the type of higher-order linguistic processing described in this Chapter, and also would need to be grounded in the world.

10.6   Conclusions and comparisons

It is suggested that it feels like something to be an organism or machine that can think about its own (syntactic and semantically grounded) thoughts.

It is suggested that qualia, raw sensory, and emotional, 'feels', arise secondarily to having evolved such a higher-order thought system, and that sensory and emotional processing feels like something because once this emotional processing has entered the planning, higher-order thought, system, it would be unparsimonious for it not to feel like something, given that all the other processing in this system I suggest does feel like something.

The adaptive value of having sensory and emotional feelings, or qualia, is thus suggested to be that such inputs are important to the long-term planning, explicit, processing system. Raw sensory feels, and subjective states associated with emotional and motivational states, may not necessarily arise first in evolution.

Reasons why the ventral visual system is more closely related to explicit than implicit processing include the fact that representations of objects and individuals need to enter the planning, hence conscious, system, and are considered in more detail by Rolls (2003) and by Rolls and Deco (2002).

Evidence that explicit, conscious, processing may have a higher threshold in sensory processing than implicit processing is considered by Rolls (2003) and Rolls (2006c), based on neurophysiological and psychophysical investigations of backward masking (Rolls and Tovee 1994, Rolls, Tovee, Purcell, Stewart and Azzopardi 1994b, Rolls, Tovee and Panzeri 1999b, Rolls 2003, Rolls 2006c). It is suggested there that part of the adaptive value of this is that if linguistic processing is inherently serial and slow, it may be maladaptive to interrupt it unless there is a high probability that the interrupting signal does not arise from noise in the system. In the psychophysical and neurophysiological studies, it was found that face stimuli presented for 16 ms and followed immediately by a masking stimulus were not consciously perceived by humans, yet produced above chance identification, and firing of inferior temporal cortex neurons in macaques for approximately 30 ms. If the mask was delayed for 20 ms, the neurons fired for approximately 50 ms, and the test face stimuli were more likely to be perceived consciously. In a similar backward masking paradigm, it was found that happy vs angry face expressions could influence how much beverage was wanted and consumed even when the faces were not consciously perceived (Winkielman and Berridge 2005, Winkielman and Berridge 2003). This is further evidence that unconscious emotional stimuli can influence behaviour.

The theory is different from some other higher-order theories of consciousness (Rosenthal 1990, Rosenthal 1993, Rosenthal 2004, Carruthers 2000, Gennaro 2004) in that it provides an account of the evolutionary, adaptive, value of a higher order thought system in helping to solve a credit assignment problem that arises in a multistep syntactic plan, links this type of processing to consciousness, and therefore emphasizes a role for syntactic processing in consciousness.

The theory described here is also different from other theories of consciousness and affect. James and Lange (James 1884, Lange 1885) held that emotional feelings arise when feedback from the periphery (about for example heart rate) reach the brain, but had no theory of why some stimuli and not others produced the peripheral changes, and thus of why some but not other events produce emotional feelings.

Moreover, the evidence that feedback from peripheral autonomic and proprioceptive systems is essential for emotions is very weak, in that for example blocking peripheral feedback does not eliminate emotions, and producing peripheral, e.g. autonomic, changes does not elicit emotion (Reisenzein 1983, Schachter and Singer 1962, Rolls 1999a) (see Section 2.6.1).

Damasio's theory of emotion (Damasio 1994, Damasio 2003) is a similar theory to the James–Lange theory (and is therefore subject to some of the same objections), but holds that the peripheral feedback is used in decision-making rather than in consciousness. He does not formally define emotions, but holds that body maps and representations are the basis of emotions. When considering consciousness, he assumes that all consciousness is self-consciousness (Damasio 2003) (p. 184), and that the foundational images in the stream of the mind are images of some kind of body event, whether the event happens in the depth of the body or in some specialized sensory device near its periphery (Damasio 2003) (p. 197). His theory does not appear to be a fully testable theory, in that he suspects that "the ultimate quality of feelings, a part of why feelings feel the way they feel, is conferred by the neural medium" (Damasio 2003) (p. 131). Thus presumably if processes he discusses (Damasio 1994, Damasio 2003) were implemented in a computer, then the computer would not have all the same properties with respect to consciousness as the real brain. In this sense he appears to be arguing for a non-functionalist position, and something crucial about consciousness being related to the particular biological machinery from which the system is made. In this respect the theory seems somewhat intangible.

LeDoux's approach to emotion (LeDoux 1992, LeDoux 1995, LeDoux 1996) is largely (to quote him) one of automaticity, with emphasis on brain mechanisms involved in the rapid, subcortical, mechanisms involved in fear. LeDoux, in line with Johnson-Laird (1988) and Baars (1988), emphasizes the role of working memory in consciousness, where he views working memory as a limited-capacity serial processor that creates and manipulates symbolic representations (p 280). He thus holds that much emotional processing is unconscious, and that when it becomes conscious it is because emotional information is entered into a working memory system. However, LeDoux (1996) concedes that consciousness, especially its phenomenal or subjective nature, is not completely explained by the computational processes that underlie working memory (p 281).

Panksepp's (1998) approach to emotion has its origins in neuroethological investigations of brainstem systems that when activated lead to behaviours like fixed action patterns, including escape, flight and fear behaviour. His views about consciousness include the postulate that "feelings may emerge when endogenous sensory and emotional systems within the brain that receive direct inputs from the outside world as well as the neurodynamics of the SELF (a Simple Ego-type Life Form) begin to reverberate with each other's changing neuronal firing rhythms" (Panksepp 1998) (p 309).

Thus the theory of consciousness described in this Chapter is different from some other theories of consciousness.

11 Conclusions, and broader issues

11.1 Conclusions

Let us evaluate where we have reached in this book, before we consider some broader issues, including the background that this biological approach to emotion provides for understanding some issues that arise in ethics, and how some of the concepts developed here may help us to understand some aspects of human emotion that are expressed in literature.

1. We have a scientific approach to emotion, its nature, and its functions (Chapters 2 and 3). It has been shown that this approach can help with classifying different emotions (Chapter 2), and in understanding what information processing systems in the brain are involved in emotion, and how they are involved (Chapters 4–8).

2. We have reached a quite specific view about how brains are designed around reward and punishment evaluation systems, because this is the way that genes can build a complex system that will produce appropriate but flexible behaviour to increase their fitness, as described in Chapter 3. The way natural selection does this is to build us with reward and punishment systems that will direct our behaviour towards goals in such a way that survival and in particular fitness are achieved. By specifying goals, rather than particular behavioural patterns of responses, genes leave much more open the possible behavioural strategies that might be required to increase their fitness. Specifying particular behavioural responses would be inefficient in terms of behavioural flexibility as environments change during evolution, and also would be more genetically costly to specify (in terms of the information to be encoded and the possibility of error). This view of the evolutionarily adaptive value for genes to build organisms using reward- and punishment-decoding and action systems in the brain places one squarely in line as a scientist from Darwin, and is a key part of my theory of emotion that will I envisage stand the test of time. It helps us to understand much of sensory information processing in the brain, followed by reward- and punishment-evaluation, followed by behaviour-selection and -execution to obtain the goals identified by the sensory/reinforcer decoding systems.

3. The importance of reward and punishment systems in brain design helps us to understand not only the significance and importance of emotion, but also of motivational behaviour, which frequently involves working to obtain goals that are specified by the current state of internal signals to achieve homeostasis (see Chapters 5 on hunger and 6 on thirst) or are influenced by internal hormonal signals (Chapter 9 on sexual behaviour). Indeed, motivation may be seen as a state in which one is working for a goal, and emotion as a state that occurs when the goal, a reinforcer, is obtained, and that may persist afterwards. The concept of gene-defined reinforcers providing the goals for action helps to understand the relation between motivational states (or desires) and emotion, as the organism must be built to be motivated to obtain the goals, and to be placed in a different state (emotion) when the goal is or is not achieved by the action. Emotional states may be motivating, as in frustrative non-reward. The close but clear relation between motivation and emotion is that both involve what humans describe as affective states (e.g. feeling hungry, liking the taste of a food, feeling happy because of a social reinforcer), and both are about goals.

4. We have outlined in Chapters 4–8 what may be the fundamental architectural and design principles of the brain for sensory, reward, and punishment information processing in primates *including humans*. These architectural principles include the following:

(a) For potential secondary reinforcers, analysis is to the stage of invariant object identi- fication before reward and punisher associations are learned. The reason for this is to enable correct generalization to other instances of the same or similar objects, even when a reward or punisher has been associated with one instance previously.

(b) The representation of the object is (appropriately) in a form that is ideal as an input to pattern associators that allow the reinforcement associations to be learned. The representations are appropriately encoded in that they can be decoded by dot product decoding of the type that is very neuronally plausible; are distributed so allowing excellent generalization and graceful degradation; have relatively independent information conveyed by different neurons in the ensemble thus allowing very high capacity; and allow much of the information to be read off very quickly, in periods of 20–50 ms (see Chapter 4, Appendix A, and Rolls and Treves (1998) and Rolls and Deco (2002)).

(c) An aim of processing in the ventral visual system (which projects to the inferior tem- poral visual cortex) is to help select the goals, or objects with reward or punisher associations, for actions. Action is concerned with the identification and selection of goals, for action, in the environment. The ventral visual system is crucially involved in this. I thus disagree with Milner and Goodale (1995) that the dorsal visual system is for the control of action, and the ventral visual system for 'perception', e.g. perceptual and cognitive representations. The ven- tral visual system is concerned with selecting the goals for action. It does this by providing invariant representations of objects, with a representation that is appropriate for interfacing to systems [such as the amygdala and orbitofrontal cortex, see Chapter 4, and Figs. 4.2 and 4.3, and 10.4 in which association cortex would correspond in vision to the inferior temporal visual cortex] which determine using pattern association the reward or punishment value of the object, as part of the process of selecting which goal is appropriate for action. Some of the evidence for this described in Chapter 4 is that large lesions of the temporal lobes (which damage the ventral visual system and some of its outputs such as the amygdala) produce the Kluver-Bucy syndrome, in which monkeys select objects indiscriminately, independently of their reward value, and place them in their mouths. The dorsal visual system helps with executing those actions, for example with shaping the hand appropriately to pick up a se- lected object. (Often this type of sensori-motor operation is performed implicitly, i.e. without conscious awareness.) In so far as explicit planning about future goals and actions requires knowledge of objects and their reward or punisher associations, it is the ventral visual system that provides the appropriate input for planning future actions. Further, for the same reason, I propose that when explicit, or conscious, planning is required, activity in the ventral visual system will be closely related to consciousness, because it is to objects, represented in the ventral visual system, that we normally apply multi-step planning processes.

(d) For primary reinforcers, the reward decoding may occur after several stages of processing, as in the primate taste system in which reward is decoded only after the primary taste cortex. The architectural principle here is that in primates there is one main taste information-processing stream in the brain, via the thalamus to the primary taste cortex, and the information about the identity of the taste is not biased by modulation of how good the taste is before this, so that the taste representation in the primary cortex can be used for purposes that are not reward-dependent. One example might be learning where a particular taste can be found in the environment, even when the primate is not hungry and therefore the taste is not currently rewarding. In the case of other sensory systems, the reinforcement value may be made explicit early on in sensory processing. This occurs, for example, in the pain system. The architectural basis of this is that there are different channels (nerve fibres) for pain and touch, so that the affective value and the identity of a tactile stimulus can be carried by separate parallel information channels, allowing separate representation and processing of each.

(e) In non-primates including, for example, rodents, the design principles may involve less sophisticated design features, partly because the stimuli being processed are simpler. For example, view-invariant object recognition is probably much less developed in non-primates, with the recognition that is possible being based more on physical similarity in terms of texture, colour, simple features, etc. (see Rolls and Deco (2002)). It may be because there is less sophisticated cortical processing of visual stimuli in this way that other sensory systems are also organized more simply, with, for example, some (but not total, only perhaps 30%) modulation of taste processing by hunger early in sensory processing in rodents (Scott, Yan and Rolls 1995, Rolls and Scott 2003). Further, while it is appropriate usually to have emotional responses to well-processed objects (e.g. the sight of a particular person), there are instances, such as a loud noise or a pure tone associated with punishment, where it may be possible to tap off a sensory representation early in sensory information processing that can be used to produce emotional responses, and this may occur, for example, in rodents, where the subcortical auditory system provides afferents to the amygdala (see Chapter 4).

(f) Another design principle is that the outputs of the reward and punishment systems must be treated by the action system as being the goals for action. The action systems must be built to try to maximize the activation of the representations produced by rewarding events, and to minimize the activation of the representations produced by punishers or stimuli associated with punishers. Drug addiction produced by the psychomotor stimulants such as amphetamine and cocaine can be seen as activating the brain at the stage where the outputs of the amygdala and orbitofrontal cortex, which provide representations of whether stimuli are associated with rewards or punishers, are fed into the ventral striatum to influence approach behaviour. The fact that addiction is persistent may be related to the fact that because the outputs of the amygdala and orbitofrontal cortex are after the stage of stimulus–reinforcer learning, the action system has to be built to interpret the representations they provide as meaning that reward actually is available.

5. Especially in primates, the visual processing in emotional and social behaviour requires sophisticated representation of individuals, and for this there are many neurons devoted to face processing. In addition, there is a separate system that encodes face gesture, movement, and view, as all are important in social behaviour, for interpreting whether a particular individual, with his or her own reinforcement associations, is producing threats or appeasements.

6. After mainly unimodal processing to the object level, sensory systems then project into convergence zones. Those especially important for reward and punishment, emotion and motivation, are the orbitofrontal cortex and amygdala, where primary reinforcers are represented. These parts of the brain appear to be especially important in emotion and motivation not only because they are the parts of the brain where in primates the primary (unlearned) reinforcing value of stimuli is represented, but also because they are the parts of the brain that perform pattern-association learning between potential secondary reinforcers and primary reinforcers. They are thus the parts of the brain involved in learning the emotional and motivational value of stimuli. The orbitofrontal cortex is involved in the rapid, one-trial, reversal of emotional behaviour when the reinforcement contingencies change, and this may be implemented by switching a rule, as described in Section 4.5.7 and Appendix 2. These orbitofrontal cortex neurons may be described as reward-predicting neurons.

7. The reward evaluation systems have tendencies to self-regulate, so that on average they can operate in a common currency that leads to the selection of different rewards with appropriately balanced probabilities, and often depending on modulation by internal motivational signals.

8. A principle that assists the selection of different behaviours is sensory-specific satiety, which builds up when a reward is repeated for a number of minutes. A principle that helps behaviour to lock on to one goal for at least a useful period is incentive motivation, the process by which early on in the presentation of a reward there is reward potentiation. There are probably simple neurophysiological bases for these time-dependent processes in the reward (as opposed to the early sensory) systems that involve synaptic habituation and (non-associative) facilitation respectively.

9. With the advances made in the last 30 years in understanding the brain mechanisms involved in reward and punishment, and emotion and motivation, the basis for addiction to drugs is becoming clearer, with dopamine playing an important role, particularly in the conditioned reinforcing effects of stimuli associated with drug usage, which influence 'wanting' for the addictive substance. Further, now that we are starting to understand how different brain systems contribute to emotion, this provides a better foundation for developing pharmacological treatments for depression and anxiety that may target particular brain areas (Chapter 8).

10. Although the architectural design principles of the brain to the stage of the representation of rewards and punishers, and thus of emotion, seems apparent, it is less clear how selection between the reward and punishment signals is made, how the costs of actions are taken into account, and how actions are selected. Some of the processes that may be involved are described in Chapters 4, 8 and 10, and decision making is considered further in Section 11.2, but much remains to be understood. The processes, which may be partly independent and performed by different brain systems (Chapter 4), include:

(a) comparison of different rewards, which may be facilitated by the representation of different rewards within a region within which lateral inhibition may operate in the human medial orbitofrontal cortex (Section 4.5.5.8);

(b) Pavlovian learning processes which enable stimuli to elicit approach or withdrawal as well as affective states which may become the goals for instrumental actions;

(c) Pavlovian learning processes which enable autonomic and endocrine responses to be elicited by conditioned stimuli (Section 4.6.1.1);

(d) action–outcome learning to obtain particular goals (Section 4.6.1.2);

(e) and stimulus–response or habit behaviour typical for overlearned responses when the goal no longer directs the behaviour, but the behaviour occurs as an automatic response to the stimulus (Sections 4.6.1.2, 8.4 and 8.9).

11. With respect to the dopamine system, it appears that the activity of the dopamine neurons does not represent reward, and is not correlated with hedonic or emotional states (see Chapter 8). Part of the evidence for this is that the dopamine neurons may fire in relation to a reward prediction error, rather than in relation to reward itself, and that damage to the dopaminergic system does not impair hedonic responses or 'liking'. Dopamine pathways do influence systems involved in Pavlovian (classically conditioned) incentive salience effects mediated by the ventral striatum, and may thereby influence 'wanting'. However, there are inconsistencies with the dopamine reward prediction error hypothesis, with respect for example to whether the dopamine system is implicated in salience vs reward prediction, whether a reward prediction error signal could facilitate the learning of stimuli associated with punishment, and how uncertainty vs reward-prediction error descriptions of the functions of dopamine neurons may be incompatible (see Chapter 8 and Section 8.4.7).

12. In addition to the implicit system for action selection, in humans and perhaps related animals there is also an explicit system that can use language to compute actions to obtain deferred rewards using a one-off plan. The language system enables one-off multistep plans that require the syntactic organization of symbols to be formulated in order to obtain rewards and avoid punishers. There are thus two separate systems for producing actions to rewarding and punishing stimuli in humans. These systems may weight different courses of action differently, and produce conflict in decision-making, in that each can produce behaviour for different goals (immediate vs deferred). Understanding our evolutionary history is useful in enabling us to understand our emotional decision-making processes, and the conflicts that may be inherent in how they operate.

13. It is possible that emotional feelings, part of the much larger problem of consciousness, arise as part of a process that involves thoughts about thoughts, which have the adaptive value of helping to correct one-off multistep plans. This is the approach described in Chapter 10, but there seems to be no clear way to choose which theory of consciousness is moving in the right direction, and caution must be exercised here.

14. Functional neuroimaging and neuropsychological data in humans (see Chapters 4 and 8) are consistent with many of the conclusions based on primate data including neurophysiology which provide the fundamental evidence needed to make computational models of how the brain functions as an information processing system exchanging information between its computing elements, the neurons (see Appendices 1 and 2 and Rolls and Deco (2002)). In addition, the human findings provide interesting new evidence on how top-down cognitive effects can influence emotions in areas such as the orbitofrontal cortex (Section 4.5.5.7). The mechanisms by which cognitive states have top-down effects on emotion are probably similar to the biased competition mechanisms that subserve top-down attentional effects (Rolls and

Deco 2002, Deco and Rolls 2003, Deco and Rolls 2005b) (see also Section 4.10).

15. In relation to animal welfare, the suggestion arises that in addition to being guided by health, it may be useful to be guided by how the animals set their priorities for different reinforcers. This follows from the hypothesis that the brain is designed round reward/punisher evaluation systems, and behaviour optimizes obtaining the goals defined by the genes. The degree to which different genes make different reinforcers important, and how they depend on for example motivational state, then directly influence the value the animal places on a provision. The value or choice of the reinforcer thus provides a useful measure of its 'importance to the animal'. When making these measures of the value of different reinforcers, it is important to be aware of the many factors that can influence the selection of a reinforcer. Examples are the fact that the choice of a reinforcer is very sensitive to incentive motivational effects, priming, delay of reinforcement, and shows rapid extinction if the reinforcer is of low value, as shown by the behaviour when tested under zero drive conditions (see Section 7.6). We may also note that the reinforcer value systems in the brain are generally different to the systems involved in autonomic and endocrine responses (see Chapter 4). The implication is that the systems (for reinforcer value vs autonomic/endocrine responses) have evolved separately, and that the autonomic/endocrine responses elicited in emotion-provoking situations may not necessarily be a good guide to the reinforcing value (as measured by choice) or 'importance' of the resource to the animal.

11.2 Decision-making

We have shown how rewards and punishers provide a basis for understanding emotion. Rewards and punishers, and emotion, are important in decision-making. I integrate some of the themes of this book by showing how there are different types of choice or decision that are made about rewards and punishers (see also Cardinal et al. (2002), Berridge and Robinson (2003) and Rolls (2007c)), and how emotion is related to these different types of decision (see Fig. 10.4).

11.2.1 Selection of mainly autonomic responses, and their classical conditioning

Responses produced by primary rewards and punishers, such as salivation, a change of heart rate, or arousal, can become classically conditioned (see Section 4.6.1.1 on page 150), and this is a form of stimulus–response (CS–UCS) learning. These responses are important for fitness, and are being selected, but hardly merit the term 'decision'. Brain regions such as the amygdala, orbitofrontal cortex, and anterior cingulate cortex are involved in these responses.

11.2.2 Selection of approach or withdrawal, and their classical conditioning

Rewards and punishers also lead to approach or withdrawal, and these effects can be classically conditioned (see Section 4.6.1.1). This is an important way in which genes can influence the behaviour that is selected, and this might be thought of as a very simple, automated, 'decision'. However, there is little flexibility in the response that is selected, in that the behaviour is either approach (e.g. to a sweet taste), or withdrawal/rejection (e.g. to a bitter taste), and in this sense behaviour is being selected by the reinforcer, but the 'decision' is essentially an automated type of behaviour. This type of approach behaviour to rewards can be classically conditioned, resulting in conditioned 'incentive salience' or 'wanting' effects (Berridge and Robinson 1998, Berridge and Robinson 2003), and this learning is implemented via the amygdala and ventral striatum, is under control of dopamine (Cardinal et al. 2002), and contributes to addiction (Robinson and Berridge 2003).

11.2.3   Selection of fixed stimulus–response habits

Stimulus–response connections can be reinforced by rewards or punishers to produce fixed habits (see Section 4.6.1.2 on page 152). Habits typically arise when behavioural responses are overlearned, and it is suggested that action–outcome learning sets up the correct stimulus–response conditions for a habit learning system to implement fixed responses to stimuli (Section 4.6.1.2). Once a habit has been learned, we may think of the behavioural selection as being a rather fixed type of 'decision'. The basal ganglia may be especially involved in habit learning (see Sections 8.4 and 8.4.7), though it does receive inputs that may be important in this process from the amygdala and orbitofrontal cortex. Reinforcement learning (see Section A.5) using reward prediction errors implemented in dopamine neuron firing may or not be important in this habit learning (see Sections 8.4 and 8.4.7).

11.2.4   Selection of arbitrary behaviours to obtain goals, action–outcome learning, and emotional learning

The real power of emotion, and rewards and punishers, occurs when goals for actions are specified by genes, and arbitrary actions can then be performed (instrumentally) to achieve the goals (see Chapters 2 and 3). The type of learning is action–outcome learning (see Sections 4.6.1.2, 4.7 and 8.9). Motivated behaviour is made to obtain, terminate or avoid the goal, and when the reward or punisher is or is not obtained, terminated, or avoided, emotional states occur that may be further motivating. Although in evolution Darwinian processes lead to gene-defined goals, it is also the case that in humans goals may be generated by other processes, including cultural processes.

The orbitofrontal cortex is important in representing the rewards and punishers, and in performing rapid stimulus–reinforcer association learning and reversal. This is the fundamental type of learning involved in producing learned emotional or affective states, and is stimulus–stimulus learning.

The orbitofrontal cortex is thus very important in emotion and affective states. The orbitofrontal cortex is not itself involved in action–outcome association learning, in that actions appear not to be represented in the orbitofrontal cortex (see Section 4.5). It is important for action–outcome learning though, in that it represents the affective outcomes. Brain regions such as the cingulate cortex may be involved in action–outcome association learning (see Section 4.7.2), and receive inputs about the outcomes, and predicted outcomes, from the orbitofrontal cortex.

11.2.5 The roles of the prefrontal cortex in decision-making and attention

First we consider the functions of the dorsolateral prefrontal cortex in short-term memory. Then we consider how this functionality enables the dorsolateral prefrontal cortex to participate in certain types of decision-making, those decision tasks that require a short-term or working memory.

A common way that the brain implements a short term memory is to maintain the firing of neurons during a short memory period after the end of a stimulus (see Fuster (2000), Goldman-Rakic (1995) and Rolls and Deco (2002); and Section A.3). In the inferior temporal cortex this firing may be maintained for a few hundred ms even when the monkey is not performing a memory task (Rolls and Tovee 1994, Rolls, Tovee, Purcell, Stewart and Azzopardi 1994b, Rolls, Tovee and Panzeri 1999b, Desimone 1996). In more ventral temporal cortical areas such as the entorhinal cortex the firing may be maintained for longer periods in delayed match to sample tasks (Suzuki, Miller and Desimone 1997), and in the prefrontal cortex for even tens of seconds (Fuster 1997, Fuster 2000). In the dorsolateral (area 46) and inferior convexity (area 12/47) prefrontal cortex (for diagram see Fig. 4.1 on page 64) the firing of the neurons may be related to the memory of spatial responses or objects (Goldman-Rakic 1996, Wilson, O'Sclaidhe and Goldman-Rakic 1993) or both (Rao, Rainer and Miller 1997), and in the principal sulcus / arcuate sulcus region to the memory of places for eye movements (Funahashi, Bruce and Goldman-Rakic 1989). The firing may be maintained by the operation of associatively modified recurrent collateral connections between nearby pyramidal cells producing attractor states in autoassociative networks (see Section A.3).

For the short term memory to be maintained during periods in which new stimuli are to be perceived, there must be separate networks for the perceptual and short term memory functions, and indeed two coupled networks (with one in the inferior temporal visual cortex for perceptual functions, and another in the prefrontal cortex for maintaining the short term memory during intervening stimuli) provide a precise model of the interaction of perceptual and short term memory systems (Renart, Parga and Rolls 2000, Renart, Moreno, Rocha, Parga and Rolls 2001) (see Fig. 11.1). In particular, this model shows how a prefrontal cortex attractor (autoassociation) network could be triggered by a sample visual stimulus represented in the inferior temporal visual cortex in a delayed match to sample task, and could keep this attractor active during a memory interval in which intervening stimuli are shown. Then when the sample stimulus reappears in the task as a match stimulus, the inferior temporal cortex module shows a large response to the match stimulus, because it is activated both by the visual incoming match stimulus, and by the consistent backprojected memory of the sample stimulus still being represented in the prefrontal cortex memory module (see Fig. 11.1).

This computational model makes it clear that in order for ongoing perception to occur unhindered in posterior cortex (parietal and temporal lobe) networks, there must be a separate set of modules that is capable of maintaining a representation over intervening stimuli. This is the fundamental understanding offered for the evolution and functions of the dorsolateral prefrontal cortex, and it is this ability to provide multiple separate short term attractor memories that provides I suggest the basis for its functions in planning.

Renart, Parga and Rolls (2000) and Renart, Moreno, Rocha, Parga and Rolls (2001) performed analyses and simulations which showed that for working memory to be implemented in this way, the connections between the perceptual and the short term memory modules (see Fig. 11.1) must be relatively weak. As a starting point, they used the neurophysiological

Inferior temporal cortex (IT)   Prefrontal cortex (PF)

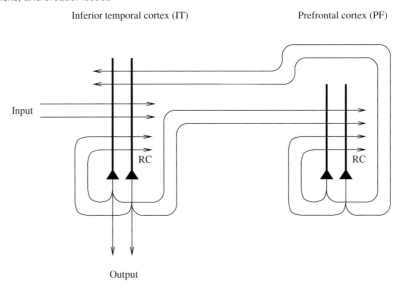

Fig. 11.1 A short term memory autoassociation network in the prefrontal cortex could hold active a working memory representation by maintaining its firing in an attractor state. The prefrontal module would be loaded with the to-be-remembered stimulus by the posterior module (in the temporal or parietal cortex) in which the incoming stimuli are represented. Backprojections from the prefrontal short term memory module to the posterior module would enable the working memory to be unloaded, to for example influence on-going perception (see text). RC - recurrent collateral connections.

data showing that in delayed match to sample tasks with intervening stimuli, the neuronal activity in the inferior temporal visual cortex (IT) is driven by each new incoming visual stimulus (Miller, Li and Desimone 1993b, Miller and Desimone 1994), whereas in the pre-frontal cortex, neurons start to fire when the sample stimulus is shown, and continue the firing that represents the sample stimulus even when the potential match stimuli are being shown (Miller, Erickson and Desimone 1996). The architecture studied by Renart, Parga and Rolls (2000) was as shown in Fig. 11.1, with both the intramodular (recurrent collateral) and the intermodular (forward IT to PF, and backward PF to IT) connections trained on the set of patterns with an associative synaptic modification rule. A crucial parameter is the strength of the intermodular connections, g, which indicates the relative strength of the intermodular to the intramodular connections. (This parameter measures effectively the relative strengths of the currents injected into the neurons by the inter-modular relative to the intra-modular connections, and the importance of setting this parameter to relatively weak values for useful interactions between coupled attractor networks was highlighted by Renart, Parga and Rolls (1999b) and Renart, Parga and Rolls (1999a), as shown in Section A.4.) The patterns themselves were sets of random numbers, and the simulation utilized a dynamical approach with neurons with continuous (hyperbolic tangent) activation functions (see (Shiino and Fukai 1990, Kuhn 1990, Kuhn, Bos and van Hemmen 1991, Amit and Tsodyks 1991)). The external current injected into IT by the incoming visual stimuli was sufficiently strong to trigger the IT module into a state representing the incoming stimulus. When the sample was shown, the initially silent PF module was triggered into activity by the weak ($g > 0.002$) intermodular connections. The PF module remained firing to the sample stimulus even when

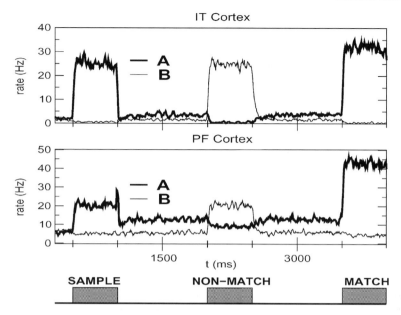

Fig. 11.2 Interaction between the prefrontal cortex (PF) and the inferior temporal cortex (IT) in a delayed match to sample task with intervening stimuli with the architecture illustrated in Fig. 11.1. Above: activity in the IT attractor module. Below: activity in the PF attractor module. The thick lines show the firing rates of the set of neurons with activity selective for the Sample stimulus (which is also shown as the Match stimulus, and is labelled **A**), and the thin lines the activity of the neurons with activity selective for the Non-Match stimulus, which is shown as an intervening stimulus between the Sample and Match stimulus and is labelled **B**. A trial is illustrated in which **A** is the Sample (and Match) stimulus. The prefrontal cortex module is pushed into an attractor state for the sample stimulus by the IT activity induced by the sample stimulus. Because of the weak coupling to the PF module from the IT module, the PF module remains in this Sample-related attractor state during the delay periods, and even while the IT module is responding to the non-match stimulus. The PF module remains in its Sample-related state even during the Non-Match stimulus because once a module is in an attractor state, it is relatively stable. When the Sample stimulus reappears as the Match stimulus, the PF module shows higher Sample stimulus-related firing, because the incoming input from IT is now adding to the activity in the PF attractor network. This in turn also produces a match enhancement effect in the IT neurons with Sample stimulus-related selectivity, because the backprojected activity from the PF module matches the incoming activity to the IT module. After Renart, Parga and Rolls, 2000 and Renart, Moreno, de la Rocha, Parga and Rolls, 2001.

IT was responding to potential match stimuli later in the trial, provided that g was less than 0.024, because then the intramodular recurrent connections could dominate the firing (see Fig. 11.2). If g was higher than this, then the PF module was pushed out of the attractor state produced by the sample stimulus. The IT module responded to each incoming potentially matching stimulus provided that g was not greater than approximately 0.024. Moreover, this value of g was sufficiently large that a larger response of the IT module was found when the stimulus matched the sample stimulus (the match enhancement effect found neurophysiologically, and a mechanism by which the matching stimulus can be identified). This simple model thus shows that the operation of the prefrontal cortex in short term memory tasks such as delayed match to sample with intervening stimuli, and its relation to posterior perceptual networks, can be understood by the interaction of two weakly coupled attractor networks, as shown in Figs. 11.1 and 11.2.

This approach emphasizes that in order to provide a good brain lesion test of prefrontal cortex short term memory functions, the task set should require a short term memory for stimuli over an interval in which other stimuli are being processed, because otherwise the posterior cortex perceptual modules could implement the short term memory function by their own recurrent collateral connections. This approach also emphasizes that there are many at least partially independent modules for short term memory functions in the prefrontal cortex (e.g. several modules for delayed saccades; one or more for delayed spatial (body) responses in the dorsolateral prefrontal cortex; one or more for remembering visual stimuli in the more ventral prefrontal cortex; and at least one in the left prefrontal cortex used for remembering the words produced in a verbal fluency task – see Section 10.3 of Rolls and Treves (1998)).

This computational approach thus provides a clear understanding of why a separate (prefrontal) mechanism is needed for working memory functions. This understanding then provides a basis for understanding the contributions of the dorsolateral prefrontal cortex to attention and decision-making (Rolls and Deco 2002, Deco and Rolls 2003, Deco and Rolls 2005a, Deco and Rolls 2005b), as summarized next.

Attention can control or influence decision-making. One way in which it does this is by a top-down influence of information held in a short term memory in the prefrontal cortex on earlier perceptual modules in the temporal and parietal lobes. The general architecture is that illustrated in Fig. 11.1 and shown in more detail in Fig. 11.3. The information to which attention must be paid, for example spatial position in a scene, is loaded into the dorsolateral prefrontal cortex short term memory, and this then biases competition between different representations in the parietal or temporal cortex (Desimone and Duncan 1995, Rolls and Deco 2002, Deco and Rolls 2004, Deco and Rolls 2005a). This *biased competition* is understood at the detailed level of an integrate-and-fire neuronal network model in which the top-down bias can have highly non-linear effects on the competition between competing perceptual representations (Deco and Rolls 2005b, Deco and Rolls 2006).

Another way in which attention can influence decision-making is by influencing the mapping from stimuli to responses. This is needed for example in tasks in which the rule is sometimes that one aspect of a stimulus, for example its spatial position, must be mapped to a particular spatial response, yet at other times the rule is that a different aspect of the stimulus, for example which object is being shown, must be mapped to a particular response. The prefrontal cortex contributes to this type of decision-making in two ways. First it provides a short term memory which holds active the current rule. Second, if there is a delay between the stimulus and the response, short term memory networks in the prefrontal cortex can bridge the delay. This type of rule-based mapping task has been studied using single neuron recording by Asaad, Rainer and Miller (1998) and Asaad, Rainer and Miller (2000), and neurons have been described that encode and hold active in the delay period the object and spatial properties of the stimuli, combinations of each of these stimulus properties with the response required, and the responses. Deco and Rolls (2003) have developed a model of this type of decision-making in which rule-encoding neurons in a short term attractor network keep the current rule active, and this operates as in attentional networks to bias the competition at the level of the stimulus-response combination neurons. The formal architecture of the model is similar to that of the model shown in Fig. 4.48, though the types of neuron are different. This biased competition operates in such a way that when the correct combination neurons are biased, the mapping automatically occurs from the correct aspect of the stimulus (its spatial position or object

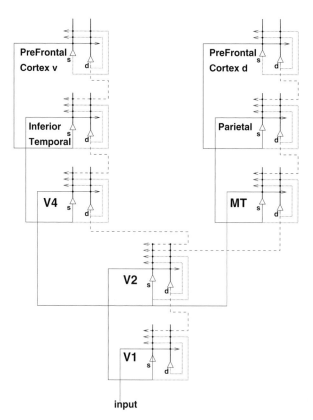

Fig. 11.3 The overall architecture of the model of object and spatial processing and attention, including the prefrontal cortical areas that provide the short term memory required to hold the object or spatial target of attention active. Forward projections between areas are shown as solid lines, and backprojections as dashed lines. The triangles represent pyramidal cell bodies, with the thick vertical line above them the dendritic trees. The cortical layers in which the cells are concentrated are indicated by s (superficial, layers 2 and 3) and d (deep, layers 5 and 6). The prefrontal cortical areas most strongly reciprocally connected to the inferior temporal cortex 'what' processing stream are labelled v to indicate that they are in the more ventral part of the lateral prefrontal cortex, area 46, close to the inferior convexity in macaques. The prefrontal cortical areas most strongly reciprocally connected to the parietal visual cortical 'where' processing stream are labelled d to indicate that they are in the more dorsal part of the lateral prefrontal cortex, area 46, in and close to the banks of the principal sulcus in macaques (see text). V1 is the primary visual cortex, and V2, V4 and MT are other visual cortical areas (see Rolls and Deco 2002 for further details).

identity) to the correct response after the delay period. One interesting aspect of this model of how the prefrontal cortex implements this type of decision-making is that the network maps from stimuli to responses by having separate attractors for the stimuli, for the combinations of stimuli and responses, and for the responses. These attractor networks are hierarchically coupled by using asymmetrical feedforward vs feedback connections from stimulus neurons, through stimulus-response combination neurons, to response neurons, to perform the desired stimulus-to-motor response transform (Deco and Rolls 2003). Another interesting aspect of this model of decision making is that it can perform reversal, which it does by altering the rule module output to bias instead a different set of stimulus-response combination neurons that implement the reverse mapping (Deco and Rolls 2005d). Another interesting aspect of the model is that it implements the short term memory functions required because it consists of a set of attractor networks (described in Section A.3). The model is also very interesting for it shows how at the start of the delay period neurons can have firing that is part of a network that holds the stimulus representation active, but later in the delay period can have firing that reflects the behavioural response that will be made (see also Takeda and Funahashi (2002)). The network model of decision-making shows that individual neurons can change their activity from stimulus-related to response-related at different times in the delay period, and that this is an interesting property of hierarchically connected attractor networks. The model itself is described in detail by Deco and Rolls (2003), and is summarized in Section B.4 (see also Deco and Rolls (2005a)). The model also provides a basis for understanding how, as the rewarded rules change in the Wisconsin card sorting task, the mapping can change from one stimulus dimension (e.g. the colour of the items on the cards) to another (e.g. the number of items on the cards), which is an example of an extradimensional shift which depends on the dorsolateral prefrontal cortex (Dias, Robbins and Roberts 1996).

If a prefrontal cortex module is to control behaviour in a working memory task, then it must be capable of assuming some type of executive control. There may be no need to have a single central executive that is additional to the control that must be capable of being exerted by short term memory modules. This is in contrast to what has traditionally been assumed for the prefrontal cortex (Shallice and Burgess 1996). The concept of executive function in the prefrontal cortex may thus be implicit in its capability to function as a short term memory that can control behaviour. Further, the role of the prefrontal cortex in executive function may be limited to situations in which a short-term or working memory functionality is required. For example, the execution of 'free-will' tasks in which subjects make decisions about which finger to raise is impaired by damage to the prefrontal cortex, and causes activation of the prefrontal cortex (Frith, Friston, Liddle and Frackowiak 1991, Jahanshahi, Jenkins, Brown, Marsden, Passingham and Brooks 1995, Jahanshahi, Dinberger, Fuller and Frith 2000), yet is a task which places demands on a working memory for previous responses, as the subjects try to make different responses from trial to trial to demonstrate their 'free will'. The impairment in verbal fluency tasks (in which a large number of different words must be produced with a given first letter) produced by left prefrontal cortex lesions (Baldo, Shimamura, Delis, Kramer and Kaplan 2001) may similarly be related to a difficulty in utilizing short term memory to remember which words have already been produced, so that further words can be different. It has also been argued that the prefrontal cortex may be especially involved in working memory in which items must be manipulated, for example in planning an optimal route or shopping expedition (Shallice 1982, Shallice and Burgess 1996, Petrides 1996). The rearrangement of items is essentially a syntactic function in which symbols must be flexibly related or linked to each other in particular ways (see Section 10.2), and this manipulation of syntactic relations may not itself be a function of the dorsolateral prefrontal cortex, damage to which does not impair syntactic and linguistic operations in general, which may depend more on specialized brain regions such as Broca's area (Kolb and Whishaw 2003, Caplan 1996). Thus the dorsolateral prefrontal cortex may provide the short term memory capability which is required when several items must be held in short term memory for manipulation by another processing region. Overall, the implication of these concepts is that the off-line short term memory functionality provided by the prefrontal cortex is fundamental to what it provides for brain computation, and that this functionality is useful in a number of tasks which are predicated on short term memory such as attention, executive function (when short term memory is required), planning, free-will, verbal fluency, and manipulation of items (which must be held in a short term memory in order to be manipulated). All of these functions use the short term memory functionality provided by the dorsolateral prefrontal cortex, but other parts of the computation depend on other brain regions. It may be noted that when decisions require not delay-related processing but instead reward and punishment evaluation, then it is the other part of the prefrontal cortex, the orbitofrontal cortex, that is involved (see Section 11.2.4).

This model (Deco and Rolls 2003) of decision-making with delays also has interesting implications for understanding disorders of attention and decision-making that follow frontal lobe damage or interference with dopamine systems. For example, Deco and Rolls (2003) simulated the effect of blockade of dopamine receptors, one effect of which is to limit the maximum current that can flow through NMDA receptor activated ion channels (Chen, Greengard and Yan 2004, Seamans and Yang 2004). The effect of this in the model of decision-making is to limit the rate of firing of the population of neurons that are in the current attractor, and this makes the attractor basin shallow (Deco and Rolls 2003). The implication of this is that attention can too easily be shifted if dopamine is low, so that the current attentional rule can not be stably maintained, and so that the biasing effect of the attentional rule does not produce such strong biasing, leading also to incorrect mappings between stimuli and responses. This is consistent with previous work showing that in simpler, single attractor, networks, D1 agonists, which can increase NMDA and GABA receptor mediated currents can increase the depth and width of basins of attraction (Durstewitz and Seamans 2002), which could affect working memory.

In the context of the effects of low NMDA receptor mediated currents produced for example by D1 receptor blockade (Chen et al. 2004) and the shallow basins of attraction in the model of decision-making produced by this manipulation (Deco and Rolls 2003), it is of considerable interest that attention and decision-making (executive function) are impaired in patients with schizophrenia, which could be related to shallow basins of attraction in dorsolateral prefrontal networks that implement the short term memory required for attention, and the weakening of the biasing effect that this normally has on the neurons that map sensory inputs to motor outputs. Consistent with this concept, NMDA receptor blockade by dissociative anesthetics (e.g. ketamine, and phencyclidine or 'angel dust') in normal subjects produces symptoms of schizophrenia including the positive symptoms such as distractability and impaired executive function, and the negative symptoms such as the flattened affect or emotion (Goff and Coyle 2001, Coyle, Tsai and Goff 2003). (Consistent with the hypothesis of shallow basins of attraction, ketamine impairs performance at the Wisconsin card sorting task, delayed word recall, and verbal fluency.) Further, agents that indirectly enhance NMDA receptor function via the glycine modulatory site reduce the negative symptoms and variably improve functioning in schizophrenic subjects receiving typical antipsychotics (Goff and Coyle 2001). This is consistent with the theory that the basins of attraction are deepened by enhancing the effects of NMDA receptor activation. Further, clozapine (an atypical antipsychotic) is a partial agonist at the glycine modulatory site (Goff and Coyle 2001). While D1 dopamine receptor mediated effects can increase NMDA mediated currents, D2 receptor mediated effects can have the opposite effects (Goff and Coyle 2001, Seamans and Yang 2004), so that dopamine

system might involve the orbitofrontal cortex, which as we have seen (Section 4.5) represents different types of reward and punisher (e.g. monetary gain and loss), and lesions of which in humans lead to impairments in changing behaviour when rewards are received less often for particular choices (Hornak, O'Doherty, Bramham, Rolls, Morris, Bullock and Polkey 2004, Berlin, Rolls and Kischka 2004), to impulsive choices (Berlin, Rolls and Iversen 2005), and to impairments in gambling tasks (Bechara et al. 1994, Bechara et al. 1998). This suggested dissociation of decision systems is the same concept as that encompassed by the hypothesis of dual routes to action considered in Section 10.3 and by Rolls (1999a) (see Fig. 10.4).

Consistent with the point being made about evolutionarily old emotion-based decision systems vs a recent rational system present in humans is that humans trade off immediate costs/benefits against cost/benefits that are delayed by as much as decades, whereas non-human primates have not been observed to engage in unpreprogrammed delay of gratification involving more than a few minutes (Rachlin 1989, Kagel et al. 1995)[42].

Moreover, individual differences in sensitivity to rewards and punishers could lead to personality differences with respect to impulsive behaviour (see Section 2.7), and indeed patients with Borderline Personality Disorder behave similarly with respect to their impulsive behaviour to patients with orbitofrontal cortex lesions (Berlin, Rolls and Kischka 2004, Berlin and Rolls 2004, Berlin, Rolls and Iversen 2005).

Consistent with dual emotional and rational bases for decisions in humans, a 'quasi-hyperbolic' time discounting function that splices together two discounting functions – an emotional one that distinguishes sharply between present and future, and a rational one that discounts exponentially and more shallowly – provides a good fit to experimental data including retirement saving, credit-card borrowing, and procrastination (Laibson 1997, Angeletos, Laibson, Repetto, Tobacman and Weinberg 2001, O'Donoghue and Rabin 1999). This dual mechanism process can be modelled formally by

$$r(t) = \beta\gamma^t r(0) \tag{11.1}$$

where $r(t)$ is the time discounted reward value at time t, and $r(0)$ is the reward value if received immediately at time $t = 0$ (McClure, Laibson, Loewenstein and Cohen 2004). β ($0 < \beta \leq 1$) (or in fact its inverse) represents the uniform downweighting of future compared to immediate rewards, and is the parameter that encompasses the effects of emotion on decision-making in this formulation. β is 1 at time zero, and is set to a value that scales a reward at any future time relative to the value at time 0. If $\beta = 0.8$, this indicates that relative to a reward of value r at time zero, the reward at any future time would have a value of 0.8. In this sense, it models the role of emotion in decision-making as down-valuing a reward at any future time compared to immediately by a uniform discounting factor β. The γ ($\gamma \leq 1$) parameter is the discount rate in the standard exponential formula that treats a given delay equivalently independently of when it occurs (i.e. in any time interval, the value decreases by a fixed proportion of the value it has already reached), and encompasses the rational route to decision-making. In the model, it produces exponential decay of the value of a reward according to how long it is delayed. It is used in the model to capture the effects of long-term economic planning for the future.

McClure, Laibson, Loewenstein and Cohen (2004) performed an fMRI investigation in which smaller immediate rewards (today) could be chosen vs larger delayed rewards (given after delays of up to six weeks). (The monetary rewards were in the range $5–$40.) Brain areas

---

[42] Seasonal food storage is not an exception, in that it appears to be stereotyped and instinctive, and hence is unlike the generalizable nature of human planning (McClure, Laibson, Loewenstein and Cohen 2004).

that showed more activation for immediate vs delayed rewards (and reflected the β emotional parameter) included the medial orbitofrontal cortex, the medial prefrontal cortex/pregenual cingulate cortex, and the ventral striatum. Brain areas where activations reflected the decisions being made and the decision difficulty but which were not preferentially activated in relation to the immediate reward parameter β included the lateral prefrontal cortex (a brain region implicated in higher level cognitive functions including working memory and executive functions (Miller and Cohen 2001, Deco and Rolls 2003)), and a part of the parietal cortex implicated in numerical processing (Dehaene, Dehaene-Lambertz and Cohen 1998). (Activations in these prefrontal and parietal areas reflect the effects of the γ^t variable in equation 11.1.) Thus emotional decisions that emphasize the importance of immediate rewards may preferentially activate reward-related areas ('β areas') such as the medial orbitofrontal cortex, pregenual cingulate cortex, and the ventral striatum, whereas difficult decisions requiring cost–benefit analysis about the value of long-term rewards preferentially activate a more cognitive system ('γ areas') that may be involved in rational thought and multistep calculation.

11.2.6.3 Reward prediction error, temporal difference error, and choice

The expected utility may alter from time to time, for example during a trial. For example, there is a reward prediction error when a reward is predicted but not obtained. Similarly, there is a reward prediction error when a reward is not expected but is obtained. The reward prediction error may be defined as the difference between the reward obtained and the reward predicted (see Section A.5.2). The firing of dopamine neurons may reflect these reward prediction errors (Schultz 1998, Schultz et al. 1997, Waelti et al. 2001, Schultz 2004) (but see Section 8.3.4).

O'Doherty et al. (2004) related reward prediction error correlated activations of the ventral striatum to a 'critic' that learns to predict a future reward because these activations occurred even when no action was required in a Pavlovian conditioning task, and reward prediction error correlated activations of the dorsal striatum to an 'actor' because it showed stronger activation during instrumental learning than Pavlovian association[43].

The hypothesis that dopamine neuron firing provides a reward prediction error signal (Schultz 1998, Schultz et al. 1997, Waelti et al. 2001, Schultz 2004) appears to be inconsistent with the evidence that dopamine neuron firing and activations of parts of the striatum are also produced by aversive, novel, or intense/salient stimuli (Zink et al. 2003, Zink et al. 2004) (see Section 8.3.4). Indeed, Zink et al. (2004) argue, from an fMRI investigation in which caudate and nucleus accumbens activations were greater when responses were made to obtain money than when money was given passively, that the activity in these regions is not related to reward value or predictions, but instead to *saliency*, that is to an arousing event to which attentional and/or behavioural resources are redirected (see further Section 8.1).

Reward prediction error encoding is in contrast to that of many neurons in the head of the caudate nucleus, which fire in relation to predicted rewards (Rolls, Thorpe and Maddison 1983c). They do this in that they start firing as soon as a cue such as a tone, or a light that precedes the tone, is given to indicate that a trial is starting, and continue to respond if a visual stimulus is shown indicating that a juice reward will be obtained, and stop responding if a different visual stimulus is shown indicating that aversive saline will be obtained (see Section 8.4.3.4).

The reward prediction error approach to changes in expected utility can be developed into a temporal difference learning approach, in which the temporal difference error depends on the

---

[43] See Section A.5.3 for a description of the functions of a 'critic' and an 'actor' in reward prediction learning.

difference in the reward value prediction at two successive time steps (see Appendix 1, Section A.5.3 and Equation A.29). This temporal difference error is useful in some temporal difference reinforcement learning algorithms for producing learning that optimizes predictions, and thus how to learn optimal actions as events unfold in time, for example during a trial (see Appendix 1, Section A.5.3). Temporal difference models have been applied to model the activity of dopamine neurons (Suri and Schultz 2001), and of fMRI activations related to the anticipation of reward (O'Doherty et al. 2003a).

Seymour et al. (2004) took the temporal difference approach in an fMRI analysis of a more complicated, second-order, pain conditioning task, with two successive visual cues to predict either low or high pain. The second cue was fully predictive of the strength of the subsequently experienced pain. The first cue only allowed a probabilistic prediction. Thus in a low proportion (18%) of the trials, the expectation evoked by the first cue was reversed by the second cue. The punisher value (pain) prediction thus alters on some trials after the second cue is delivered, generating a temporal difference prediction error. After many conditioning trials, the punisher prediction value becomes good on the 82% of trials where the first cue does predict the second cue, and during the learning the temporal difference error at the time the second cue is shown becomes low. However, on the 18% of trials where the first cue makes the incorrect prediction of the second cue, temporal difference prediction errors remain when the second cue is presented. The temporal difference error was correlated with activations in the ventral putamen (a part of the ventral striatum), the right insular cortex (probably providing a somatosensory representation of the left hand to which the pain was delivered), the right head of the caudate nucleus, and the substantia nigra (a region where dopamine neurons are located), suggesting that these areas are involved in learning expectations of pain. It should be noted that this was a conditioning procedure, and that although pain expectations were being learned, decisions were not being made by the subjects.

The temporal difference approach was taken in an fMRI study of a decision task by Rolls, McCabe and Redoute (2007b) described in Section 8.4.3.1. They showed in a probabilistic decision task in which the expected utility was systematically varied that temporal difference (reward prediction) errors were reflected in activity in the ventral striatum (see Fig. 8.10 on page 330). However, the findings showed that care is needed in interpreting fMRI signals as related to temporal difference (reward prediction) errors, for the correlation with TD error was related to the fact that in the ventral striatum, the activations were related to the reward actually obtained on each trial, and changed at the point in each trial on which this information was made available to the participant (see Section 8.4.3.1). Thus the ventral striatal activation was related to decision-making in so far as its activation reflected the reward actually provided on a given trial.

11.2.7 Selection of optimal actions by explicit rational thought

In Section 10.3 the hypothesis was developed that an explicit rational planning system allows immediate rewards encoded by an implicit emotional reward evaluation to be deferred. In this sense there are dual routes to action, one emotional, and the second rational and syntactic (see Fig. 10.4). Further evidence for these two types of decision-making was described in Section 11.2.6.2 in which the influence of immediate vs delayed rewards was considered. In delayed reward decisions, a rational, logic-based, system requiring syntactic manipulation of symbols that can treat each moment of delay equally, and calculate choice based on an exponential decrease of reward value with increasing delay, is involved. This rational decision system might involve language or mathematical systems in the brain, and the ability to hold several items in a working memory while the trade-offs of different long-term courses of action are compared.

A different more emotion-based system might operate according to heuristics that have become built into the system during evolution that might disproportionately value immediate rewards compared to delayed rewards.

Consistent with the point being made about evolutionarily old emotion-based decision systems vs a recent rational system present in humans is that humans trade off immediate costs/benefits against cost/benefits that are delayed by as much as decades, whereas non-human primates have not been observed to engage in unpreprogrammed delay of gratification involving more than a few minutes (Rachlin 1989, Kagel et al. 1995). Moreover, as described in Section 11.2.6.2, there appear to be different systems involved in these types of decision, with the orbitofrontal and pregenual cingulate cortices implicated in immediate emotion-related reward-based decision-making, and the lateral prefrontal cortex and parietal cortex implicated in long-term cost–benefit planning-related decision-making.

11.3   Emotion and ethics

I have argued in this book that much of the foundation of our emotional behaviour arises from specification by genes of primary reinforcers that provide goals for our actions. We have emotional reactions in certain circumstances, such as when we see that we are about to suffer pain, when we fall in love, or if someone does not return a favour in a reciprocal interaction. What is the relation between our emotions, and what we think is right, that is our ethical principles? If we think something is right, such as returning something that has been on loan, is this a fundamental and absolute ethical principle, or might it have arisen from deep-seated biologically-based systems shaped to be adaptive by natural selection operating in evolution to select genes that tend to promote the survival of those genes?

Many principles that we regard as ethical principles *might* arise in this way. For example, as noted in Chapter 2, guilt might arise when there is a conflict between an available reward and a rule or law of society. Jealousy is an emotion that might be aroused in a male if the faithfulness of his partner seems to be threatened by her liaison (e.g. flirting) with another male. In this case the reinforcement contingency that is operating is produced by a punisher, and it may be that males are specified genetically to find this punishing because it indicates a potential threat to their paternity and parental investment, as described in Chapters 9 and 3. Similarly, a female may become jealous if her partner has a liaison with another female, because the resources available to the 'wife' useful to bring up her children are threatened. Again, the punisher here may be gene-specified, as described in Chapter 3. Such emotional responses might influence what we build into some of the ethical principles that surround marriage and partnerships for raising children.

Many other similar examples can be surmised from the area of evolutionary psychology (see e.g. Ridley (1993b), Ridley (1996), and Buss (1999)). For example, there may be a set of reinforcers that are genetically specified to help promote social cooperation and even reciprocal altruism, and that might thus influence what we regard as ethical, or at least what we are willing to accept as ethical principles. Such genes might specify that emotion should be elicited, and behavioural changes should occur, if a cooperating partner defects or 'cheats' (Cosmides and Tooby 1999). Moreover, the genes may build brains with genetically specified rules that are useful heuristics for social cooperation, such as acting with a strategy of 'generous tit-for tat', which can be more adaptive than strict 'tit-for-tat', in that being generous occasionally is a good strategy to help promote further cooperation that has failed when both partners defect in a strict 'tit-for-tat' scenario (Ridley 1996). Genes that specify good heuristics to promote social cooperation may thus underlie such complex emotional states as feeling forgiving.

It is suggested that many apparently complex emotional states have their origins in designing animals to perform well in such sociobiological and socioeconomic situations (Ridley 1996, Glimcher 2003, Glimcher 2004). In this way, many principles that humans accept as ethical may be closely related to strategies that are useful heuristics for promoting social cooperation, and emotional feelings associated with ethical behaviour may be at least partly related to the adaptive value of such gene-specified strategies.

The situation is clarified by the ideas I have advanced in Chapter 10 and in this Chapter about a rational syntactically based reasoning system and how this interacts with an evolutionarily older emotional system with gene-specified rewards. The rational system enables us for example to defer immediate gene-specified rewards, and make longer-term plans for actions that in the long term may have more useful outcomes. This rational system enables us to make reasoned choices, and to reason about what is right. Indeed, it is because of the linguistic system that the naturalistic fallacy become an issue. In particular, we should not believe that what is right is what is natural (*the naturalistic fallacy*), because we have a rational system that can go beyond simpler gene-specified rewards and punishers that may influence our actions through brain systems that operate at least partly implicitly, i.e. unconsciously. I now consider further the relation between the biological underpinnings to emotion, and ethics, morals, and morality.

There are many reasons why people have particular moral beliefs, and believe that it is good to act in particular ways. It is possible that biology can help to explain why certain types of behaviour are adopted perhaps implicitly by humans, and become incorporated for consistency into explicit rules for conduct. This approach does not, of course, replace other approaches to what is moral, but it may help in implementing moral beliefs held for other reasons to have some insight into some of the directions that the biological underpinnings of human behaviour might lead. Humans may be better able to decide explicitly what to do when they have knowledge and insight into the biological underpinnings. It is in this framework that the following points are made, with no attempt made to lead towards any suggestions about what is 'right' or 'wrong'. The arguments that follow are based on the hypothesis that there are biological underpinnings based on the types of reward and punishment systems that have been built into our genes during evolution for at least some of the types of behaviour held to be moral.

One type of such biological underpinning is kin selection. This would tend to produce supportive behaviour towards individuals likely to be related, especially towards children, grandchildren, siblings etc., depending on how closely they are genetically related. This does tend to occur in human societies, and is part of what is regarded as 'right', and indeed it is a valued 'right' to be able to pass on goods, possessions, wealth, etc., to children. The underlying basis here would be genes for kin altruism[44].

---

[44] Kin selection genes spread because of kin altruism. Such genes direct their bodies to aid relatives because those relatives have a high chance of having the same relative-helping gene. This is a specific mechanism, and it happens to be incorrect to think that genes direct their bodies to aid relatives because those bodies 'share genes' in general

Another such underpinning might be the fact that many animals, and especially primates, co-operate with others in order to achieve ends which turn out to be on average to their advantage, including genetic advantage. One example includes the coalitions formed by groups of males in order to obtain a female for one of the groups, followed by reciprocation of the good turn later (see Ridley (1996)). This is an example of altruism, in this case by groups of primates, which is to the advantage of both groups or individuals provided that neither individual or group cheats, in which case the rules for social interaction must change to keep the strategy stable. Another such underpinning, in this case for property 'rights', might be the territory guarding behaviour that is so common from fish to primates. Another such underpinning might be the jealousy and guarding of a partner shown by males who invest parental care in their partner's offspring. This occurs in many species of birds, and also in humans, with both exemplars showing male parental investment because of the immaturity of the children. This might be a biological underpinning to the 'right' to fidelity in a female partner.

The suggestion I make is that in all these cases, and in many others, there are biological underpinnings that determine what we find rewarding or punishing, designed into genes by evolution to lead to appropriate behaviour that helps to increase the fitness of the genes. When these implicit systems for rewards and punishers start to be expressed explicitly (in language) in humans, the explicit rules, rights, and laws that are formalized are those that set out in language what the biological underpinnings 'want' to occur[45]. Clearly in formulating the explicit rights and laws, some compromise is necessary in order to keep the society stable. When the rights and laws are formulated in small societies, it is likely that individuals in that society will have many of the same genes, and rules such as 'help your neighbour' (but 'make war with "foreigners" ') will probably be to the advantage of one's genes. However, when the society increases in size beyond a small village (in the order of 1000), then the explicitly formalized rules, rights, and laws may no longer produce behaviour that turns out to be to the advantage of an individual's genes. In addition, it may no longer be possible to keep track of individuals in order to maintain the stability of 'tit-for-tat' co-operative social strategies (Dunbar 1996, Ridley 1996)[46]. In such cases, other factors doubtless come into play to additionally influence what groups hold to be right. For example, a group of subjects in a society might demand the 'right' to free speech because it is to their economic advantage.

Thus overall it is suggested that many aspects of what a society holds as right and moral, and of what becomes enshrined in explicit 'rights' and laws, are related to biological underpinnings, which have usually evolved because of the advantage to the individual's genes, but that as societies develop other factors also start to influence what is believed to be 'right' by groups of individuals, related to socioeconomic factors. In both cases, the laws and rules of the society develop so that these 'rights' are protected, but often involve compromise in such a way that a large proportion of the society will agree to, or can be made subject to, what is held as right.

(see Hamilton (1964); and the Chapter on inclusive fitness in Dawkins (1995)).

[45] Before the rules are explicitly formalized, conventions may be developed and spread using language, for example in the form of verbal traditions handed down from generation to generation that may provide possible models for behaviour, such as Homer's Odyssey.

[46] A limit on the size of the group for reciprocal altruism might be set by the ability both to have direct evidence for and remember person–reinforcer associations for large numbers of different individual people. In this situation, reputation passed on verbally from others who have the direct experience of whether an individual can be trusted to reciprocate might be a factor in the adaptive value of language and gossip (Dunbar 1996, Dunbar 1993).

To conclude this discussion, we note that what is natural does not necessarily imply what is 'right' (the naturalistic fallacy, pointed out by G. E. Moore) (see, e.g., Singer (1981)). However, our notions of what we think of as right may be related to biological underpinnings, and the point of this discussion is that it can only give helpful insight into human behaviour to realize this. Other ways in which a biological approach, based on what our brains have evolved to treat as rewarding or punishing, can illuminate moral issues, and rights, follow.

'Pain is a worse state than no pain'. This is a statement held as true by some moral philosophers, and is said to hold with no reference to biological underpinnings. It is a self-evident truth, and certain implications for behaviour may follow from the proposition. A biological approach to pain is that the elicitation of pain has to be punishing (in the sense that animals will work to escape or avoid it), as pain is the state elicited by stimuli signalling a dimension of environmental conditions that reduces survival and therefore gene fitness.

'Incest is morally wrong. One should not marry a brother or sister. One should not have intercourse with any close relation.' The biological underpinning is that children of close relations have an increased chance of having double-recessive genes, which are sometimes harmful to the individual and reduce fitness. In addition, breeding out may produce hybrid vigour. It is presumably for this reason that many animals as well as humans have behavioural strategies (influenced by the properties of reward systems) that reduce inbreeding (e.g. philopatry, that is only one sex remaining in the natal unit at the time of puberty; and mate selection influenced by the olfactory receptor/major histocompatibility genes as described in Section 9.8). At the same time, it may be adaptive (for genes) to pair with another animal that has many of the same genes, for this may help complex gene sequences to be passed intact into the next generation. This may underlie the fact that quails have mechanisms that enable them to recognize their cousins, and make them appear attractive, an example of kin selection (Bateson 1983). In humans, if one were part of a strong society (in which one's genes would have a good chance not to be eliminated by other societies), then it could be advantageous (whether male or female) to invest resources with someone else who would provide maximum genetic and resource potential for one's children, which on average across a society of relatively small size and not too mobile would be a person with relatively similar genes and resources (wealth, status etc.) to oneself. In an exception to this, in certain societies there has been a tradition of marrying close relations (e.g. the Pharaohs of Egypt), and part of the reason for this could be maintaining financial and other resources within the (genetic) family.

There may be several reasons why particular behavioural conduct may be selected. A first is that the conduct may be good for the individual and for the genes of the individual, at least on average. An example might be a prohibition on killing others in the same society (while at the same time defending that kin group in times of war). The advantage here could be for one's own genes, which would be less at risk in a society without large numbers of killings. A second reason is that particular codes of conduct might effectively help one's genes by making society stable. An example here might be a prohibition on theft, which would serve to protect property. A third reason is that the code of conduct might actually be to other, powerful, individuals' advantage, and might have been made for that reason into a rule that others in society are persuaded to follow. A general rule in society might be that honesty is a virtue, but the rule might be given a special interpretation or ignored by members of society too powerful to challenge. As discussed in Chapter 9, different aspects of behaviour could have different importance for males and females. This could lead men and women to put different stress on different rules of society, because they have different importance for men and women. One example might be being unfaithful. Because this could be advantageous to men's genes, this may be treated by men as a less serious error of conduct than by women. However, within men there could be differential condemnation, with men predisposed to being faithful being more concerned about infidelity in other men, because it is a potential threat to them. In the same way, powerful men who can afford to have liaisons with many women may be less concerned about infidelity than less powerful men, whose main genetic investment may be with one woman.

Society may set down certain propositions of what is 'right'. One reason for this is that it may be too difficult on every occasion, and for everyone, to work out explicitly what all the payoffs of each rule of conduct are. A second reason is that what is promulgated as 'right' could actually be to someone else's advantage, and it would not be wise to expose this fully. One way to convince members of society not to do what is apparently in their immediate interest is to promise a reward later. Such deferred rewards are often offered by religions. The ability to work for a deferred reward using a one-off plan in this way becomes possible, it was suggested earlier in this Chapter, with the evolution of the explicit, propositional, system.

The overall view that one is led to is that some of our moral beliefs may be explicit, verbal, formulations of what may reflect factors built genetically by kin selection into behaviour, namely a tendency to favour kin, because they are likely to share some of an individual's genes. In a small society this explicit formulation may be 'appropriate' (from the point of view of the genes), in that many members of that society will be related to that individual. When the society becomes larger, the relatedness may decrease, yet the explicit formulation of the rules or laws of society may not change. In such a situation, it is presumably appropriate for society to make it clear to its members that its rules for what is acceptable and 'right' behaviour are set in place so that individuals can live in safety, and with some expectation of help from society in general.

Other factors that can influence what is held to be right might reflect socioeconomic advantage to groups or alliances of individuals. It would be then in a sense up to individuals to decide whether they wished to accept the rules, with the costs and benefits provided by the rules of that society, in a form of Social Contract. Individuals who did not agree to the social contract might wish to transfer to another society with a different place on the continuum of costs and potential benefits to the individuals, or to influence the laws and policies of their own society. Individuals who attempt to cheat the system would be expected to pay a cost in terms of punishment meted out by the society in accordance with its rules.

11.4   Emotion and literature

Those interested in literature are sometimes puzzled by the following situation, which can perhaps be clarified by the theory of emotion developed here. The puzzle is that emotions often seem very intense in humans, indeed sometimes so intense that they produce behaviour that does not seem to be adaptive, such as fainting instead of producing an active escape response, or freezing instead of avoiding, or vacillating endlessly about emotional situations and decisions, or falling hopelessly in love even when it can be predicted to be without hope or to bring ruin. The puzzle is not only that the emotion is so intense, but also that even with our rational, reasoning, capacities, humans still find themselves in these situations, and may find it difficult to produce reasonable and effective decisions and behaviour for resolving the situation. The reasons for this include, I suggest, the following.

In humans, the reward and punishment systems may operate implicitly in comparable ways to those in other animals. But in addition to this, humans have the explicit system, which enables us consciously to look and predict many steps ahead (using language and syntax) the consequences of environmental events, and also to reflect on previous events (see Chapter 10). The consequence of this explicit processing is that we can see the full impact of rewarding and punishing events, both looking ahead to see how this will impact us, and reflecting back to previous situations that we can see may never be repeated. For example, in humans grief occurs with the loss of a loved one, and this may be much more intense than might occur simply because of failure to receive a positively reinforcing stimulus, because we can look ahead to see that the person will never be present again, can process all the possible consequences of that, and can remember all the previous occasions with that person. In another example, someone may faint at the sight of blood, and this is more likely to occur in humans because we appreciate the full consequences of major loss of blood, which we all know is life-threatening.

Thus what happens is that reinforcing events can have a very much greater reinforcing value in humans than in other animals, because we have so much cognitive, especially linguistic, processing that leads us to evaluate and appreciate many reinforcing events far more fully than can other animals. Thus humans may decode reinforcers to have supernormal intensity relative to what is usual in other animals, and the supernormal appreciated intensity of the decoded reinforcers leads to super-strong emotions. The emotional states can then be so strong that they are not necessarily adaptive, and indeed language has brought humans out of the environmental conditions under which our emotional systems evolved. For example, the autonomic responses to the sight of blood may be so strong, given that we know the consequences of loss of blood, that we faint rather than helping. Another example is that panic and anxiety states can be exacerbated by feeling the heart pounding, because we are able to use our explicit processing system to think and worry about all the possible causes. One can think of countless other examples from life, and indeed make up other examples, which of course is part of what novelists do.

A second reason for such strong emotions in humans is that the stimuli that produce emotions may be much stronger than those in which our emotional systems evolved. For example, with man-made artefacts (such as cars and guns which may injure many people simultaneously, or a large bus speeding towards one, both of which produce super-normal stimuli), the sights and related stimuli that can be produced in terms of damage to humans are much more intense that those present when our emotional systems evolved. In this way, the things we see can in some cases produce super-strong emotions. Indeed, the strength and sometimes maladaptive consequences of human emotions have preoccupied literature and literary theorists for the last 2,400 years, since Aristotle.

A third reason for the intensely mobilizing, and sometimes immobilizing, effects of emotions in humans is that we can evaluate linguistically, with reasoning, the possible courses of action open to us in emotional situations. Because we can evaluate the possible effects of reinforcers many steps ahead in our plans, and because language enables us to produce flexible one-off plans for actions, and enables us to work for deferred rewards based on one-off plans (see Chapter 10), the ways in which reinforcers are used in decision-making becomes much more complex than in those animals that cannot produce similar one-off plans using language. The consequence of this is that decision-making can become very difficult, with so many potential but uncertain reinforcement outcomes, that humans may vacillate. They are trying to compute by this explicit method the most favourable outcome of each plan in terms of the net reinforcements received, rather than using reinforcement implicitly to select the highest currently available reinforcer.

A fourth reason for complexity in the human emotional system is that there are, it is suggested, two routes to action for emotions in humans, an implicit (unconscious) and an explicit route (see Chapter 10). These systems may not always agree. The implicit system may tend to produce one type of behaviour, typically for immediately available rewards. The explicit system may tend to produce another planned course of action to produce better deferred rewards. Conflict between these systems can lead to many difficult situations, will involve conscience (what is right as conceived by the explicit system) and the requirement to abide by laws (which assume a rational explicit system responsible for our actions). It appears that the implicit system does often control our behaviour, as shown by the effects of frontal lobe damage in humans, which may produce deficits in reward-reversal tasks, even when the human can explicitly state the correct behaviour in the situation (see Chapters 4 and 10). The conflicts that arise between these implicit and explicit systems are again some of the very stuff on which literature often capitalizes.

A fifth reason for complexity in the human emotional system is that we, as social animals, with major investments in our children who benefit from long-term parental co-operation, and with advantages to be gained from social alliances if the partners can be trusted, may be built to try to estimate the goals and reliability of those we know. For example, it may matter to a woman with children whether her partner has been attracted by / is in love with / a different woman, as this could indicate a reduction of help and provision. Humans may thus be very interested in the emotional lives of each other, as this may impact on their own lives. Indeed, humans will, for this sort of reason, be very interested in who is co-operating with whom, and gossip about this may even have acted as a selective pressure for the evolution of language (Dunbar 1996, Dunbar 1993). In these circumstances, fascination with unravelling the thoughts and emotions of others (using the capacity described as theory of mind (Frith and Frith 2003, Gallagher and Frith 2003)), and empathy which may facilitate this (Singer, Seymour, O'Doherty, Kaube, Dolan and Frith 2004), would have adaptive value, though it is difficult computationally to model the minds and interactions of groups of other people, and to keep track of who knows what about whom, as this requires many levels of nested syntactical reference. Our resulting fascination with this, and perhaps the value of experience of as wide a range of situations as possible, may then be another reason why human emotions, and guessing others' emotions in complex social situations, may also be part of the stuff of novelists, playwrights, and poets. Indeed, it may be important for us to find it attractive to engage in this type of processing because of its potential adaptive value, and this may be part of the reason why we find drama, novels, and poetry so fascinating.

A sixth reason for complexity in the human emotional system is that high level cognitive processing can reach down in to the emotional systems and influence how they respond. This was demonstrated in the experiment by DeAraujo, Rolls et al. (2005) in which it was shown that processing at the linguistic level, in the form of a word label, can influence processing as far down in sensory processing as the secondary olfactory cortex in the orbitofrontal cortex, the first stage in cortical processing at which the reward- or punishment-related (hence affective) significance of stimuli is made explicit in the neuronal representations of stimuli (see Figs. 4.40–4.43). An implication of this is that cognitive factors such as the current cultural, cognitive, interpretation of literature or music may influence how the literature or music is perceived emotionally (Reddy 2001). Correspondingly, when in the 18th and 19th centuries sentiment developed as a cultural aspect of emotion in literature, the great cognitive emphasis on sentiment can be predicted to have influenced how people responded emotionally to novels written at that time. Thus the current cognitive and cultural context may have an effect not just on the high-level cognitive processing involved in emotion, but may also reach down into the systems (such as the orbitofrontal cortex) where emotion is first made explicit in brain processing, and influence at that level the emotional feelings that occur.

When at the performance of a drama or when reading a novel, the emotional feelings that occur may be partly related to the empathetic states that are being elicited as part of the way in which we are built to try to understand the feelings of others, so as better to predict their behaviour. Of course at the drama or when reading a novel, we know with our explicit system that these are not real events that have direct consequences for us, and top-down cognitive attentional processes (see Section 4.5.5.7) may influence to what extent we allow the incoming events to elicit emotional responses in us, using probably a biased competition attentional mechanism (Rolls and Deco 2002, Deco and Rolls 2003, Deco and Rolls 2005b).

11.5 Close

This book started by raising the following questions. What are emotions? Why do we have emotions? What is their adaptive value? What are the brain mechanisms of emotion, and how can disorders of emotion be understood? Why does it feel like something to have an emotion? Why do emotions sometimes feel so intense? When we know what emotions are, why we have them, how they are produced by our brains, and why it feels like something to have an emotion, we will have a broad-ranging explanation of emotion. It is in this sense that the title of this book is *Emotion Explained*. How close have we come to this?

This book provides answers to these questions. The 'why' question is answered by a Darwinian, evolutionary, theory of the adaptive value of emotion in terms of the design of animals and the brain, for the book shows that if genes specify a range of rewards and punishers (primary reinforcers) as the goals for action, then this is an efficient way for genes to influence adaptively the behaviour of the organism to promote fitness (of the genes). Part of the adaptive value, simplicity, and efficiency of this design is that the behaviour itself is not determined or specified by the genes, which need to specify just the goals for actions. This means that during the lifetime of the organism, appropriate actions to obtain the goals can be learned, allowing great flexibility of the behaviour. Another part of the adaptive value of the design is that arbitrary, previously neutral, stimuli can become associated with a primary reinforcer by stimulus–reinforcer association learning, so that there is great flexibility in learning in the lifetime of the organism about which stimuli are associated with primary reinforcers, and should also act as emotional stimuli, and lead towards attainment of the goals specified by the primary reinforcers. This is I believe a fundamental approach to understanding why we have emotions.

This Darwinian account of the 'why' question fits naturally with the operational definition of emotions as states (with particular functions) elicited by reinforcers (Chapter 2), for the reinforcers define the goals for action, that is rewards and punishers, and it is the rewards and punishers that are operationally related to emotional states. The definition thus should not be thought of as a behaviourist definition of emotion, but as a definition linked to the deep biological adaptive value of designing animals around reward and punishment systems. In addition, the definition is not behaviourist in the sense that cognitive states can elicit emotions, and that emotions can influence cognitive states (see for example Sections 2.8 and 4.10). Further, the definition is not limited to an account of a narrow range of emotions, but can encompass a very wide range of emotions, as outlined in Chapter 2. An advantage of the approach is that it clearly specifies what emotions are, and what their adaptive value is.

The 'how' question about the implementation of emotion in the brain is addressed not only by a wealth of data from neuroscience, but also by a set of principles of the brain organization for emotion set out at the start of this Chapter. An advantage of the approach to emotion described here is that it leads to well formulated questions about how to investigate the brain mechanisms that underlie emotion, for the approach indicates that it is important to understand where primary reinforcers are decoded and represented in the brain, how and where stimulus–reinforcer association learning occurs in the brain, how action–outcome (i.e. action-reinforcer) learning occurs, and the ways in which rewards and punishers influence decision-making as outlined in Section 11.2.

In relation to decision-making, it is shown that there are multiple routes via which rewards and punishers, that is emotion-provoking stimuli and the states they elicit, can influence behaviour (see Section 11.2). An important division is into the implicit ways in which rewards directly influence choice via processes such as Pavlovian approach and action–outcome learning, and an explicit route via which immediate rewards can be deferred using a long-term one-off explicit plan which may enable alternative rewards to be obtained in the long term. This is the 'dual routes to action' account developed in Chapter 10 and Section 11.2. Further approaches to decision-making are described by Rolls (2007c).

In relation to emotional feelings, it is emphasized that this is part of the much larger problem of consciousness. My own approach to this is described in Chapter 10, but it is pointed out that this is just one approach, that there do not seem to be clear criteria by which any particular theory can be confirmed, and that in the circumstances such theories should not be taken to have practical implications. Nevertheless, these are interesting issues.

It is also shown how a scientific approach to emotion can illuminate some of the biological underpinnings on top of which ethical and moral principles are developed (Section 11.3). A scientific approach to emotion also provides comments about the role of emotion in literature (Section 11.4).

This approach to emotion also fits well with the development of a precise and quantitative understanding of how emotion is implemented, using the computational approaches illustrated in Appendix 1 and Appendix 2.

Thus we may suggest that we are getting closer to a scientific understanding and explanation of emotion; and that we have some useful guidelines for investigations that will further enhance our understanding[47].

---

[47]The front cover, Psyche Opening the Door into Cupid's Garden painted in 1903 by J.W.Waterhouse, is a metaphor for this approach.

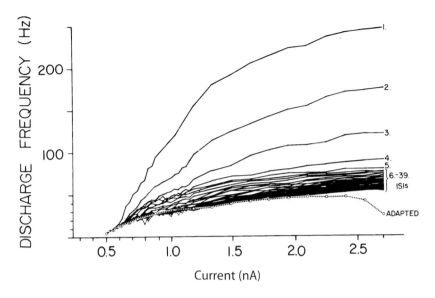

Fig. A.4 Frequency current plot (the closest experimental analogue of the activation function) for a CA1 pyramidal cell. The firing frequency (in Hz) in response to the injection of 1.5 s long, rectangular depolarizing current pulses has been plotted against the strength of the current pulses (in nA) (abscissa). The first 39 interspike intervals (ISIs) are plotted as instantaneous frequency (1/ISI, where ISI is the inter-stimulus interval), together with the average frequency of the adapted firing during the last part of the current injection (circles and broken line). The plot indicates a current threshold at approximately 0.5 nA, a linear range with a tendency to saturate, for the initial instantaneous rate, above approximately 200 Hz, and the phenomenon of adaptation, which is not reproduced in simple non-dynamical models (see further Appendix A5 of Rolls and Treves, 1998). (Reprinted with permission from Lanthorn, Storn and Andersen, 1984.)

computations to be performed in neuronal networks, including removing interfering effects of similar memories, and enabling neurons to perform logical operations, such as firing only if several inputs are present simultaneously.

A property implied by equation A.1 is that the postsynaptic membrane is electrically short, and so summates its inputs irrespective of where on the dendrite the input is received. In real neurons, the transduction of current into firing frequency (the analogue of the transfer function of equation A.2) is generally studied not with synaptic inputs but by applying a steady current through an electrode into the soma. Examples of the resulting curves, which illustrate the additional phenomenon of firing rate adaptation, are reproduced in Fig. A.4.

A.1.4 Synaptic modification

For a neuronal network to perform useful computation, that is to produce a given output when it receives a particular input, the synaptic weights must be set up appropriately. This is often performed by synaptic modification occurring during learning.

A simple learning rule that was originally presaged by Donald Hebb (1949) proposes that synapses increase in strength when there is conjunctive presynaptic and postsynaptic activity. The Hebb rule can be expressed more formally as follows:

$$\delta w_{ij} = \alpha y_i x_j. \tag{A.3}$$

where δw_{ij} is the change of the synaptic weight w_{ij} that results from the simultaneous (or conjunctive) presence of presynaptic firing x_j and postsynaptic firing y_i (or strong depolarization), and α is a learning rate constant that specifies how much the synapses alter on any one pairing. The presynaptic and postsynaptic activity must be present approximately simultaneously (to within perhaps 100–500 ms in the real brain).

The Hebb rule is expressed in this multiplicative form to reflect the idea that both presynaptic and postsynaptic activity must be present for the synapses to increase in strength. The multiplicative form also reflects the idea that strong pre- and postsynaptic firing will produce a larger change of synaptic weight than smaller firing rates. The Hebb rule thus captures what is typically found in studies of associative Long-Term Potentiation (LTP) in the brain, described in Section A.1.5.

One useful property of large neurons in the brain, such as cortical pyramidal cells, is that with their short electrical length, the postsynaptic term, y_i, is available on much of the dendrite of a cell. The implication of this is that once sufficient postsynaptic activation has been produced, any active presynaptic terminal on the neuron will show synaptic strengthening. This enables associations between coactive inputs, or correlated activity in input axons, to be learned by neurons using this simple associative learning rule.

A.1.5 Long-Term Potentiation and Long-Term Depression as models of synaptic modification

Long-Term Potentiation (LTP) and Long-Term Depression (LTD) provide useful models of some of the synaptic modifications that occur in the brain. The synaptic changes found appear to be synapse–specific, and to depend on information available locally at the synapse. LTP and LTD may thus provide a good model of the biological synaptic modifications involved in real neuronal network operations in the brain. We next therefore describe some of the properties of LTP and LTD, and evidence that implicates them in learning in at least some brain systems. Even if they turn out not to be the basis for the synaptic modifications that occur during learning, they have many of the properties that would be needed by some of the synaptic modification systems used by the brain.

Long-term potentiation (LTP) is a use-dependent and sustained increase in synaptic strength that can be induced by brief periods of synaptic stimulation. It is usually measured as a sustained increase in the amplitude of electrically evoked responses in specific neural pathways following brief trains of high-frequency stimulation (see Fig. A.5b). For example, high frequency stimulation of the Schaffer collateral inputs to the hippocampal CA1 cells results in a larger response recorded from the CA1 cells to single test pulse stimulation of the pathway. LTP is long-lasting, in that its effect can be measured for hours in hippocampal slices, and in chronic in vivo experiments in some cases it may last for months. LTP becomes evident rapidly, typically in less than 1 minute. LTP is in some brain systems associative. This is illustrated in Fig. A.5c, in which a weak input to a group of cells (e.g. the commissural input to CA1) does not show LTP unless it is given at the same time as (i.e. associatively with) another input (which could be weak or strong) to the cells. The associativity arises because it is only when sufficient activation of the postsynaptic neuron to exceed the threshold of NMDA receptors (see below) is produced that any learning can occur. The two weak inputs summate to produce sufficient depolarization to exceed the threshold. This associative

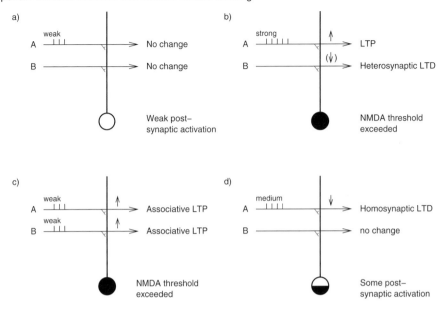

Fig. A.5 Schematic illustration of synaptic modification rules as revealed by Long-Term Potentiation (LTP) and Long-Term Depression (LTD). The activation of the postsynaptic neuron is indicated by the extent to which its soma is black. There are two sets of inputs to the neuron: A and B. (a) A weak input (indicated by 3 spikes) on the set A of input axons produces little postsynaptic activation, and there is no change in synaptic strength. (b) A strong input (indicated by 5 spikes) on the set A of input axons produces strong postsynaptic activation, and the active synapses increase in strength. This is LTP. It is homosynaptic in that the synapses that increase in strength are the same as those through which the neuron is activated. LTP is synapse–specific, in that the inactive axons, B, do not show LTP. They either do not change in strength, or they may weaken. The weakening is called heterosynaptic LTD, because the synapses that weaken are other than those through which the neuron is activated (hetero- is Greek for other). (c) Two weak inputs present simultaneously on A and B summate to produce strong postsynaptic activation, and both sets of active synapses show LTP. (d) Intermediate strength firing on A produces some activation, but not strong activation, of the postsynaptic neuron. The active synapses become weaker. This is homosynaptic LTD, in that the synapses that weaken are the same as those through which the neuron is activated (homo- is Greek for same).

property is shown very clearly in experiments in which LTP of an input to a single cell only occurs if the cell membrane is depolarized by passing current through it at the same time as the input arrives at the cell. The depolarization alone or the input alone is not sufficient to produce the LTP, and the LTP is thus associative. Moreover, in that the presynaptic input and the postsynaptic depolarization must occur at about the same time (within approximately 500 ms), the LTP requires temporal contiguity. LTP is also synapse-specific, in that for example an inactive input to a cell does not show LTP even if the cell is strongly activated by other inputs (Fig. A.5b, input B).

These spatiotemporal properties of LTP can be understood in terms of actions of the inputs on the postsynaptic cell, which in the hippocampus has two classes of receptor, NMDA (N-methyl-D-aspartate) and K–Q (kainate–quisqualate), both activated by the glutamate released by the presynaptic terminals. The NMDA receptor channels are normally blocked by Mg^{2+}, but when the cell is strongly depolarized by strong tetanic stimulation of the type necessary to

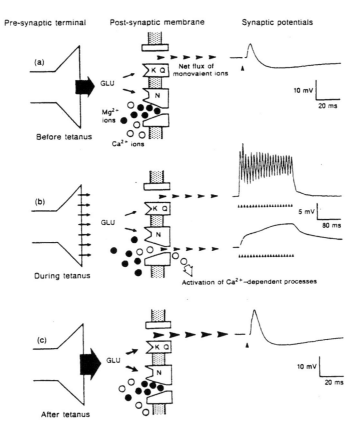

Pre-synaptic terminal   Post-synaptic membrane   Synaptic potentials

Fig. A.6 The mechanism of induction of LTP in the CA1 region of the hippocampus. (a) Neurotransmitter (e.g. L-glutamate) is released and acts upon both K–Q (kainate–quisqualate) and NMDA (N) receptors. The NMDA receptors are blocked by magnesium and the excitatory synaptic response (EPSP) is
therefore mediated primarily by ion flow through the channels associated with K–Q receptors. (b) During
high-frequency activation, the magnesium block of the ion channels associated with NMDA receptors is
released by depolarization. Activation of the NMDA receptor by transmitter now results in ions moving
through the channel. In this way, calcium enters the postsynaptic region to trigger various intracellular
mechanisms that eventually result in an alteration of synaptic efficacy. (c) Subsequent low-frequency stimulation results in a greater EPSP. See text for further details. (Reprinted with permission from Collingridge
and Bliss, 1987.)

induce LTP, the Mg^{2+} block is removed, and Ca^{2+} entering via the NMDA receptor channels
triggers events that lead to the potentiated synaptic transmission (see Fig. A.6). Part of the
evidence for this is that NMDA antagonists such as AP5 (D-2-amino-5-phosphonopentanoate)
block LTP. Further, if the postsynaptic membrane is voltage clamped to prevent depolarization
by a strong input, then LTP does not occur. The voltage-dependence of the NMDA receptor
channels introduces a threshold and thus a non-linearity that contributes to a number of the
phenomena of some types of LTP, such as cooperativity (many small inputs together produce
sufficient depolarization to allow the NMDA receptors to operate), associativity (a weak
input alone will not produce sufficient depolarization of the postsynaptic cell to enable the

NMDA receptors to be activated, but the depolarization will be sufficient if there is also a strong input), and temporal contiguity between the different inputs that show LTP (in that if inputs occur non-conjunctively, the depolarization shows insufficient summation to reach the required level, or some of the inputs may arrive when the depolarization has decayed). Once the LTP has become established (which can be within one minute of the strong input to the cell), the LTP is expressed through the K–Q receptors, in that AP5 blocks only the establishment of LTP, and not its subsequent expression (Bliss and Collingridge 1993, Nicoll and Malenka 1995, Fazeli and Collingridge 1996).

There are a number of possibilities about what change is triggered by the entry of Ca^{2+} to the postsynaptic cell to mediate LTP. One possibility is that somehow a messenger reaches the presynaptic terminals from the postsynaptic membrane and, if the terminals are active, causes them to release more transmitter in future whenever they are activated by an action potential. Consistent with this possibility is the observation that, after LTP has been induced, more transmitter appears to be released from the presynaptic endings. Another possibility is that the postsynaptic membrane changes just where Ca^{2+} has entered, so that K–Q receptors become more responsive to glutamate released in future. Consistent with this possibility is the observation that after LTP, the postsynaptic cell may respond more to locally applied glutamate (using a microiontophoretic technique).

The rule that underlies associative LTP is thus that synapses connecting two neurons become stronger if there is conjunctive presynaptic and (strong) postsynaptic activity. This learning rule for synaptic modification is sometimes called the Hebb rule, after Donald Hebb of McGill University who drew attention to this possibility, and its potential importance in learning (Hebb 1949).

In that LTP is long-lasting, develops rapidly, is synapse-specific, and is in some cases associative, it is of interest as a potential synaptic mechanism underlying some forms of memory. Evidence linking it directly to some forms of learning comes from experiments in which it has been shown that the drug AP5, infused so that it reaches the hippocampus to block NMDA receptors, blocks spatial learning mediated by the hippocampus (see Morris (1989), Martin, Grimwood and Morris (2000)). The task learned by the rats was to find the location relative to cues in a room of a platform submerged in an opaque liquid (milk). Interestingly, if the rats had already learned where the platform was, then the NMDA infusion did not block performance of the task. This is a close parallel to LTP, in that the learning, but not the subsequent expression of what had been learned, was blocked by the NMDA antagonist AP5. Although there is still some uncertainty about the experimental evidence that links LTP to learning (see for example Martin, Grimwood and Morris (2000)), there is a need for a synapse-specific modifiability of synaptic strengths on neurons if neuronal networks are to learn (see Section A.2). If LTP is not always an exact model of the synaptic modification that occurs during learning, then something with many of the properties of LTP is nevertheless needed, and is likely to be present in the brain given the functions known to be implemented in many brain regions (see Rolls and Treves (1998)).

In another model of the role of LTP in memory, Davis (2000) has studied the role of the amygdala in learning associations to fear-inducing stimuli. He has shown that blockade of NMDA synapses in the amygdala interferes with this type of learning, consistent with the idea that LTP also provides a useful model of this type of learning (see further Chapter 4).

Long-Term Depression (LTD) can also occur. It can in principle be associative or non-associative. In associative LTD, the alteration of synaptic strength depends on the pre- and postsynaptic activities. There are two types. Heterosynaptic LTD occurs when the postsynaptic neuron is strongly activated, and there is low presynaptic activity (see Fig. A.5b input B, and Table A.1). Heterosynaptic LTD is so-called because the synapse that weakens is other than (hetero-) the one through which the postsynaptic neuron is activated. Heterosynaptic LTD is important in associative neuronal networks, and in competitive neuronal networks (see Chapter 7 of Rolls and Deco (2002)). In competitive neural networks it would be helpful if the degree of heterosynaptic LTD depended on the existing strength of the synapse, and there is some evidence that this may be the case (see Chapter 7 of Rolls and Deco (2002)). Homosynaptic LTD occurs when the presynaptic neuron is strongly active, and the postsynaptic neuron has some, but low, activity (see Fig. A.5d and Table A.1). Homosynaptic LTD is so-called because the synapse that weakens is the same as (homo-) the one that is active. Heterosynaptic and homosynaptic LTD are found in the neocortex (Artola and Singer 1993, Singer 1995, Frégnac 1996) and hippocampus (Christie 1996), and in many cases are dependent on activation of NMDA receptors (see also Fazeli and Collingridge (1996)). LTD in the cerebellum is evident as weakening of active parallel fibre to Purkinje cell synapses when the climbing fibre connecting to a Purkinje cell is active (Ito 1984, Ito 1989, Ito 1993b, Ito 1993a).

An interesting time-dependence of LTP and LTD has been observed, with LTP occurring especially when the presynaptic spikes precede by a few ms the postsynaptic activation, and LTD occurring when the presynaptic spikes follow the postsynaptic activation by a few ms (Markram, Lübke, Frotscher and Sakmann 1997, Bi and Poo 1998). This type of temporally asymmetric Hebbian learning rule, demonstrated in the neocortex and the hippocampus, can induce associations over time, and not just between simultaneous events. Networks of neurons with such synapses can learn sequences (Minai and Levy 1993), enabling them to predict the future state of the postsynaptic neuron based on past experience (Abbott and Blum 1996) (see further Koch (1999), Markram, Pikus, Gupta and Tsodyks (1998) and Abbott and Nelson (2000)). This mechanism, because of its apparent time-specificity for periods in the range of tens of ms, could also encourage neurons to learn to respond to temporally synchronous presynaptic firing (Gerstner, Kreiter, Markram and Herz 1997), and indeed to decrease the synaptic strengths from neurons that fire at random times with respect to the synchronized group. This mechanism might also play a role in the normalization of the strength of synaptic connection strengths onto a neuron. Under the somewhat steady state conditions of the firing of neurons in the higher parts of the ventral visual system on the 10 ms timescale that are observed not only when single stimuli are presented for 500 ms (see Fig. 4.11), but also when macaques have found a search target and are looking at it (in the experiments described in Section 4.4.5.3), the average of the presynaptic and postsynaptic rates are likely to be the important determinants of synaptic modification. Part of the reason for this is that correlations between the firing of simultaneously recorded inferior temporal cortex neurons are not common, and if present are not very strong or typically restricted to a short time window in the order of 10 ms (see Rolls and Deco (2002), Franco, Rolls, Aggelopoulos and Treves (2004) and Aggelopoulos, Franco and Rolls (2005)). This point is also made in the context that each neuron has thousands of inputs, several tens of which are normally likely to be active when a cell is firing above its spontaneous firing rate and is strongly depolarized. This may make it unlikely statistically that there will be a strong correlation between a particular presynaptic spike and postsynaptic firing, and thus that this is likely to be a main determinant of synaptic strength under these natural conditions.

A.1.6 Distributed representations

When considering the operation of many neuronal networks in the brain, it is found that many useful properties arise if each input to the network (arriving on the axons as a firing rate vector **x**) is encoded in the activity of an ensemble or population of the axons or input lines (distributed encoding), and is not signalled by the activity of a single input, which is called local encoding. We start with some definitions, and then highlight some of the differences, and summarize some evidence that shows the type of encoding used in some brain regions. Then in Section A.2.8 (e.g. Table A.2), we show how many of the useful properties of the neuronal networks described depend on distributed encoding. Rolls and Deco (2002) (in Chapter 5) review evidence on the encoding actually found in visual cortical areas.

A.1.6.1 Definitions

A *local representation* is one in which all the information that a particular stimulus or event occurred is provided by the activity of one of the neurons. In a famous example, a single neuron might be active only if one's grandmother was being seen. An implication is that most neurons in the brain regions where objects or events are represented would fire only very rarely. A problem with this type of encoding is that a new neuron would be needed for every object or event that has to be represented. There are many other disadvantages of this type of encoding, many of which are made apparent in this book. Moreover, there is evidence that objects are represented in the brain by a different type of encoding.

A *fully distributed representation* is one in which all the information that a particular stimulus or event occurred is provided by the activity of the full set of neurons. If the neurons are binary (e.g. either active or not), the most distributed encoding is when half the neurons are active for any one stimulus or event.

A *sparse distributed representation* is a distributed representation in which a small proportion of the population of neurons is active at any one time. In a sparse representation with binary neurons, less than half of the neurons are active for any one stimulus or event. For binary neurons, we can use as a measure of the sparseness the proportion of neurons in the active state. For neurons with real, continuously variable, values of firing rates, the sparseness a of the representation can be measured, by extending the binary notion of the proportion of neurons that are firing, as

$$a = \frac{(\sum_{i=1}^{N} y_i/N)^2}{\sum_{i=1}^{N} y_i^2/N} \tag{A.4}$$

where y_i is the firing rate of the ith neuron in the set of N neurons (Treves and Rolls 1991).

Coarse coding utilizes overlaps of receptive fields, and can compute positions in the input space using differences between the firing levels of coactive cells (e.g. colour-tuned cones in the retina). The representation implied is very distributed. Fine coding (in which for example a neuron may be 'tuned' to the exact orientation and position of a stimulus) implies more local coding.

A.1.6.2 Advantages of different types of coding

One advantage of distributed encoding is that the similarity between two representations can be reflected by the correlation between the two patterns of activity that represent the different stimuli. We have already introduced the idea that the input to a neuron is represented by the activity of its set of input axons x_j, where j indexes the axons, numbered from $j = 1, C$ (see Fig. A.2 and equation A.1). Now the set of activities of the input axons is a vector (a vector is an ordered set of numbers; Appendix 1 of Rolls and Treves (1998) and of Rolls and Deco (2002) provides a summary of some of the concepts involved). We can denote as x_1 the vector of axonal activity that represents stimulus 1, and x_2 the vector that represents stimulus 2. Then the similarity between the two vectors, and thus the two stimuli, is reflected by the correlation between the two vectors. The correlation will be high if the activity of each axon in the two representations is similar; and will become more and more different as the activity of more and more of the axons differs in the two representations. Thus the similarity of two inputs can be represented in a graded or continuous way if (this type of) distributed encoding is used. This enables generalization to similar stimuli, or to incomplete versions of a stimulus (if it is for example partly seen or partly remembered), to occur. With a local representation, either one stimulus or another is represented, and similarities between different stimuli are not encoded.

Another advantage of distributed encoding is that the number of different stimuli that can be represented by a set of C components (e.g. the activity of C axons) can be very large. A simple example is provided by the binary encoding of an 8-element vector. One component can code for which of two stimuli has been seen, 2 components (or bits in a computer byte) for 4 stimuli, 3 components for 8 stimuli, 8 components for 256 stimuli, etc. That is, the number of stimuli increases exponentially with the number of components (or in this case, axons) in the representation. (In this simple binary illustrative case, the number of stimuli that can be encoded is 2^C.) Put the other way round, even if a neuron has only a limited number of inputs (e.g. a few thousand), it can nevertheless receive a great deal of information about which stimulus was present. This ability of a neuron with a limited number of inputs to receive information about which of potentially very many input events is present is probably one factor that makes computation by the brain possible. With local encoding, the number of stimuli that can be encoded increases only linearly with the number C of axons or components (because a different component is needed to represent each new stimulus). (In our example, only 8 stimuli could be represented by 8 axons.)

In the real brain, there is now good evidence that in a number of brain systems, including the high-order visual and olfactory cortices, and the hippocampus, distributed encoding with the above two properties, of representing similarity, and of exponentially increasing encoding capacity as the number of neurons in the representation increases, is found (Rolls and Tovee 1995b, Abbott, Rolls and Tovee 1996a, Rolls, Treves and Tovee 1997b, Rolls, Treves, Robertson, Georges-François and Panzeri 1998b, Rolls, Aggelopoulos, Franco and Treves 2004). For example, in the primate inferior temporal visual cortex, the number of faces or objects that can be represented increases approximately exponentially with the number of neurons in the population (see Chapter 4). If we consider instead the information about which stimulus is seen, we see that this rises approximately linearly with the number of neurons in the representation (see Chapter 4). This corresponds to an exponential rise in the number of stimuli encoded, because information is a log measure (see Appendix B of Rolls and Deco (2002)). A similar result has been found for the encoding of position in space by the primate hippocampus (Rolls, Treves, Robertson, Georges-François and Panzeri 1998b). It is particularly important that the information can be read from the ensemble of neurons using a simple measure of the similarity of vectors, the correlation (or dot product) between two vectors. The importance of this is that it is essentially vector similarity operations that characterize

where **x** or the conditioned stimulus (CS) is 101010, and **y** or the firing produced by the unconditioned stimulus (UCS) is 1100. (The arrows indicate the flow of signals.) The synaptic weights are initially all 0.

After pairing the CS with the UCS during one learning trial, some of the synaptic weights will be incremented according to Eqn A.6, so that after learning this pair the synaptic weights will become as shown in Fig. A.9:

		U	C	S	
		1	1	0	0
		↓	↓	↓	↓
CS					
1 →		1	1	0	0
0 →		0	0	0	0
1 →		1	1	0	0
0 →		0	0	0	0
1 →		1	1	0	0
0 →		0	0	0	0

Fig. A.9 Pattern association: after synaptic modification. The synapses where there is conjunctive pre- and post-synaptic activity have been strengthened to value 1.

We can represent what happens during recall, when, for example, we present the CS that has been learned, as shown in Fig. A.10:

CS				
1 →	1	1	0	0
0 →	0	0	0	0
1 →	1	1	0	0
0 →	0	0	0	0
1 →	1	1	0	0
0 →	0	0	0	0
	↓	↓	↓	↓
	3	3	0	0 Activation h_i
	1	1	0	0 Firing y_i

Fig. A.10 Pattern association: recall. The activation h_i of each neuron i is converted with a threshold of 2 to the binary firing rate y_i (1 for high, and 0 for low).

The activation of the four output neurons is 3300, and if we set the threshold of each output neuron to 2, then the output firing is 1100 (where the binary firing rate is 0 if below threshold, and 1 if above). The pattern associator has thus achieved recall of the pattern 1100, which is correct.

We can now illustrate how a number of different associations can be stored in such a pattern associator, and retrieved correctly. Let us associate a new CS pattern 110001 with the UCS 0101 in the same pattern associator. The weights will become as shown next in Fig. A.11 after learning:

```
                    U  C  S
                    0  1  0  1
                    ↓  ↓  ↓  ↓
         CS
         1 →        1  2  0  1
         1 →        0  1  0  1
         0 →        1  1  0  0
         0 →        0  0  0  0
         0 →        1  1  0  0
         1 →        0  1  0  1
```

Fig. A.11 Pattern association: synaptic weights after learning a second pattern association.

If we now present the second CS, the retrieval is as shown in Fig. A.12:

```
         CS
         1 →        1  2  0  1
         1 →        0  1  0  1
         0 →        1  1  0  0
         0 →        0  0  0  0
         0 →        1  1  0  0
         1 →        0  1  0  1
                    ↓  ↓  ↓  ↓

                    1  4  0  3  Activation $h_i$
                    0  1  0  1  Firing $y_i$
```

Fig. A.12 Pattern association: recall with the second CS.

The binary output firings were again produced with the threshold set to 2. Recall is perfect.

This illustration shows the value of some threshold non-linearity in the activation function of the neurons. In this case, the activations did reflect some small cross-talk or interference from the previous pattern association of CS1 with UCS1, but this was removed by the threshold operation, to clean up the recall firing. The example also shows that when further associations are learned by a pattern associator trained with the Hebb rule, Eqn A.6, some synapses will reflect increments above a synaptic strength of 1. It is left as an exercise to the reader to verify that recall is still perfect to CS1, the vector 101010. (The activation vector **h** is 3401, and the output firing vector **y** with the same threshold of 2 is 1100, which is perfect recall.)

A.2.3 The vector interpretation

The way in which recall is produced, equation A.7, consists for each output neuron i of multiplying each input firing rate x_j by the corresponding synaptic weight w_{ij} and summing the products to obtain the activation h_i. Now we can consider the firing rates x_j where j varies from 1 to N', the number of axons, to be a vector. (A vector is simply an ordered set of numbers – see Appendix 1 of Rolls and Deco (2002).) Let us call this vector $\mathbf{x}$. Similarly, on a neuron i, the synaptic weights can be treated as a vector, $\mathbf{w}_i$. (The subscript i here indicates that this is the weight vector on the ith neuron.) The operation we have just described to obtain the activation of an output neuron can now be seen to be a simple multiplication operation of two vectors to produce a single output value (called a scalar output). This is the inner product or dot product of two vectors, and can be written

$$h_i = \mathbf{x} \cdot \mathbf{w}_i. \tag{A.9}$$

The inner product of two vectors indicates how similar they are. If two vectors have corresponding elements the same, then the dot product will be maximal. If the two vectors are similar but not identical, then the dot product will be high. If the two vectors are completely different, the dot product will be 0, and the vectors are described as orthogonal. (The term orthogonal means at right angles, and arises from the geometric interpretation of vectors, which is summarized in Appendix 1 of Rolls and Deco (2002).) Thus the dot product provides a direct measure of how similar two vectors are.

It can now be seen that a fundamental operation many neurons perform is effectively to compute how similar an input pattern vector $\mathbf{x}$ is to their stored weight vector $\mathbf{w}_i$. The similarity measure they compute, the dot product, is a very good measure of similarity, and indeed, the standard (Pearson product-moment) correlation coefficient used in statistics is the same as a normalized dot product with the mean subtracted from each vector, as shown in Appendix 1 of Rolls and Deco (2002). (The normalization used in the correlation coefficient results in the coefficient varying always between $+1$ and -1, whereas the actual scalar value of a dot product clearly depends on the length of the vectors from which it is calculated.)

With these concepts, we can now see that during learning, a pattern associator adds to its weight vector a vector $\delta\mathbf{w}_i$ that has the same pattern as the input pattern $\mathbf{x}$, if the postsynaptic neuron i is strongly activated. Indeed, we can express equation A.6 in vector form as

$$\delta\mathbf{w}_i = \alpha y_i \mathbf{x}. \tag{A.10}$$

We can now see that what is recalled by the neuron depends on the similarity of the recall cue vector $\mathbf{x}_r$ to the originally learned vector $\mathbf{x}$. The fact that during recall the output of each neuron reflects the similarity (as measured by the dot product) of the input pattern $\mathbf{x}_r$ to each of the patterns used originally as $\mathbf{x}$ inputs (conditioned stimuli in Fig. A.7) provides a simple way to appreciate many of the interesting and biologically useful properties of pattern associators, as described next.

A.2.4 Properties

A.2.4.1 Generalization

During recall, pattern associators generalize, and produce appropriate outputs if a recall cue vector $\mathbf{x}_r$ is similar to a vector that has been learned already. This occurs because the recall operation involves computing the dot (inner) product of the input pattern vector $\mathbf{x}_r$ with the synaptic weight vector $\mathbf{w}_i$, so that the firing produced, y_i, reflects the similarity of the current input to the previously learned input pattern $\mathbf{x}$. (Generalization will occur to input cue or conditioned stimulus patterns $\mathbf{x}_r$ that are incomplete versions of an original conditioned stimulus $\mathbf{x}$, although the term completion is usually applied to the autoassociation networks described in Section A.3.)

This is an extremely important property of pattern associators, for input stimuli during recall will rarely be absolutely identical to what has been learned previously, and automatic generalization to similar stimuli is extremely useful, and has great adaptive value in biological systems.

Generalization can be illustrated with the simple binary pattern associator considered above. (Those who have appreciated the vector description just given might wish to skip this illustration.) Instead of the second CS, pattern vector 110001, we will use the similar recall cue 110100, as shown in Fig. A.13:

```
      CS
      1 →    1  2  0  1
      1 →    0  1  0  1
      0 →    1  1  0  0
      1 →    0  0  0  0
      0 →    1  1  0  0
      0 →    0  1  0  1
             ↓  ↓  ↓  ↓

             1  3  0  2  Activation h_i
             0  1  0  1  Firing y_i
```

Fig. A.13 Pattern association: generalization using an input vector similar to the second CS.

It is seen that the output firing rate vector, 0101, is exactly what should be recalled to CS2 (and not to CS1), so correct generalization has occurred. Although this is a small network trained with few examples, the same properties hold for large networks with large numbers of stored patterns, as described more quantitatively in the section on capacity below and in Appendix A3 of Rolls and Treves (1998).

A.2.4.2 Graceful degradation or fault tolerance

If the synaptic weight vector $\mathbf{w}_i$ (or the weight matrix, which we can call $\mathbf{W}$) has synapses missing (e.g. during development), or loses synapses, then the activation h_i or $\mathbf{h}$ is still reasonable, because h_i is the dot product (correlation) of $\mathbf{x}$ with $\mathbf{w}_i$. The result, especially after passing through the activation function, can frequently be perfect recall. The same property arises if for example one or some of the conditioned stimulus (CS) input axons are lost or damaged. This is a very important property of associative memories, and is not a property of conventional computer memories, which produce incorrect data if even only 1 storage location (for 1 bit or binary digit of data) of their memory is damaged or cannot be accessed. This property of graceful degradation is of great adaptive value for biological systems.

We can illustrate this with a simple example. If we damage two of the synapses in Fig. A.12 to produce the synaptic matrix shown in Fig. A.14 (where x indicates a damaged synapse which has no effect, but was previously 1), and now present the second CS, the retrieval is as follows:

CS

1 →	1	2	0	1	
1 →	0	1	0	x	
0 →	1	1	0	0	
0 →	0	0	0	0	
0 →	1	x	0	0	
1 →	0	1	0	1	
	↓	↓	↓	↓	
	1	4	0	2	Activation h_i
	0	1	0	1	Firing y_i

Fig. A.14 Pattern association: graceful degradation when some synapses are damaged (x).

The binary output firings were again produced with the threshold set to 2. The recalled vector, 0101, is perfect. This illustration again shows the value of some threshold non-linearity in the activation function of the neurons. It is left as an exercise to the reader to verify that recall is still perfect to CS1, the vector 101010. (The output activation vector **h** is 3301, and the output firing vector **y** with the same threshold of 2 is 1100, which is perfect recall.)

A.2.4.3 The importance of distributed representations for pattern associators

A distributed representation is one in which the firing or activity of all the elements in the vector is used to encode a particular stimulus. For example, in a conditioned stimulus vector CS1 that has the value 101010, we need to know the state of all the elements to know which stimulus is being represented. Another stimulus, CS2, is represented by the vector 110001. We can represent many different events or stimuli with such overlapping sets of elements, and because in general any one element cannot be used to identify the stimulus, but instead the information about which stimulus is present is distributed over the population of elements or neurons, this is called a distributed representation (see Section A.1.6). If, for binary neurons, half the neurons are in one state (e.g. 0), and the other half are in the other state (e.g. 1), then the representation is described as fully distributed. The CS representations above are thus fully distributed. If only a smaller proportion of the neurons is active to represent a stimulus, as in the vector 100001, then this is a sparse representation. For binary representations, we can quantify the sparseness by the proportion of neurons in the active (1) state.

In contrast, a local representation is one in which all the information that a particular stimulus or event has occurred is provided by the activity of one of the neurons, or elements in the vector. One stimulus might be represented by the vector 100000, another stimulus by the vector 010000, and a third stimulus by the vector 001000. The activity of neuron or element 1 would indicate that stimulus 1 was present, and of neuron 2, that stimulus 2 was present. The representation is local in that if a particular neuron is active, we know that the stimulus represented by that neuron is present. In neurophysiology, if such cells were present, they might be called 'grandmother cells' (cf. Barlow (1972), (1995)), in that one neuron might represent a stimulus in the environment as complex and specific as one's grandmother. Where the activity of a number of cells must be taken into account in order to represent a stimulus (such as an individual taste), then the representation is sometimes described as using ensemble encoding.

The properties just described for associative memories, generalization, and graceful degradation are only implemented if the representation of the CS or x vector is distributed. This occurs because the recall operation involves computing the dot (inner) product of the input pattern vector x_r with the synaptic weight vector w_i. This allows the activation h_i to reflect the similarity of the current input pattern to a previously learned input pattern x only if several or many elements of the x and x_r vectors are in the active state to represent a pattern. If local encoding were used, e.g. 100000, then if the first element of the vector (which might be the firing of axon 1, i.e. x_1, or the strength of synapse $i1$, w_{i1}) is lost, the resulting vector is not similar to any other CS vector, and the activation is 0. In the case of local encoding, the important properties of associative memories, generalization and graceful degradation do not thus emerge. Graceful degradation and generalization are dependent on distributed representations, for then the dot product can reflect similarity even when some elements of the vectors involved are altered. If we think of the correlation between Y and X in a graph, then this correlation is affected only a little if a few X, Y pairs of data are lost (see Appendix 1 of Rolls and Deco (2002)).

A.2.5 Prototype extraction, extraction of central tendency, and noise reduction

If a set of similar conditioned stimulus vectors x are paired with the same unconditioned stimulus e_i, the weight vector w_i becomes (or points towards) the sum (or with scaling, the average) of the set of similar vectors x. This follows from the operation of the Hebb rule in equation A.6. When tested at recall, the output of the memory is then best to the average input pattern vector denoted $< x >$. If the average is thought of as a prototype, then even though the prototype vector $< x >$ itself may never have been seen, the best output of the neuron or network is to the prototype. This produces 'extraction of the prototype' or 'central tendency'. The same phenomenon is a feature of human memory performance (see McClelland and Rumelhart (1986) Chapter 17), and this simple process with distributed representations in a neural network accounts for the psychological phenomenon.

If the different exemplars of the vector x are thought of as noisy versions of the true input pattern vector $< x >$ (with incorrect values for some of the elements), then the pattern associator has performed 'noise reduction', in that the output produced by any one of these vectors will represent the output produced by the true, noiseless, average vector $< x >$.

A.2.6 Speed

Recall is very fast in a real neuronal network, because the conditioned stimulus input firings x_j ($j = 1, C$ axons) can be applied simultaneously to the synapses w_{ij}, and the activation h_i can be accumulated in one or two time constants of the dendrite (e.g. 10–20 ms). Whenever the threshold of the cell is exceeded, it fires. Thus, in effectively one step, which takes the brain no more than 10–20 ms, all the output neurons of the pattern associator can be firing with rates that reflect the input firing of every axon. This is very different from a conventional digital computer, in which computing h_i in equation A.7 would involve C multiplication and addition operations occurring one after another, or $2C$ time steps.

The brain performs parallel computation in at least two senses in even a pattern associator. One is that for a single neuron, the separate contributions of the firing rate x_j of each axon j multiplied by the synaptic weight w_{ij} are computed in parallel and added in the same time step. The second is that this can be performed in parallel for all neurons $i = 1, N$ in the network, where there are N output neurons in the network. It is these types of parallel processing that enable these classes of neuronal network in the brain to operate so fast, in effectively so few steps.

Learning is also fast ('one-shot') in pattern associators, in that a single pairing of the conditioned stimulus $\mathbf{x}$ and the unconditioned stimulus (UCS) $\mathbf{e}$ which produces the unconditioned output firing $\mathbf{y}$ enables the association to be learned. There is no need to repeat the pairing in order to discover over many trials the appropriate mapping. This is extremely important for biological systems, in which a single co-occurrence of two events may lead to learning that could have life-saving consequences. (For example, the pairing of a visual stimulus with a potentially life-threatening aversive event may enable that event to be avoided in future.) Although repeated pairing with small variations of the vectors is used to obtain the useful properties of prototype extraction, extraction of central tendency, and noise reduction, the essential properties of generalization and graceful degradation are obtained with just one pairing. The actual time scales of the learning in the brain are indicated by studies of associative synaptic modification using long-term potentiation paradigms (LTP, see Section A.1.5). Co-occurrence or near simultaneity of the CS and UCS is required for periods of as little as 100 ms, with expression of the synaptic modification being present within typically a few seconds.

A.2.7 Local learning rule

The simplest learning rule used in pattern association neural networks, a version of the Hebb rule, is, as shown in equation A.6 above,

$$\delta w_{ij} = \alpha y_i x_j.$$

This is a local learning rule in that the information required to specify the change in synaptic weight is available locally at the synapse, as it is dependent only on the presynaptic firing rate x_j available at the synaptic terminal, and the postsynaptic activation or firing y_i available on the dendrite of the neuron receiving the synapse (see Fig. A.15b). This makes the learning rule biologically plausible, in that the information about how to change the synaptic weight does not have to be carried from a distant source, where it is computed, to every synapse. Such a non-local learning rule would not be biologically plausible, in that there are no appropriate connections known in most parts of the brain to bring in the synaptic training or teacher signal to every synapse.

Evidence that a learning rule with the general form of equation A.6 is implemented in at least some parts of the brain comes from studies of long-term potentiation, described in Section A.1.5. Long-term potentiation (LTP) has the synaptic specificity defined by equation A.6, in that only synapses from active afferents, not those from inactive afferents, become strengthened. Synaptic specificity is important for a pattern associator, and most other types of neuronal network, to operate correctly. The number of independently modifiable synapses

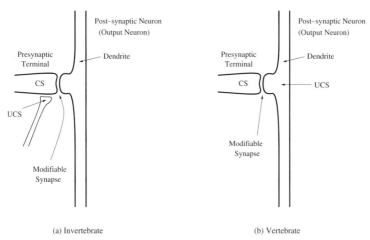

Fig. A.15 (b) In vertebrate pattern association learning, the unconditioned stimulus (UCS) may be made available at all the conditioned stimulus (CS) terminals onto the output neuron because the dendrite of the postsynaptic neuron is electrically short, so that the effect of the UCS spreads for long distances along the dendrite. (a) In contrast, in at least some invertebrate association learning systems, the unconditioned stimulus or teaching input makes a synapse onto the presynaptic terminal carrying the conditioned stimulus.

on each neuron is a primary factor in determining how many different memory patterns can be stored in associative memories (see Sections A.2.7.1 and A.3.3.6).

Another useful property of real neurons in relation to equation A.6 is that the postsynaptic term, y_i, is available on much of the dendrite of a cell, because the electrotonic length of the dendrite is short. In addition, active propagation of spiking activity from the cell body along the dendrite may help to provide a uniform postsynaptic term for the learning. Thus if a neuron is strongly activated with a high value for y_i, then any active synapse onto the cell will be capable of being modified. This enables the cell to learn an association between the pattern of activity on all its axons and its postsynaptic activation, which is stored as an addition to its weight vector $\mathbf{w}_i$. Then later on, at recall, the output can be produced as a vector dot product operation between the input pattern vector $\mathbf{x}$ and the weight vector $\mathbf{w}_i$, so that the output of the cell can reflect the correlation between the current input vector and what has previously been learned by the cell.

It is interesting that at least many invertebrate neuronal systems may operate very differently from those described here, as described by Rolls and Treves (1998) (see Fig. A.15a).

A.2.7.1 Capacity

The question of the storage capacity of a pattern associator is considered in detail in Appendix A3 of Rolls and Treves (1998). It is pointed out there that, for this type of associative network, the number of memories that it can hold simultaneously in storage has to be analysed together with the retrieval quality of each output representation, and then only for a given quality of the representation provided in the input. This is in contrast to autoassociative nets (Section A.3), in which a critical number of stored memories exists (as a function of various parameters of the network), beyond which attempting to store additional memories results in it becoming impossible to retrieve essentially anything. With a pattern associator, instead, one will always retrieve something, but this something will be very small (in information or correlation terms) if too many associations are simultaneously in storage and/or if too little is provided as input.

The conjoint quality-capacity input analysis can be carried out, for any specific instance of a pattern associator, by using formal mathematical models and established analytical procedures (see e.g. Treves (1995)). This, however, has to be done case by case. It is anyway useful to develop some intuition for how a pattern associator operates, by considering what its capacity would be in certain well-defined simplified cases.

Linear associative neuronal networks These networks are made up of units with a linear activation function, which appears to make them unsuitable to represent real neurons with their positive-only firing rates. However, even purely linear units have been considered as provisionally relevant models of real neurons, by assuming that the latter operate sometimes in the linear regime of their transfer function. (This implies a high level of spontaneous activity, and may be closer to conditions observed early on in sensory systems rather than in areas more specifically involved in memory.) As usual, the connections are trained by a Hebb (or similar) associative learning rule. The capacity of these networks can be defined as the total number of associations that can be learned independently of each other, given that the linear nature of these systems prevents anything more than a linear transform of the inputs. This implies that if input pattern C can be written as the weighted sum of input patterns A and B, the output to C will be just the same weighted sum of the outputs to A and B. If there are N' input axons, then there can be only at most N' mutually independent input patterns (i.e. none able to be written as a weighted sum of the others), and therefore the capacity of linear networks, defined above, is just N', or equal to the number of inputs to each neuron. In general, a random set of less than N' vectors (the CS input pattern vectors) will tend to be mutually independent but not mutually orthogonal (at $90 \deg$ to each other) (see Appendix 1 of Rolls and Deco (2002)). If they are not orthogonal (the normal situation), then the dot product of them is not 0, and the output pattern activated by one of the input vectors will be partially activated by other input pattern vectors, in accordance with how similar they are (see equations A.9 and A.10). This amounts to interference, which is therefore the more serious the less orthogonal, on the whole, is the set of input vectors.

Since input patterns are made of elements with positive values, if a simple Hebbian learning rule like the one of equation A.6 is used (in which the input pattern enters directly with no subtraction term), the output resulting from the application of a stored input vector will be the sum of contributions from all other input vectors that have a non-zero dot product with it (see Appendix 1 of Rolls and Deco (2002)), and interference will be disastrous. The only situation in which this would not occur is when different input patterns activate completely different input lines, but this is clearly an uninteresting circumstance for networks operating with distributed representations. A solution to this issue is to use a modified learning rule of the following form:

$$\delta w_{ij} = \alpha y_i (x_j - x) \tag{A.11}$$

where x is a constant, approximately equal to the average value of x_j. This learning rule includes (in proportion to y_i) increasing the synaptic weight if $(x_j - x) > 0$ (long-term potentiation), and decreasing the synaptic weight if $(x_j - x) < 0$ (heterosynaptic long-term depression). It is useful for x to be roughly the average activity of an input axon x_j across patterns, because then the dot product between the various patterns stored on the weights and the input vector will tend to cancel out with the subtractive term, except for the pattern equal to (or correlated with) the input vector itself. Then up to N' input vectors can still be learned by the network, with only minor interference (provided of course that they are mutually independent, as they will in general tend to be).

Table A.1 Effects of pre- and post-synaptic activity on synaptic modification

	Post-synaptic activation	
	0	high
Presynaptic firing 0	No change	Heterosynaptic LTD
high	Homosynaptic LTD	LTP

This modified learning rule can also be described in terms of a contingency table (Table A.1) showing the synaptic strength modifications produced by different types of learning rule, where LTP indicates an increase in synaptic strength (called Long-Term Potentiation in neurophysiology), and LTD indicates a decrease in synaptic strength (called Long-Term Depression in neurophysiology). Heterosynaptic long-term depression is so-called because it is the decrease in synaptic strength that occurs to a synapse that is other than that through which the postsynaptic cell is being activated. This heterosynaptic long-term depression is the type of change of synaptic strength that is required (in addition to LTP) for effective subtraction of the average presynaptic firing rate, in order, as it were, to make the CS vectors appear more orthogonal to the pattern associator. The rule is sometimes called the Singer–Stent rule, after work by Singer (1987) and Stent (1973), and was discovered in the brain by Levy (Levy (1985); Levy and Desmond (1985); see Brown, Kairiss and Keenan (1990)). Homosynaptic long-term depression is so-called because it is the decrease in synaptic strength that occurs to a synapse which is (the same as that which is) active. For it to occur, the postsynaptic neuron must simultaneously be inactive, or have only low activity. (This rule is sometimes called the BCM rule after the paper of Bienenstock, Cooper and Munro (1982); see Rolls and Deco (2002), Chapter 7).

Associative neuronal networks with non-linear neurons With non-linear neurons, that is with at least a threshold in the activation function so that the output firing y_i is 0 when the activation h_i is below the threshold, the capacity can be measured in terms of the number of different clusters of output pattern vectors that the network produces. This is because the non-linearities now present (one per output neuron) result in some clustering of the outputs produced by all possible (conditioned stimulus) input patterns **x**. Input patterns that are similar to a stored input vector can produce, due to the non-linearities, output patterns even closer to the stored output; and vice versa sufficiently dissimilar inputs can be assigned to different output clusters thereby increasing their mutual dissimilarity. As with the linear counterpart, in order to remove the correlation that would otherwise occur between the patterns because the elements can take only positive values, it is useful to use a modified Hebb rule of the form shown in equation A.11.

With fully distributed output patterns, the number p of associations that leads to different clusters is of order C, the number of input lines (axons) per output neuron (that is, of order N' for a fully connected network), as shown in Appendix A3 of Rolls and Treves (1998). If sparse patterns are used in the output, or alternatively if the learning rule includes a non-linear postsynaptic factor that is effectively equivalent to using sparse output patterns, the coefficient of proportionality between p and C can be much higher than one, that is, many more patterns can be stored than inputs onto each output neuron (see Appendix A3 of Rolls and Treves (1998)). Indeed, the number of different patterns or prototypes p that can be stored can be derived for example in the case of binary units (Gardner 1988) to be

$$p \approx C/[a_o log(1/a_o)] \tag{A.12}$$

where a_o is the sparseness of the output firing pattern **y** produced by the unconditioned stimulus. p can in this situation be much larger than C (see Rolls and Treves (1990), and Appendix A3 of Rolls and Treves (1998)). This is an important result for encoding in pattern associators, for it means that provided that the activation functions are non-linear (which is the case with real neurons), there is a very great advantage to using sparse encoding, for then many more than C pattern associations can be stored. Sparse representations may well be present in brain regions involved in associative memory (see Chapter 12 of Rolls and Treves (1998)) for this reason.

The non-linearity inherent in the NMDA receptor-based Hebbian plasticity present in the brain may help to make the stored patterns more sparse than the input patterns, and this may be especially beneficial in increasing the storage capacity of associative networks in the brain by allowing participation in the storage of especially those relatively few neurons with high firing rates in the exponential firing rate distributions typical of neurons in sensory systems (see Rolls and Deco (2002)).

A.2.7.2 Interference

Interference occurs in linear pattern associators if two vectors are not orthogonal, and is simply dependent on the angle between the originally learned vector and the recall cue or CS vector (see Appendix 1 of Rolls and Deco (2002)), for the activation of the output neuron depends simply on the dot product of the recall vector and the synaptic weight vector (equation A.9). Also in non-linear pattern associators (the interesting case for all practical purposes), interference may occur if two CS patterns are not orthogonal, though the effect can be controlled with sparse encoding of the UCS patterns, effectively by setting high thresholds for the firing of output units. In other words, the CS vectors need not be strictly orthogonal, but if they are too similar, some interference will still be likely to occur.

The fact that interference is a property of neural network pattern associator memories is of interest, for interference is a major property of human memory. Indeed, the fact that interference is a property of human memory and of neural network association memories is entirely consistent with the hypothesis that human memory is stored in associative memories of the type described here, or at least that network associative memories of the type described represent a useful exemplar of the class of parallel distributed storage network used in human memory.

It may also be suggested that one reason that interference is tolerated in biological memory is that it is associated with the ability to generalize between stimuli, which is an invaluable feature of biological network associative memories, in that it allows the memory to cope with

Input A	1	0	1
Input B	0	1	1

Required Output	1	1	0

Fig. A.16 A non-linearly separable mapping.

stimuli that will almost never be identical on different occasions, and in that it allows useful analogies that have survival value to be made.

A.2.7.3 Expansion recoding

If patterns are too similar to be stored in associative memories, then one solution that the brain seems to use repeatedly is to expand the encoding to a form in which the different stimulus patterns are less correlated, that is, more orthogonal, before they are presented as CS stimuli to a pattern associator. The problem can be highlighted by a non-linearly separable mapping (which captures part of the eXclusive OR (XOR) problem), in which the mapping that is desired is as shown in Fig. A.16. The neuron has two inputs, A and B.

This is a mapping of patterns that is impossible for a one-layer network, because the patterns are not linearly separable[49]. A solution is to remap the two input lines A and B to three input lines 1–3, that is to use expansion recoding, as shown in Fig. A.17. This can be performed by a competitive network (see Rolls and Deco (2002) Chapter 7). The synaptic

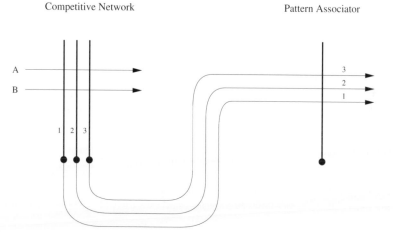

Fig. A.17 Expansion recoding. A competitive network followed by a pattern associator that can enable patterns that are not linearly separable to be learned correctly.

weights on the dendrite of the output neuron could then learn the following values using a simple Hebb rule, equation A.6, and the problem could be solved as in Fig. A.18. The whole

---

[49] See Appendix 1 of Rolls and Deco (2002). There is no set of synaptic weights in a one-layer net that could solve the problem shown in Fig. A.16. Two classes of patterns are not linearly separable if no hyperplane can be positioned in their N-dimensional space so as to separate them (see Appendix 1 of Rolls and Deco (2002)). The XOR problem has the additional constraint that $A = 0, B = 0$ must be mapped to Output = 0.

	Synaptic weight
Input 1 (A=1, B=0)	1
Input 2 (A=0, B=1)	1
Input 3 (A=1, B=1)	0

Fig. A.18 Synaptic weights on the dendrite of the output neuron in Fig. A.17.

network would look like that shown in Fig. A.17.

Rolls and Treves (1998) show that competitive networks could help with this type of recoding, and could provide very useful preprocessing for a pattern associator in the brain. It is possible that the lateral nucleus of the amygdala performs this function, for it receives inputs from the temporal cortical visual areas, and may preprocess them before they become the inputs to associative networks at the next stage of amygdala processing (see Fig. 4.52).

A.2.8 Implications of different types of coding for storage in pattern associators

Throughout this Section, we have made statements about how the properties of pattern associators – such as the number of patterns that can be stored, and whether generalization and graceful degradation occur – depend on the type of encoding of the patterns to be associated. (The types of encoding considered, local, sparse distributed, and fully distributed, are described above.) We draw together these points in Table A.2.

Table A.2 Coding in associative memories*

	Local	Sparse distributed	Fully distributed
Generalization, Completion, Graceful degradation	No	Yes	Yes
Number of patterns that can be stored	N (large)	of order $C/[a_o \log(1/a_o)]$ (can be larger)	of order C (usually smaller than N)
Amount of information in each pattern (values if binary)	Minimal ($\log(N)$ bits)	Intermediate ($Na_o \log(1/a_o)$ bits)	Large (N bits)

* N refers here to the number of output units, and C to the average number of inputs to each output unit. a_o is the sparseness of output patterns, or roughly the proportion of output units activated by a UCS pattern. Note: logs are to the base 2.

The amount of information that can be stored in each pattern in a pattern associator is considered in Appendix A3 of Rolls and Treves (1998).

In conclusion, the architecture and properties of pattern association networks make them very appropriate for stimulus–reinforcer association learning. Their high capacity enables them to learn the correct reinforcement associations for very large numbers of different stimuli.

A.3 Autoassociation memory: attractor networks

In this Section an introduction to autoassociation or attractor networks is given, as this type of network may be relevant to understanding how mood states are maintained.

Autoassociative memories, or attractor neural networks, store memories, each one of which is represented by a different set of the neurons firing. The memories are stored in the recurrent synaptic connections between the neurons of the network, for example in the recurrent collateral connections between cortical pyramidal cells. Autoassociative networks can then recall the appropriate memory from the network when provided with a fragment of one of the memories. This is called completion. Many different memories can be stored in the network and retrieved correctly. A feature of this type of memory is that it is content addressable: that is, the information in the memory can be accessed if just the contents of the memory (or a part of the contents of the memory) are used. This is in contrast to a conventional computer, in which the address of what is to be accessed must be supplied, and used to access the contents of the memory. Content addressability is an important simplifying feature of this type of memory, which makes it suitable for use in biological systems. The issue of content addressability will be amplified below.

An autoassociation memory can be used as a short-term memory, in which iterative processing round the recurrent collateral connections between the principal neurons in the network keeps a representation active by continuing, persistent, neuronal firing. Used in this way, attractor networks provide the basis for the implementation of short-term memory in the dorsolateral prefrontal cortex. In this cortical area, the short-term memory provides the basis for keeping a memory active even while perceptual areas such as the inferior temporal visual cortex must respond to each incoming visual stimulus in order for it to be processed, to produce behavioural responses, and for it to be perceived (Renart, Moreno, Rocha, Parga and Rolls 2001). The implementation of short-term memory in the prefrontal cortex which can maintain neuronal firing even across intervening stimuli provides an important foundation for attention, in which an item or items must be held in mind for a period and during this time bias other brain areas by top-down processing using cortico-cortical backprojections (Rolls and Deco 2002, Deco and Rolls 2004, Deco and Rolls 2005b), or determine how stimuli are mapped to responses (Deco and Rolls 2003) or to rewards (see Appendix 2 and Deco and Rolls (2005d)) with rapid, one-trial, task switching and decision making. This dorsolateral prefrontal cortex short-term memory system also provides a computational foundation for executive function, in which several items must be held in a working memory so that they can be performed with the correct priority and order (Rolls and Deco 2002). In brain areas involved in emotion, attractor networks may play a role in maintaining a mood state, at least in the short-term after for example frustrative non-reward (see Chapters 2 and 3), and possibly in the longer term. Other functions for autoassociation networks including perceptual short-term memory which may be used in the learning of invariant representations, constraint satisfaction, and episodic memory are described by Rolls and Treves (1998) and Rolls and Deco (2002).

A.3.1 Architecture and operation

The prototypical architecture of an autoassociation memory is shown in Fig. A.19. The external input e_i is applied to each neuron i by unmodifiable synapses. This produces firing y_i of each neuron, or a vector of firing on the output neurons $\mathbf{y}$. Each output neuron i is connected by a recurrent collateral connection to the other neurons in the network, via modifiable connection

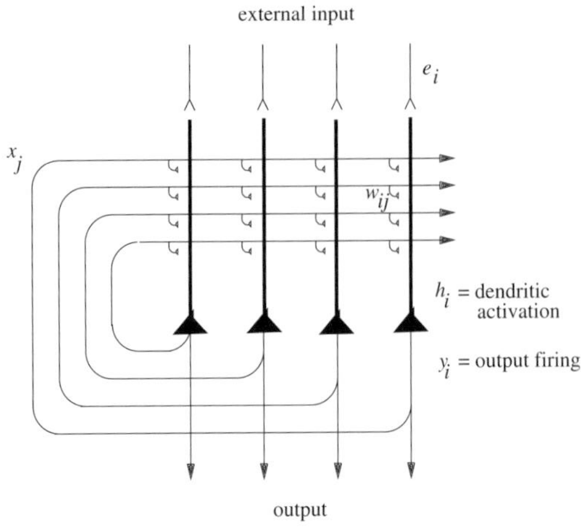

external input

e_i

x_j

w_{ij}

h_i = dendritic activation

y_i = output firing

output

Fig. A.19 The architecture of an autoassociative neural network.

weights w_{ij}. This architecture effectively enables the output firing vector **y** to be associated during learning with itself. Later on, during recall, presentation of part of the external input will force some of the output neurons to fire, but through the recurrent collateral axons and the modified synapses, other neurons in **y** can be brought into activity. This process can be repeated a number of times, and recall of a complete pattern may be perfect. Effectively, a pattern can be recalled or recognized because of associations formed between its parts. This of course requires distributed representations.

Next we introduce a more precise and detailed description of the above, and describe the properties of these networks. Ways to analyse formally the operation of these networks are introduced in Appendix A4 of Rolls and Treves (1998) and by Amit (1989).

A.3.1.1 Learning

The firing of every output neuron i is forced to a value y_i determined by the external input e_i. Then a Hebb-like associative local learning rule is applied to the recurrent synapses in the network:

$$\delta w_{ij} = \alpha y_i y_j. \tag{A.13}$$

(The term y_j in this equation is the presynaptic term shown as x_j in Fig. A.19, and this is due to the fact that the recurrent collateral connections connect the outputs of the network back as inputs.) It is notable that in a fully connected network, this will result in a symmetric matrix of synaptic weights, that is the strength of the connection from neuron 1 to neuron 2 will be the same as the strength of the connection from neuron 2 to neuron 1 (both implemented via recurrent collateral synapses).

It is a factor that is sometimes overlooked that there must be a mechanism for ensuring that during learning y_i does approximate e_i, and must not be influenced much by activity in the recurrent collateral connections, otherwise the new external pattern **e** will not be stored in the network, but instead something will be stored that is influenced by the previously stored memories. Mechanisms that may facilitate this are described by Rolls and Treves (1998) and Rolls and Deco (2002).

A.3.1.2 Recall

During recall, the external input e_i is applied, and produces output firing, operating through the non-linear activation function described below. The firing is fed back by the recurrent collateral axons shown in Fig. A.19 to produce activation of each output neuron through the modified synapses on each output neuron. The activation h_i produced by the recurrent collateral effect on the ith neuron is, in the standard way, the sum of the activations produced in proportion to the firing rate of each axon y_j operating through each modified synapse w_{ij}, that is,

$$h_i = \sum_j y_j w_{ij} \qquad \text{(A.14)}$$

where $\sum_j$ indicates that the sum is over the C input axons to each neuron, indexed by j.

The output firing y_i is a function of the activation h_i produced by the recurrent collateral effect (internal recall) and by the external input (e_i):

$$y_i = \mathrm{f}(h_i + e_i) \qquad \text{(A.15)}$$

The activation function should be nonlinear, and may be for example binary threshold, linear threshold, sigmoid, etc (see Fig. A.3). The threshold at which the activation function operates is set in part by the effect of the inhibitory neurons in the network (not shown in Fig. A.19). The connectivity is that the pyramidal cells have collateral axons that excite the inhibitory interneurons, which in turn connect back to the population of pyramidal cells to inhibit them by a mixture of shunting (divisive) and subtractive inhibition using GABA (gamma-amino-butyric acid) synaptic terminals, as described by Rolls and Deco (2002). There are many fewer inhibitory neurons than excitatory neurons (in the order of 5–10%, and of connections to and from inhibitory neurons, and partly for this reason the inhibitory neurons are considered to perform generic functions such as threshold setting, rather than to store patterns by modifying their synapses (see Rolls and Deco (2002))). The non-linear activation function can minimize interference between the pattern being recalled and other patterns stored in the network, and can also be used to ensure that what is a positive feedback system remains stable. The network can be allowed to repeat this recurrent collateral loop a number of times. Each time the loop operates, the output firing becomes more like the originally stored pattern, and this progressive recall is usually complete within 5–15 iterations.

A.3.2 Introduction to the analysis of the operation of autoassociation networks

With complete connectivity in the synaptic matrix, and the use of a Hebb rule, the matrix of synaptic weights formed during learning is symmetric. The learning algorithm is fast, 'one-shot', in that a single presentation of an input pattern is all that is needed to store that pattern.

During recall, a part of one of the originally learned stimuli can be presented as an external input. The resulting firing is allowed to iterate repeatedly round the recurrent collateral system, gradually on each iteration recalling more and more of the originally learned pattern. Completion thus occurs. If a pattern is presented during recall that is similar but not identical to any of the previously learned patterns, then the network settles into a stable recall state in which the firing corresponds to that of the most similar previously learned pattern. The network can thus generalize in its recall to the most similar previously learned pattern. The activation function of the neurons should be non-linear, since a purely linear system would not produce any categorization of the input patterns it receives, and therefore would not be able to effect anything more than a trivial (i.e. linear) form of completion and generalization.

Recall can be thought of in the following way, relating it to what occurs in pattern associators. The external input $\mathbf{e}$ is applied, produces firing $\mathbf{y}$, which is applied as a recall cue on the recurrent collaterals as $\mathbf{y}^T$. (The notation $\mathbf{y}^T$ signifies the transpose of $\mathbf{y}$, which is implemented by the application of the firing of the neurons $\mathbf{y}$ back via the recurrent collateral axons as the next set of inputs to the neurons.) The activity on the recurrent collaterals is then multiplied with the synaptic weight vector stored during learning on each neuron to produce the new activation h_i which reflects the similarity between $\mathbf{y}^T$ and one of the stored patterns. Partial recall has thus occurred as a result of the recurrent collateral effect. The activations h_i after thresholding (which helps to remove interference from other memories stored in the network, or noise in the recall cue) result in firing y_i, or a vector of all neurons $\mathbf{y}$, which is already more like one of the stored patterns than, at the first iteration, the firing resulting from the recall cue alone, $\mathbf{y} = f(\mathbf{e})$. This process is repeated a number of times to produce progressive recall of one of the stored patterns.

Autoassociation networks operate by effectively storing associations between the elements of a pattern. Each element of the pattern vector to be stored is simply the firing of a neuron. What is stored in an autoassociation memory is a set of pattern vectors. The network operates to recall one of the patterns from a fragment of it. Thus, although this network implements recall or recognition of a pattern, it does so by an association learning mechanism, in which associations between the different parts of each pattern are learned. These memories have sometimes been called autocorrelation memories (Kohonen 1977), because they learn correlations between the activity of neurons in the network, in the sense that each pattern learned is defined by a set of simultaneously active neurons. Effectively each pattern is associated by learning with itself. This learning is implemented by an associative (Hebb-like) learning rule.

Formal approaches to the operation of these networks have been described by Hopfield (1982), Amit (1989), Hertz, Krogh and Palmer (1991), and Rolls and Treves (1998).

A.3.3 Properties

The internal recall in autoassociation networks involves multiplication of the firing vector of neuronal activity by the vector of synaptic weights on each neuron. This inner product vector multiplication allows the similarity of the firing vector to previously stored firing vectors to be provided by the output (as effectively a correlation), if the patterns learned are distributed. As a result of this type of 'correlation computation' performed if the patterns are distributed, many important properties of these networks arise, including pattern completion (because part of a pattern is correlated with the whole pattern), and graceful degradation (because a damaged synaptic weight vector is still correlated with the original synaptic weight vector). Some of these properties are described next.

A.3.3.1 Completion

One important and useful property of these memories is that they complete an incomplete input vector, allowing recall of a whole memory from a small fraction of it. The memory recalled in response to a fragment is that stored in the memory that is closest in pattern similarity (as measured by the dot product, or correlation). Because the recall is iterative and progressive, the recall can be perfect.

A.3.3.2 Generalization

The network generalizes in that an input vector similar to one of the stored vectors will lead to recall of the originally stored vector, provided that distributed encoding is used. The principle by which this occurs is similar to that described for a pattern associator.

A.3.3.3 Graceful degradation or fault tolerance

If the synaptic weight vector $\mathbf{w}_i$ on each neuron (or the weight matrix) has synapses missing (e.g. during development), or loses synapses (e.g. with brain damage or aging), then the activation h_i (or vector of activations $\mathbf{h}$) is still reasonable, because h_i is the dot product (correlation) of $\mathbf{y}^T$ with $\mathbf{w}_i$. The same argument applies if whole input axons are lost. If an output neuron is lost, then the network cannot itself compensate for this, but the next network in the brain is likely to be able to generalize or complete if its input vector has some elements missing, as would be the case if some output neurons of the autoassociation network were damaged.

A.3.3.4 Speed

The recall operation is fast on each neuron on a single iteration, because the pattern $\mathbf{y}^T$ on the axons can be applied simultaneously to the synapses $\mathbf{w}_i$, and the activation h_i can be accumulated in one or two time constants of the dendrite (e.g. 10–20 ms). If a simple implementation of an autoassociation net such as that described by Hopfield (1982) is simulated on a computer, then 5–15 iterations are typically necessary for completion of an incomplete input cue $\mathbf{e}$. This might be taken to correspond to 50–200 ms in the brain, rather too slow for any one local network in the brain to function. However, it transpires (see Rolls and Deco (2002), Treves (1993), Battaglia and Treves (1998), Appendix A5 of Rolls and Treves (1998), and Panzeri, Rolls, Battaglia and Lavis (2001)) that if the neurons are treated not as McCulloch-Pitts neurons which are simply 'updated' at each iteration, or cycle of time steps (and assume the active state if the threshold is exceeded), but instead are analysed and modelled as 'integrate-and-fire' neurons in real continuous time, then the network can effectively 'relax' into its recall state very rapidly, in one or two time constants of the synapses[50]. This corresponds to perhaps 20 ms in the brain. One factor in this rapid dynamics of autoassociative networks with brain-like 'integrate-and-fire' membrane and synaptic properties is that with some spontaneous activity, some of the neurons in the network are close to threshold already before the recall cue is applied, and hence some of the neurons are very quickly pushed by the recall cue into firing, so that information starts to be exchanged very rapidly (within 1–2 ms of brain time) through the modified synapses by the neurons in the network. The progressive exchange of information starting early on within what would otherwise be thought of as an iteration period (of perhaps 20 ms, corresponding to a neuronal firing rate of 50 spikes/s), is the mechanism accounting for rapid recall in an autoassociative neuronal network made biologically realistic in this way. Further analysis of the fast dynamics of these networks if they are implemented in a biologically plausible way with 'integrate-and-fire' neurons is provided in Appendix A5 of Rolls and Treves (1998), by Rolls and Deco (2002), and by Treves (1993).

Learning is fast, 'one-shot', in that a single presentation of an input pattern $\mathbf{e}$ (producing $\mathbf{y}$) enables the association between the activation of the dendrites (the postsynaptic term h_i)

---

[50]Integrate-and-fire neurons are described in Appendix 2.

(without increasing the number of connections per neuron) does not increase the number of different patterns that can be stored (see Rolls and Treves (1998) Appendix A4), although it may enable simpler encoding of the firing patterns, for example more orthogonal encoding, to be used. This latter point may account in part for why there are generally in the brain more neurons in a recurrent network than there are connections per neuron. Another advantage of having many neurons in the network may be related to the fact that within any integration time period of 20 ms not all neurons will have fired a spike if the average firing rate is less than 50 Hz. Having large numbers of neurons may enable the vector of neuronal firing to contribute to recall efficiently even though not every neuron can contribute in a short time period.

The non-linearity inherent in the NMDA receptor-based Hebbian plasticity present in the brain may help to make the stored patterns more sparse than the input patterns, and this may be especially beneficial in increasing the storage capacity of associative networks in the brain by allowing participation in the storage of especially those relatively few neurons with high firing rates in the exponential firing rate distributions typical of neurons in sensory systems (see Rolls and Treves (1998) and Rolls and Deco (2002)).

A.3.3.7 Context

The environmental context in which learning occurs can be a very important factor that affects retrieval in humans and other animals. Placing the subject back into the same context in which the original learning occurred can greatly facilitate retrieval.

Context effects arise naturally in association networks if some of the activity in the network reflects the context in which the learning occurs. Retrieval is then better when that context is present, for the activity contributed by the context becomes part of the retrieval cue for the memory, increasing the correlation of the current state with what was stored. (A strategy for retrieval arises simply from this property. The strategy is to keep trying to recall as many fragments of the original memory situation, including the context, as possible, as this will provide a better cue for complete retrieval of the memory than just a single fragment.)

The effects that mood has on memory including visual memory retrieval may be accounted for by backprojections from brain regions such as the amygdala in which the current mood, providing a context, is represented, to brain regions involved in memory such as the perirhinal cortex, and in visual representations such as the inferior temporal visual cortex (see Rolls and Stringer (2001b) and Section 4.10). The very well-known effects of context in the human memory literature could arise in the simple way just described. An implication of the explanation is that context effects will be especially important at late stages of memory or information processing systems in the brain, for there information from a wide range of modalities will be mixed, and some of that information could reflect the context in which the learning takes place. One part of the brain where such effects may be strong is the hippocampus, which is implicated in the memory of recent episodes, and which receives inputs derived from most of the cortical information processing streams, including those involved in spatial representations (see Chapter 6 of Rolls and Treves (1998), Rolls (1996b), and Rolls (1999c)).

It is now known that reward-related information is associated with place-related information in the primate hippocampus, and this provides a particular neural system in which mood context can influence memory retrieval (Rolls and Xiang 2005).

A.3.3.8 Memory for sequences

One of the first extensions of the standard autoassociator paradigm that has been explored in the literature is the capability to store and retrieve not just individual patterns, but whole sequences of patterns. Hopfield (1982) suggested that this could be achieved by adding to the standard connection weights, which associate a pattern with itself, a new, asymmetric component, that associates a pattern with the next one in the sequence. In practice this scheme does not work very well, unless the new component is made to operate on a slower time scale than the purely autoassociative component (Kleinfeld 1986, Sompolinsky and Kanter 1986). With two different time scales, the autoassociative component can stabilize a pattern for a while, before the heteroassociative component moves the network, as it were, into the next pattern. The heteroassociative retrieval cue for the next pattern in the sequence is just the previous pattern in the sequence. A particular type of 'slower' operation occurs if the asymmetric component acts after a delay τ. In this case, the network sweeps through the sequence, staying for a time of order τ in each pattern.

If implemented with integrate-and-fire neurons with biologically plausible dynamics, this type of sequence memory will either step through its remembered sequence with uncontrollable speed, or not step through the sequence. A proposal that attractor networks with adapting synapses could be used to retain memory sequences is an interesting alternative (Deco and Rolls 2005c).

A.4 Coupled attractor networks

In this Section A.4 an introduction to how attractor networks can interact is given, as this may be relevant to understanding how mood states influence cognitive processing, and vice versa.

It is prototypical of the cerebral neocortical areas that there are recurrent collateral connections between the neurons within an area or module, and forward connections to the next cortical area in the hierarchy, which in turn sends backprojections (see Rolls and Deco (2002)). This architecture, made explicit in Fig. 4.66 on page 199, immediately suggests, given that the recurrent connections within a module, and the forward and backward connections, are likely to be associatively modifiable, that the operation incorporates at least to some extent interactions between coupled attractor (autoassociation) networks. For these reasons, it is important to analyse the rules that govern the interactions between coupled attractor networks. This has been done using the formal type of model described in Section 12.1.2 of Rolls and Deco (2002) introduced here (see also Renart, Parga and Rolls (1999b), Renart, Parga and Rolls (1999a), Renart, Parga and Rolls (2000), Renart, Moreno, Rocha, Parga and Rolls (2001), and Deco and Rolls (2003)).

One boundary condition is when the coupling between the networks is so weak that there is effectively no interaction. This holds when the coupling parameter g between the networks is less than approximately 0.002, where the coupling parameter indicates the relative strength of the intermodular to the intramodular connections, and measures effectively the relative strengths of the currents injected into the neurons by the inter-modular relative to the intramodular (recurrent collateral) connections (Renart, Parga and Rolls 1999b). At the other extreme, if the coupling parameter is strong, all the networks will operate as a single attractor network, together able to represent only one state (Renart, Parga and Rolls 1999b). This critical value of the coupling parameter (at least for reciprocally connected networks with symmetric synaptic strengths) is relatively low, in the region of 0.024 (Renart, Parga and Rolls 1999b). This is one reason why cortico-cortical backprojections are predicted to be quantitatively relatively weak, and for this reason it is suggested end on the apical parts of the dendrites of cortical pyramidal cells (see Section 1.11 of Rolls and Deco (2002)). In the strongly coupled regime when the system of networks operates as a single attractor, the total storage capacity (the number of patterns that can be stored and correctly retrieved) of all the networks will be set just by the number of synaptic connections received from other neurons in the network, a number in the order of a few thousand. This is one reason why connected cortical networks are thought not to act in the strongly coupled regime, because the total number of memories that could be represented in the whole of the cerebral cortex would be so small, in the order of a few thousand, depending on the sparseness of the patterns (see equation A.18) (O'Kane and Treves 1992).

Between these boundary conditions, that is in the region where the inter-modular coupling parameter g is in the range 0.002–0.024, it has been shown that interesting interactions can occur (Renart, Parga and Rolls 1999b, Renart, Parga and Rolls 1999a). In a bimodular archi-tecture, with forward and backward connections between the modules, the capacity of one module can be increased, and an attractor is more likely to be found under noisy conditions, if there is a consistent pattern in the coupled attractor. By consistent we mean a pattern that during training was linked associatively by the forward and backward connections, with the pattern being retrieved in the first module. This provides a quantitative model for understand-ing some of the effects that backprojections can produce by supporting particular states in earlier cortical areas (Renart, Parga and Rolls 1999b). The total storage capacity of the two networks is however in line with O'Kane and Treves (1992), not a great deal greater than the storage capacity of one of the modules alone. Thus the help provided by the attractors in falling into a mutually compatible global retrieval state (in e.g. the scenario of a hierarchical system) is where the utility of such coupled attractor networks must lie. Another interesting application of such weakly coupled attractor networks is in coupled perceptual and short-term memory systems in the brain, described in Section 12.1 of Rolls and Deco (2002). Thus the most interesting scenario for coupled attractor networks is when they are weakly coupled, for then interactions occur whereby how well one module responds to its own inputs can be influ-enced by the states of the other modules, but it can retain partly independent representations. This emphasizes the importance of weak interactions between coupled modules in the brain (Renart, Parga and Rolls 1999b, Renart, Parga and Rolls 1999a, Renart, Parga and Rolls 2000).

If a multimodular architecture is trained with each of many patterns (which might be visual stimuli) in one module associated with one of a few patterns (which might be mood states) in a connected module, then interesting effects due to this asymmetry are found, as described in Section 4.10 and by Rolls and Stringer (2001b).

An interesting issue that arises is how rapidly a system of interacting attractor networks such as that illustrated in Fig. 4.66 settles into a stable state. Is it sufficiently rapid for the interacting attractor effects described to contribute to cortical information processing? It is likely that the settling of the whole system is quite rapid, if it is implemented (as it is in the brain) with synapses and neurons that operate with continuous dynamics, where the time constant of the synapses dominates the retrieval speed, and is in the order of 15 ms for each module, as described in Section 7.6 of Rolls and Deco (2002) and by Panzeri, Rolls, Battaglia and Lavis (2001). It is shown there that a multimodular attractor network architecture can process information in approximately 15 ms per module (assuming an inactivation time constant for the synapses of 10 ms).

Attractor networks can be coupled together with stronger forward than backward connec-tions. This provides a model of how the prefrontal cortex could map sensory inputs (in one attractor), through intermediate attractors that respond to combinations of sensory inputs and the behavioural responses being made, to further attractors that encode the response to be made (Deco and Rolls 2003). Having attractors at each stage enables the prefrontal cortex to bridge delays between parts of a task. The hierarchical organization of the attractors achieved by the stronger forward than backward connections enables the mapping to be from sensory input to motor output. The presence of intermediate attractors with neurons that respond to combinations of the stimuli and the behavioural responses to be made allows a top-down attentional input to bias the competition implemented by the intermediate level attractors to enable the behaviour to be switched from one cognitive mapping to another (Deco and Rolls 2003). The whole architecture has been modelled at the integrate-and-fire neuronal level, and simulates the activity of the different populations of neurons just described which are types of neuron recorded in the prefrontal cortex when monkeys are performing this decision task (see Deco and Rolls (2003)).

The cortico-cortical backprojection connectivity described can be interpreted as a system that allows the forward-projecting neurons in one cortical area to be linked autoassociatively with the backprojecting neurons in the next cortical area (see Fig. 4.66 and Rolls and Deco (2002)). It is interesting to note that if the forward and backprojection synapses were associatively modifiable, but there were no recurrent connections in each of the modules, then the whole system could still operate (with the right parameters) as an attractor network.

A.5 Reinforcement learning

In supervised networks, an error signal is provided for each output neuron in the network, and whenever an input to the network is provided, the error signals specify the magnitude and direction of the error in the output produced by each neuron. These error signals are then used to correct the synaptic weights in the network in such a way that the output errors for each input pattern to be learned gradually diminish over trials (see Rolls and Deco (2002)). These networks have an architecture that might be similar to that of the pattern associator shown in Fig. A.7, except that instead of an unconditioned stimulus, there is an error correction signal provided for each output neuron. Such a network trained by an error-correcting (or delta) rule is known as a one-layer perceptron. The architecture is not very plausible for most brain regions, in that it is not clear how an individual error signal could be computed for each of thousands of neurons in a network, and fed into each neuron as its error signal and then used in a delta rule synaptic correction (see Rolls and Treves (1998) and Rolls and Deco (2002)).

The architecture can be generalized to a multilayer feedforward architecture with many layers between the input and output (Rumelhart, Hinton and Williams 1986), but the learning is very non-local and rather biologically implausible (see Rolls and Treves (1998) and Rolls and Deco (2002)), in that an error term (magnitude and direction) for each neuron in the network must be computed from the errors and synaptic weights of all subsequent neurons in the network that any neuron influences, usually on a trial-by-trial basis, by a process known as error backpropagation. Thus although computationally powerful, an issue with perceptrons and multilayer perceptrons that makes them generally biologically implausible for many brain regions is that a separate error signal must be supplied for each output neuron, and that with multilayer perceptrons, computed error backpropagation must occur.

When operating in an environment, usually a simple binary or scalar signal representing success or failure of the whole network or organism is received. This is usually action-dependent feedback that provides a single evaluative measure of the success or failure. Eval-

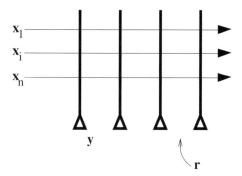

Fig. A.20 A network trained by a single reinforcement input r. The inputs to each neuron are $x_j, j = 1, C$; and y is the output of one of the output neurons.

uative feedback tells the learner whether or not, and possibly by how much, its behaviour has improved; or it provides a measure of the 'goodness' of the behaviour. Evaluative feedback does not directly tell the learner what it should have done, and although it may provide an index of the degree (i.e. magnitude) of success, it does not include directional information telling the learner how to change its behaviour towards a target, as does error-correction learning (see Barto (1995)). Partly for this reason, there has been some interest in networks that can be taught with such a single reinforcement signal. In this Section, approaches to such networks are described. It is noted that such networks are classified as reinforcement networks in which there is a single teacher, and that these networks attempt to perform an optimal mapping between an input vector and an output neuron or set of neurons. They thus solve the same class of problems as single layer and multilayer perceptrons. They should be distinguished from pattern-association networks in the brain, which might learn associations between previously neutral stimuli and primary reinforcers such as taste (signals which might be interpreted appropriately by a subsequent part of the brain), but do not attempt to produce arbitrary mappings between an input and an output, using a single reinforcement signal.

A class of problems to which such reinforcement networks might be applied are motor-control problems. It was to such a problem that Barto and Sutton (Barto 1985, Sutton and Barto 1981) applied a reinforcement learning algorithm, the associative reward–penalty algorithm described next. The algorithm can in principle be applied to multilayer networks, and the learning is relatively slow. The algorithm is summarized by Rolls and Treves (1998) and Hertz, Krogh and Palmer (1991). More recent developments in reinforcement learning are described by Sutton and Barto (1998) and reviewed by Dayan and Abbott (2001), and some of these developments are described in Section A.5.3.

A.5.1 Associative reward–penalty algorithm of Barto and Sutton

The terminology of Barto and Sutton is followed here (see Barto (1985)).

A.5.1.1 Architecture

The architecture, shown in Fig. A.20, uses a single reinforcement signal, r, = +1 for reward, and –1 for penalty. The inputs x_i take real (continuous) values. The output of a neuron, y, is binary, +1 or –1. The weights on the output neuron are designated w_i.

A.5.1.2 Operation

1. An input vector is applied to the network, and produces activation, h, in the normal way as follows:

$$h = \sum_{j=1}^{C} x_j w_j \qquad (A.19)$$

where $\sum_{j=1}^{C}$ indicates that the sum is over the C input axons (or connections) indexed by j to each neuron.

2. The output y is calculated from the activation with a noise term η included. The principle of the network is that if the added noise on a particular trial helps performance, then whatever change it leads to should be incorporated into the synaptic weights, in such a way that the next time that input occurs, the performance is improved.

$$y = \begin{cases} +1 & \text{if } h + \eta \geq 0, \\ -1 & \text{else.} \end{cases} \qquad (A.20)$$

where η = the noise added on each trial.

3. Learning rule. The weights are changed as follows:

$$\delta w_j = \begin{cases} \rho(y - E[y|h])x_j & \text{if } r = +1, \\ \rho\lambda(-y - E[y|h])x_j & \text{if } r = -1. \end{cases} \qquad (A.21)$$

ρ and λ are learning-rate constants. (They are set so that the learning rate is higher when positive reinforcement is received than when negative reinforcement is received.) $E[y|h]$ is the expectation of y given h (usually a sigmoidal function of h with the range ± 1). $E[y|h]$ is a (continuously varying) indication of how the neuron usually responds to the current input pattern, i.e. if the actual output y is larger than normally expected, by computing $h = \sum w_j x_j$, because of the noise term, and the reinforcement is +1, increase the weight from x_j; and vice versa. The expectation could be the prediction generated before the noise term is incorporated.

This network combines an associative capacity with its properties of generalization and graceful degradation, with a single 'critic' or error signal for the whole network (Barto 1985). [The term $y - E[y|h]$ in Equation A.21 can be thought of as an error for the output of the neuron: it is the difference between what occurred, and what was expected to occur. The synaptic weight is adjusted according to the sign and magnitude of the error of the postsynaptic firing, multiplied by the presynaptic firing, and depending on the reinforcement r received. The rule is similar to a Hebb synaptic modification rule (Equation A.6), except that the postsynaptic term is an error instead of the postsynaptic firing rate, and the learning is modulated by the reinforcement.] The network can solve difficult problems (such as balancing a pole by moving a trolley that supports the pole from side to side, as the pole starts to topple). Although described for single-layer networks, the algorithm can be applied to multilayer networks. The learning rate is very slow, for there is a single reinforcement signal on each trial for the whole network, not a separate error signal for each neuron in the network as is the case in a perceptron trained with an error rule (see Rolls and Deco (2002) and Rolls and Treves (1998)).

This associative reward–penalty reinforcement-learning algorithm is certainly a move towards biological relevance, in that learning with a single reinforcer can be achieved. That single reinforcer might be broadcast throughout the system by a general projection system. It is not clear yet how a biological system might store the expected output $E[y|h]$ for comparison with the actual output when noise has been added, and might take into account the sign and magnitude of this difference. Nevertheless, this is an interesting algorithm, which is related to the temporal difference reinforcement learning algorithm described in Section A.5.3.

A.5.2 Error correction or delta rule learning, and classical conditioning

In classical or Pavlovian associative learning, a number of different types of association may be learned (see Section 4.6.1.1). This type of associative learning may be performed by networks with the general architecture and properties of pattern associators (see Section A.2 and Fig. A.7). However, the time course of the acquisition and extinction of these associations can be expressed concisely by a modified type of learning rule in which an error correction term is used (introduced in Section A.5.1), rather than the postsynaptic firing y itself as in Equation A.6. Use of this modified, error correction, type of learning also enables some of the properties of classical conditioning to be explained (see Dayan and Abbott (2001) for review), and this type of learning is therefore described briefly here. The rule is known in learning theory as the Rescorla–Wagner rule, after Rescorla and Wagner (1972).

The Rescorla–Wagner rule is a version of error correction or delta-rule learning, and is based on a simple linear prediction of the expected reward value, denoted by v, associated with a stimulus representation x ($x = 1$ if the stimulus is present, and $x = 0$ if the stimulus is absent). The expected reward value v is expressed as the input stimulus variable x multiplied by a weight w

$$v = wx. \tag{A.22}$$

The error in the reward prediction is the difference between the expected reward v and the actual reward obtained r, i.e.

$$\Delta = r - v \tag{A.23}$$

where Δ is the reward prediction error. The value of the weight w is learned by a rule designed to minimize the expected squared error $<(r - v)^2>$ between the actual reward r and the predicted reward v. The angle brackets indicate an average over the presentations of the stimulus and reward. The delta rule will perform the required type of learning:

$$\delta w = k(r - v)x \tag{A.24}$$

where δw is the change of synaptic weight, k is a constant that determines the learning rate, and the term $(r - v)$ is the error Δ in the output (equivalent to the error in the postsynaptic firing, rather than the postsynaptic firing y itself as in Equation A.6). Application of this rule during conditioning with the stimulus x presented on every trial results in the weight w approaching the asymptotic limit $w = r$ exponentially over trials as the error Δ becomes zero. In extinction, when $r = 0$, the weight (and thus the output of the system) exponentially decays to $w = 0$. This rule thus helps to capture the time course over trials of the acquisition and extinction of conditioning. The rule also helps to account for a number of properties of classical conditioning, including blocking, inhibitory conditioning, and overshadowing (see Dayan and Abbott (2001)).

How this functionality is implemented in the brain is not yet clear. We consider one suggestion (Schultz et al. 1995b, Schultz 2004) after we introduce a further sophistication of reinforcement learning which allows the time course of events within a trial to be taken into account.

A.5.3 Temporal Difference (TD) learning

An important advance in the area of reinforcement learning was the introduction of algorithms that allow for learning to occur when the reinforcement is delayed or received over a number of time steps, and which allow effects within a trial to be taken into account (Sutton and Barto 1998, Sutton and Barto 1990). A solution to these problems is the addition of an adaptive critic that learns through a time difference (TD) algorithm how to predict the future value of the reinforcer. The time difference algorithm takes into account not only the current reinforcement just received, but also a temporally weighted average of errors in predicting future reinforcements. The temporal difference error is the error by which any two temporally adjacent error predictions are inconsistent (see Barto (1995)). The output of the critic is used as an effective reinforcer instead of the instantaneous reinforcement being received (see Sutton and Barto (1998), Sutton and Barto (1990) and Barto (1995)). This is a solution to the temporal credit assignment problem, and enables future rewards to be predicted. Summaries are provided by Doya (1999), Schultz et al. (1997) and Dayan and Abbott (2001).

In reinforcement learning, a learning agent takes an *action* $\mathbf{u}(t)$ in response to the *state* $\mathbf{x}(t)$ of the environment, which results in the change of the state

$$\mathbf{x}(t + 1) = F(\mathbf{x}(t), \mathbf{u}(t)), \tag{A.25}$$

and the delivery of the reinforcement signal, or *reward*

$$r(t + 1) = R(\mathbf{x}(t), \mathbf{u}(t)). \tag{A.26}$$

In the above equations, $\mathbf{x}$ is a vector representation of inputs x_j, and equation A.25 indicates that the next state $\mathbf{x}(t + 1)$ at time $(t + 1)$ is a function F of the state at the previous time step of the inputs and actions at that time step in a closed system. In equation A.26 the reward at the next time step is determined by a reward function R which uses the current sensory inputs and action taken. The time t may refer to time within a trial.

The goal is to find a *policy* function G which maps sensory inputs $\mathbf{x}$ to actions

$$\mathbf{u}(t) = G(\mathbf{x}(t)) \tag{A.27}$$

which maximizes the cumulative sum of the rewards based on the sensory inputs.

The current action $\mathbf{u}(t)$ affects all future states and accordingly all future rewards. The maximization is realized by the use of the *value function* V of the states to predict, given the sensory inputs $\mathbf{x}$, the cumulative sum (possibly discounted as a function of time) of all future rewards $V(\mathbf{x})$ (possibly within a learning trial) as follows:

$$V(\mathbf{x}) = E[r(t + 1) + \gamma r(t + 2) + \gamma^2 r(t + 3) + ...] \tag{A.28}$$

where $r(t)$ is the reward at time t, and $E[\cdot]$ denotes the expected value of the sum of future rewards up to the end of the trial. $0 \leq \gamma \leq 1$ is a discount factor that makes rewards that arrive sooner more important than rewards that arrive later, according to an exponential decay function. (If $\gamma = 1$ there is no discounting.) It is assumed that the presentation of future cues and rewards depends only on the current sensory cues and not the past sensory cues. The right hand side of equation A.28 is evaluated for the dynamics in equations A.25–A.27 with the initial condition $\mathbf{x}(t) = \mathbf{x}$. The two basic ingredients in reinforcement learning are the estimation (which we term $\hat{V}$) of the value function V, and then the improvement of the policy or action $\mathbf{u}$ using the value function (Sutton and Barto 1998).

The basic algorithm for learning the value function is to minimize the *temporal difference* (TD) *error* $\Delta(t)$ for time t within a trial, and this is computed by a 'critic' for the estimated value predictions $\hat{V}(\mathbf{x}(t))$ at successive time steps as

$$\Delta(t) = [r(t) + \gamma\hat{V}(\mathbf{x}(t))] - \hat{V}(\mathbf{x}(t-1)) \tag{A.29}$$

where $\hat{V}(\mathbf{x}(t)) - \hat{V}(\mathbf{x}(t-1))$ is the difference in the reward value prediction at two successive time steps, giving rise to the terminology temporal difference learning. If we introduce the term $\hat{v}$ as the estimate of the cumulated reward by the end of the trial, we can define it as a function $\hat{V}$ of the current sensory input $\mathbf{x}(t)$, i.e. $\hat{v} = \hat{V}(\mathbf{x})$, and we can also write equation A.29 as

$$\Delta(t) = r(t) + \gamma\hat{v}(t) - \hat{v}(t-1) \tag{A.30}$$

which draws out the fact that it is differences at successive timesteps in the reward value predictions $\hat{v}$ that are used to calculate Δ.

$\Delta(t)$ is used to improve the estimates $\hat{v}(t)$ by the 'critic', and can also be used (by an 'actor') to choose appropriate actions.

For example, when the value function is represented (in the critic) as

$$\hat{V}(\mathbf{x}(t)) = \sum_{j=1}^{n} w_j^C x_j(t) \tag{A.31}$$

the learning algorithm for the (value) weight w_j^C in the critic is given by

$$\delta w_j^C = k_c\Delta(t)x_j(t-1) \tag{A.32}$$

where δw_j^C is the change of synaptic weight, k_c is a constant that determines the learning rate for the sensory input x_j, and $\Delta(t)$ is the Temporal Difference error at time t. Under certain conditions this learning rule will cause the estimate $\hat{v}$ to converge to the true value (Dayan and Sejnowski 1994).

A simple way of improving the policy of the actor is to take a stochastic action

$$u_i(t) = g(\sum_{j=1}^{n} w_{ij}^A x_j(t) + \mu_i(t)), \tag{A.33}$$

where g() is a scalar version of the policy function G, w_{ij}^A is a weight in the actor, and $\mu_i(t)$ is a noise term. The TD error $\Delta(t)$ as defined in equation A.29 then signals the unexpected delivery of the reward $r(t)$ or the increase in the state value $\hat{V}(\mathbf{x}(t))$ above expectation, possibly due to the previous choice of action $u_i(t-1)$. The learning algorithm for the action weight w_{ij}^A in the actor is given by

$$\delta w_{ij}^A = k_a\Delta(t)(u_i(t-1) - <u_i>)x_j(t-1), \tag{A.34}$$

where $<u_i>$ is the average level of the action output, and k_a is a learning rate constant in the actor.

Thus, the TD error $\Delta(t)$, which signals the error in the reward prediction at time t, works as the main teaching signal in both learning the value function (implemented in the critic), and the selection of actions (implemented in the actor). The usefulness of a separate critic is that it enables the TD error to be calculated based on the difference in reward value predictions at two successive time steps as shown in equation A.29.

The algorithm has been applied to modelling the time course of classical conditioning (Sutton and Barto 1990). The algorithm effectively allows the future reinforcement predicted from past history to influence the responses made, and in this sense allows behaviour to be guided not just by immediate reinforcement, but also by 'anticipated' reinforcements. Different types of temporal difference learning are described by Sutton and Barto (1998). An application is to the analysis of decisions when future rewards are discounted with respect to immediate rewards (Dayan and Abbott 2001, Tanaka, Doya, Okada, Ueda, Okamoto and Yamawaki 2004). Another application is to the learning of sequences of actions to take within a trial (Suri and Schultz 1998).

The possibility that dopamine neuron firing may provide an error signal useful in training neuronal systems to predict reward has been discussed in Section 8.3.4. It has been proposed that the firing of the dopamine neurons can be thought of as an error signal about reward prediction, in that the firing occurs in a task when a reward is given, but then moves forward in time within a trial to the time when a stimulus is presented that can be used to predict when the taste reward will be obtained (Schultz et al. 1995b) (see Fig. 8.5). The argument is that there is no prediction error when the taste reward is obtained if it has been signalled by a preceding conditioned stimulus, and that is why the dopamine midbrain neurons do not respond at the time of taste reward delivery, but instead, at least during training, to the onset of the conditioned stimulus (Waelti, Dickinson and Schultz 2001). If a different conditioned stimulus is shown that normally predicts that no taste reward will be given, there is no firing of the dopamine neurons to the onset of that conditioned stimulus.

This hypothesis has been built into models of learning in which the error signal is used to train synaptic connections in dopamine pathway recipient regions (such as presumably the striatum and orbitofrontal cortex) (Houk et al. 1995, Schultz 2004, Schultz et al. 1997, Waelti et al. 2001, Dayan and Abbott 2001). Some difficulties with the hypothesis are discussed in Section 8.3.4. The difficulties include the fact that dopamine is released in large quantities by aversive stimuli (see Section 8.3.4); that error computations for differences between the expected reward and the actual reward received on a trial are computed in the primate orbitofrontal cortex, where expected reward, actual reward, and error neurons are all found, and lesions of which impair the ability to use changes in reward contingencies to reverse behaviour (see Section 4.5.5.5); that the tonic, sustained, firing of the dopamine neurons in the delay period of a task with probabilistic rewards reflects reward uncertainty, and not the expected reward, nor the magnitude of the prediction error (see Section 8.3.4 and Shizgal and Arvanitogiannis (2003)); and that reinforcement learning is suited to setting up connections that might be required in fixed tasks such as motor habit or sequence learning, for reinforcement learning algorithms seek to set weights correctly in an 'actor', but are not suited to tasks where rules must be altered flexibly, as in rapid one trial reversal, for which a very different type of mechanism is described in Appendix B.

Overall, reinforcement learning algorithms are certainly a move towards biological relevance, in that learning with a single reinforcer can be achieved in systems that might learn motor habits or fixed sequences. Whether a single prediction error is broadcast throughout a neural system by a general projection system, such as the dopamine pathways in the brain, which distribute to large parts of the striatum and the prefrontal cortex, remains to be clearly established.

Appendix 2 Reward reversal in the orbitofrontal cortex – a model

This Appendix provides a formal model of how one-trial reward reversal, which is a property of orbitofrontal cortex neurons, could be implemented in the orbitofrontal cortex. The model and its properties have been described in outline in Section 4.5.7. This Appendix provides a more detailed description of how the model is implemented, and has the broader aim of showing how one can make models that can proceed to the level of the spiking of neurons for direct comparison with neuronal data. The type of model described here is an integrate-and-fire model of each neuron, and there are several different coupled networks of such neurons. The model includes the detailed dynamics and properties of the synapses on each neuron and the ion channels that they affect, and thus allows predictions of the effects of pharmacological agents on the operation of the whole network (and thus on emotion). The model also for the same reason allows quantitative explorations of how different types of receptor (e.g. AMPA vs NMDA) are involved in the operation of the network, and thus allows predictions of selective interference with these different receptors. Because the model includes the ion flows across the neuronal membrane that influence the depolarization of the postsynaptic cells, it is possible to integrate across the relevant ion flows which require energy to be pumped back across the cell membranes, and because this has metabolic implications which increase the local blood flow, to predict the fMRI signal.

The model described thus shows how it is possible to relate the low-level details of the operation of parts of the brain at the receptor and ion channel levels, through models of the spiking of different neurons in different coupled networks, to the psychological function of each network, and the fMRI neuroimaging signals that would be recorded from the system. Models of this type will become increasingly important for understanding how the brain functions and implements processes such as emotion, for these models provide quantitative links between the different levels of neuroscience investigations, show how the global collective properties of populations of neurons produce important psychological effects, and provide a coherent and rigorous model of brain function.

This particular model was described by Deco and Rolls (2005d), but is prototypical of a number of detailed dynamical models of brain and psychological functions (Deco and Rolls 2003, Deco, Rolls and Horwitz 2004, Deco and Rolls 2005c, Deco and Rolls 2005b, Deco and Rolls 2005a). Further background to this type of integrate-and-fire model is provided by Rolls and Deco (2002), Brunel and Wang (2001), Dayan and Abbott (2001), Wilson (1999), and Gerstner and Kistler (2002).

B.1 Introduction

Higher brain functions, such as *cognitive flexibility*, require associative cortical areas that mediate the coordination between working memory, attention, whether expected rewards are obtained, and the alteration of behaviour if the reinforcers are not obtained as expected. Brain regions such as the orbitofrontal cortex, amygdala, and anterior cingulate cortex have been implicated in this remarkable ability of primates to learn associations between sensory stimuli and rewarding or punishing reinforcers that can rapidly and flexibly alter the probability of behaviour, as described in Chapter 4. The ability to respond rapidly to changing reinforcement contingencies is fundamental to an understanding of emotion, given that emotion can be at least operationally defined in terms of states elicited by rewards and punishers (see Chapter 2). The first computational issue addressed here (and by Deco and Rolls (2005d)) is how the rapid reversal of neuronal responses that code for the reward associations of visual stimuli could occur. Rapid stimulus–reinforcer association learning is the type of learning involved in the elicitation of emotional states.

The second computational issue addressed here is how rewards can rapidly control the way that stimuli are mapped to behavioural responses. This remapping is shown for example in *conditional object-response tasks* in which when one object is seen, one response (e.g. a right oculomotor saccade) must be made to obtain reward, and when a second object is seen, a different response (e.g. a left oculomotor saccade) must be made to obtain reward. In this type of task, stimulus–reward association learning alone is insufficient, because each stimulus is equally associated with reward. To account for the performance of and the rapid reversal of this task, and the types of neuron recorded in the prefrontal cortex in this task (Asaad et al. 1998), Deco and Rolls (2003) proposed and investigated a network in which the mapping between the stimuli and the responses could be switched by a rule or contextual input operating to bias competition in stimulus–response combination neurons in an intermediate layer between the sensory inputs and the motor outputs. Deco and Rolls (2003) described a network using biased competition produced by a rule or contextual input that could make a hierarchically organized set of integrate-and-fire networks change the mapping from sensory inputs to motor outputs on the basis of either the conditional object-response rule or a delayed spatial response rule (requiring attention to switch from objects to the spatial position of the objects), accounting for the neurophysiological data obtained in this task switching by Asaad et al. (2000). In modelling these two tasks, Deco and Rolls (2003) postulated but did not explicitly model the rule or contextual input (acting as a bias) that could be reversed when the reinforcement contingencies in the tasks changed. This is the second computational issue addressed by Deco and Rolls (2005d) and described here, namely how the change in the rewards being received could implement a switch from one rule to another for this rule or contextual representation. This leads to a full model of how the changing reinforcement contingencies could switch between the different types of stimulus-to-motor response mapping required in these tasks. The issues addressed here are part of the large and important area of reinforcement learning, that is how behaviour is altered on the basis of reinforcement (see Section A.5).

I note that stimulus–reinforcer learning can be implemented by a pattern association network (where the unconditioned stimulus forcing the output neurons to respond is the reinforcer, and the conditioned stimulus becomes associated with this by associatively modifiable synapses) (Rolls and Treves 1998, Rolls 1999a, Rolls and Deco 2002) (see Section A.2). Such a pattern association network could in principle unlearn the association by using associative synapses that incorporate long term depression (Rolls and Treves 1998, Rolls and Deco 2002) (see Fig. 4.5 on page 74). Although reversal might be implemented by having long-term synaptic depression (LTD) for synapses that represented the reward-associated stimulus before the reversal, and long-term potentiation (LTP) of the synapses for the new stimulus that after reversal is associated with reward, this would require one-trial LTP and one-trial heterosynaptic LTD to account for one-trial stimulus–reward reversal (Thorpe, Rolls and Maddison 1983, Rolls, Critchley, Mason and Wakeman 1996b, Rolls 2000e). Moreover, this mechanism would not provide a source for the contextual, rule-based input with persistent (continuing) activity required for the biased competition solution to rapid remapping of stimuli to responses (Deco and Rolls 2003). Nor would it account for the non-associative process illustrated in Fig. 4.36 on page 117 which shows that after reversal learning set is acquired, the visual stimulus that was associated with a punisher before the reversal contingency was applied is now chosen, even though it has not been recently associated with reward.

Deco and Rolls (2005d) therefore investigated a mechanism that by utilizing an attractor recurrent autoassociative network (Hopfield 1982, Rolls and Treves 1998, Rolls and Deco 2002) can maintain the rule that is current in a continuing active state of firing until the rule is reversed by punishment or the failure to receive an expected reward. To implement this model in a way that can be compared directly with neurophysiology, the processes occurring at the AMPA, NMDA, and GABA synapses are dynamically modelled in an integrate-and-fire implementation to produce realistic spiking dynamics (Brunel and Wang 2001, Deco and Rolls 2003). This also enables the synaptic adaptation that is part of the rule reversal mechanism to be realistically implemented. The stimulus-to-reward part of the model contains different populations of neurons in attractor networks that respond selectively to the sensory stimulus, to a combination of a particular sensory stimulus and whether it currently signifies reward or punishment (conditional reward neurons), and reward, all of which are present in the primate orbitofrontal cortex (Thorpe, Rolls and Maddison 1983, Rolls, Critchley, Mason and Wakeman 1996b) (see below). The neuronal populations or pools are arranged hierarchically, and have global inhibition through inhibitory interneurons to implement competition. The hierarchical structure is organized within the general framework of the biased competition model of attention (Moran and Desimone 1985, Spitzer, Desimone and Moran 1988, Motter 1993, Miller, Gochin and Gross 1993a, Chelazzi, Miller, Duncan and Desimone 1993, Reynolds and Desimone 1999, Chelazzi 1998, Rolls and Deco 2002). Rolls and Deco (2002) added to this framework by introducing a neurodynamical theoretical framework for biased competition, which assumes that multiple activated populations of neurons engage in competitive interactions, and that top-down interactions with other cortical modules bias this competition in favour of specific neurons.

B.2 The model of stimulus–reinforcer association reversal

In order to investigate the neurodynamics underlying the rapid stimulus–reward reversal in the context of the findings of Thorpe, Rolls and Maddison (1983) and Rolls, Critchley, Mason and Wakeman (1996b) (see Section 4.5), Deco and Rolls (2005d) explicitly modelled the level of processes occurring at the AMPA, NMDA and GABA synapses in the integrate-and-fire implementation to produce realistic spiking dynamics. They followed the biased competition based neurodynamical framework (Rolls and Deco 2002, Deco and Zihl 2001, Deco and Lee 2002, Corchs and Deco 2002), and also the integrate-and-fire neuronal framework introduced and studied by Brunel and Wang (2001). They incorporated shunting inhibition (Rolls and Treves 1998, Battaglia and Treves 1998) and inhibitory-to-inhibitory cell synaptic connections (Brunel and Wang 2001) which are useful in maintaining stability of the dynamical system, and incorporated appropriate currents to achieve low firing rates (Amit and Brunel 1997, Brunel and Wang 2001). In accordance with the neurophysiological evidence of Thorpe, Rolls and Maddison (1983) and Rolls, Critchley, Mason and Wakeman (1996b), the network architecture investigated assumed the existence of different types of neuronal populations or pools. One type shows object-tuned sensory neuronal responses (selective visual responses). A second type of neuron responds to a combination of a particular object and it being associated with reward, or a particular object and it being associated with punishment. (They are the conditional reward neurons described in Section 4.5.5.4 and illustrated in Fig. 4.32 on page 112, and shown in Table 4.1 on page 112 as neurons showing conditional reversal.) A third type of neuron is reward-tuned in that it responds whenever a visual stimulus is decoded as reward regardless of whether the contingencies are reversed or not; or is punisher-tuned in that it responds whenever a stimulus is decoded as punishment-associated regardless of whether the contingencies are reversed or not. (These are the neurons that show full reversal, and are indicated in Table 4.1 as neurons showing reversal.) Local synaptic connections (which could be set up by development and learning) between these neuronal pools are sufficient for operation of the model. First the architecture and operation of the model are described, and then a full mathematical specification of the model and the neuronal parameters used are given in Section B.6.

A conceptual overview of the architecture, illustrated in Fig. 4.48 on page 143, is that in the lower module, stimuli are mapped from sensory neurons (level 1, at the bottom), through an intermediate layer of object-reward combination neurons with rule-dependent activity, to layer 3 which contains Reward/Punisher neurons. The mapping through the intermediate layer can be biased by the rule module inputs to perform a direct or reversed mapping. The activity in the rule module can be reversed by the error signal in the orbitofrontal cortex that occurs when an expected reward is not obtained (see Section 4.5.5.5). The reversal occurs because the attractor state in the rule module is shut down by inhibition arising from the effects of the error signal, and restarts in the opposite attractor state because of partial synaptic or neuronal adaptation of the previously active rule neurons.

B.2.1 The network

The network is composed of two modules: a rule module, and a sensory – intermediate neuron – reward module, as shown in Fig. 4.48. Each module contains N_E (excitatory) pyramidal cells and N_I inhibitory interneurons. In the simulations, Deco and Rolls (2005d) used $N_E = 1600$ and $N_I = 400$ for the sensory – intermediate neuron – reward module; and $N_E = 1000$ and $N_I = 200$ for the rule module, consistent with the neurophysiologically observed proportion of 80% pyramidal cells versus 20% interneurons (Abeles 1991, Rolls and Deco 2002). In each module, the neurons are fully connected (with synaptic strengths as specified below). Neurons in the orbitofrontal cortical network shown in Fig. 4.48 are clustered into populations or pools. Each pool of selective excitatory cells contains $f N_E$ neurons. In the simulations $f = 0.05$ for the associative module (where there are thus 80 neurons in each selective pool); and $f = 0.1$ for the rule module (where there are thus 100 neurons in each selective pool). There are two different types of pool: excitatory and inhibitory.

In the sensory – intermediate neuron – reward module, there are four subtypes of excitatory pool, namely: object-tuned (visual sensory pools); object-and-expected-reward-tuned (i.e. conditional reward neurons) (intermediate or associative pools); reward (vs punisher)-tuned pools; and nonselective pools. Object pools are feature-specific, encoding for example the identity of an object (in our case two object-specific pools: syringe and other object, or triangle vs square). The Reward/Punisher pools represent whether the visual stimulus being presented is currently associated with Reward (and for other neurons, with Punishment). Reward neurons are envisaged as naturally leading to an approach response, such as Go, and Punisher neurons as naturally leading to escape or avoidance behaviour, characterized as NoGo behaviour. The intermediate or associative pools (in that they are between the sensory and Reward/Punisher association representing pools) are context-specific and perform the mapping between the sensory stimuli to the anticipated reward/punishment pool. (In our case there are four pools at the intermediate level, two for the direct rewarding context: object 1–rewarding, object 2–punishing, and two for the reversal condition: object 1–punishing, object 2–rewarding). These intermediate pools respond to combinations of the sensory stimuli and the expected reward, e.g. to object 1 and an expected reward (glucose obtained after licking). The sensory – intermediate – reward module consists of three hierarchically organized levels of attractor network, with stronger synaptic connections in the forward than the backprojection direction. The rule module acts as a biasing input to bias the competition between the object–reward combination neurons at the intermediate level of the sensory – intermediate – reward module. It is an important part of the architecture that at the intermediate level of the sensory – intermediate – reward module one set of neurons fire if an object being presented is currently associated with reward, and a different set if the object being presented is currently associated with punishment. This representation means that these neurons can be used for different functions, such as the elicitation of emotional or autonomic responses, which occur for example to stimuli associated with particular reinforcers (see Chapters 4–6).

In the rule module, there are two different subtypes of excitatory pools: context-tuned (rule pools), and the non-selective pools. The rule pools encode the context (in our case, one pool represents: object 1 is rewarding (in that glucose taste reward is obtained if a lick is made) and object 2 is punishing (associated with aversive saline taste so that licking should be avoided); and the other pool represents that the reverse contingencies apply currently.

In both modules, the remaining excitatory neurons do not have specific sensory, response or biasing inputs, and are in a nonselective pool. (They have some spontaneous firing, and help to introduce some noise into the simulation, which aids in generating the almost Poisson spike firing patterns of neurons in the simulation that are a property of many neurons recorded in the brain (Brunel and Wang 2001).) All the inhibitory neurons are clustered into a common inhibitory pool for each module, so that there is global competition throughout each module.

We assume that the synaptic coupling strengths between any two neurons in the network act as if they were established by Hebbian learning, i.e. the coupling will be strong if the pair of neurons have correlated activity, and weak if they are activated in an uncorrelated way. As a consequence of this, neurons within a specific excitatory pool are mutually coupled with a strong weight $w_s = 2.1$. Neurons in the inhibitory pool are mutually connected with an intermediate weight $w = 1$ (forming the inhibitory to inhibitory connections that are useful in achieving non-oscillatory firing). They are also connected with all excitatory neurons with the same intermediate weight $w = 1$. The connection strength between two neurons in two different specific excitatory pools is weak and given by $w_w = 1 - 2f(w_s - 1)/(1 - 2f)$ unless otherwise specified (see next paragraph) (where f is the fraction of the excitatory neurons that are in each pool as described above, e.g. $f = 0.05$ for the sensory – intermediate neuron – reward module). Neurons in a specific excitatory pool are connected to neurons in the nonselective pool with a feedforward synaptic weight $w = 1$ and a feedback synaptic connection of weight w_w.

The connections between the different pools are set up so that each specific intermediate or associative pool is connected with the corresponding specific sensory-tuned pool, reward rule context-tuned pool from the rule module, and reward/punishment-tuned pool, as if they were based on Hebbian learning of the activity of individual pools while the different tasks are being performed. The strengths of the feedforward and feedback connections between different pools are indicated in Table B.1 for the associative module and in Table B.2 for the rule module. The connection between the rule-pools of the rule module and the associative-pools of the associative module were $w_{\mathrm{intermodule}} = 1.1$ and used only AMPA synapses.

Table B.1 Neuronal connectivity between different neuronal pools in the stimulus – intermediate – Reward/Punishment modules

Pools	O1	O2	O1-R	O2-P	O1-P	O2-R	R	P	Unsp.	Inh.
O1	w_s	w_w	w_{ff}	w_w	w_{ff}	w_w	w_w	w_w	1	1
O2	w_w	w_s	w_w	w_{ff}	w_w	w_{ff}	w_w	w_w	1	1
O1-R	w_{fb}	w_w	w_s	w_w	w_w	w_w	w_s	w_w	1	1
O2-P	w_w	w_{fb}	w_w	w_s	w_w	w_w	w_w	w_s	1	1
O1-P	w_{fb}	w_w	w_w	w_w	w_s	w_w	w_w	w_s	1	1
O2-R	w_w	w_{fb}	w_w	w_w	w_w	w_s	w_s	w_w	1	1
R	w_w	w_w	w_w	w_w	w_w	w_w	w_s	w_w	1	1
P	w_w	w_w	w_w	w_w	w_w	w_w	w_w	w_s	1	1
Unsp.	w_w	w_w	w_w	w_w	w_w	w_w	w_w	w_w	1	1
Inh.	1	1	1	1	1	1	1	1	1	1

O1: Object 1 sensory pool (Syringe, or triangle); O2: Object 2 sensory pool (other object, or square); O1-R: intermediate pool for object 1 associated with reward; O2-P: intermediate pool for object 2 associated with punishment; O1-P: intermediate pool for object 1 associated with punishment; O2-R: intermediate pool for object 2 associated with reward; R: Reward (Go) pool; P: Punishment (NoGo) pool; Unsp: non-specific neuronal pool; Inh: inhibitory neuron pool. w_w: weak synaptic strength (0.878). w_s: strong synaptic strength (=2.1). w_{ff}: feedforward synaptic strength (=2.1). w_{fb}: feedback synaptic strength (=1.7).

Each neuron (pyramidal cells and interneurons) receives $N_{\mathrm{ext}} = 800$ excitatory AMPA synaptic connections from outside the network. These connections provide two different types of external interactions: 1) a background noise due to the spontaneous firing activity of neurons outside the network; 2) a sensory-related input (object-specific). The external inputs are given by a Poisson train of spikes. In order to model the background spontaneous activity of neurons in the network (Brunel and Wang 2001), we assume that Poisson spikes arrive at each external synapse with a rate of 3 Hz, consistent with the spontaneous activity observed in the cerebral cortex (Wilson, O'Scalaidhe and Goldman-Rakic 1994, Rolls and Treves 1998). In other words, the effective external spontaneous background input rate of spikes to each cell summed across all synapses is $\nu_{\mathrm{ext}} = N_{\mathrm{ext}} \times 3$ Hz = 2.4 kHz. The sensory input is encoded by increasing the external input Poisson rate ν_{ext} to $\nu_{\mathrm{ext}} + \lambda_{\mathrm{input}}$ to the neurons in the appropriate specific sensory pools (Brunel and Wang 2001). λ_{input} is 200 Hz, which corresponds across n synapses to an average increase of $200/n$ Hz at each synapse, or on

Table B.2 Neuronal connectivity between different neuronal pools in the rule module

Pools	Rule Direct (O1-R)	Rule Reversal (O1-P)	Unsp.	Inh.
Rule Direct (O1-R)	w_s	w_w	1	1
Rule Reversal (O1-P)	w_w	w_s	1	1
Unsp.	w_w	w_w	1	1
Inh.	1	1	1	1

Rule Direct (O1-R): Object 1 is currently associated with Reward; Rule Reversal (O1-P): Object 1 is currently associated with Punishment; Unsp: non-specific neuronal pool; Inh: inhibitory neuron pool. w_w: weak synaptic strength (0.878). w_s: strong synaptic strength (=2.1).

average a change of rate at the 800 excitatory synapses from 3 to 3.25 Hz on each synapse.

The cortical architecture introduced above for the sensory – intermediate neuron – reward module presents the characteristic that its different global attractors corresponding to the different sensory cue – reward context – response situations, are each composed of a set of single pool attractors, where the single pools that are active represent a particular combination of sensory, associative and reward/punishment pools. (Attractor autoassociation networks are described in Appendix 1.) The cue stimulus, and the biasing top-down rule or context information from the rule module, drive the system into the corresponding attractor. In fact, the system is dynamically driven according to the biased competition hypothesis (Moran and Desimone 1985, Spitzer et al. 1988, Motter 1993, Miller et al. 1993a, Chelazzi et al. 1993, Reynolds and Desimone 1999, Chelazzi 1998, Rolls and Deco 2002). Multiple excitatory pools of neurons activated by the sensory cue stimulus engage in competitive interactions using the interneurons to implement the global competition within the sensory – intermediate – reward module. The top-down interactions bias this competition in favour of specific pools, resulting in the build up of the global attractor that corresponds to the context-specific stimulus – reward mapping required.

Care is needed when simulating these continuous dynamical systems on digital computers. In this research, all neuronal and synaptic equations were integrated using the second-order Runge-Kutta method, with an integration step of $dt = 0.1$ ms. Checks were performed to show that this was sufficiently small. For the neural membrane potential equations, interpolation of the spike times and their use in the synaptic currents and potentials were taken into account following the prescription of Hansel, Mato, Meunier and Neltner (1998), in order to avoid numerical problems due to the discontinuity of the membrane potential and its derivative at the spike firing time. The external trains of Poisson spikes were generated randomly and independently.

B.2.2 Reward reversal: the operation of the rule module neurons

The cue-response mapping required under a specific context is achieved via the biasing effect of the spiking information coming from the rule-pools. For a specific context a specific rule-pool will be activated, and the other rule-pools are inactive. When a reward reversal occurs, the rule pools switch their activity, i.e. the previously activated context-specific rule pool is inactivated, and a new rule pool (that was inactive) is now activated, to encode the new context. Switching the rule-pools switches the bias being applied to the intermediate pools, which effectively represent when a stimulus is shown whether it is (in the context of the current rule) associated with reward or with aversive saline. From the intermediate pool, the mapping is then straightforward to the reward/punishment pools (which have implied connections to produce a Go response (of licking) if a currently reward-associated visual stimulus is being shown, and a NoGo response of not licking if a stimulus currently associated with aversive saline is shown.

To achieve the reversal in the rule module, (which is at the heart of the process), we assumed that the attractor state in the rule-module is reset via a nonspecific global inhibitory signal, which is received after each punishment or absence of an expected reward. Neurons that respond in just this way, i.e. when an expected reward is not obtained, and a stimulus–reinforcement reversal must occur, were found in the orbitofrontal cortex by Thorpe, Rolls and Maddison (1983). These neurons can be described as error neurons (Section 4.5.5.5). Deco and Rolls (2005d) implemented the effects of this error signal by increasing for 50 ms the external AMPA-input to the inhibitory pool of the rule module (see Fig. 4.48). (The increase was from ν_{ext} to $\nu_{\text{ext}} + \lambda_{\text{Punish}}$ with $\lambda_{\text{Punish}} = 900$ Hz, which corresponds to an increase of 1.125 Hz to each of the 800 external synapses impinging on the neurons of the inhibitory pool. This compares to the mean value of the spontaneous external input of 3 Hz per synapse.) This increased the global inhibition of the rule module, and suppressed the activity of all the excitatory neuronal pools in the rule module. Effectively, the firing of the error neurons activated the inhibitory neurons in the rule module. (The effect could be implemented in the brain by the active error neurons activating inhibitory interneurons that influence, among other neurons, the rule-module excitatory neurons. The system would work just as well if this inhibitory feedback was applied to both the modules shown in Fig. 4.48, not just the rule module, and this might be more parsimonious in terms of the connectivity required in the brain.)

Deco and Rolls (2005d) incorporated into the excitatory synaptic connections between the neurons in the rule module the property that they show some spike-frequency-adaptation process (with details provided below). This provides a mechanism that implements a temporal memory of the previously activated pool. When the attractor state of the rule module is shut down by the inhibitory input, then the attractor state that subsequently emerges when firing starts again will be different from the state that has just been present, because of the synaptic adaptation in the synapses that supported the previous attractor state. In order to assure that one of the rule-pools was active, and to promote high competition between the possible reward contexts, we excited externally all rule-pools with the same non-specific input by increasing the external input Poisson firing rate impinging on the excitatory pools of the rule module (from ν_{ext} to $\nu_{\text{ext}} + B$ with $B = 200$ Hz).

The implementations of different spike-frequency-adaptation mechanisms used in the rule-module are now described.

One implementation (used for the simulations shown in Figs. B.3, B.4 and B.5) was a sodium inactivation based spike-frequency-adaptation mechanism. A full statistical analysis of a model of sodium inactivation in the framework of integrate-and-fire models was introduced by Giugliano, La Camera, Rauch, Luescher and Fusi (2002) as a realistic candidate for long lasting non-monotonic effects in current-to-rate response functions observed in vitro (Rauch, La Camera, Luescher, Senn and Fusi 2003) and associated with spike-frequency-

mechanisms. The model was called an integrate-and-may-fire (IMF) model, and takes into account the inactivation of sodium channels after spike generation. The integrate-and-fire model is modified, by changing the condition that when the membrane potential reaches the threshold θ, the emission of a spike at that time is an event occurring with an activity-dependent probability q. After the spike emission, the membrane potential is clamped to the value $V_{\text{reset}} = -55$ mV, for an absolute refractory time, after which the current integration starts again. However, each time the excitability threshold θ is crossed and no spike has been generated (i.e. an event with probability $1 - q$), the membrane potential is reset to $H_2 (0 < V_{\text{reset}} < H_2 < \theta)$ and no refractoriness occurs. Additionally, q is a decreasing function of a slow voltage-dependent variable ω $(0 < \omega < 1)$, reminiscent of the sigmoidal voltage dependence of the fast inactivation state variables that characterize conductance-based model neurons:

$$q = \left[1 + e^{\frac{(\omega - \omega_0)}{\sigma_\omega}} \right]^{-1} \tag{B.1}$$

where ω evolves by,

$$\tau_\omega \frac{d\omega(t)}{dt} = \frac{V(t)}{\theta} - \omega \tag{B.2}$$

which corresponds to a first approximation to the average transmembrane electric field experienced by individual ion channels and affecting their population-level activation and inactivation. In our simulations we utilized $\tau_\omega = 10,000$ ms, $\sigma_\omega = 0.01$, $\omega_0 = 0.87$, and $H_2 = -52$ mV.

Deco and Rolls (2005d) also tried other spike-frequency adapting mechanisms, including Ca^{++}-activated K^+ hyper-polarizing currents (Liu and Wang 2001), and short-term synaptic depression (Abbott and Nelson 2000). Both of them were successfully used for producing the desired reward reversal based context-switching. The synaptic depression mechanism was used for Fig. 4.49, and the details were after Dayan and Abbott (2001) page 185. In particular, the probability of release P_{rel} was decreased after each presynaptic spike by a factor $P_{\text{rel}} = P_{\text{rel}}.f_{\text{D}}$ with $f_{\text{D}} = 0.994$. Between presynaptic action potentials the release probability P_{rel} is updated by

$$\tau_P \frac{dP_{\text{rel}}}{dt} = P_0 - P_{\text{rel}} \tag{B.3}$$

with $P_0 = 1$.

B.2.3   The neurons in the model

Deco and Rolls (2005d) used leaky integrate-and-fire neurons for modelling the excitatory pyramidal cells and the inhibitory interneurons. Fig. B.1 shows graphically the synaptic and membrane processes. The basic circuit of an integrate-and-fire model consists of the cell membrane capacitance C_{m} in parallel with the cell membrane resistance R_{m} driven by a synaptic current which produces excitatory or inhibitory postsynaptic potentials (EPSPs or IPSPs). The incoming presynaptic δ-pulse from other neurons is basically low-pass filtered first by the synaptic and membrane time constants, before it is utilized to produce the EPSPs or IPSPs in the one-compartment neuronal model. These potentials are integrated by the cell, and if a threshold θ is reached, a δ-pulse (spike) is fired and transmitted to other neurons, and the potential of the neuron is reset. Biologically realistic parameters (McCormick, Connors, Lighthall and Prince 1985) are used. For example, for both excitatory and inhibitory neurons a resting potential $V_{\text{L}} = -70$ mV, a firing threshold $\theta = -50$ mV, and a reset potential

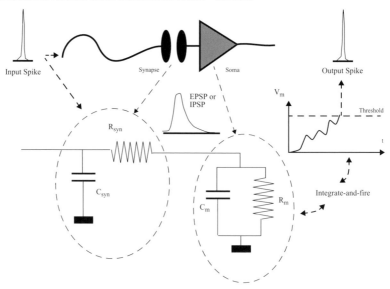

Fig. B.1 Integrate-and-fire neuron. The basic circuit of an integrate-and-fire model consists of the neuron's membrane capacitance C_m in parallel with the membrane's resistance R_m driven by a synaptic current with a conductance and time constant determined by the synaptic resistance R_{syn} and capacitance C_{syn} shown in the Figure. These effects produce excitatory or inhibitory postsynaptic potentials, EPSPs or IPSPs. These potentials are integrated by the cell, and if a threshold θ is reached a δ-pulse (spike) is fired and transmitted to other neurons, and the membrane potential is reset. (After Deco and Rolls 2003.)

$V_{\text{reset}} = -55$ mV were used. The membrane capacitance C_{m} was 0.5 nF for the pyramidal neurons and 0.2 nF for the inhibitory interneurons. The membrane leak conductance g_{m} was 25 nS for pyramidal cells, and 20 nS for interneurons. The refractory period τ_{ref} was 2 ms for pyramidal cells, and 1 ms for interneurons. Hence, the membrane time constant $\tau_{\text{m}} = C_{\text{m}}/g_{\text{m}}$ was 20 ms for pyramidal cells, and 10 ms for interneurons.

B.2.4   The synapses in the model

The synaptic current flows into the cells are mediated by three different families of receptors. The recurrent excitatory postsynaptic EPSPs are mediated by AMPA and NMDA (N-methyl-D-aspartate) receptors. These two glutamatergic excitatory synapses are on the pyramidal cells and on the interneurons. The external inputs (background, sensory input, or external top-down interaction from other areas) are mediated by AMPA synapses on pyramidal cells and interneurons. Inhibitory GABAergic synapses on pyramidal cells and interneurons yield the corresponding IPSPs. The mathematical descriptions of each synaptic channel are provided in Section B.6, and the corresponding parameters are also specified there. We consider that the NMDA currents have a voltage dependence that is controlled by the extracellular magnesium concentration (Jahr and Stevens 1990), $C_{\text{Mg}^{++}} = 1$ mM. We neglect the rise time of both AMPA and GABA synaptic currents because they are typically very short (< 1 ms). The rise time for NMDA synapses is $\tau_{\text{NMDA,rise}} = 2$ ms (Spruston, Jonas and Sakmann 1995, Hestrin, Sah and Nicoll 1990). All synapses have a synaptic delay of 0.5 ms. The time constant for AMPA synapses is $\tau_{\text{AMPA}} = 2$ ms (Spruston et al. 1995, Hestrin et al. 1990), for NMDA

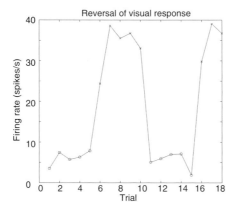

Fig. B.2 Simulation of the experimental results of Thorpe, Rolls and Maddison, 1983, on the reversal of visual responses in an orbitofrontal cortex single neuron illustrated in Fig. 4.31. On trials 1–5, no response of the neuron occurred to the sight of a syringe from which the monkey had been given orally glucose reward solution to drink on the previous trial. On trials 6–9, the neuron responded to the sight of the same syringe from which he had been given aversive hypertonic saline drink on the previous trial. Two more reversals (trials 10–15, and 16–17) were performed. In the simulated results, the firing rate is shown of the neurons in the Punishment pool of the orbitofrontal cortex final (Reward/Punishment) neuronal pools in the sensory – intermediate – reward module. The neuron signalled punishment only when the object, O1 (the syringe used to feed the monkey), predicted punishment, and the neuronal response reversed in one trial. (After Deco and Rolls 2005d.)

synapses $\tau_{NMDA,decay} = 100$ ms (Spruston et al. 1995, Hestrin et al. 1990), and for GABA synapses $\tau_{GABA} = 10$ ms (Salin and Prince 1996, Xiang, Huguenard and Prince 1998). The synaptic conductivities for each receptor type were taken from Brunel and Wang (2001), and were adjusted using a mean field analysis to be approximately 1 nS in magnitude, and were consistent with experimentally observed values (Destexhe, Mainen and Sejnowski 1998) (see Section B.6). As was noted by Brunel and Wang (2001), Wang (1999) and Lisman, Fellous and Wang (1998), the recurrent excitation was assumed to be largely mediated by the NMDA receptors, in order to provide more robust persistent activity during the short-term memory related delay period; and the amplitude of recurrent excitation was smaller than that of feedback inhibition, and therefore the net recurrent input (i.e. the sum of these two terms) to a neuron was hyperpolarizing during spontaneous activity (i.e. without external inputs) (Brunel and Wang 2001, Amit and Brunel 1997). Fig. 4.48 shows schematically the synaptic structure assumed in the orbitofrontal cortical network.

B.3 Single neuron visual discrimination reversal in the orbitofrontal cortex: operation of the model

Deco and Rolls (2005d) simulated, with the architecture described in the preceding section and shown in Fig. 4.48, the experimental set-up utilized by Thorpe, Rolls and Maddison (1983) and Rolls, Critchley, Mason and Wakeman (1996b) in order to analyse theoretically the neuronal activity in the primate orbitofrontal cortex underlying the execution of a visual

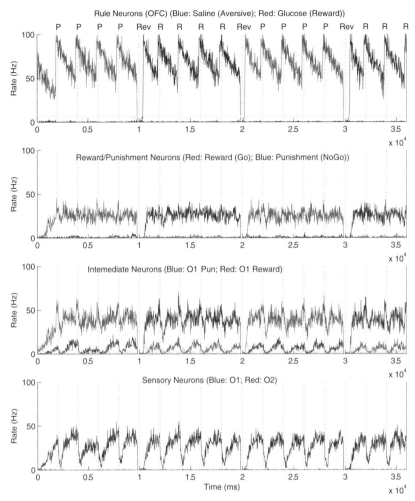

Fig. B.3 Temporal evolution of the averaged population activity for all neural pools (sensory, intermediate (stimulus–reward/punishment), and Reward/Punishment) in the stimulus – intermediate – reward module and the rule module during the execution of the reversal of the Go/NoGo visual discrimination task shown in Fig. 4.31. Each vertical line indicates a new trial. The yellow curve in the top graph shows the average activity of the inhibitory interneurons in the rule module. O1 was the syringe used to present the stimuli in Fig. 4.31. R: Reward trial; P: Punishment Trial; Rev: Reversal trial, i.e. the first trial after the reward contingency was reversed when Reward was expected but Punishment was obtained. (After Deco and Rolls 2005d.) (See colour plates section.)

discrimination reward reversal task. The model was able to reverse the behavioural responses quickly, so that if it obtained a non-reward signal (saline for licking) to a stimulus that had previously been associated with reward, it subsequently only produced a lick to the previously punished stimulus which now indicated that reward was available.

Fig. B.2 shows the reversal of visual responses in the orbitofrontal pool corresponding to the 'object 1-aversive' association. This figure can be compared with the neurophysiological results shown in Fig. 4.31 on page 111. Because the significance of the visual stimuli had been

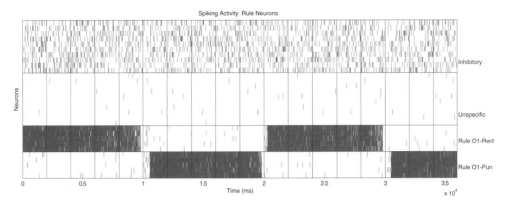

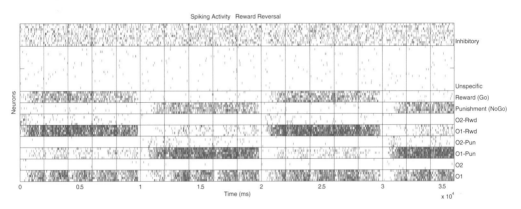

Fig. B.4 Rastergrams of randomly selected neurons for each pool in the OFC network from the simulation shown in Figs. B.2 and B.3 during the execution and reversal of the Go/NoGo visual discrimination task of Thorpe, Rolls and Maddison (1983). Each vertical line indicates a new trial. O1, object 1 (the syringe) was used throughout this experiment. O1-Rwd is the intermediate pool responding to O1 when it is associated with reward. O1-Pun is the intermediate pool responding to O1 when it is associated with punishment. The final pools are denoted Reward (which implies a Go response) and Punishment (which signifies a NoGo response). (After Deco and Rolls 2005d.)

altered, the neurons in the 'object 1-aversive' associative pool responded only in the cases where visual object 1 was shown, and the model did not perform a lick response because a saline solution was being expected. In fact, in this case, the 'object 1' sensory pool and the 'Punishment (NoGo)' pool of the Reward/Punishment pool were also co-activated as parts of the same global attractor. On the other hand, during the trials where object 1 was associated with a glucose reward, then the 'object 1-reward' associative pool responded with high activation, together with the sensory 'object 1' pool and the 'Reward (Go)' Reward/Punishment pool. These three pools formed the global attractor under this rewarding condition, and therefore the former attractors corresponding to the reversal condition were suppressed through inhibition within the global attractor. The rule input thus biased the competition in the correct direction.

Figs. B.3 and B.4 show the whole spatio-temporal picture by plotting the firing rates and the corresponding rastergrams. The rastergrams (Fig. B.4) show randomly selected neurons for each pool in the stimulus – intermediate – reward module (5 for each sensory, intermediate and Reward (Go)/Punishment(NoGo) pool, 20 for the non-selective excitatory pool, and 10 for the inhibitory pool), and in the rule module (5 for each rule pool, 10 for the non-selective excitatory pool, and 10 for the inhibitory pool). The spatio-temporal spiking activity shows both attractors described above, i.e. those that were present when the task was run non-reversed and reversed. The cue stimulus, and the biasing rule top-down synaptic connections applied to the associative neurons, drive the system into the corresponding global attractor utilizing biased competition mechanisms. The activity of the rule pools was switched correctly by the external non-reward signal. It is of interest that although the inputs produced by the error signal were applied only to the inhibitory neurons in the rule module (via their AMPA receptors), most of these inhibitory neurons in fact decreased their firing rates on the coarse time scale. This is because there are inhibitory to inhibitory neuron connections, and because the inhibition produced in the excitatory neurons itself caused less drive to the inhibitory neurons. Although the total firing in the modules thus was decreased, the synaptic activity produced at least by the inhibitory external input was strong. This is of interest, for total synaptic activity, rather than average firing rate, may be reflected in fMRI signals (Deco, Rolls and Horwitz 2004). In any case, the switching of the attractor in the rule module acts as a reversal of the biasing context input to the stimulus–reward-response module, and therefore a switching of the attractors in the associative module. This is a biased competition operation. As shown in Figs. B.3 and B.4, this switching is very fast, within one trial of when a non-reward signal was obtained.

Fig. 4.49 on page 145 shows the results of a simulation of the more usual Go/NoGo task design with a pseudorandom sequence of trials. On each trial, either Object 1 (a triangle) or Object 2 (a square) was shown. In Fig. 4.49, on trial 1 the rule network was operating in the direct mapping state, the sensory pool responded to the triangle, the intermediate pool that was selected based on this sensory input and the direct rule bias was the triangle-reward pool (O1R in Fig. 4.48), this pool led to activation of the Reward (or Go) pool, and a reward (R) was obtained. On trial 2 the sensory pool for the square (O1) responded, and this with the direct rule bias led to the intermediate square-Non-reward (O2P) pool to be selected, and this in turn led to Punishment neurons being active, leading to a NoGo response (i.e. no action). On trial 3 the sensory triangle pool was activated, leading because of the direct rule to activation of the intermediate triangle-reward pool, and Reward was decoded (leading to a Go response being made). However, because this was a reversal trial, punishment was obtained, leading to activation of the error input, which increased the inhibition in the rule module, and quenching of the rule module attractor. When the rule module attractor started up again, it started with the reverse rule neurons active, as they won the competition with the direct rule neurons, whose excitatory synapses had adapted during the previous few trials. On trial 4 the sensory-square input neurons were activated, and the intermediate neurons representing square-reward were activated (due to the biasing influence of the reversed rule input to these intermediate neurons), the Reward neurons in the third layer were activated (leading to a Go response), and reward was obtained. On trial 5 the sensory-triangle neurons activated the triangle-Non-reward intermediate neurons under the biasing influence of the reversed rule input, and Punishment was decoded by the third layer (resulting in a NoGo response). On trial 6, the sensory-square neurons were activated leading to activation of the intermediate square-reward neurons, and Reward (and a Go response) was produced. However, this was another reversal trial, non-reward or punishment activated the error inputs, and the rule neurons in the rule module were quenched, and started up again with the direct rule neurons active in the rule module, due to the synaptic depression of the synapses between the reversed rule neurons.

B.4   A model of reversal of a conditional object-response task by the dorsolateral prefrontal cortex

So far, we have considered the reversal of a stimulus–reinforcer association, which is the type involved in emotional states. However, other types of mapping can be reversed. One example is the mapping of stimuli to behavioural responses. It is of interest to consider the reversal of this type of mapping, partly because it is an important to contrast stimulus–response mapping from that involved in producing emotional states, and partly because the underlying neural substrates may be analogous, providing supporting evidence for the theory presented here of rapid reversals.

The experiment we consider will be the reversal of a *conditional object–visuomotor response task*, because there is evidence on the types of neuronal activity in the dorsolateral prefrontal cortex (PFC) during this task (Asaad, Rainer and Miller 1998), and neuronal data are important for providing a firm foundation for the computational model. The task required the monkeys to make one response (e.g. a left oculomotor saccade) after a delay following the presentation of one object (e.g. A) at the fovea, and a different response (e.g. a right oculomotor saccade) after a delay following the presentation of another object (e.g. B) at the fovea. The cue period was 500 ms, and the short-term memory delay period separating the cue and response was 1,000 ms. Asaad et al. (1998) trained the monkeys under two different conditions, namely: 1) direct association, and 2) reverse association. The direct condition corresponded to the association of one object, for example A, with a leftward eye motor response, and the other object, for example B, with a rightward eye motor response. The reverse condition corresponded to the reversed association of cue and responses, i.e. object A was now associated with a rightward eye motor response, and object B with a leftward eye motor response.

We adapted the network structure to simulate this task. The architecture is similar to that shown in Fig. 4.48, but what is coded in the intermediate layer of the lower module, which is now a stimulus – stimulus–response combination – response module is different. The sensory pools now encode information about objects. The object or feature-based sensory pools are feature-specific, encoding for example the identity of an object (e.g. form, colour, etc.). The premotor pools encode the motor response (in our case the leftward or rightward oculomotor saccade), and replace the Reward/Punishment pools in the third layer in Fig. 4.48. The intermediate pools (in that they are between the sensory and premotor pools) are task-specific and perform the mapping between the sensory stimuli and the required motor response. The intermediate pools respond to combinations of the sensory stimuli and the response required, e.g. to object A requiring a left oculomotor saccade. The intermediate (or associative) pools receive a top-down biasing input that comes from the rule module, where now the two rule pools correspond to the direct and reversed conditional response association.

Figure B.5A shows the simulation results corresponding to Fig. 5a in the paper of Asaad et al. (1998) (of which we show an example in Fig. B.5B). Fig. B.5A plots the average firing activity of the two motor direction-selective response pools around the time of reversal at trial zero. The stars show the responses to the object that, having indicated a saccade in the neuron's preferred direction before the reversal, starts after the reversal at trial zero to

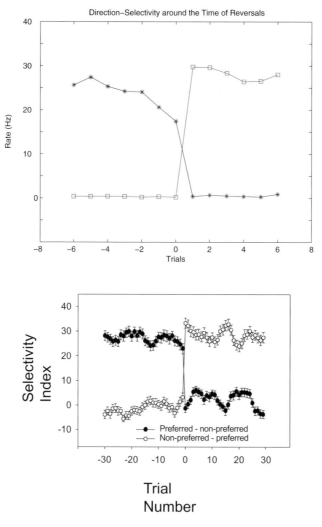

Fig. B.5 Reversal of a conditional object–response task with a delay. Average firing activity of the two motor direction-selective pools around the time of reversal which occurred at trial zero. (A, above) Simulation results. The stars show the responses to the object that, having indicated a saccade in the neuron's preferred direction, begins at trial zero to indicate a saccade in the neuron's non-preferred direction. The squares show the opposite, namely the activity produced by the object that before reversal cued a saccade in the non-preferred direction, and after reversal required an eye movement in the neuron's preferred direction. After Deco and Rolls (2005d). (B, below) Neurophysiological results obtained in the experiment of Asaad et al. (1998) during reversal.

indicate a saccade in the neuron's non-preferred direction. The squares show the opposite, namely the activity produced by the object that before reversal at trial 0 cued a saccade in the neuron's non-preferred direction, and after reversal required an eye movement in the preferred direction. The simulation results show the same rapid reversal context switching observed in the experiments, which corresponds dynamically with a change in the whole attractor structure due to the non-rewarding inhibitory signal provided at the time of reversal. This error signal resets the whole rule module to zero firing, and, because of the intrinsic temporal memory associated with the spike-frequency adaptation mechanism or short term depression, when the rule module network starts up again, the opposite rule pool is active. This reverses the bias on the associative module, and the stimulus–response associations there are reversed.

B.5   Evaluation of the models

The model of Section B.2 shows how rapid stimulus–reinforcer association reversal learning could occur. It is an important part of the architecture that at the intermediate level of the sensory – intermediate neuron – reward module one set of neurons (conditional reward neurons) fire if a particular object being presented (but not other objects) is currently associated with reward. This is in line with what is found in the primate orbitofrontal cortex (Thorpe, Rolls and Maddison 1983), as illustrated for a conditional reward neuron in Fig. 4.32 on page 112. This representation means that these intermediate neurons can be used for different functions, such as the elicitation of emotional or autonomic responses, which occur for example to stimuli associated with particular reinforcers (Rolls 1999a). For example, this allows different emotional responses to occur to different cognitive stimuli, even if the same primary reinforcer is associated with both stimuli.

This property makes the architecture quite functionally different to that of the dorsolateral prefrontal network architecture modelled by Deco and Rolls (2003), and described in Section B.4 which performs a stimulus to motor response mapping using neurons at the intermediate level that respond to combinations of stimuli and motor responses, which is the type of neuron recorded in that region (Asaad, Rainer and Miller 1998, Asaad, Rainer and Miller 2000). The dorsolateral prefrontal network thus operates by switching between two habits (stimulus–response associations). In contrast, the orbitofrontal cortex architecture described here in Section B.2 maps stimuli to expected rewards. The expected rewards then provide the goal for any appropriate behavioural response. This introduces flexibility into the response selection, and this flexible choice provides a fundamental evolutionary advantage of emotion in brain design (see Chapter 3, Rolls (1999a), and Rolls (2004e)).

After the conditional reward layer of intermediate neurons, the next layer represents the reward (or punishment) value of the stimulus independently of whether the current rule is direct or reversed. This third layer is thus the layer at which emotional states and responses can be elicited, as it is this layer that represents the current reward (or punishment) value of the stimulus independently of reversal. These third layer neurons will then in the real brain tend to elicit approach, which is an unlearnt behaviour to a reward, and escape or avoidance, which is the natural behaviour to a punisher. However, the utility of a reward representation, which can be rapidly reversed in one trial as described here, is that any instrumental action can then be performed to obtain the reward, or avoid or escape the punisher. This is how the flexibility of behaviour arises that was referred to above as a fundamental evolutionary advantage of designing the brain with reward and punisher systems (see Chapter 3, Rolls (1999a), and Rolls (2004e)).

It is worth noting that the neurons described by Asaad et al. (1998) and Asaad et al. (2000) in the dorsolateral prefrontal cortex that respond to combinations of particular visual stimuli and responses are analogous to those orbitofrontal cortex conditional reward neurons that respond to combinations of particular visual stimuli and rewards (Thorpe, Rolls and Maddison 1983).

The rapid switch of the rule in the model is produced by a single error without any synaptic modification. To set up the networks that hold the different rules, some learning is needed, and the learning of the appropriate rule pools with the correct connections to the intermediate pools is what I suggest is occurring while the reversal learning set is being acquired. Acquisition of the learning set can take a number of reversals, during which the number of trials for the reversal to occur gradually decreases to one trial. The actual implementation described here, of using an attractor network to hold the current rule, which then biases intermediate conditional neurons to achieve the correct mapping to reward (or, in the case of the dorsolateral prefrontal cortex, to responses) does appear to be quite fundamental, because an active short-term (rule) memory implemented by persistent firing in an attractor does provide the necessary source of bias input for the biased competition stimulus – intermediate – reward mapping network. A synaptic modification process occurring in a pattern association stimulus–reward network when an error indicated that the rule had been reversed would require large and one-trial synaptic depression to prevent the former reward-associated stimulus from still producing reward. Instead, in the approach taken by Deco and Rolls (2005d), it has been shown that by reversing the state of a dynamical system when the error comes, and using this reversed state (of the rule module) to provide an active bias input to a mapping network, then very rapid, one-trial, reversal can be obtained. We note that the rule has to be available for many trials (until the next reversal). The intermediate neurons in the mapping module that respond to combinations of stimuli and reward are only active when the stimulus is applied. Thus they could not hold the current rule in any short-term memory. This is why a separate rule module is required.

The model makes predictions that can be tested neurophysiologically. One prediction is that there will be rule neurons in the orbitofrontal cortex, which have high firing when one rule applies and low firing when a different rule applies. These neurons should reverse their state when the monkey reverses in the visual discrimination reversal task, and should maintain their state of firing for as long as the rule applies. Second, the rule neurons should, immediately after reversal to the high-firing state, have somewhat higher firing than later, reflecting some adaptation in their state. It will be of interest to measure the time course of this alteration of firing rate, which is predicted to take 10–100 sec to develop, and should last for at least 60 sec. Third, it should be possible if a long delay occurs during testing, or if the monkey is allowed to sleep for a few minutes, to predict from the state of firing of the rule neurons which rule the monkey will use to interpret the stimuli (in terms of whether reversal applies or not). Fourth, there should be different rule neurons for different stimulus pairs if several stimulus pairs are used simultaneously, and the pairs are reversed independently. Further, the rule neurons may be not only visual stimulus-specific, but also task- or context-specific, in that reversal of the association in one task need not imply the reversal of the interpretation of the stimuli in all tasks. Some topological segregation within the orbitofrontal cortex of different localized neuronal pools would provide appropriate underpinning for this fourth point to be realized.

The mechanism described here involves *no modulation of synaptic weights* by the non-reward signal known to be present in the orbitofrontal cortex (Thorpe, Rolls and Maddison 1983) (where it is probably computed from the visual neurons that respond to expected reward and the taste neurons that signal the reward or punishment actually obtained (Thorpe, Rolls and Maddison 1983, Rolls, Critchley, Mason and Wakeman 1996b, Rolls 1997c, Deco and

Rolls 2005d). Instead, the mechanism for reversal of the rule neurons described here involves just non-specific, probably feedback, inhibition to quench the recurrently connected neurons that implement the current rule attractor, and partial synaptic adaptation which has been taking place since the previous rule change to ensure that the attractor restarts with the neurons that represent the alternative rule being active. Because the rule neurons act as a biased competition gating input to the stimulus–reward combination neurons that map the sensory input to the reward neurons, the very next time after an error trial that the other stimulus is presented, it is correctly mapped as being reward-related (Thorpe, Rolls and Maddison 1983), *even though it has not been recently associated with delivery of a reward.*

Third, the model described here provides an explanation for the conditional visual stimulus–reward combination neurons in the orbitofrontal cortex described by Thorpe, Rolls and Maddison (1983), and olfactory stimulus–reward combination neurons described in primates by Rolls, Critchley, Mason and Wakeman (1996b) (see Section 4.5.5.4) and reported as also being present in what may or may not be an anatomically and functionally homologous area in rats by Schoenbaum, Chiba and Gallagher (1999). These conditional stimulus–reward combination neurons respond to one stimulus when it is associated with reward, and not to a different stimulus when it is associated with reward. These neurons are important to how the model described here functions, for these combination neurons receive the biasing input from the rule module, and enable the mapping from stimulus to reward to be changed immediately when the reward rule module changes its state, because this is a biased competition mechanism with operates dynamically when the biasing input changes with no need for any further synaptic modification. This biased competition switching of the stimulus–reward mapping by the rule module is at the heart of the process described here, and it is a strength of the theory presented here that it gives an account of the presence and need for the conditional stimulus–reward combination neurons in a part of the brain important in implementing rapid, one-trial, stimulus–reward switching, the orbitofrontal cortex (Thorpe, Rolls and Maddison 1983, Rolls, Critchley, Mason and Wakeman 1996b, Rolls, Hornak, Wade and McGrath 1994a, Hornak, O'Doherty, Bramham, Rolls, Morris, Bullock and Polkey 2004, Deco and Rolls 2005d).

In the model described here, there is no reliance on other brain systems such as the basal ganglia or ventral tegmental dopamine neurons to compute and/or represent the non-reward signal (cf Rolls (1999a)), for this error signal is already explicitly represented in the primate orbitofrontal cortex by neurons that we have shown respond whenever an expected reward is not obtained (Thorpe, Rolls and Maddison 1983), as are the signals required to compute this of whether a reward is expected on any given trial given the visual stimulus shown (Thorpe, Rolls and Maddison 1983), and whether the reward is obtained as shown by the firing of taste neurons (Thorpe, Rolls and Maddison 1983, Rolls, Yaxley and Sienkiewicz 1990). Indeed, the neurons that change their mappings in the striatum during reward reversal (Rolls, Thorpe and Maddison 1983c, Setlow, Schoenbaum and Gallagher 2003, Schoenbaum and Setlow 2003) (cf. Divac et al. (1967) and Cools, Clark, Owen and Robbins (2002)) appear to reflect the change of mapping received from direct inputs from the orbitofrontal cortex to the striatum rather than the computation that a change of mapping is required. Indeed, this was suggested in the original paper of Rolls, Thorpe and Maddison (1983c) in which the neuronal recordings in the caudate nucleus were made in the same task and in some of the same macaques as those used in the original orbitofrontal cortex recordings of Thorpe, Rolls and Maddison (1983). Whereas all the signals required for the computation were present in the orbitofrontal cortex, they were not in the striatum (Thorpe, Rolls and Maddison 1983, Rolls, Thorpe and

Maddison 1983c). Taking these findings and the connectional anatomy together, it is much more likely that neuronal activity in the basal ganglia, including the dopamine neurons in the tegmentum (which receive inputs from the striatum), reflects activity in the orbitofrontal cortex, rather than being computed in the basal ganglia, and this has important implications for understanding the functions of the orbitofrontal cortex vs the basal ganglia (see Chapter 8 and Rolls (1999a)).

The implementation of the model goes right to the level of synaptic and spiking dynamics, and can therefore describe the dynamics accurately and can allow the neuronal spiking activity in the model to be directly compared to single neuron recordings. This is related to the fact that the model utilizes explicit and realistic biophysical processes, namely an explicit description of the synaptic dynamics (AMPA, NMDA and GABA) and spiking mechanisms, constrained by the experimentally measured biophysical parameters (e.g. latencies, synaptic and membrane conductances, reversal potential etc.). In fact, firing rate-based approaches, are not necessarily consistent with spiking level approaches, as has been thoroughly analysed recently (Brunel and Wang 2001). Even more, rate-based approaches are only valid under stationary conditions, and are not able to describe the non-stationary temporal dynamics, which is the main goal of the model of Deco and Rolls (2005d), and is part of the reason why this class of model is included here. The use of rate-based approaches has been recently extensively studied (Del Giudice, Fusi and Mattia 2003, Brunel and Wang 2001), and the importance of deriving rate-response function that are consistent with the spiking and dynamics background has been stressed, a procedure which we used here to find the parameters of the model. In order to do this, a mean-field approach has to be used. The essence of the mean-field approximation is to simplify the integrate-and-fire equations by replacing, after the diffusion approximation (Tuckwell 1988), the sums of the synaptic components by the average DC component and a fluctuation term (see Rolls and Deco (2002)). The stationary dynamics of each population can be described by the *population transfer function*, which provides the average population rate as a function of the average input current. The set of stationary, self-reproducing rates ν_i for the different populations i in the network can be found by solving a set of coupled self-consistency equations. This enables a posteriori selection of the parameter region which shows in the state space the emergent behaviour that is to be investigated (e.g. biased competition) (see Deco and Rolls (2005b) and Deco and Rolls (2005a) for a detailed analysis of this approach). After that, with this set of parameters, we perform the full non-stationary simulations using the *true dynamics* only described by the full integrate-and-fire scheme. The mean field study assures us that this dynamics will converge to a stationary attractor that is consistent with what is to be investigated (Del Giudice, Fusi and Mattia 2003, Brunel and Wang 2001). Therefore in the work described here Deco and Rolls (2005d) used a mean-field approximation to explore how the different operational regimes of the network depend on the values of certain parameters. The mean-field analysis performed in this work uses the formulation derived in Brunel and Wang (2001), which is consistent with the network of neurons used. Their formulation departs from the equations describing the dynamics of one neuron to provide a stochastic analysis of the mean-first passage time of the membrane potentials, which results in a description of the population spiking rates as functions of the model parameters.

In conclusion, the only way to perform a non-stationary analysis of the temporal dynamics, for direct comparison with the neuronal recording results, is via the 'explicit' use of the synaptic and spiking mechanisms as incorporated in the integrate-and-fire model described here, after a prior analysis of a consistent mean-field derived approach for the analysis of the stationary attractors.

B.6 Integrate-and-Fire model equations and parameters

In this Section the mathematical equations that describe the spiking activity and synapse dynamics in the network are provided, following in general the formulation described by Brunel and Wang (2001).

Each neuron is described by an integrate-and-fire model. The subthreshold membrane potential $V(t)$ of each neuron evolves according to the following equation:

$$C_m \frac{dV(t)}{dt} = -g_m(V(t) - V_L) - I_{\text{syn}}(t) \tag{B.4}$$

where $I_{\text{syn}}(t)$ is the total synaptic current flow into the cell, V_L is the resting potential, C_m is the membrane capacitance, and g_m is the membrane conductance. When the membrane potential $V(t)$ reaches the threshold θ a spike is generated, and the membrane potential is reset to V_{reset}. The neuron is unable to spike during the first τ_{ref} which is the absolute refractory period.

The total synaptic current is given by the sum of glutamatergic excitatory components (NMDA and AMPA) and inhibitory components (GABA). As described above, in the model the external excitatory contributions are produced through AMPA receptors ($I_{\text{AMPA,ext}}$), while the excitatory recurrent synapses operate through AMPA and NMDA receptors ($I_{\text{AMPA,rec}}$ and $I_{\text{NMDA,rec}}$). The total synaptic current is therefore given by:

$$I_{\text{syn}}(t) = I_{\text{AMPA,ext}}(t) + I_{\text{AMPA,rec}}(t) + I_{\text{NMDA,rec}}(t) + I_{\text{GABA}}(t) \tag{B.5}$$

where

$$I_{\text{AMPA,ext}}(t) = g_{\text{AMPA,ext}}(V(t) - V_E) \sum_{j=1}^{N_{\text{ext}}} s_j^{\text{AMPA,ext}}(t) \tag{B.6}$$

$$I_{\text{AMPA,rec}}(t) = g_{\text{AMPA,rec}}(V(t) - V_E) \sum_{j=1}^{N_E} w_j s_j^{\text{AMPA,rec}}(t) \tag{B.7}$$

$$I_{\text{NMDA,rec}}(t) = \frac{g_{\text{NMDA}}(V(t) - V_E)}{(1 + C_{Mg^{++}} \exp(-0.062V(t)/3.57))} \sum_{j=1}^{N_E} w_j s_j^{\text{NMDA}}(t) \tag{B.8}$$

In the preceding equations $V_E = 0$ mV and $V_I = -70$ mV. The synaptic strengths w_j are specified above and in Table B.1. The fractions of open channels s are given by:

$$\frac{ds_j^{\text{AMPA,ext}}(t)}{dt} = -\frac{s_j^{\text{AMPA,ext}}(t)}{\tau_{\text{AMPA}}} + \sum_k \delta(t - t_j^k) \tag{B.9}$$

$$\frac{ds_j^{\text{AMPA,rec}}(t)}{dt} = -\frac{s_j^{\text{AMPA,rec}}(t)}{\tau_{\text{AMPA}}} + \sum_k \delta(t - t_j^k) \tag{B.10}$$

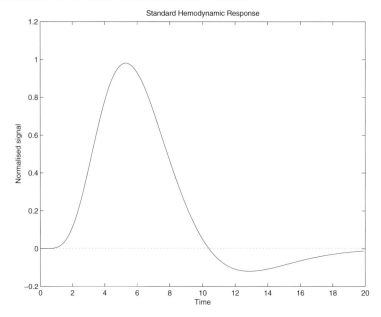

Fig. B.6 Haemodynamic response function, shown as a function of time in s.

$$\frac{ds_j^{\text{NMDA}}(t)}{dt} = -\frac{s_j^{\text{NMDA}}(t)}{\tau_{\text{NMDA,decay}}} + \alpha x_j(t)(1 - s_j^{\text{NMDA}}(t)) \tag{B.11}$$

$$\frac{dx_j(t)}{dt} = -\frac{x_j(t)}{\tau_{\text{NMDA,rise}}} + \sum_k \delta(t - t_j^k) \tag{B.12}$$

$$\frac{ds_j^{\text{GABA}}(t)}{dt} = -\frac{s_j^{\text{GABA}}(t)}{\tau_{\text{GABA}}} + \sum_k \delta(t - t_j^k) \tag{B.13}$$

where the sums over k represent a sum over spikes emitted by presynaptic neuron j at time t_j^k. The value of $\alpha = 0.5\text{ms}^{-1}$.

The values of the conductances for pyramidal neurons in the associative module were: $g_{\text{AMPA,ext}} = 2.08$, $g_{\text{AMPA,rec}} = 0.052$, $g_{\text{NMDA}} = 0.164$ and $g_{\text{GABA}} = 0.72$; and for interneurons: $g_{\text{AMPA,ext}} = 1.62$, $g_{\text{AMPA,rec}} = 0.0405$, $g_{\text{NMDA}} = 0.129$ and $g_{\text{GABA}} = 0.487$ nS.

The values of the conductances for pyramidal neurons in the rule module were: $g_{\text{AMPA,ext}} = 2.08$, $g_{\text{AMPA,rec}} = 0.104$ $g_{\text{NMDA}} = 0.328$ and $g_{\text{GABA}} = 1.44$; and for interneurons: $g_{\text{AMPA,ext}} = 1.62$, $g_{\text{AMPA,rec}} = 0.081$, $g_{\text{NMDA}} = 0.258$ and $g_{\text{GABA}} = 0.973$ nS.

B.7   Simulation of fMRI signals: haemodynamic convolution of synaptic activity

An important advantage of the type of integrate-and-fire model of networks of neurons described in this Appendix is that predictions can be made about functional neuroimaging signals that will result from the operation of the network. The reason that this close relation can be drawn is that the synaptic currents in the neurons are directly modelled in the type of integrate-and-fire network described, and it is the energy required to pump the ions back against their potentials that is a major factor in generating fMRI signals. This is described next.

The functional magnetic resonance neuroimaging (fMRI) BOLD (blood oxygen level-dependent) signal, which is likely to reflect the total synaptic activity in an area (as ions need to be pumped back across the cell membrane) rather than the spiking neuronal activity (Logothetis, Pauls, Augath, Trinath and Oeltermann 2001), is spatially and temporally filtered. The filtering reflects the inherent spatial resolution with which the blood flow changes, as well as the resolution of the scanner, and filtering which may be applied for statistical purposes, and the slow temporal response of the blood flow changes (Glover 1999, Buxton and Frank 1997, Buxton, Wong and Frank 1998). Glover (1999) demonstrated that a good fitting of the haemodynamical response $h(t)$ can be achieved by the following analytic function:

$$h(t) = c_1 t^{n_1} e^{-\frac{t}{t_1}} - a_2 c_2 t^{n_2} e^{-\frac{t}{t_2}} \tag{B.14}$$

$$c_i = \max(t^{n_i} e^{-\frac{t}{t_i}}) \tag{B.15}$$

where t is the time, and c_1, c_2, a_2, n_1, and n_2 are parameters that are adjusted to fit the experimentally measured haemodynamical response. Fig. B.6 plots the haemodynamic standard response $h(t)$ for a biologically realistic set of parameters (see Deco, Rolls and Horwitz (2004)).

The temporal evolution of fMRI signals can be simulated from an integrate-and-fire population of neurons by convolving the total synaptic activity in the simulated population of neurons with the standard haemodynamic response formulation of Glover (1999) presented above (Deco, Rolls and Horwitz 2004, Horwitz and Tagamets 1999)). The total synaptic current (I_{syn}) is given by the sum of the absolute values of the glutamatergic excitatory components (implemented through NMDA and AMPA receptors) and inhibitory components (GABA) (Tagamets and Horwitz 1998, Horwitz, Tagamets and McIntosh 1999, Rolls and Deco 2002, Deco, Rolls and Horwitz 2004). In our simulations (Deco, Rolls and Horwitz 2004) the external excitatory contributions are produced through AMPA receptors ($I_{AMPA,ext}$), while the excitatory recurrent synaptic currents are produced through AMPA and NMDA receptors ($I_{AMPA,rec}$ and $I_{NMDA,rec}$). The GABA inhibitory currents are denoted by I_{GABA}. Consequently, the simulated fMRI signal activity S_{fMRI} is calculated by the following convolution equation:

$$S_{fMRI}(t) = \int_0^\infty h(t - t') I_{syn}(t') \, dt'. \tag{B.16}$$

This procedure has been used to simulate fMRI signals produced by the activity of neurons in the dorsolateral prefrontal cortex during object and spatial working memory tasks in humans, and one interesting finding is that the level of inhibition in the network can change the signal from one that is typical of spatial working memory to one that is typical of object working memory (Deco, Rolls and Horwitz 2004).

Thus integrate-and-fire models of the type described in this Appendix are important in allowing precise quantitative models to be made of the spiking of neurons in well defined networks for direct comparison with recordings of neuronal activity in neurophysiological investigations; and also allow direct predictions about signals measured in fMRI experiments. These models thus provide a principled and fundamental way of testing theories of brain function, for they make detailed predictions at different levels (e.g. neuronal firing and fMRI signals), and indeed allow brain function, including that involved in emotion, to be understood at levels that span from transmitter effects via different types of receptor on ion channels, through neuronal firing, to functional brain imaging signals (see further Rolls and Deco (2002) and Deco, Rolls and Horwitz (2004)).

Appendix 3 Glossary

Instrumental reinforcers are stimuli that, if their occurrence, termination, or omission is made contingent upon the making of an action, alter the probability of the future emission of that action (Gray 1975, Mackintosh 1983, Dickinson 1980, Lieberman 2000). Rewards and punishers are instrumental reinforcing stimuli. The notion of an action here is that an arbitrary action, e.g. turning right vs turning left, will be performed in order to obtain the reward or avoid the punisher, so that there is no pre-wired connection between the response and the reinforcer. Some stimuli are **primary (unlearned) reinforcers** (e.g., the taste of food if the animal is hungry, or pain); while others may become reinforcing by learning, because of their association with such primary reinforcers, thereby becoming 'secondary reinforcers'. This type of learning may thus be called 'stimulus–reinforcer association learning', and occurs via a stimulus–stimulus associative learning process.

A **positive reinforcer** (such as food) increases the probability of emission of a response on which it is contingent, the process is termed **positive reinforcement**, and the outcome is a **reward** (such as food).

A **negative reinforcer** (such as a painful stimulus) increases the probability of emission of a response that causes the negative reinforcer to be omitted (as in **active avoidance**) or terminated (as in **escape**), and the procedure is termed **negative reinforcement**.

Punishment refers to procedures in which the probability of an action is decreased. Punishment thus describes procedures in which an action decreases in probability if it is followed by a painful stimulus, as in **passive avoidance**. Punishment can also be used to refer to a procedure involving the omission or termination of a reward ('**extinction**' and '**time out**' respectively), both of which decrease the probability of responses (Gray 1975, Mackintosh 1983, Dickinson 1980, Lieberman 2000).

A **punisher** when delivered acts instrumentally to decrease the probability of responses on which it is contingent, or when not delivered (escaped from or avoided) acts as a negative reinforcer in that it then increases the probability of the action on which its non-delivery is contingent. Note that my definition of a punisher, which is similar to that of an aversive stimulus, is of a stimulus or event that can either decrease the probability of actions on which it is contingent, or increase the probability of actions on which its non-delivery is contingent. The term **punishment** is restricted to situations where the probability of an action is being decreased.

Emotions are states elicited by reinforcers, where the states have the set of functions described in Chapter 3. My argument is that an affectively positive or 'appetitive' stimulus (which produces a state of pleasure) acts operationally as a **reward**, which when delivered acts instrumentally as a positive reinforcer, or when not delivered (omitted or terminated) acts to decrease the probability of responses on which it is contingent. Conversely I argue that an affectively negative or aversive stimulus (which produces an unpleasant state) acts operationally as a **punisher**, which when delivered acts instrumentally to decrease the probability of responses on which it is contingent, or when not delivered (escaped from or avoided) acts as a negative reinforcer in that it then increases the probability of the action on which its non-delivery is contingent[51].

Classical conditioning or **Pavlovian conditioning**. When a **conditioned stimulus (CS)** (such as a tone) is paired with a primary reinforcer or **unconditioned stimulus (US)** (such as a painful stimulus), then there are opportunities for a number of types of association to be formed. Some of these involve 'classical conditioning' or 'Pavlovian conditioning', in which no action is performed that affects the contingency between the conditioned stimulus and the unconditioned stimulus. Typically an **unconditioned response (UR)**, for example an alteration of heart rate, is produced by the US, and will come to be elicited by the CS as a **conditioned response (CR)**. These responses are typically autonomic (such as the heart beating faster), or endocrine (for example the release of adrenaline (epinephrine in American usage) by the adrenal gland). In addition, the organism may learn to perform an instrumental response with the skeletal muscles in order to alter the probability that the primary reinforcer will be obtained. In our example, the experimenter might alter the contingencies so that when the tone sounded, if the organism performed a response such as pressing a lever, then the painful stimulus could be avoided. In the instrumental learning situation there are still opportunities for many classically conditioned responses, including emotional states such as fear, to occur. The associative processes involved in classical conditioning, and the influences that these processes may have on instrumental performance, are described in Section 4.6.1.

Motivated behaviour occurs when an animal will perform an instrumental (i.e. arbitrary operant) response to obtain a reward or to escape from or avoid a punisher. If this criterion of an arbitrary operant response is not met, and only a fixed response can be performed, then the term **drive** can be used to describe the state of the animal when it will work to obtain or escape from the stimulus.

Fitness is the reproductive potential of genes. Through the process of natural selection and reproduction, fit genes are selected for the next generation.

Long-term potentiation (LTP) is the increase in synaptic strength that can occur during learning. It is typically associative, depending on conjunctive presynaptic activity and postsynaptic depolarization.

---

[51]Note that my definition of a punisher, which is similar to that of an aversive stimulus, is of a stimulus or event that can either decrease the probability of actions on which it is contingent, or increase the probability of actions on which its non-delivery is contingent. The term punishment is restricted to situations where the probability of an action is being decreased.

Long-term depression (LTP) is the decrease in synaptic strength that can occur during learning. It is typically associative, occurring when the presynaptic activity is low and the postsynaptic depolarization is high (heterosynaptic long-term depression), or when the presynaptic activity is high, and the postsynaptic activity is only moderate (homosynaptic long-term depression) (see Fig. A.5).

References

Abbott, L. F. and Blum, K. I. (1996). Functional significance of long-term potentiation for sequence learning and prediction, *Cerebral Cortex* **6**: 406–416.

Abbott, L. F. and Nelson, S. B. (2000). Synaptic plasticity: taming the beast, *Nature Neuroscience* **3**: 1178–1183.

Abbott, L. F., Rolls, E. T. and Tovee, M. J. (1996a). Representational capacity of face coding in monkeys, *Cerebral Cortex* **6**: 498–505.

Abbott, L. F., Varela, J. A., Sen, K. and Nelson, S. B. (1996b). Synaptic depression and cortical gain control, *Cerebral Cortex* **6**: 498–505.

Abeles, M. (1991). *Corticonics: Neural Circuits of the Cerebral Cortex*, Cambridge University Press, Cambridge.

Abercrombie, E. D., Keefe, K. A., DiFrischia, D. S. and Zigmond, M. J. (1989). Differential effect of stress on in vivo dopamine release in striatum, nucleus accumbens, and medial frontal cortex, *Journal of Neurochemistry* **52**: 1655–1658.

Adams, C. D. (1982). Variations in the sensitivity of instrumental responding to reinforcer devaluation, *Quarterly Journal of Experimental Psychology B* **34**: 77–98.

Adams, C. D. and Dickinson, A. (1981). Instrumental responding following reinforcer devaluation, *Quarterly Journal of Experimental Psychology B* **33**: 109–121.

Adams, J. E. (1976). Naloxone reversal of analgesia produced by brain stimulation in the human, *Pain* **2**: 161–166.

Adelmann, P. K. and Zajonc, R. B. (1989). Facial efference and the experience of emotion, *Annual Review of Psychology* **40**: 249–280.

Adolphs, R., Tranel, D., Damasio, H. and Damasio, A. R. (1994). Impaired recognition of emotion in facial expressions following bilateral damage to the human amygdala, *Nature* **372**: 669–672.

Adolphs, R., Tranel, D., Damasio, H. and Damasio, A. R. (1995). Fear and the human amygdala, *Journal of Neuroscience* **15**: 5879–5891.

Adolphs, R., Tranel, D., Hamann, S., Young, A. W., Calder, A. J., Phelps, E. A., Anderson, A., Lee, G. P. and Damasio, A. R. (1999). Recognition of facial emotion in nine individuals with bilateral amygdala damage, *Neuropsychologia* **37**: 1111–1117.

Adolphs, R., Tranel, D. and Denburg, N. (2000). Impaired emotional declarative memory following unilateral amygdala damage, *Learning and Memory* **7**: 180–186.

Adolphs, R., Tranel, D. and Baron-Cohen, S. (2002). Amygdala damage impairs recognition of social emotions from facial expressions, *Journal of Cognitive Neuroscience* **14**: 1–11.

Adolphs, R., Gosselin, F., Buchanan, T. W., Tranel, D., Schyns, P. and Damasio, A. R. (2005). A mechanism for impaired fear recognition after amygdala damage, *Nature* **433**: 68–72.

Aggelopoulos, N. C. and Rolls, E. T. (2005). Natural scene perception: inferior temporal cortex neurons encode the positions of different objects in the scene, *European Journal of Neuroscience* **22**: 2903–2916.

Aggelopoulos, N. C., Franco, L. and Rolls, E. T. (2005). Object perception in natural scenes: encoding by inferior temporal cortex simultaneously recorded neurons, *Journal* of *Neurophysiology* **93**: 1342–1357.

Aggleton, J. P. (1992). The functional effects of amygdala lesions in humans, a comparison with findings from monkeys, *in* J. P. Aggleton (ed.), *The Amygdala*, Wiley-Liss, New York, chapter 19, pp. 485–503.

Aggleton, J. P. and Passingham, R. E. (1981). Syndrome produced by lesions of the amygdala in monkeys (Macaca mulatta), *Journal of Comparative and Physiological Psychology* **95**: 961–977.

Aggleton, J. P. and Passingham, R. E. (1982). An assessment of the reinforcing properties of foods after amygdaloid lesions in rhesus monkeys, *Journal of Comparative and Physiological Psychology* **96**: 71–77.

Aggleton, J. P. (ed.) (2000). *The Amygdala, A Functional Analysis*, 2nd edn, Oxford University Press, Oxford.

Aggleton, J. P., Burton, M. J. and Passingham, R. E. (1980). Cortical and subcortical afferents to the amygdala in the rhesus monkey (Macaca mulatta), *Brain Research* **190**: 347–368.

Aiello, L. C. and Wheeler, P. (1995). The expensive-tissue hypothesis: the brain and the digestive system in human and primate evolution, *Current Anthropology* **36**: 199–221.

Aigner, T. G., Mitchell, S. J., Aggleton, J. P., DeLong, M. R., Struble, R. G., Price, D. L., Wenk, G. L., Pettigrew, K. D. and Mishkin, M. (1991). Transient impairment of recognition memory following ibotenic acid lesions of the basal forebrain in macaques, *Experimental Brain Research* **86**: 18–26.

Ainslie, G. (1992). *Picoeconomics*, Cambridge Univeristy Press, Cambridge.

Akert, K., Gruesen, R. A., Woolsey, C. N. and Meyer, D. R. (1961). Kluver-Bucy syndrome in monkeys with neocortical ablations of temporal lobe, *Brain* **84**: 480–498.

Akil, H., Mayer, D. J. and Liebeskind, J. C. (1976). Antagonism of stimulation-produced analgesia by naloxone, a narcotic antagonist, *Science* **191**: 961–962.

Alexander, G. E., Crutcher, M. D. and DeLong, M. R. (1990). Basal ganglia thalamo-cortical circuits: parallel substrates for motor, oculomotor, 'prefrontal' and 'limbic' functions, *Progress in Brain Research* **85**: 119–146.

Alexander, R. D. (1975). The search for a general theory of behavior, *Behavioral Sciences* **20**: 77–100.

Alexander, R. D. (1979). *Darwinism and Human Affairs*, University of Washington Press, Seattle.

Allport, A. (1988). What concept of consciousness?, *in* A. J. Marcel and E. Bisiach (eds), *Consciousness in Contemporary Science*, Oxford University Press, Oxford, pp. 159–182.

Amaral, D. G. (2003). The amygdala, social behavior, and danger detection, *Annals of the New York Academy of Sciences* **1000**: 337–347.

Amaral, D. G. and Price, J. L. (1984). Amygdalo-cortical projections in the monkey (Macaca fascicularis), *Journal of Comparative Neurology* **230**: 465–496.

Amaral, D. G., Price, J. L., Pitkanen, A. and Carmichael, S. T. (1992). Anatomical organization of the primate amygdaloid complex, *in* J. P. Aggleton (ed.), *The Amygdala*, Wiley-Liss, New York, chapter 1, pp. 1–66.

Amaral, D. G., Bauman, M. D., Capitanio, J. P., Lavenex, P., Mason, W. A., Mauldin-Jourdain, M. L. and Mendoza, S. P. (2003). The amygdala: is it an essential component of the neural network for social cognition?, *Neuropsychologia* **41**: 517–522.

Amit, D. J. (1989). *Modelling Brain Function*, Cambridge University Press, New York.

Amit, D. J. and Brunel, N. (1997). Model of global spontaneous activity and local structured activity during delay periods in the cerebral cortex, *Cerebral Cortex* **7**: 237–252.

Amit, D. J. and Tsodyks, M. V. (1991). Quantitative study of attractor neural network retrieving at low spike rates. I. substrate – spikes, rates and neuronal gain, *Network* **2**: 259–273.

Amit, D. J., Gutfreund, H. and Sompolinsky, H. (1987). Statistical mechanics of neural networks near saturation, *Annals of Physics (New York)* **173**: 30–67.

Amsel, A. (1958). The role of frustrative non-reward in non-continuous reward situations, *Psychological Bulletin* **55**: 102–119.

Amsel, A. (1962). Frustrative non-reward in partial reinforcement and discrimination learning: some recent history and a theoretical extension, *Psychological Review* **69**: 306–328.

Anand, B. K. and Brobeck, J. R. (1951). Localization of a feeding center in the hypothalamus of the rat, *Proceedings of the Society for Experimental Biology and Medicine* **77**: 323–324.

Anderson, A. K. and Phelps, E. A. (2001). Lesions of the human amygdala impair enhanced perception of emotionally salient events, *Nature* **17**: 305–309.

Anderson, A. K., Christoff, K., Stappen, I., Panitz, D., Ghahremani, D. G., Glover, G., Gabrieli, J. D. and Sobel, N. (2003). Dissociated neural representations of intensity and valence in human olfaction, *Nature Neuroscience* **6**: 196–202.

Anderson, J. R. (1996). ACT: a simple theory of complex cognition, *American Psychologist* **51**: 355–365.

Anderson, M. E. (1978). Discharge patterns of basal ganglia neurons during active maintenance of postural stability and adjustment to chair tilt, *Brain Research* **143**: 325–338.

Anderson, S. W., Bechara, A., Damasio, H., Tranel, D. and Damasio, A. R. (1999). Impairment of social and moral behaviour related to early damage in human prefrontal cortex, *Nature Neuroscience* **2**: 1032–1037.

Andrew, R. J. (1963). Evolution of facial expression, *Science* **142**: 1034–1041.

Angeletos, G.-M., Laibson, D., Repetto, A., Tobacman, J. and Weinberg, S. (2001). The hyperbolic buffer stock model: calibration, simulation, and empirical evaluation, *Journal of Economic Perspectives* **15**: 47–68.

Antelman, S. M. and Szechtman, H. (1975). Tail pinch induces eating in sated rats which appears to depend on nigrostriatal dopamine, *Science* **189**: 731–733.

Aou, S., Oomura, Y., Lenard, L., Nishino, H., Inokuchi, A., Minami, T. and Misaki, H. (1984). Behavioral significance of monkey hypothalamic glucose-sensitive neurons, *Brain Research* **302**: 69–74.

Apanius, V., Penn, D., Slev, P. R., Ruff, L. R. and Potts, W. K. (1997). The nature of selection on the major histocompatibility complex, *Critical Reviews in Immunology* **17**: 179–224.

Armstrong, D. M. and Malcolm, M. (1984). *Consciousness and Causality*, Blackwell, Oxford.

Aron, A. R., Fletcher, P. C., Bullmore, E. T., Sahakian, B. J. and Robbins, T. W. (2003). Stop-signal inhibition disrupted by damage to inferior frontal gyrus in humans, *Nature Neuroscience* **6**: 115–116.

Artola, A. and Singer, W. (1993). Long term depression: related mechanisms in cerebellum, neocortex and hippocampus, *in* M. Baudry, R. F. Thompson and J. L. Davis (eds), *Synaptic Plasticity: Molecular, Cellular and Functional Aspects*, MIT Press, Cambridge, MA, chapter 7, pp. 129–146.

Asaad, W. F., Rainer, G. and Miller, E. K. (1998). Neural activity in the primate prefrontal cortex during associative learning, *Neuron* **21**: 1399–1407.

Asaad, W. F., Rainer, G. and Miller, E. K. (2000). Task-specific neural activity in the primate prefrontal cortex, *Journal of Neurophysiology* **84**: 451–459.

Avena, N. M. and Hoebel, B. G. (2003a). Amphetamine-sensitised rats show sugar-induced hyperactivity (cross-sensitization) and sugar hyperphagia, *Pharmacology, Biochemistry and Behaviour* **74**: 635–639.

Avena, N. M. and Hoebel, B. G. (2003b). A diet promoting sugar dependency causes behavioural cross-sensitisation to a low dose of amphetamine, *Neuroscience* **122**: 17–20.

Baars, B. J. (1988). *A Cognitive Theory of Consciousness*, Cambridge University Press, New York.

Baddeley, R. J., Abbott, L. F., Booth, M. J. A., Sengpiel, F., Freeman, T., Wakeman, E. A. and Rolls, E. T. (1997). Responses of neurons in primary and inferior temporal visual cortices to natural scenes, *Proceedings of the Royal Society B* **264**: 1775–1783.

Bailer, U. F. and Kaye, W. H. (2003). A review of neuropeptide and neuroendocrine dysregulation in anorexia and bulimia nervosa, *Current Drug Targets - CNS and Neurological Disorders* **2**: 53–59.

Baker, R. R. (1996). *Sperm Wars*, Fourth Estate, London.

Baker, R. R. and Bellis, M. A. (1993). Human sperm competition: ejaculate manipulation by females and a function for the female orgasm, *Animal Behaviour* **46**: 887–909.

Baker, R. R. and Bellis, M. A. (1995). *Human Sperm Competition: Copulation, Competition and Infidelity*, Chapman and Hall, London.

Baldo, J. V., Shimamura, A. P., Delis, D. C., Kramer, J. and Kaplan, E. (2001). Verbal and design fluency in patients with frontal lobe lesions, *Journal of the International Neuropsychological Society* **7**: 586–596.

Ballard, D. H. (1993). Subsymbolic modelling of hand-eye co-ordination, *in* D. E. Broadbent (ed.), *The Simulation of Human Intelligence*, Blackwell, Oxford, chapter 3, pp. 71–102.

Balleine, B. W. (1992). Instrumental performance following a shift in primary motivation depends upon incentive learning, *Journal of Experimental Psychology* **18**: 236–250.

Balleine, B. W. (1994). Asymmetrical interactions between thirst and hunger in Pavlovian-instrumental transfer, *Quarterly Journal of Experimental Psychology B* **47**: 211–231.

Balleine, B. W. and Dickinson, A. (1991). Instrumental performance following reinforcer devaluation depends upon incentive learning, *Quarterly Journal of Experimental Psychology B* **43**: 279–296.

Balleine, B. W. and Dickinson, A. (1998). The role of incentive learning in instrumental outcome revaluation by sensory-specific satiety, *Animal Learning and Behavior* **26**: 46–59.

Bar-On, R. (1997). *The Emotional Intelligence Inventory (EQ-i): Technical Manual*, Multi-Health Systems, Toronto.

Barbarich, N. C., Kaye, W. H. and Jimerson, D. (2003). Neurotransmitter and imaging studies in anorexia nervosa: new targets for treatment, *Current Drug Targets - CNS and Neurological Disorders* **2**: 61–72.

Barbas, H. (1988). Anatomic organization of basoventral and mediodorsal visual recipient prefrontal regions in the rhesus monkey, *Journal of Comparative Neurology* **276**: 313–342.

Barbas, H. (1993). Organization of cortical afferent input to the orbitofrontal area in the rhesus monkey, *Neuroscience* **56**: 841–864.

Barbas, H. (1995). Anatomic basis of cognitive-emotional interactions in the primate prefrontal cortex, *Neuroscience and Biobehavioral Reviews* **19**: 499–510.

Barbas, H. and Pandya, D. N. (1989). Architecture and intrinsic connections of the prefrontal cortex in the rhesus monkey, *Journal of Comparative Neurology* **286**: 353–375.

Barlow, H. (1995). The neuron doctrine in perception, *in* M. S. Gazzaniga (ed.), *The Cognitive Neurosciences*, MIT Press, Cambridge, MA, chapter 26, pp. 415–435.

Barlow, H. (1997). Single neurons, communal goals, and consciousness, *in* M. Ito, Y. Miyashita and E. T. Rolls (eds), *Cognition, Computation, and Consciousness*, Oxford University Press, Oxford, chapter 7, pp. 121–136.

Barlow, H. B. (1972). Single units and sensation: A neuron doctrine for perceptual psychology, *Perception* **1**: 371–394.

Baron-Cohen, S., Wheelwright, S. and Joliffe, T. (1997). Is there a 'language of the eyes'? Evidence from normal adults, and adults with autism or Asperger syndrome, *Visual Cognition* **4**: 311–331.

Baron-Cohen, S., Ring, H. A., Bullmore, E. T., Wheelwright, S., Ashwin, C. and Williams, S. C. R. (2000). The amygdala theory of autism, *Neuroscience and Biobehavioral Reviews* **24**: 355–364.

Barrett, L., Dunbar, R. and Lycett, J. (2002). *Human Evolutionary Psychology*, Palgrave, Basingstoke.

Barsh, G. S. and Schwartz, M. W. (2002). Genetic approaches to studying energy balence: perception and integration, *Nature Reviews Genetics* **3**: 589–600.

Barsh, G. S., Farooqi, I. S. and O'Rahilly, S. (2000). Genetics of body weight regulation, *Nature* **404**: 644–651.

Barto, A. G. (1985). Learning by statistical cooperation of self-interested neuron-like computing elements, *COINS Tech. Rep., University of Massachusetts, Department of Computer and Information Science, Amherst.*

Barto, A. G. (1995). Adaptive critics and the basal ganglia, *in* J. C. Houk, J. L. Davis and D. G. Beiser (eds), *Models of Information Processing in the Basal Ganglia*, MIT Press, Cambridge, MA, chapter 11, pp. 215–232.

Barton, R. A. and Aggleton, J. P. (2000). Primate evolution and the amygdala, *in* J. P. Aggleton (ed.), *The Amygdala: A Functional Analysis*, 2nd edn, Oxford University Press, Oxford, pp. 479–508.

Bateson, P. (1983). *Mate Choice*, Cambridge University Press, Cambridge.

Battaglia, F. and Treves, A. (1998). Stable and rapid recurrent processing in realistic autoassociative memories, *Neural Computation* **10**: 431–450.

Baum, M. J., Everitt, B. J., Herbert, J. and Keverne, E. B. (1977). Hormonal basis of proceptivity and receptivity in female primates, *Archives of Sexual Behavior* **6**: 173–192.

Bauman, M. D., Lavenex, P., Mason, W. A., Capitanio, J. P. and Amaral, D. G. (2004). The development of social behaviour following neonatal amygdala lesions in rhesus monkeys, *Journal of Cognitive Neuroscience* **16**: 1388–1411.

Baxter, M. G. and Murray, E. A. (2000). Reinterpreting the behavioural effects of amygdala lesions in non-human primates, *in* J. P. Aggleton (ed.), *The Amygdala: a Functional Analysis*, 2nd edn, Oxford University Press, Oxford, chapter 16, pp. 545–568.

Baxter, M. G. and Murray, E. A. (2002). The amygdala and reward, *Nature Reviews Neuroscience* **3**: 563–573.

Baxter, R. D. and Liddle, P. F. (1998). Neuropsychological deficits associated with schizophrenic syndromes, *Schizophrenia Research* **30**: 239–249.

Baylis, G. C. and Rolls, E. T. (1987). Responses of neurons in the inferior temporal cortex in short term and serial recognition memory tasks, *Experimental Brain Research* **65**: 614–622.

Baylis, G. C., Rolls, E. T. and Leonard, C. M. (1985). Selectivity between faces in the responses of a population of neurons in the cortex in the superior temporal sulcus of the monkey, *Brain Research* **342**: 91–102.

Baylis, G. C., Rolls, E. T. and Leonard, C. M. (1987). Functional subdivisions of temporal lobe neocortex, *Journal of Neuroscience* **7**: 330–342.

Baylis, L. L. and Gaffan, D. (1991). Amygdalectomy and ventromedial prefrontal ablation produce similar deficits in food choice and in simple object discrimination learning for an unseen reward, *Experimental Brain Research* **86**: 617–622.

Baylis, L. L. and Rolls, E. T. (1991). Responses of neurons in the primate taste cortex to glutamate, *Physiology and Behavior* **49**: 973–979.

Baylis, L. L., Rolls, E. T. and Baylis, G. C. (1994). Afferent connections of the orbitofrontal cortex taste area of the primate, *Neuroscience* **64**: 801–812.

Bear, M. F. and Singer, W. (1986). Modulation of visual cortical plasticity by acetylcholine and noradrenaline, *Nature* **320**: 172–176.

Beauchamp, G. K. and Yamazaki, K. (2003). Chemical signalling in mice, *Biochemical Society Transactions* **31**: 147–151.

Bechara, A., Damasio, A. R., Damasio, H. and Anderson, S. W. (1994). Insensitivity to future consequences following damage to human prefrontal cortex, *Cognition* **50**: 7–15.

Bechara, A., Tranel, D., Damasio, H. and Damasio, A. R. (1996). Failure to respond autonomically to anticipated future outcomes following damage to prefrontal cortex, *Cerebral Cortex* **6**: 215–225.

Bechara, A., Damasio, H., Tranel, D. and Damasio, A. R. (1997). Deciding advantageously before knowing the advantageous strategy, *Science* **275**: 1293–1295.

Bechara, A., Damasio, H., Tranel, D. and Anderson, S. W. (1998). Dissociation of working memory from decision making within the human prefrontal cortex, *Journal of Neuroscience* **18**: 428–437.

Bechara, A., Damasio, H., Damasio, A. R. and Lee, G. P. (1999). Different contributions of the human amygdala and ventromedial prefrontal cortex to decision making, *Journal of Neurosience* **19**: 5473–5481.

Bechara, A., Damasio, H., Tranel, D. and Damasio, A. R. (2005). The Iowa Gambling Task and the somatic marker hypothesis: some questions and answers, *Trends in Cognitive Sciences* **9**: 159–162.

Beckstead, R. M. and Norgren, R. (1979). An autoradiographic examination of the central distribution of the trigeminal, facial, glossopharyngeal, and vagal nerves in the monkey, *Journal of Comparative Neurology* **184**: 455–472.

Beckstead, R. M., Morse, J. R. and Norgren, R. (1980). The nucleus of the solitary tract in the monkey: projections to the thalamus and brainstem nuclei, *Journal of Comparative Neurology* **190**: 259–282.

Beluzzi, J. D., Grant, N., Garsky, V., Sarantakis, D., Wise, C. D. and Stein, L. (1976). Analgesia induced in vivo by central administration of enkephalin in rat, *Nature* **260**: 625–626.

Ben-Ari, E. T. (2000). Choosy females, *BioScience* **50**: 7–12.

Ben-Ze'ev, A. (2000). *The Subtlety of Emotions*, MIT Press, Cambridge, MA.

Benabou, R. and Pycia, M. (2002). Dynamic inconsistency and self-control: a planner-doer interpretation, *Economics Letters* **77**: 419–424.

Berglund, A. and Rosenqvist, G. (2001). Male pipefish prefer ornamented females, *Animal Behaviour* **61**: 345–350.

Berlin, H. and Rolls, E. T. (2004). Time perception, impulsivity, emotionality, and personality in self-harming borderline personality disorder patients, *Journal of Personality Disorders* **18**: 358–378.

Berlin, H., Rolls, E. T. and Kischka, U. (2004). Impulsivity, time perception, emotion, and reinforcement sensitivity in patients with orbitofrontal cortex lesions, *Brain* **127**: 1108–1126.

Berlin, H., Rolls, E. T. and Iversen, S. D. (2005). Borderline Personality Disorder, impulsivity, and the orbitofrontal cortex, *American Journal of Psychiatry* **58**: 234—-245.

Berliner, D. L., Monti-Bloch, L., Jennings-White, C. and Diaz-Sanchez, V. (1996). The functionality of the human vomeronasal organ (VNO): evidence for steroid receptors, *Journal of Steroid Biochemistry and Molecular Biology* **58**: 259–265.

Bermond, B., Fasotti, L., Niewenhuyse, B. and Schuerman, J. (1991). Spinal cord lesions, peripheral feedback and intensities of emotional feelings, *Cognition and Emotion* **5**: 201–220.

Berridge, K. C. and Robinson, T. E. (1998). What is the role of dopamine in reward: hedonic impact, reward learning, or incentive salience?, *Brain Research Reviews* **28**: 309–369.

Berridge, K. C. and Robinson, T. E. (2003). Parsing reward, *Trends in Neurosciences* **26**: 507–513.

Berridge, K. C., Flynn, F. W., Schulkin, J. and Grill, H. J. (1984). Sodium depletion enhances salt palatability in rats, *Behavioral Neuroscience* **98**: 652–660.

Bertino, M., Beauchamp, G. K. and Engelman, K. (1991). Naltrexone, an opioid blocker, alters taste perception and nutrient intake in humans, *American Journal of Physiology* **261**: 59–63.

Bertram, B. C. R. (1975). Social factors influencing reproduction in wild lions, *Journal of Zoology* **177**: 463–482.

Betzig, L. L. (1986). *Despotism and Differential Reproduction*, Aldine, New York.

Betzig, L. L. (ed.) (1997). *Human Nature: a Critical Reader*, Oxford University Press, New York.

Beumont, P. J. V., Burrows, G. D. and Caspar, R. C. (eds) (1987). *Handbook of Eating Disorders. Part 1: Anorexia and Bulimia Nervosa*, Elsevier, Amsterdam.

Bi, G.-Q. and Poo, M.-M. (1998). Activity-induced synaptic modifications in hippocampal culture, dependence on spike timing, synaptic strength and cell type, *Journal of Neuroscience* **18**: 10464–10472.

Bienenstock, E. L., Cooper, L. N. and Munro, P. W. (1982). Theory for the development of neuron selectivity: orientation specificity and binocular interaction in visual cortex, *Journal of Neuroscience* **2**: 32–48.

Birkhead, T. (2000). *Promiscuity*, Faber and Faber, London.

Birkhead, T. R. and Moller, A. P. (1992). *Sperm Competition in Birds*, Academic Press, London.

Birkhead, T. R. and Pizzari, T. (2002). Postcopulatory sexual selection, *Nature Reviews Genetics* **3**: 262–273.

Birkhead, T. R., Chaline, N., Biggins, J. D., Burke, T. and Pizzari, T. (2004). Nontransivity of paternity in a bird, *Evolution* **58**: 416–420.

Bishop, M. P., Elder, S. T. and Heath, R. G. (1963). Intracranial self-stimulation in man, *Science* **140**: 394–395.

Bjorklund, A. and Lindvall, O. (1986). Catecholaminergic brainstem regulatory systems, *in* V. B. Mountcastle, F. E. Bloom and S. R. Geiger (eds), *Handbook of Physiology: the Nervous System*, Vol. 4, Intrinsic systems of the Brain, American Psychological Society, Bethesda, pp. 155–236.

Blair, H. T., Schafe, G. E., Bauer, E. P., Rodrigues, S. M. and LeDoux, J. E. (2001). Synaptic plasticity in the lateral amygdala: a cellular hypothesis of fear conditioning, *Learning and Memory* **8**: 229–242.

Blair, H. T., Tinkelman, A., Moita, M. A. P. and LeDoux, J. E. (2003). Associative plasticity in neurons of the lateral amygdala during auditory fear conditioning, *Annals of the New York Academy of Science* **985**: 485–487.

Blair, R. J., Morris, J. S., Frith, C. D., Perrett, D. I. and Dolan, R. J. (1999). Dissociable neural responses to facial expressions of sadness and anger, *Brain* **122**: 883–893.

Blair, R. J. R. (2003). Facial expressions, their communicatory functions and neuro-cognitive substrates, *Philosophical Transactions of the Royal Society of London B* **358**: 561–572.

Blaney, P. H. (1986). Affect and memory: a review, *Psychological Bulletin* **99**: 229–246.

Blass, E. M. and Epstein, A. N. (1971). A lateral preoptic osmosensitive zone for thirst in the rat, *Journal of Comparative and Physiological Psychology* **76**: 378–394.

Blaustein, J. D. and Erskine, M. S. (2002). Feminine sexual behavior, *in* D. W. Pfaff, A. P. Arnold, A. M. Etgen, S. E. Fahrbach and R. T. Rubin (eds), *Hormones, Brain and Behavior*, Vol. 1, Academic Press, San Diego, CA, chapter 2, pp. 139–214.

Bliss, T. V. P. and Collingridge, G. L. (1993). A synaptic model of memory: long-term potentiation in the hippocampus, *Nature* **361**: 31–39.

Block, N. (1995a). On confusion about a function of consciousness, *Behavioral and Brain Sciences* **18**: 22–47.

Block, N. (1995b). Two neural correlates of consciousness, *Trends in Cognitive Sciences* **9**: 46–52.

Blood, A. J., Zatorre, R. J., Bermudez, P. and Evans, A. C. (1999). Emotional responses to pleasant and unpleasant music correlate with activity in paralimbic brain regions, *Nature Neuroscience* **2**: 382–387.

Blood, A. J.and Zatorre, R. J. (2001). Intensely pleasureable responses to music correlate with activity of brain regions implicated in reward and emotion, *Proceedings of the National Academy of Sciences USA* **98**: 11818–11823.

Boden, M. A. (ed.) (1996). *The Philosophy of Artificial Life*, Oxford University Press, Oxford.

Booth, D. A. (1985). Food-conditioned eating preferences and aversions with interoceptive elements: learned appetites and satieties, *Annals of the New York Academy of Sciences* **443**: 22–37.

Booth, M. C. A. and Rolls, E. T. (1998). View-invariant representations of familiar objects by neurons in the inferior temporal visual cortex, *Cerebral Cortex* **8**: 510–523.

Borsini, F. and Rolls, E. T. (1984). Role of noradrenaline and serotonin in the basolateral region of the amygdala in food preferences and learned taste aversions in the rat, *Physiology and Behavior* **33**: 37–43.

Boussaoud, D., Desimone, R. and Ungerleider, L. G. (1991). Visual topography of area TEO in the macaque, *Journal of Computational Neurology* **306**: 554–575.

Bowlby, J. (1969). *Attachment and Loss: Volume 1 Attachment*, Hogarth Press, London.

Bowlby, J. (1973). *Attachment and Loss: Volume 2 Separation*, Hogarth Press, London.

Bowlby, J. (1980). *Attachment and Loss: Volume 3 Loss*, Hogarth Press, London.

Bowles, S. and Gintis, H. (2005). Prosocial emotions, *in* L. E. Blume and S. N. Durlauf (eds), *The Economy As an Evolving Complex System III*, Santa Fe Institute, Santa Fe, NM.

Boyd, E. S. and Gardner, L. C. (1967). Effect of some brain lesions on intracranial self-stimulation in the rat, *American Journal of Physiology* **213**: 1044–1052.

Boyd, R., Gintis, H., Bowles, S. and Richerson, P. J. (2003). The evolution of altruistic punishment, *Proceedings of the National Academy of Sciences* **100**: 3531–3535.

Bray, G. A., Inoue, S. and Nishizawa, Y. (1981). Hypothalamic obesity: the autonomic hypothesis and the lateral hypothalamus, *Diabetologia* **20 (Suppl.)**: 366–378.

Brebner, K., Childress, A. R. and Roberts, D. C. (2002). A potential role for GABA (B) agonists in the treatment of psychostimulant addiction, *Alcohol and Alcoholism* **37**: 478–484.

Bremner, J. D., Vythilingam, M., Vermetten, E., Nazeer, A., Adil, J., Khan, S., Staib, L. H. and Charney, D. S. (2002). Reduced volume of orbitofrontal cortex in major depression, *Biological Psychiatry* **51**: 273–279.

Brothers, L. and Ring, B. (1993). Mesial temporal neurons in the macaque monkey with responses selective for aspects of social stimuli, *Behavioural Brain Research* **57**: 53–61.

Brown, T. H., Kairiss, E. W. and Keenan, C. L. (1990). Hebbian synapses: biophysical mechanisms and algorithms, *Annual Review of Neuroscience* **13**: 475–511.

Brown, V. J., Desimone, R. and Mishkin, M. (1995). Responses of cells in the tail of the caudate nucleus during visual discrimination learning, *Journal of Neurophysiology* **74**: 1083–1094.

Brownell, K. D. and Fairburn, C. (1995). *Eating Disorders and Obesity: a Comprehensive Handbook*, Guildford Press, New York.

Brunel, N. and Wang, X. (2001). Effects of neuromodulation in a cortical networks model of object working memory dominated by recurrent inhibition, *Journal of Computational Neuroscience* **11**: 63–85.

Brunello, N., Mendlewicz, J., Kasper, S., Leonard, B., Montgomery, S., Craig Nelson, J., Paykel, E., Versiani, M. and Racagni, G. (2002). The role of noradrenaline and selective noradrenaline reuptake inhibition in depression, *European Neuropsychopharmacology* **12**: 461–475.

Buck, L. (2000). Smell and taste: the chemical senses, *in* E. Kandel, J. H. Schwartz and T. H. Jessel (eds), *Principles of Neural Science*, 4 th edn, McGraw-Hill, New York, chapter 32, pp. 625–647.

Buck, L. and Axel, R. (1991). A novel multigene family may encode odorant receptors: a molecular basis for odor recognition, *Cell* **65**: 175–187.

Buggy, J. and Johnson, A. (1977a). Anteroventral third ventricle periventricular ablation: temporary adipsia and persisting thirst deficits, *Neuroscience Letters* **5**: 177–182.

Buggy, J. and Johnson, A. (1977b). Preoptic-hypothalamic periventricular lesions: thirst deficits and hypernatremia, *American Journal of Physiology* **23**: R44–R52.

Bunney, B. S. and Aghajanian, G. K. (1976). Dopamine and norepinephrine innervated cells in the rat prefrontal cortex: pharmacological differentiation using micro-iontophoretic techniques, *Life Sciences* **19**: 1783–1792.

Burton, M. J., Rolls, E. T. and Mora, F. (1976). Effects of hunger on the responses of neurones in the lateral hypothalamus to the sight and taste of food, *Experimental Neurology* **51**: 668–677.

Bush, G., Luu, P. and Posner, M. I. (2000). Cognitive and emotional influences in anterior cingulate cortex, *Trends in Cognitive Sciences* **4**: 215–222.

Bush, G., Vogt, B. A., Holmes, J., Dales, A. M., Greve, D., Jenike, M. A. and Rosen, B. R. (2002). Dorsal anterior cingulate cortex: a role in reward-based decision making, *Proceedings of the National Academy of Sciences* **99**: 523–528.

Buss, D. M. (1989). Sex differences in human mate preferences: evolutionary hypotheses tested in 37 cultures, *Behavioural and Brain Sciences* **12**: 1–14.

Buss, D. M. (1994). *The Evolution of Desire: Strategies of Human Mating*, Basic Books, New York.

Buss, D. M. (1999). *Evolutionary Psychology: The New Science of the Mind*, Allyn and Bacon, Boston, MA.

Buss, D. M. and Schmitt, D. P. (1993). Sexual strategies theory: an evolutionary perspective on human mating, *Psychological Review* **100**: 204–232.

Buss, D. M., Abbott, M., Angeleitner, A., Asherian, A., Biaggio, A., Blancovillasenor, A., Bruchonschweitzer, M., Chu, H., Czapinski, J., DeRaad, B., Ekehammar, B., Ellohamy, N., Fioravanti, M., Georgas, J., Gjerde, P., Guttman, R., Hazan, F., Iwawaki, S., Janakiramaiah, N., Khosroshani, F., Kreitler, S., Lachenicht, L., Lee, M., Liik, K., Little, B., Mika, S., Moadelshahid, M., Moane, G., Montero, M., Mundycastle, A. C., Niit, T., Nsenduluka, E., Pienkowski, R., Pirttila-Backman, A. M., Deleon, J. P., Rousseau, J., Runco, M. A., Safir, M. P., Samuels, C., Sanitioso, R., Serpell, R., Smid, N., Spencer, C., Tadinac, M., Todorova, E. N., Troland, K., Vandenbrande, L., Van Heck, G., Vanlangenhove, L. and Yang, K. S. (1990). International preferences in selecting mates: a study of 37 cultures, *Journal of Cross-Cultural Psychology* **21**: 5–47.

Bussey, T. J. and Everitt, B. J. (1997). Dissociable effects of cingulate and medial frontal cortex lesions on stimulus–reward learning using a novel Pavlovian autoshaping procedure for the rat: implications for the neurobiology of emotion, *Behavioral Neuroscience* **111**: 908–919.

Bussey, T. J., Muir, J. L., Everitt, B. J. and Robbins, T. W. (1997). Triple dissociation of anterior cingulate, posterior cingulate, and medial frontal cortices on visual discrimination tasks using a touchscreen testing procedure for the rat, *Behavioral Neuroscience* **111**: 920–936.

Butter, C. M. (1969). Perseveration in extinction and in discrimination reversal tasks following selective prefrontal ablations in Macaca mulatta, *Physiology and Behavior* **4**: 163–171.

Butter, C. M. and Snyder, D. R. (1972). Alterations in aversive and aggressive behaviors following orbitofrontal lesions in rhesus monkeys, *Acta Neurobiologica Experimentalis* **32**: 525–565.

Butter, C. M., McDonald, J. A. and Snyder, D. R. (1969). Orality, preference behavior, and reinforcement value of non-food objects in monkeys with orbital frontal lesions, *Science* **164**: 1306–1307.

Butter, C. M., Snyder, D. R. and McDonald, J. A. (1970). Effects of orbitofrontal lesions on aversive and aggressive behaviors in rhesus monkeys, *Journal of Comparative Physiology and Psychology* **72**: 132–144.

Buxton, R. B. and Frank, L. R. (1997). A model for the coupling between cerebral blood flow and oxygen metabolism during neural stimulation, *Journal of Cerebral Blood Flow and Metabolism* **17**: 64–72.

Buxton, R. B., Wong, E. C. and Frank, L. R. (1998). Dynamics of blood flow and oxygenation changes during brain activation: the balloon model, *Magnetic Resonance in Medicine*

39: 855–864.

Byrne, R. W. and Whiten, A. (1988). *Machiavellian Intelligence: Social Expertise and the Evolution of Intellect in Monkeys, Apes and Humans*, Clarendon, Oxford.

Caan, W., Perrett, D. I. and Rolls, E. T. (1984). Responses of striatal neurons in the behaving monkey. 2. Visual processing in the caudal neostriatum, *Brain Research* **290**: 53–65.

Cabanac, M. (1971). Physiological role of pleasure, *Science* **173**: 1103–1107.

Cabanac, M. and Duclaux, R. (1970). Specificity of internal signals in producing satiety for taste stimuli, *Nature* **227**: 966–967.

Cabanac, M. and Fantino, M. (1977). Origin of olfacto-gustatory alliesthesia: Intestinal sensitivity to carbohydrate concentration?, *Physiology and Behavior* **10**: 1039–1045.

Cacioppo, J. T., Klein, D. J., Berntson, G. C. and Hatfield, E. (1993). The psychophysiology of emotion, *in* M. Lewis and J. M. Hatfield (eds), *Handbook of Emotions*, Guildford, New York, pp. 119–145.

Cador, M., Robbins, T. W. and Everitt, B. J. (1989). Involvement of the amygdala in stimulus–reward associations: interaction with the ventral striatum, *Neuroscience* **30**: 77–86.

Caggiula, A. R. (1970). Analysis of the copulation-reward properties of posterior hypothalamic stimulation in male rats, *Journal of Comparative and Physiological Psychology* **70**: 399–412.

Cahusac, P. M. B., Rolls, E. T., Miyashita, Y. and Niki, H. (1993). Modification of the responses of hippocampal neurons in the monkey during the learning of a conditional spatial response task, *Hippocampus* **3**: 29–42.

Calabresi, P., Maj, R., Pisani, A., Mercuri, N. B. and Bernardi, G. (1992). Long-term synaptic depression in the striatum: physiological and pharmacological characterization, *Journal of Neuroscience* **12**: 4224–4233.

Calder, A. J., Young, A. W., Rowland, D., Perrett, D. I., Hodges, J. R. and Etcoff, N. L. (1996). Facial emotion recognition after bilateral amygdala damage: differentially severe impairment of fear, *Cognitive Neuropsycology* **13**: 699–745.

Calder, A. J., Keane, J., Manes, F., Antoun, N. and Young, A. W. (2000). Impaired recognition and experience of disgust following brain injury, *Nature Neuroscience* **3**: 1077–1078.

Calder, A. J., Keane, J., Lawrence, A. D. and Manes, F. (2004). Impaired recognition of anger following damage to the ventral striatum, *Brain* **127**: 1958–1969.

Campfield, L. A. and Smith, F. J. (1990). Systemic factors in the control of food intake: evidence for patterns as signals, *in* E. M. Stricker (ed.), *Handbook of Behavioral Neurobiology*, Vol. 10, Neurobiology of Food and Fluid Intake, Plenum, New York.

Campfield, L. A., Smith, F. J., Guisez, Y., Devos, R. and Burn, P. (1995). Recombinant mouse ob protein: evidence for a peripheral signal linking adiposity and central neural networks, *Science* **269**: 546–549.

Canli, T., Zhao, Z., Desmond, J. E., Kang, E., Gross, J. and Gabrieli, J. D. (2001). An fMRI study of personality influences on brain reactivity to emotional stimuli, *Behavioral Neuroscience* **115**: 33–42.

Canli, T., Sivers, H., Whitfield, S. L., Gotlib, I. H. and Gabrieli, J. D. (2002). Amygdala response to happy faces as a function of extraversion, *Science* **296**: 2191.

Cannistraro, P. A. and Rauch, S. L. (2003). Neural circuitry of anxiety: evidence from structural and functional neuroimaging studies, *Psychopharmacology Bulletin* **37**: 8–25.

Cannon, W. B. (1927). The James–Lange theory of emotion: a critical examination and an alternative theory, *American Journal of Psychology* **39**: 106–124.

Cannon, W. B. (1929). *Bodily Changes in Pain, Hunger, Fear and Rage*, 2nd edn, Appleton, New York.

Cannon, W. B. (1931). Again the James–Lange theory of emotion: a critical examination and an alternative theory, *Psychological Review* **38**: 281–295.

Caplan, D. (1996). *Language: Structure, Processing and Disorders*, MIT Press, Cambridge, MA.

Cardinal, N. and Everitt, B. J. (2004). Neural and psychological mechanisms underlying appetitive learning: links to drug addiction, *Current Opinion in Neurobiology* **14**: 156–162.

Cardinal, N., Pennicott, D. R., Sugathapala, C. L., Robbins, T. W. and Everitt, B. J. (2001). Impulsive choice induced in rats by lesions of the nucleus accumbens core, *Science* **292**: 2499–2501.

Cardinal, N., Parkinson, J. A., Hall, J. and Everitt, B. J. (2002). Emotion and motivation: the role of the amygdala, ventral striatum, and prefrontal cortex, *Neuroscience and Biobehavioral Reviews* **26**: 321–352.

Carlson, N. R. (2004). *Physiology of Behavior*, 8th edn, Pearson, Boston.

Carmichael, S. T. and Price, J. L. (1994). Architectonic subdivision of the orbital and medial prefrontal cortex in the macaque monkey, *Journal of Comparative Neurology* **346**: 366–402.

Carmichael, S. T. and Price, J. L. (1995a). Limbic connections of the orbital and medial prefrontal cortex in macaque monkeys, *Journal of Comparative Neurology* **363**: 615–641.

Carmichael, S. T. and Price, J. L. (1995b). Sensory and premotor connections of the orbital and medial prefrontal cortex of macaque monkeys, *Journal of Comparative Neurology* **363**: 642–664.

Carmichael, S. T., Clugnet, M.-C. and Price, J. L. (1994). Central olfactory connections in the macaque monkey, *Journal of Comparative Neurology* **346**: 403–434.

Carruthers, P. (1996). *Language, Thought and Consciousness*, Cambridge University Press, Cambridge.

Carruthers, P. (2000). *Phenomenal Consciousness*, Cambridge University Press, Cambridge.

Carter, S. C. (1998). Neuroendocrine perpectives on social attachment and love, *Psychoneuroendocrinology* **23**: 779–818.

Celada, P., Puig, M. V., Armagos-Bosch, M., Adell, A. and Artigas, F. (2004). The therapeutic role of 5-HT$_{1A}$ and 5-HT$_{2A}$ receptors in depression, *Journal of Psychiatry and Neuroscience* **29**: 252–265.

Chalmers, D. J. (1996). *The Conscious Mind*, Oxford University Press, Oxford.

Chaudhari, N. and Roper, S. D. (1998). Molecular and physiological evidence for glutamate (umami) taste transduction via a G protein-coupled receptor, *Annals of the New York Academy of Sciences* **855**: 398–406.

Chaudhari, N., Yang, H., Lamp, C., Delay, E., Cartford, C., Than, T. and Roper, S. (1996). The taste of monosodium glutamate: membrane receptors in taste buds, *Journal of Neuroscience* **16**: 3817–3826.

Chaudhari, N., Landin, A. M. and Roper, S. (2000). A metabolic glutamate receptor variant functions as a taste receptor, *Nature Neuroscience* **3**: 113–119.

Chelazzi, L. (1998). Serial attention mechanisms in visual search: a critical look at the evidence, *Psychological Research* **62**: 195–219.

Chelazzi, L., Miller, E., Duncan, J. and Desimone, R. (1993). A neural basis for visual search in inferior temporal cortex, *Nature (London)* **363**: 345–347.

Chen, G., Greengard, P. and Yan, Z. (2004). Potentiation of NMDA receptor currents by dopamine D1 receptors in prefrontal cortex, *Proceedings of the National Academy of Sciences USA* **101**: 2596–2600.

Cheney, D. L. and Seyfarth, R. M. (1990). *How Monkeys See the World*, University of Chicago Press, Chicago.

Chevalier-Skolnikoff, S. (1973). Facial expression of emotion in non-human primates, *in* P. Ekman (ed.), *Darwin and Facial Expression*, Academic Press, New York, pp. 11–89.

Chiavaras, M. M. and Petrides, M. (2001). Three-dimensional probabilistic atlas of the human orbitofrontal sulci in standardised stereotaxic space, *Neuroimage* **13**: 479–496.

Childress, A. R., Mozley, P. D., McElgin, W., Fitzgerald, J., Reivich, M. and O'Brien, C. P. (1999). Limbic activation during cue-induced cocaine craving, *American Journal of Psychiatry* **156**: 11–18.

Christie, B. R. (1996). Long-term depression in the hippocampus, *Hippocampus* **6**: 1–2.

Clark, D. A. and Beck, A. T. (1999). *Scientific Foundations of Cognitive Theory and Therapy of Depression*, Wiley, New York.

Clark, J. M., Clark, A. J. M., Bartle, A. and Winn, P. (1991). The regulation of feeding and drinking in rats with lesions of the lateral hypothalamus made by N-methyl-D-aspartate, *Neuroscience* **45**: 631–640.

Clark, L., Cools, R. and Robbins, T. W. (2004). The neuropsychology of ventral prefrontal cortex: decision-making and reversal learning, *Brain and Cognition* **55**: 41–53.

Clavier, R. M. (1976). Brain stem self-stimulation: catecholamine or non-catecholamine mediation?, *in* A. Wauquier and E. T. Rolls (eds), *Brain-Stimulation Reward*, North-Holland, Amsterdam, pp. 239–250.

Clavier, R. M. and Routtenberg, A. (1976). Brain stem self-stimulation attenuated by lesions of medial forebrain bundle but not by lesions of locus coeruleus or the caudal ventral norepinephrine bundle, *Brain Research* **101**: 251–271.

Coghill, R. C., Talbot, J. D., Evans, A. C., Meyer, E., Gjedde, A., Bushnell, M. C. and Duncan, G. H. (1994). Distributed processing of pain and vibration in the human brain, *Journal of Neuroscience* **14**: 4095–4108.

Colantuoni, C., Rada, P., McCarthy, J., Patten, C., Avena, N. M., Chadeayne, A. and Hoebel, B. G. (2002). Evidence that intermittent, excessive sugar intake causes endogenous opioid dependence, *Obesity Research* **10**: 478–488.

Collingridge, G. L. and Bliss, T. V. P. (1987). NMDA receptors: their role in long-term potentiation, *Trends in Neurosciences* **10**: 288–293.

Colwill, R. M. and Rescorla, R. A. (1985). Postconditioning devaluation of a reinforcer affects instrumental responding, *Journal of Experimental Psychology* **11**: 120–132.

Colwill, R. M. and Rescorla, R. A. (1988). Associations between the discriminative stimulus and the reinforcer in instrumental learning, *Journal of Experimental Psychology* **14**: 155–164.

Colwill, R. M. and Rescorla, R. A. (1990). Evidence for the hierarchical structure of instrumental learning, *Animal Learning and Behaviour* **18**: 71–82.

Cone, R. D. (2005). Anatomy and regulation of the central melanocortin system, *Nature Neuroscience* **8**: 571–578.

Cools, R., Clark, L., Owen, A. M. and Robbins, T. W. (2002). Defining the neural mechnisms of probablistic reversal learning using event-related functional magnetic resonance imaging, *Journal of Neuroscience* **22**: 4563–4567.

Cooper, J. R., Bloom, F. E. and Roth, R. H. (2003). *The Biochemical Basis of Neuropharmacology*, 8th edn, Oxford University Press, Oxford.

Corchs, S. and Deco, G. (2002). Large-scale neural model for visual attention: integration of experimental single cell and fMRI data, *Cerebral Cortex* **12**: 339–348.

Cornell, C. E., Rodin, J. and Weingarten, H. (1989). Stimulus-induced eating when satiated, *Physiology and Behavior* **45**: 695–704.

Corwin, R. L. and Buda-Levin, A. (2004). Behavioral models of binge-type eating, *Physiology and Behavior* **82**: 123–130.

Cosmides, I. and Tooby, J. (1999). Evolutionary psychology, *in* R. Wilson and F. Keil (eds), *MIT Encyclopedia of the Cognitive Sciences*, MIT Press, Cambridge, MA, pp. 295–298.

Cowley, J. J. and Brooksbank, B. W. L. (1991). Human exposure to putative pheromones and changes in aspects of social behaviour, *Journal of Steroid Biochemistry and Molecular Biology* **39**: 647–659.

Coyle, J. T., Tsai, G. and Goff, D. (2003). Converging evidence of NMDA receptor hypofunction in the pathophysiology of schizophrenia, *Annals of the New York Academy of Sciences* **1003**: 318–327.

Craig, A. D., Chen, K., Bandy, D. and Reiman, E. M. (2000). Thermosensory activation of insular cortex, *Nature Neuroscience* **3**: 184–190.

Crick, F. H. C. and Koch, C. (1990). Towards a neurobiological theory of consciousness, *Seminars in the Neurosciences* **2**: 263–275.

Critchley, H. D. and Rolls, E. T. (1996a). Hunger and satiety modify the responses of olfactory and visual neurons in the primate orbitofrontal cortex, *Journal of Neurophysiology* **75**: 1673–1686.

Critchley, H. D. and Rolls, E. T. (1996b). Olfactory neuronal responses in the primate orbitofrontal cortex: analysis in an olfactory discrimination task, *Journal of Neurophysiology* **75**: 1659–1672.

Critchley, H. D. and Rolls, E. T. (1996c). Responses of primate taste cortex neurons to the astringent tastant tannic acid, *Chemical Senses* **21**: 135–145.

Cromwell, H. C. and Schultz, W. (2003). Effects of expectations for different reward magnitudes on neuronal activity in primate striatum, *Journal of Neurophysiology* **89**: 2823–2838.

Crow, T. J. (1976). Specific monoamine systems as reward pathways, *in* A. Wauquier and E. T. Rolls (eds), *Brain-Stimulation Reward*, North-Holland, Amsterdam, pp. 211–238.

Crow, T. J., Spear, P. J. and Arbuthnott, G. W. (1972). Intracranial self-stimulation with electrodes in the region of the locus coeruleus, *Brain Research* **36**: 275–287.

Crutcher, M. D. and DeLong, M. R. (1984a). Single cell studies of the primate putamen. I. Functional organisation, *Experimental Brain Research* **53**: 233–243.

Crutcher, M. D. and DeLong, M. R. (1984b). Single cell studies of the primate putamen. II. Relations to direction of movements and pattern of muscular activity, *Experimental Brain Research* **53**: 244–258.

Cullen, E. (1957). Adaptations in the kittiwake to cliff-nesting, *Ibis* **99**: 275–302.

Cummings, D. E. and Schwartz, M. W. (2003). Genetics and pathophysiology of human obesity, *Annual Reviews of Medicine* **54**: 453–471.

Cummings, D. E., Frayo, R. S., Marmonier, C., Aubert, R. and Chapolet, D. (2004). Plasma ghrelin levels and hunger scores in humans initiating meals voluntarily without time- and food-related cues, *American Journal of Physiology - Endocrinology and Metabolism* **287**: 297–304.

Cunningham, M. R., Roberts, A. R., Barbee, A. P. and Druen, P. B. (1995). Their ideas of beauty are, on the whole, the same as ours: consistency and variability in the cross-cultural perception of female physical attractiveness, *Journal of Personality and Social Psychology* **68**: 261–279.

Dahlström, A. and Fuxe, K. (1965). Evidence for the existence of monoamine-containing neurons in the central nervous system: demonstration of monoamines in the cell bodies of brain stem neurons, *Acta Physiologia Scandinavica* **62**: 1–55.

Daly, M. and Wilson, M. (1988). *Homicide*, Aldine De Gruyter, New York.

Damasio, A. R. (1994). *Descartes' Error: Emotion, Reason, and the Human Brain*, Grosset/Putnam, New York.

Damasio, A. R. (2003). *Looking for Spinoza*, Heinemann, London.

Damasio, H., Grabowski, T., Frank, R., Galaburda, A. M. and Damasio, A. R. (1994). The return of Phineas Gage: clues about the brain from the skull of a famous patient, *Science* **264**: 1102–1105.

Darwin, C. (1859). *The Origin of Species*, John Murray. [reprinted (1982) by Penguin Books Ltd], London.

Darwin, C. (1871). *The Descent of Man, and Selection in Relation to Sex*, John Murray. [reprinted (1981) by Princeton University Press], London.

Darwin, C. (1872). *The Expression of the Emotions in Man and Animals*, University of Chicago Press. [reprinted (1998) (3rd edn) ed. P. Ekman. Harper Collins], Glasgow.

Davidson, R. J. (1992). Anterior cerebral asymmetry and the nature of emotion, *Brain and Cognition* **6**: 245–268.

Davidson, R. J. (2003). Affective neuroscience and psychophysiology: toward a synthesis, *Psychophysiology* **40**: 655–665.

Davidson, R. J., Ekman, P., Saron, C., Senulis, J. and Friesen, W. V. (1990). Approach/withdrawal and cerebral asymmetry, *Journal of Personality and Social Research* **58**: 330–341.

Davis, M. (1992). The role of the amygdala in conditioned fear, *in* J. P. Aggleton (ed.), *The Amygdala*, Wiley-Liss, New York, chapter 9, pp. 255–306.

Davis, M. (1994). The role of the amygdala in emotional learning, *International Review of Neurobiology* **36**: 225–266.

Davis, M. (2000). The role of the amygdala in conditioned and unconditioned fear and anxiety, *in* J. P. Aggleton (ed.), *The Amygdala: a Functional Analysis*, 2nd edn, Oxford University Press, Oxford, chapter 6, pp. 213–287.

Davis, M., Campeau, S., Kim, M. and Falls, W. A. (1995). Neural systems and emotion: the amygdala's role in fear and anxiety, *in* J. L. McGaugh, N. M. Weinberger and G. Lynch (eds), *Brain and Memory: Modulation and Mediation of Neuroplasticity*, Oxford University Press, New York, pp. 3–40.

Dawkins, M. S. (1986a). *Unravelling Animal Behaviour*, 1st edn, Longman, Harlow.

Dawkins, M. S. (1990). From an animal's point of view: motivation, fitness, and animal welfare, *Behavioral and Brain Sciences* **13**: 1–61.

Dawkins, M. S. (1993). *Through Our Eyes Only? The Search for Animal Consciousness*, Freeman, Oxford.

Dawkins, M. S. (1995). *Unravelling Animal Behaviour*, 2nd edn, Longman, Harlow.

Dawkins, R. (1976). *The Selfish Gene*, Oxford University Press, Oxford.

Dawkins, R. (1982). *The Extended Phenotype*, Freeman, Oxford.

Dawkins, R. (1986b). *The Blind Watchmaker*, Longman, Harlow.

Dawkins, R. (1989). *The Selfish Gene*, 2nd edn, Oxford University Press, Oxford.

Dayan, P. and Abbott, L. F. (2001). *Theoretical Neuroscience*, MIT Press, Cambridge, MA.

Dayan, P. and Sejnowski, T. J. (1994). TD(λ) converges with probability 1, *Machine Learning* **14**: 295–301.

De Araujo, I. E. T. and Rolls, E. T. (2004). Representation in the human brain of food texture and oral fat, *Journal of Neuroscience* **24**: 3086–3093.

De Araujo, I. E. T., Rolls, E. T. and Stringer, S. M. (2001). A view model which accounts for the response properties of hippocampal primate spatial view cells and rat place cells, *Hippocampus* **11**: 699–706.

De Araujo, I. E. T., Kringelbach, M. L., Rolls, E. T. and Hobden, P. (2003a). Representation of umami taste in the human brain, *Journal of Neurophysiology* **90**: 313–319.

De Araujo, I. E. T., Kringelbach, M. L., Rolls, E. T. and McGlone, F. (2003b). Human cortical responses to water in the mouth, and the effects of thirst, *Journal of Neurophysiology* **90**: 1865–1876.

De Araujo, I. E. T., Rolls, E. T., Kringelbach, M. L., McGlone, F. and Phillips, N. (2003c). Taste-olfactory convergence, and the representation of the pleasantness of flavour in the human brain, *European Journal of Neuroscience* **18**: 2059–2068.

De Araujo, I. E. T., Rolls, E. T., Velazco, M. I., Margot, C. and Cayeux, I. (2005). Cognitive modulation of olfactory processing, *Neuron* **46**: 671–679.

De Gelder, B., Vroomen, J., Pourtois, G. and Weiskrantz, L. (1999). Non-conscious recognition of affect in the absence of striate cortex, *NeuroReport* **10**: 3759–3763.

Deadwyler, S., Hayashizaki, S., Cheer, J. and Hampson, R. E. (2004). Reward, memory and substance abuse: functional neuronal circuits in the nucleus accumbens, *Neuroscience and Biobehavioral Reviews* **27**: 703–711.

Deco, G. and Lee, T. (2002). A unified model of spatial and object attention based on inter-cortical biased competition, *Neurocomputing* **44–46**: 775–781.

Deco, G. and Rolls, E. T. (2003). Attention and working memory: a dynamical model of neuronal activity in the prefrontal cortex, *European Journal of Neuroscience* **18**: 2374–2390.

Deco, G. and Rolls, E. T. (2004). A neurodynamical cortical model of visual attention and invariant object recognition, *Vision Research* **44**: 621–644.

Deco, G. and Rolls, E. T. (2005a). Attention, short term memory, and action selection: a unifying theory, *Progress in Neurobiology* **76**: 236–256.

Deco, G. and Rolls, E. T. (2005b). Neurodynamics of biased competition and cooperation for attention: a model with spiking neurons, *Journal of Neurophysiology* **94**: 295–313.

Deco, G. and Rolls, E. T. (2005c). Sequential memory: a putative neural and synaptic dynamical mechanism, *Journal of Cognitive Neuroscience* **17**: 294–307.

Deco, G. and Rolls, E. T. (2005d). Synaptic and spiking dynamics underlying reward reversal in the orbitofrontal cortex, *Cerebral Cortex* **15**: 15–30.

Deco, G. and Rolls, E. T. (2006). A neurophysiological model of decision-making and Weber's law, *European Journal of Neuroscience* **24**: 901–916.

Deco, G. and Zihl, J. (2001). Top-down selective visual attention: a neurodynamical approach,

Visual Cognition **8**: 119–140.

Deco, G., Rolls, E. T. and Horwitz, B. (2004). 'What' and 'where' in visual working memory: a computational neurodynamical perspective for integrating fMRI and single-neuron data, *Journal of Cognitive Neuroscience* **16**: 683–701.

Dehaene, S., Dehaene-Lambertz, G. and Cohen, L. (1998). Abstract representations of numbers in the animal and human brain, *Trends in Neurosciences* **21**: 355–361.

Del Giudice, P., Fusi, S. and Mattia, M. (2003). Modeling the formation of working memory with networks of integrate-and-fire neurons connected by plastic synapses, *Journal of Physiology (Paris)* **97**: 659–681.

Delgado, J. M. R. (1976). New orientations in brain stimulation in man, *in* A. Wauquier and E. T. Rolls (eds), *Brain-Stimulation Reward*, North-Holland, Amsterdam, pp. 481–504.

Delgado, M. R., Nystrom, L. E., Fissell, C., Noll, D. C. and Fiez, J. A. (2000). Tracking the human hemodynamic responses to reward and punishment in the striatum, *Journal of Neurophysiology* **84**: 3072–3077.

DeLong, M. R., Georgopoulos, A. P., Crutcher, M. D., Mitchell, S. J., Richardson, R. T. and Alexander, G. E. (1984). Functional organization of the basal ganglia: Contributions of single-cell recording studies, *Functions of the Basal Ganglia. CIBA Foundation Symposium*, Pitman, London, pp. 64–78.

Dennett, D. C. (1991). *Consciousness Explained*, Penguin, London.

Derbyshire, S. W. G., Vogt, B. A. and Jones, A. K. P. (1998). Pain and Stroop interference tasks activate separate processing modules in anterior cingulate cortex, *Experimental Brain Research* **118**: 52–60.

Desimone, R. (1996). Neural mechanisms for visual memory and their role in attention, *Proceedings of the National Academy of Sciences USA* **93**: 13494–13499.

Desimone, R. and Duncan, J. (1995). Neural mechanisms of selective visual attention, *Annual Review of Neuroscience* **18**: 193–222.

Destexhe, A., Mainen, Z. and Sejnowski, T. (1998). Kinetic models of synaptic transmission, *in* C. Koch and I. Segev (eds), *Methods in Neural Modeling: From Ions to Networks*, 2nd edn, MIT Press, Cambridge, MA, pp. 1–25.

Deutsch, J. A. and Di Cara, L. (1967). Hunger and extinction in intracranial self-stimulation, *Journal of Comparative and Physiological Psychology* **63**: 344–347.

Devinsky, O., Morrell, M. J. and Vogt, B. A. (1995). Contributions of anterior cingulate cortex to behaviour, *Brain* **118**: 279–306.

DeVries, A. C., DeVries, M. B., Taymans, S. E. and Carter, C. S. (1996). The effects of stress on social preferences are sexually dimorphic in prairie voles, *Proceedings of the National Academy of Science USA* **93**: 11980–11984.

Di Marzo, V. and Matias, I. (2005). Endocannabinoid control of food intake and energy balance, *Nature Neuroscience* **8**: 585–590.

Diamond, J. (1997). *Why is Sex Fun?*, Weidenfeld and Nicholson, London.

Dias, R., Robbins, T. W. and Roberts, A. C. (1996). Dissociation in prefrontal cortex of affective and attentional shifts, *Nature* **380**: 69–72.

DiChiara, G. (2002). Nucleus accumbens shell and core dopamine: differential role in behaviour and addiction, *Behavioural Brain Research* **137**: 75–114.

DiChiara, G., Acquas, E. and Carboni, E. (1992). Drug motivation and abuse: a neurobiological perspective, *Annals of the New York Academy of Sciences* **654**: 207–219.

Dickinson, A. (1980). *Contemporary Animal Learning Theory*, Cambridge University Press,

Cambridge.

Dickinson, A. (1985). Actions and habits - the development of behavioural autonomy, *Philosophical Transactions of the Royal Society of London B* **308**: 67–78.

Dickinson, A. (1986). Re-examination of the role of the instrumental contingency in the sodium-appetitive irrelevant incentive effect, *Quarterly Journal of Experimental Psychology B* **38**: 161–172.

Dickinson, A. (1994). Instrumental conditioning, *in* N. J. Mackintosh (ed.), *Animal Learning and Cognition*, Academic Press, San Diego, pp. 45–80.

Dickinson, A. and Balleine, B. (1994). Motivational control of goal-directed action, *Animal Learning and Behaviour* **22**: 1–18.

Dickinson, A. and Dawson, G. R. (1987a). Pavlovian processes in the motivational control of instrumental performance, *Quarterly Journal of Experimental Psychology B* **39**: 201–213.

Dickinson, A. and Dawson, G. R. (1987b). The role of the instrumental contigency in the motivational control of performance, *Quarterly Journal of Experimental Psychology B* **39**: 77–93.

Dickinson, A. and Dearing, M. F. (1979). Appetitive-aversive interactions and inhibitory processes, *in* A. Dickinson and R. A. Boakes (eds), *Mechanisms of Learning and Motivation*, Erlbaums, Hillsdale, NJ, pp. 203–231.

Dickinson, A., Nicholas, D. J. and Adams, C. D. (1983). The effects of the instrumental training contingency on susceptibility to reinforcer devaluation, *Quarterly Journal of Experimental Psychology B* **35**: 35–51.

Dickinson, A., Balleine, B., Watt, A., Gonzalez, F. and Boakes, R. A. (1995). Motivational control after extended instrumental training, *Animal Learning and Behaviour* **23**: 197–206.

Divac, I. (1975). Magnocellular nuclei of the basal forebrain project to neocortex, brain stem, and olfactory bulb. Review of some functional correlates, *Brain Research* **93**: 385–398.

Divac, I. and Oberg, R. G. E. (1979). Current conceptions of neostriatal functions, *in* I. Divac and R. G. E. Oberg (eds), *The Neostriatum*, Pergamon, New York, pp. 215–230.

Divac, I., Rosvold, H. E. and Szwarcbart, M. K. (1967). Behavioral effects of selective ablation of the caudate nucleus, *Journal of Comparative and Physiological Psychology* **63**: 184–190.

Dixson, A. F. (1998). Sexual behaviour and evolution of the seminal vesicles in primates, *Folia Primatologica* **69**: 300–306.

Dolan, R. J. (1997). Mood disorders and abnormal cingulate cortex, *Trends in Cognitive Sciences* **1**: 283–284.

Dolan, R. J. (1999). On the neurology of morals, *Nature Neuroscience* **15**: 5999–6013.

Dolan, R. J., Bench, C. J., Brown, R. G., Scott, L. C., Friston, K. J. and Frackowiak, C. S. (1992). Regional cerebral blood flow abnormalities in depressed patients with cognitive impairment, *Journal of Neurology, Neurosurgery, and Psychiatry* **55**: 768–773.

Dolan, R. J., Fletcher, P., Morris, J., Kapur, N., Deakin, J. F. W. and Frith, C. D. (1996). Neural activation during covert processing of positive emotional facial expressions, *Neuroimage* **4**: 194–200.

Dolan, R. J., Fink, G. R., Rolls, E. T., Booth, M., Holmes, A., Frackowiak, R. S. J. and Friston, K. J. (1997). How the brain learns to see objects and faces in an impoverished context, *Nature* **389**: 596–599.

Doya, K. (1999). What are the computations of the cerebellum, the basal ganglia and the cerebral cortex?, *Neural Networks* **12**: 961–974.

Drevets, W. C. and Raichle, M. E. (1992). Neuroanatomical circuits in depression: implications for treatment mechanisms, *Psychopharmacology Bulletin* **28**: 261–274.

Drevets, W. C., Price, J. L., Simpson, J. R. J., Todd, R. D., Reich, T., Vannier, M. and Raichle, M. (1997). Subgenual prefrontal cortex abnormalities in mood disorders, *Nature* **386**: 824–847.

Dulac, C. and Torello, A. T. (2003). Molecular detection of pheromone signals in mammals: from genes to behaviour, *Nature Reviews Neuroscience* **4**: 551–562.

Dunbar, R. (1993). Co-evolution of neocortex size, group size and language in humans, *Behavioural and Brain Sciences* **16**: 681–735.

Dunbar, R. (1996). *Grooming, Gossip, and the Evolution of Language*, Faber and Faber, London.

Dunn, L. T. and Everitt, B. J. (1988). Double dissociations of the effects of amygdala and insular cortex lesions on conditioned taste aversion, passive avoidance, and neophobia in the rat using the excitotoxin ibotenic acid, *Behavioral Neuroscience* **102**: 3–23.

Dunnett, S. B. and Iversen, S. D. (1982a). Neurotoxic lesions of ventrolateral but not antero-medial neostriatum impair differential reinforcement of low rates (DRL) performance, *Behavioural Brain Research* **6**: 213–226.

Dunnett, S. B. and Iversen, S. D. (1982b). Sensorimotor impairments following localised kainic acid and 6-hydroxydopamine lesions of the neostriatum, *Brain Research* **248**: 121–127.

Dunnett, S. B., Lane, D. M. and Winn, P. (1985). Ibotenic acid lesions of the lateral hypothalamus: comparison with 6-hydroxydopamine-induced sensorimotor deficits, *Neuroscience* **14**: 509–518.

Durstewitz, D. and Seamans, J. K. (2002). The computational role of dopamine D1 receptors in working memory, *Neural Networks* **15**: 561–572.

Easton, A. and Gaffan, D. (2000). Amygdala and the memory of reward: the importance of fibres of passage from the basal forebrain, *in* J. P. Aggleton (ed.), *The Amygdala: a Functional Analysis*, 2nd edn, Oxford University Press, Oxford, chapter 17, pp. 569–586.

Easton, A., Ridley, R. M., Baker, H. F. and Gaffan, D. (2002). Unilateral lesions of the cholinergic basal forebrain and fornix in one hemisphere and inferior temporal cortex in the opposite hemisphere produce severe learning impairments in rhesus monkeys, *Cerebral Cortex* **12**: 729–736.

Edmonds, D. E. and Gallistel, C. R. (1977). Reward vs. performance in self-stimulation: electrode-specific effects of AMPT on reward, *Journal of Comparative and Physiological Psychology* **91**: 962–974.

Eggert, F., Holler, C., Luszyk, D., Muller-Ruchholtz, W. and Ferstl, R. (1996). MHC-associated and MHC-independent urinary chemosignals in mice, *Physiology and Behavior* **59**: 57–62.

Eisenberger, N. I. and Lieberman, M. D. (2004). Why rejection hurts: a common neural alarm system for physical and social pain, *Trends in Cognitive Neuroscience* **8**: 294–300.

Ekman, P. (1982). *Emotion in the Human Face*, 2nd edn, Cambridge University Press, Cambridge.

Ekman, P. (1992). An argument for basic emotions, *Cognition and Emotion* **6**: 169–200.

Ekman, P. (1993). Facial expression and emotion, *American Psychologist* **48**: 384–392.

Ekman, P. (1998). Introduction, *C.Darwin: The Expression of the Emotions in Man and Animals, 1872, 3rd Edition 1998*, Harper Collins, Glasgow, pp. xxi–xxxvi.

Ekman, P. (2003). *Emotions Revealed : Understanding Faces and Feelings*, Weidenfeld and Nicolson, London.

Ekman, P., Friesen, W. V. and Ellsworth, P. C. (1972). *Emotion in the Human Face: Guidelines for Research and Integration of Findings*, Pergamon Press.

Ekman, P., Levenson, R. W. and Friesen, W. V. (1983). Autonomic nervous system activity distinguishes between the emotions, *Science* **221**: 1208–1210.

Elithorn, A., Piercy, M. F. and Crosskey, M. A. (1955). Prefrontal leucotomy and the anticipation of pain, *Journal of Neurology, Neurosurgery and Psychiatry* **18**: 34–43.

Elliffe, M. C. M., Rolls, E. T. and Stringer, S. M. (2002). Invariant recognition of feature combinations in the visual system, *Biological Cybernetics* **86**: 59–71.

Ellis, B. J. and Symons, D. (1990). Sex differences in sexual fantasy: an evolutionary psychological approach, *Journal of Sex Research* **27**: 527–555.

Elmquist, J. K., Elias, C. F. and Saper, C. B. (1999). From lesions to leptin: hypothalamic control of food intake and body weight, *Neuron* **22**: 221–232.

Engelhardt, A., Pfeifer, J.-B., Heistermann, M., Niemitz, C., Van Hoof, J. A. R. A. M. and Jodges, J. K. (2004). Assessment of females' reproductive status by male longtailed macques, Macaca fascicularis, under natural conditions, *Animal Behaviour* **67**: 915–924.

Epstein, A. N. (1960). Water intake without the act of drinking, *Science* **131**: 497–498.

Epstein, A. N., Fitzsimons, J. T. and Rolls, B. J. (1970). Drinking induced by injection of angiotensin into the brain of the rat, *Journal of Physiology (London)* **210**: 457–474.

Eslinger, P. and Damasio, A. (1985). Severe disturbance of higher cognition after bilateral frontal lobe ablation: patient EVR, *Neurology* **35**: 1731–1741.

Estes, W. K. (1948). Discriminative conditioning II Effects of Pavlovian conditioned stimulus upon a subsequently established operant response, *Journal of Experimental Psychology* **38**: 173–177.

Etcoff, N. L. (1989). Asymmetries in recognition of emotion, *in* F. Boller and F. Grafman (eds), *Handbook of Psychology*, Vol. 3, Elsevier, Amsterdam, pp. 363–382.

Evarts, E. V. and Wise, S. P. (1984). Basal ganglia outputs and motor control, *Functions of the Basal Ganglia. CIBA Foundation Symposium*, Vol. 107, Pitman, London, pp. 83–96.

Everitt, B. (1997). Craving cocaine cues: cognitive neuroscience meets drug addiction research, *Trends in Cognitive Sciences* **1**: 1–2.

Everitt, B. J. (1990). Sexual motivation: a neural and behavioural analysis of the mechanisms underlying appetitive and copulatory responses of male rats, *Neuroscience and Biobehavioral Reviews* **14**: 217–232.

Everitt, B. J. and Robbins, T. W. (1992). Amygdala-ventral striatal interactions and reward-related processes, *in* J. P. Aggleton (ed.), *The Amygdala*, Wiley, Chichester, chapter 15, pp. 401–429.

Everitt, B. J., Cador, M. and Robbins, T. W. (1989). Interactions between the amygdala and ventral striatum in stimulus–reward association: studies using a second order schedule of sexual reinforcement, *Neuroscience* **30**: 63–75.

Everitt, B. J., Morris, K. A., O'Brien, A. and Robbins, T. W. (1991). The basolateral amygdala-ventral striatal system and conditioned place preference: further evidence of limbic-striatal interactions underlying reward-related processes, *Neuroscience* **42**: 1–18.

Everitt, B. J., Cardinal, R. N., Hall, J., Parkinson, J. A. and Robbins, T. W. (2000). Differential involvement of amygdala subsystems in appetitive conditioning and drug addiction, *in* J. P. Aggleton (ed.), *The Amygdala: a Functional Analysis*, 2nd edn, Oxford University Press, Oxford, chapter 10, pp. 353–390.

Everitt, B. J., Cardinal, R. N., Parkinson, J. A. and Robbins, T. W. (2003). Appetitive behaviour: impact of amygdala-dependent mechanisms of emotional learning, *Annals of the New York Academy of Science* **985**: 233–250.

Ewart, W. (1993). Hepatic and other parenteral visceral afferents affecting ingestive behaviour, *in* D. A. Booth (ed.), *The Neurophysiology of Ingestion*, Manchester University Press, Manchester.

Eysenck, H. J. and Eysenck, S. B. G. (1968). *Personality Structure and Measurement*, R. R. Knapp, San Diego.

Eysenck, H. J. and Eysenck, S. B. G. (1985). *Personality and Individual Differences: a Natural Science Approach*, Plenum, New York.

Farooqi, I. S., Keogh, J. M., Kamath, S., Jones, S., Gibson, W. T., Trussell, R., Jebb, S. A., Lip, G. Y. H. and O'Rahilly, S. (2001). Partial leptin deficiency and human adiposity, *Nature* **414**: 34–35.

Farrow, T. F., Zheng, Y., Wilkinson, I. D., Spence, S. A., Deakin, J. F., Tarrier, N., Griffiths, P. D. and Woodruff, P. W. (2001). Investigating the functional anatomy of empathy and forgiveness, *NeuroReport* **12**: 2433–2438.

Fazeli, M. S. and Collingridge, G. L. (eds) (1996). *Cortical Plasticity: LTP and LTD*, Bios, Oxford.

Fellows, L. K. and Farah, M. J. (2003). Ventromedial frontal cortex mediates affective shifting in humans: evidence from a reversal learning paradigm, *Brain* **126**: 1830–1837.

Fellows, L. K. and Farah, M. J. (2005). Different underlying impairments in decision-making after ventromedial and dorsolateral frontal lobe damage in humans, *Cerebral Cortex* **15**: 58–63.

Ferguson, J. N., Aldag, J. M., Insel, T. R. and Young, L. J. (2001). Oxytocin in the medial amygdala is essential for social recognition in the mouse, *Journal of Neuroscience* **21**: 8278–8285.

Fibiger, H. C. (1978). Drugs and reinforcement mechanisms: a critical review of the catecholamine theory, *Annual Review of Pharmacology and Toxicology* **18**: 37–56.

Fibiger, H. C., LePiane, F. G., Jakubovic, A. and Phillips, A. G. (1987). The role of dopamine in intracranial self-stimulation of the ventral tegmental area, *Journal of Neuroscience* **7**: 3888–3896.

File, S. E. (1987). The contribution of behavioural studies to the neuropharmacology of anxiety, *Neuropharmacology* **26**: 877–886.

Fiorillo, C. D., Tobler, P. N. and Schultz, W. (2003). Discrete coding of reward probability and uncertainty by dopamine neurons, *Science* **299**: 1898–1902.

Fiorino, D. F., Coury, A., Fibiger, H. C. and Phillips, A. G. (1993). Electrical stimulation of reward sites in the ventral tegmental area increases dopamine transmission in the nucleus accumbens of the rat, *Behavioural Brain Research* **55**: 131–141.

Fiorino, D. F., Coury, A. and Phillips, A. G. (1997). Dynamic changes in nucleus accumbens dopamine efflux during the Coolidge effect in male rats, *Journal of Neuroscience* **17**: 4849–4855.

Fisher, R. A. (1930). *The Genetical Theory of Natural Selection*, Clarendon Press, Oxford.

Fisher, R. A. (1958). *The Genetical Theory of Natural Selection*, 2nd edn, Dover, New York.

Fitzsimons, J. T. (1992). Physiology and pathophysiology of thirst and sodium appetite, *in* D. W. Seldin and G. Giebisch (eds), *The Kidney: Physiology and Pathophysiology*, 2nd edn, Raven, New York, chapter 44, pp. 1615–1648.

Fitzsimons, J. T. and Moore-Gillon, M. J. (1980). Drinking and antidiuresis in response to reductions in venous return in the dog: neural and endocrine mechanisms, *Journal of Physiology* **308**: 403–416.

Fitzsimons, J. T. and Simons, B. J. (1969). The effects on drinking in the rat of intravenous infusion of angiotensin, given alone or in combination with other stimuli of thirst, *Journal of Physiology* **203**: 45–57.

Fodor, J. A. (1994). *The Elm and the Expert: Mentalese and its Semantics*, MIT Press, Cambridge, MA.

Francis, S., Rolls, E. T., Bowtell, R., McGlone, F., O'Doherty, J., Browning, A., Clare, S. and Smith, E. (1999). The representation of pleasant touch in the brain and its relationship with taste and olfactory areas, *NeuroReport* **10**: 453–459.

Franco, L., Rolls, E. T., Aggelopoulos, N. C. and Treves, A. (2004). The use of decoding to analyze the contribution to the information of the correlations between the firing of simultaneously recorded neurons, *Experimental Brain Research* **155**: 370–384.

Franco, L., Rolls, E. T., Aggelopoulos, N. C. and Jerez, J. M. (2007). Neuronal selectivity, population sparseness, and ergodicity in the inferior temporal visual cortex.

Frederick, S., Loewenstein, T. and O'Donoghue (2002). Time discounting and time preference: a critical review, *Journal of Economic Literature* **40**: 351–401.

Freeman, W. J. and Watts, J. W. (1950). *Psychosurgery in the Treatment of Mental Disorders and Intractable Pain*, 2nd edn, Thomas, Springfield, Illinois.

Frégnac, Y. (1996). Dynamics of cortical connectivity in visual cortical networks: an overview, *Journal of Physiology, Paris* **90**: 113–139.

Frey, S. and Petrides, M. (2002). Orbitofrontal cortex and memory formation, *Neuron* **36**: 171–176.

Frey, S., Kostopoulos, P. and Petrides, M. (2000). Orbitofrontal involvement in the processing of unpleasant auditory information, *European Journal of Neuroscience* **12**: 3709–3712.

Friedman, D. P., Murray, E. A., O'Neill, J. B. and Mishkin, M. (1986). Cortical connections of the somatosensory fields of the lateral sulcus of macaques: evidence for a corticolimbic pathway for touch, *Journal of Comparative Neurology* **252**: 323–347.

Frijda, N. H. (1986). *The Emotions*, Cambridge University Press, Cambridge.

Frith, C. D., Friston, K., Liddle, P. F. and Frackowiak, R. S. (1991). Willed action and the prefrontal cortex in man: a study with PET, *Proceedings of the Royal Society of London B* **244**: 241–246.

Frith, U. (2001). Mind blindness and the brain in autism, *Neuron* **32**: 969–979.

Frith, U. and Frith, C. D. (2003). Development and neurophysiology of mentalizing, *Philosophical Transactions of the Royal Society London B* **358**: 459–473.

Fulton, J. F. (1951). *Frontal Lobotomy and Affective Behavior. A Neurophysiological Analysis*, W. W. Norton, New York.

Funahashi, S., Bruce, C. and Goldman-Rakic, P. (1989). Mnemonic coding of visual space in monkey dorsolateral prefrontal cortex, *Journal of Neurophysiology* **61**: 331–349.

Fuster, J. (1997). *The Prefrontal Cortex*, 3rd edn, Raven Press, New York.

Fuster, J. (2000). *Memory Systems in the Brain*, Raven Press, New York.

Fuster, J. M. (1973). Unit activity in prefrontal cortex during delayed-response performance: neuronal correlates of transient memory, *Joural of Neurophysiology* **36**: 61–78.

Fuster, J. M. (1996). *The Prefrontal Cortex*, 3rd edn, Raven Press, New York.

Fuster, J. M. and Jervey, J. P. (1982). Neuronal firing in the inferotemporal cortex of the monkey in a visual memory task, *Journal of Neuroscience* **2**: 361–375.

Gabbott, P. L., Warner, T. A., Jays, P. R. and Bacon, S. J. (2003). Areal and synaptic inter-connectivity of prelimbic (area 32), infralimbic (area 25) and insular cortices in the rat, *Brain Research* **993**: 59–71.

Gaffan, D. (1992). Amygdala and the memory of reward, *in* J. P. Aggleton (ed.), *The Amygdala*, Wiley-Liss, New York, chapter 18, pp. 471–483.

Gaffan, D. and Harrison, S. (1987). Amygdalectomy and disconnection in visual learning for auditory secondary reinforcement by monkeys, *Journal of Neuroscience* **7**: 2285–2292.

Gaffan, D., Saunders, R. C., Gaffan, E. A., Harrison, S., Shields, C. and Owen, M. J. (1984). Effects of fornix section upon associative memory in monkeys: role of the hippocampus in learned action, *Quarterly Journal of Experimental Psychology* **36B**: 173–221.

Gaffan, D., Gaffan, E. A. and Harrison, S. (1989). Visual-visual associative learning and reward-associative learning in monkeys; the role of the amygdala, *Journal of Neuroscience* **9**: 558–564.

Gaffan, E. A., Gaffan, D. and Harrison, S. (1988). Disconnection of the amygdala from visual association cortex impairs visual reward-association learning in monkeys, *Journal of Neuroscience* **8**: 3144–3150.

Gallagher, H. L. and Frith, C. D. (2003). Functional imaging of 'theory of mind', *Trends in Cognitive Neuroscience* **7**: 77–83.

Gallagher, M. (2000). The amygdala and associative learning, *in* J. P. Aggleton (ed.), *The Amygdala: a Functional Analysis*, 2nd edn, Oxford University Press, Oxford, chapter 6, pp. 213–287.

Gallagher, M. and Holland, P. C. (1992). Understanding the function of the central nucleus: is simple conditioning enough?, *in* J. P. Aggleton (ed.), *The Amygdala: Neurobiological Aspects of Emotion, Memory, and Mental Dysfunction*, Wiley-Liss, New York, pp. 307–321.

Gallagher, M. and Holland, P. C. (1994). The amygdala complex: multiple roles in associative learning and attention, *Proceedings of the National Academy of Sciences USA* **91**: 11771–11776.

Gallant, J. L., Connor, C. E. and Van-Essen, D. C. (1998). Neural activity in areas V1, V2 and V4 during free viewing of natural scenes compared to controlled viewing, *NeuroReport* **9**: 85–90.

Gallistel, C. R. (1969). The incentive of brain-stimulation reward, *Journal of Comparative and Physiological Psychology* **69**: 713–721.

Gallistel, C. R. and Beagley, G. (1971). Specificity of brain-stimulation reward in the rat, *Journal of Comparative and Physiological Psychology* **76**: 199–205.

Gangestad, S. W. and Simpson, J. A. (2000). The evolution of human mating: trade-offs and strategic pluralism, *Behavioural and Brain Sciences* **23**: 573–644.

Gangestad, S. W. and Thornhill, R. (1999). Individual differences in developmental precision and fluctuating asymmetry: a model and its implications, *Journal of Evolutionary Biology* **12**: 402–416.

Garcia, J. (1989). Food for Tolman: cognition and cathexis in context, *in* T. Archer and L.-G.

Nilsson (eds), *Aversion, Avoidance and Anxiety*, Erlbaum, Hillsdale, NJ, pp. 45–85.

Gardner, E. (1988). The space of interactions in neural network models, *Journal of Physics A* **21**: 257–270.

Garrow, J. S. (1988). *Obesity and Related Diseases*, Churchill Livingstone, London.

Gawin, F. H. (1991). Cocaine addiction: psychology and neurophysiology, *Science* **251**: 1580–1586.

Gazzaniga, M. S. (1988). Brain modularity: towards a philosophy of conscious experience, *in* A. J. Marcel and E. Bisiach (eds), *Consciousness in Contemporary Science*, Oxford University Press, Oxford, chapter 10, pp. 218–238.

Gazzaniga, M. S. (1995). Consciousness and the cerebral hemispheres, *in* M. S. Gazzaniga (ed.), *The Cognitive Neurosciences*, MIT Press, Cambridge, MA, chapter 92, pp. 1392–1400.

Gazzaniga, M. S. and LeDoux, J. (1978). *The Integrated Mind*, Plenum, New York.

Gemba, H., Sasaki, K. and Brooks, V. B. (1986). Error potentials in limbic cortex (anterior cingulate area 24) of monkeys during motor learning, *Neuroscience Letters* **8**: 223–227.

Gennaro, R. J. (2004). *Higher Order Theories of Consciousness*, John Benjamins, Amsterdam.

George, M. S., Ketter, T. A., Parekh, P. I., Herscovitch, P. and Post, R. M. (1996). Gender differences in regional cerebral blood flow during transient self-induced sadness or happiness, *Biological Psychiatry* **40**: 859–871.

Georges-François, P., Rolls, E. T. and Robertson, R. G. (1999). Spatial view cells in the primate hippocampus: allocentric view not head direction or eye position or place, *Cerebral Cortex* **9**: 197–212.

Gerstner, W. and Kistler, W. (2002). *Spiking Neuron Models: Single Neurons, Populations and Plasticity*, Cambridge University Press, Cambridge.

Gerstner, W., Kreiter, A. K., Markram, H. and Herz, A. V. (1997). Neural codes: firing rates and beyond, *Proceedings of the National Academy of Sciences USA* **94**: 12740–12741.

Gewirtz, J. C. and Davis, M. (1998). Application of Pavlovian higher-order conditioning to the analysis of the neural substrates of fear conditioning, *Neuropharmacology* **37**: 453–459.

Gibbs, J., Fauser, D. J., Rowe, E. A., Rolls, B. J., Rolls, E. T. and Maddison, S. P. (1979). Bombesin suppresses feeding in rats, *Nature* **282**: 208–210.

Gibbs, J., Maddison, S. P. and Rolls, E. T. (1981). Satiety role of the small intestine examined in sham-feeding rhesus monkeys, *Journal of Comparative and Physiological Psychology* **95**: 1003–1015.

Gibbs, J., Rolls, B. J. and Rolls, E. T. (1986). Preabsorptive and postabsorptive factors in the termination of drinking in the rhesus monkey, *in* G. De Caro, A. Epstein and M. Massi (eds), *Physiology of Thirst and Sodium Appetite*, Plenum, New York and London, pp. 287–294.

Gibson, W. E., Reid, L. D., Sakai, M. and Porter, P. B. (1965). Intracranial reinforcement compared with sugar-water reinforcement, *Science* **148**: 1357–1359.

Gintis, H. (2003). The hitchhiker's guide to altruism: genes, culture, and the internalization of norms, *Journal of Theoretical Biology* **220**: 407–418.

Gintis, H. (2007). Towards a unified behavioral science, *Behavioral and Brain Sciences, in press*.

Giugliano, M., La Camera, G., Rauch, A., Luescher, H.-R. and Fusi, S. (2002). Non-monotonic current-to-rate response function in a novel integrate-and-fire model neuron, *in* J. Dorronsoro (ed.), *Proceedings of ICANN 2002, LNCS 2415*, Springer, New York, pp. 141–

146.

Glickman, S. E. and Schiff, B. B. (1967). A biological theory of reinforcement, *Psychological Review* **74**: 81–109.

Glimcher, P. (2003). The neurobiology of visual-saccadic decision making, *Annual Reviews of Neuroscience* **26**: 133–179.

Glimcher, P. (2004). *Decisions, Uncertainty, and the Brain*, MIT Press, Cambridge, MA.

Glover, G. H. (1999). Deconvolution of impulse response in event-related BOLD fMRI, *Neuroimage* **9**: 416–429.

Goff, D. C. and Coyle, J. T. (2001). The emerging role of glutamate in the pathophysiology and treatment of schizophrenia, *American Journal of Psychiatry* **158**: 1367–1377.

Goldman, P. S. and Nauta, W. J. H. (1977). An intricately patterned prefronto-caudate projection in the rhesus monkey, *Journal of Comparative Neurology* **171**: 369–386.

Goldman-Rakic, P. (1995). Cellular basis of working memory, *Neuron* **14**: 477–485.

Goldman-Rakic, P. S. (1996). The prefrontal landscape: implications of functional architecture for understanding human mentation and the central executive, *Philosophical Transactions of the Royal Society B* **351**: 1445–1453.

Goleman, D. (1995). *Emotional Intelligence*, Bantam, New York.

Goodglass, H. and Kaplan, E. (1979). Assessment of cognitive deficit in brain-injured patient, *in* M. S. Gazzaniga (ed.), *Handbook of Behavioural Neurobiology*, Vol. 2, Neuropsychology, Plenum, New York, pp. 3–22.

Gould, S. J. (1985). *Ontogeny and Phylogeny*, Harvard University Press, Boston.

Gould, S. J. and Lewontin, R. C. (1979). The spandrels of San Marco and the Panglossian paradigm; a critique of the adaptationist programme, *Proceedings of the Royal Society of London B* **205**: 581–598.

Grafen, A. (1990a). Biological signals as handicaps, *Journal of Theoretical Biology* **144**: 517–546.

Grafen, A. (1990b). Sexual selection unhandicapped by the Fisher process, *Journal of Theoretical Biology* **144**: 473–516.

Graham, H. N. (1992). Green tea composition, consumption and polyphenol chemistry, *Preventative Medicine* **21**: 334–350.

Gray, J. A. (1970). The psychophysiological basis of introversion-extraversion, *Behaviour Research and Therapy* **8**: 249–266.

Gray, J. A. (1975). *Elements of a Two-Process Theory of Learning*, Academic Press, London.

Gray, J. A. (1981). Anxiety as a paradigm case of emotion, *British Medical Bulletin* **37**: 193–197.

Gray, J. A. (1987). *The Psychology of Fear and Stress*, 2nd edn, Cambridge University Press, Cambridge.

Gray, J. A., Young, A. M. J. and Joseph, M. H. (1997). Dopamine's role, *Science* **278**: 1548–1549.

Gray, T. S., Piechowski, R. A., Yracheta, J. M., Rittenhouse, P. A., Betha, C. L. and Van der Kar, L. D. (1993). Ibotenic acid lesions in the bed nucleus of the stria terminalis attenuate conditioned stress-induced increases in prolactin, ACTH and corticosterone, *Neuroendocrinology* **57**: 517–524.

Graybiel, A. M. and Kimura, M. (1995). Adaptive neural networks in the basal ganglia, *in* J. C. Houk, J. L. Davis and D. G. Beiser (eds), *Models of Information Processing in the Basal Ganglia*, MIT Press, Cambridge, MA, chapter 5, pp. 103–116.

Greenberg, B. D., Li, Q., Lucas, F. R., Hu, S., Sirota, L. A., Benjamin, J., Lesch, K. P., Hamer, D. and Murphy, D. L. (2000). Association between the serotonin transporter promoter polymorphism and personality traits in a primarily female population sample, *American Journal of Medical Genetics* **96**: 202–216.

Greenberg, D., Smith, G. P. and Gibbs, J. (1990). Intraduodenal infusions of fats elicit satiety in sham-feeding rats, *American Journal of Physiology* **259**: 110–118.

Griffin, D. R. (1992). *Animal Minds*, University of Chicago Press, Chicago.

Grill, H. J. and Norgren, R. (1978). Chronically decerebrate rats demonstrate satiation but not bait shyness, *Science* **201**: 267–269.

Groenewegen, H. J., Berendse, H. W., Meredith, G. E., Haber, S. N., Voorn, P., Wolters, J. G. and Lohman, A. (1991). Functional anatomy of the ventral, limbic system-innervated striatum, *in* P. Willner and J. Scheel-Kruger (eds), *The Mesolimbic Dopamine System: from Motivation to Action*, Vol. 79, Wiley, Chichester, pp. 19–60.

Gross, C. G., Bender, D. B. and Gerstein, G. L. (1979). Activity of inferior temporal neurons in behaving monkeys, *Neuropsychologia* **17**: 215–229.

Gross, C. G., Desimone, R., Albright, T. D. and Schwartz, E. L. (1985). Inferior temporal cortex and pattern recognition, *Experimental Brain Research* **Suppl. 11**: 179–201.

Grossberg, S. (1988). Non-linear neural networks: principles, mechanisms, and architectures, *Neural Networks* **1**: 17–61.

Grossman, S. P. (1967). *A Textbook of Physiological Psychology*, Wiley, New York.

Grossman, S. P. (1973). *Essentials of Physiological Psychology*, Wiley, New York.

Grossman, S. P. (1990). *Thirst and Sodium Appetite*, Academic Press, London.

Groves, P. M. (1983). A theory of the functional organization of the neostriatum and the neostriatal control of voluntary movement, *Brain Research Reviews* **5**: 109–132.

Groves, P. M., Garcia-Munoz, M., Linder, J. C., Manley, M. S., Martone, M. E. and Young, S. J. (1995). Elements of the intrinsic organization and information processing in the neostriatum, *in* J. C. Houk, J. L. Davis and D. G. Beiser (eds), *Models of Information Processing in the Basal Ganglia*, MIT Press, Cambridge, MA, chapter 4, pp. 51–96.

Grueninger, W. E., Kimble, D. P., Grueninger, J. and Levine, S. (1965). GSR and corticosteroid response in monkeys with frontal ablations, *Neuropsychologia* **3**: 205–216.

Gurney, K., Prescott, T. J. and Redgrave, P. (2001a). A computational model of action selection in the basal ganglia I: A new functional anatomy, *Biological Cybernetics* **84**: 401–410.

Gurney, K., Prescott, T. J. and Redgrave, P. (2001b). A computational model of action selection in the basal ganglia II: Analysis and simulation of behaviour, *Biological Cybernetics* **84**: 411–423.

Hadland, K. A., Rushworth, M. F. S., Gaffan, D. and Passingham, R. E. (2003). The effect of cingulate lesions on social behaviour and emotion, *Neuropsychologia* **41**: 919–931.

Hailman, J. P. (1967). How an instinct is learned, *Scientific American* **221(6)**: 98–108.

Halgren, E. (1992). Emotional neurophysiology of the amygdala within the context of human cognition, *in* J. P. Aggleton (ed.), *The Amygdala*, Wiley-Liss, New York, chapter 7, pp. 191–228.

Hamann, S. and Canli, T. (2004). Individual differnces in emotion processing, *Current Opinion in Neurobiology* **14**: 233–238.

Hamer, D. H. and Copeland, P. (1998). *Living with our Genes: Why they matter more than you think*, Doubleday, New York.

Hamilton, W. D. (1964). The genetical evolution of social behaviour, *Journal of Theoretical*

Biology **7**: 1–52.

Hamilton, W. D. (1996). *Narrow Roads of Gene Land*, W. H. Freeman, New York.

Hamilton, W. D. and Zuk, M. (1982). Heritable true fitness and bright birds: a role for parasites, *Science* **218**: 384–387.

Hansel, D., Mato, G., Meunier, C. and Neltner, L. (1998). On numerical simulations of integrate-and-fire neural networks, *Neural Computation* **10**: 467–483.

Harcourt, A. H., Harvey, P. H., Larson, S. G. and Short, R. V. (1981). Testis weight, body weight and breeding system in primates, *Nature* **293**: 55–57.

Harcourt, A. H., Purvis, A. and Liles, L. (1995). Sperm competition: mating system, not breeding season, affects testes size of primates, *Functional Ecology* **9**: 468–476.

Harlow, C. M. (1986). *Learning to Love: The Selected Papers of HF Harlow*, Praeger, New York.

Harlow, H. F. and Stagner, R. (1933). Psychology of feelings and emotion, *Psychological Review* **40**: 84–194.

Harlow, J. M. (1848). Passage of an iron rod though the head, *Boston Medical and Surgical Journal* **39**: 389–393.

Hasselmo, M. E. and Bower, J. M. (1993). Acetylcholine and memory, *Trends in Neurosciences* **16**: 218–222.

Hasselmo, M. E., Rolls, E. T. and Baylis, G. C. (1989a). The role of expression and identity in the face-selective responses of neurons in the temporal visual cortex of the monkey, *Behavioural Brain Research* **32**: 203–218.

Hasselmo, M. E., Rolls, E. T., Baylis, G. C. and Nalwa, V. (1989b). Object-centered encoding by face-selective neurons in the cortex in the superior temporal sulcus of the monkey, *Experimental Brain Research* **75**: 417–429.

Hasselmo, M. E., Schnell, E. and Barkai, E. (1995). Learning and recall at excitatory recurrent synapses and cholinergic modulation in hippocampal region CA3, *Journal of Neuroscience* **15**: 5249–5262.

Hatfield, T., Han, J. S., Conley, M., Gallagher, M. and Holland, P. (1996). Neurotoxic lesions of basolateral, but not central, amygdala interfere with Pavlovian second-order conditioning and reinforcer devaluation effects, *Journal of Neuroscience* **16**: 5256–5265.

Hauser, M. D. (1996). *The Evolution of Communication*, MIT Press, Cambridge, MA.

Haxby, J. V., Hoffman, E. A. and Gobbini, M. I. (2002). Human neural systems for face recognition and social communication, *Biological Psychiatry* **51**: 59–67.

Heath, R. G. (1954). *Studies in Schizophrenia. A Multidisciplinary Approach to Mind-Brain Relationship*, Harvard University Press, Cambridge, MA.

Heath, R. G. (1963). Electrical self-stimulation of the brain in man, *American Journal of Psychiatry* **120**: 571–577.

Heath, R. G. (1972). Pleasure and brain activity: deep and surface encephalograms during orgasm, *Journal of Nervous and Mental Disorders* **154**: 3–18.

Hebb, D. O. (1949). *The Organization of Behavior: a Neuropsychological Theory*, Wiley, New York.

Hebert, M. A., Ardid, D., Henrie, J. A., Tamashiro, K., Blanchard, D. C. and Blanchard, R. J. (1999). Amygdala lesions produce analgesia in a novel, ethologically relevant acute pain test, *Physiology and Behavior* **67**: 99–105.

Heimer, L. and Alheid, G. F. (1991). Piecing together the puzzle of basal forebrain anatomy, *Advances in Experimental Biology and Medicine* **295**: 1–42.

Heimer, L., Switzer, R. D. and Van Hoesen, G. W. (1982). Ventral striatum and ventral pallidum. Components of the motor system?, *Trends in Neurosciences* **5**: 83–87.

Heims, H. C., Critchley, H. D., Dolan, R., Mathias, C. J. and Cipolotti, L. (2004). Social and motivational functioning is not critically dependent on feedback of autonomic responses: neuropsychological evidence from patients with pure autonomic failure, *Neuropsychologia* **42**: 1979–1988.

Heistermann, M., Ziegler, T., van Schaik, C. P., Launhardt, K., Winkler, P. and Hodges, J. K. (2001). Loss of oestrus, concealed ovulation and paternity confusion in free-ranging Hanuman langurs, *Proceedings of the Royal Society of London B* **268**: 2445–2451.

Hertz, J. A., Krogh, A. and Palmer, R. G. (1991). *Introduction to the Theory of Neural Computation*, Addison-Wesley, Wokingham, UK.

Herz, R. S. and von Clef, J. (2001). The influence of verbal labeling on the perception of odors: evidence for olfactory illusions?, *Perception* **30**: 381–391.

Herzog, A. G. and Van Hoesen, G. W. (1976). Temporal neocortical afferent connections to the amygdala in the rhesus monkey, *Brain Research* **115**: 57–69.

Hestrin, S., Sah, P. and Nicoll, R. (1990). Mechanisms generating the time course of dual component excitatory synaptic currents recorded in hippocampal slices, *Neuron* **5**: 247–253.

Hikosaka, K. and Watanabe, M. (2000). Delay activity of orbital and lateral prefrontal neurons of the monkey varying with different rewards, *Cerebral Cortex* **10**: 263–271.

Hladik, C. M. (1978). Adaptive strategies of primates in relation to leaf-eating, *in* G. G. Montgomery (ed.), *The Ecology of Arboreal Folivores*, Smithsonian Institute Press, Washington, DC, pp. 373–395.

Hoebel, B. G. (1969). Feeding and self-stimulation, *Annals of the New York Academy of Sciences* **157**: 757–778.

Hoebel, B. G. (1976). Brain-stimulation reward and aversion in relation to behavior, *in* A. Wauquier and E. T. Rolls (eds), *Brain-Stimulation Reward*, North-Holland, Amsterdam, pp. 335–372.

Hoebel, B. G. (1997). Neuroscience, and appetitive behavior research: 25 years, *Appetite* **29**: 119–133.

Hoebel, B. G., Rada, P., Mark, G. P., Parada, M., Puig de Parada, M., Pothos, E. and Hernandez, L. (1996). Hypothalamic control of accumbens dopamine: a system for feeding reinforcement, *in* G. Bray and D. Ryan (eds), *Molecular and Genetic Aspects of Obesity*, Vol. 5, Louisiana State University Press, Baton Rouge, LA, pp. 263–280.

Hohmann, G. W. (1966). Some effects of spinal cord lesions on experienced emotional feelings, *Psychophysiology* **3**: 143–156.

Holland, P. C. and Gallagher, M. (1999). Amygdala circuitry in attentional and representational processes, *Trends in Cognitive Sciences* **3**: 65–73.

Holland, P. C. and Gallagher, M. (2003). Double disosociation of the effects of lesions of basolateral and central amygdala on conditioned stimulus-potentiated feeding and Pavlovian-instrumental transfer, *European Journal of Neuroscience* **17**: 1680–1694.

Holland, P. C. and Gallagher, M. (2004). Amygdala-frontal interactions and reward expectancy, *Current Opinion in Neurobiology* **14**: 148–155.

Holland, P. C. and Straub, J. J. (1979). Differential effects of two ways of devaluing the unconditioned stimulus after pavlovian appetitive conditioning, *Journal of Experimental Psychology* **5**: 65–78.

Holman, J. G. and Mackintosh, N. J. (1981). The control of appetitive instrumental responding does not depend on classical conditioning to the discriminative stimulus, *Quarterly Journal of Experimental Psychology B* **33**: 21–31.

Hölscher, C. and Rolls, E. T. (2002). Perirhinal cortex neuronal activity is actively related to working memory in the macaque, *Neural Plasticity* **9**: 41–51.

Hölscher, C., Jacob, W. and Mallot, H. A. (2003a). Reward modulates neuronal activity in the hippocampus of the rat, *Behavioural Brain Research* **142**: 181–191.

Hölscher, C., Rolls, E. T. and Xiang, J. Z. (2003b). Perirhinal cortex neuronal activity related to long term familiarity memory in the macaque, *European Journal of Neuroscience* **18**: 2037–2046.

Hopfield, J. J. (1982). Neural networks and physical systems with emergent collective computational abilities, *Proceedings of the National Academy of Sciences of the U.S.A.* **79**: 2554–2558.

Hornak, J., Rolls, E. T. and Wade, D. (1996). Face and voice expression identification in patients with emotional and behavioural changes following ventral frontal lobe damage, *Neuropsychologia* **34**: 247–261.

Hornak, J., Bramham, J., Rolls, E. T., Morris, R. G., O'Doherty, J., Bullock, P. R. and Polkey, C. E. (2003). Changes in emotion after circumscribed surgical lesions of the orbitofrontal and cingulate cortices, *Brain* **126**: 1691–1712.

Hornak, J., O'Doherty, J., Bramham, J., Rolls, E., Morris, R., Bullock, P. and Polkey, C. (2004). Reward-related reversal learning after surgical excisions in orbitofrontal and dorsolateral prefrontal cortex in humans, *Journal of Cognitive Neuroscience* **16**: 463–478.

Hornykiewicz, O. (1973). Dopamine in the basal ganglia: its role and therapeutic implications including the use of L-Dopa, *British Medical Bulletin* **29**: 172–178.

Horvath, T. L. (2005). The hardship of obesity: a soft-wired hypothalamus, *Nature Neuroscience* **8**: 561–565.

Horvitz, J. C. (2000). Mesolimbocortical and nigrostriatal dopamine responses to salient non-reward events, *Neuroscience* **96**: 651–656.

Horwitz, B. and Tagamets, M.-A. (1999). Predicting human functional maps with neural net modeling, *Human Brain Mapping* **8**: 137–142.

Horwitz, B., Tagamets, M.-A. and McIntosh, A. R. (1999). Neural modeling, functional brain imaging, and cognition, *Trends in Cognitive Sciences* **3**: 85–122.

Houk, J. C., Adams, J. L. and Barto, A. C. (1995). A model of how the basal ganglia generates and uses neural signals that predict reinforcement, *in* J. C. Houk, J. L. Davies and D. G. Beiser (eds), *Models of Information Processing in the Basal Ganglia*, MIT Press, Cambridge, MA, chapter 13, pp. 249–270.

Howarth, C. I. and Deutsch, J. A. (1962). Drive decay: the cause of fast 'extinction' of habits learned for brain stimulation, *Science* **137**: 35–36.

Hoyle, R. H., Fejfar, M. C. and Miller, J. D. (2000). Personality and sexual risk taking: a quantitative review, *Journal of Personality* **68**: 1203–1231.

Hrdy, S. B. (1996). The evolution of female orgasms: logic please but no atavism, *Animal Behaviour* **52**: 851–852.

Hrdy, S. B. (1999). *Mother Nature: Natural Selection and the Female of the Species*, Chatto and Windus, London.

Huang, Y. H. and Mogenson, G. J. (1972). Neural pathways mediating drinking and feeding in rats, *Experimental Neurology* **37**: 269–86.

Hughes, J. (1975). Isolation of an endogenous compound from the brain with pharmacological properties similar to morphine, *Brain Research* **88**: 293–308.

Hughes, J., Smith, T. W., Kosterlitz, H. W., Fothergill, L. A., Morgan, B. A. and Morris, H. R. (1975). Identification of two related pentapeptides from the brain with potent opiate antagonist activity, *Nature* **258**: 577–579.

Hull, E. M., Meisel, R. L. and Sachs, B. D. (2002). Male sexual behavior, *in* D. W. Pfaff, A. P. Arnold, A. M. Etgen, S. E. Fahrbach and R. T. Rubin (eds), *Hormones, Brain and Behavior*, Vol. 1, Academic Press, San Diego, CA, chapter 1, pp. 3–137.

Humphrey, N. K. (1980). Nature's psychologists, *in* B. D. Josephson and V. S. Ramachandran (eds), *Consciousness and the Physical World*, Pergamon, Oxford, pp. 57–80.

Humphrey, N. K. (1986). *The Inner Eye*, Faber, London.

Hunt, J. N. (1980). A possible relation between the regulation of gastric emptying and food intake, *American Journal of Physiology* **239**: G1–G4.

Hunt, J. N. and Stubbs, D. F. (1975). The volume and energy content of meals as determinants of gastric emptying, *Journal of Physiology* **245**: 209–225.

Hunt, S. P. and Mantyh, P. W. (2001). The molecular dynamics of pain control, *Nature Reviews Neuroscience* **2**: 83–91.

Huston, J. P. and Borbely, A. A. (1973). Operant conditioning in forebrain ablated rats by use of rewarding hypothalamic stimulation, *Brain Research* **50**: 467–472.

Ikeda, K. (1909). On a new seasoning, *Journal of the Tokyo Chemistry Society* **30**: 820–836.

Imamura, K., Mataga, N. and Mori, K. (1992). Coding of odor molecules by mitral/tufted cells in rabbit olfactory bulb. I. Aliphatic compounds, *Journal of Neurophysiology* **68**: 1986–2002.

Insausti, R., Amaral, D. G. and Cowan, W. M. (1987). The entorhinal cortex of the monkey. II. Cortical afferents, *Journal of Comparative Neurology* **264**: 356–395.

Ishai, A., Ungerleider, L. G., Martin, A. and Haxby, J. V. (2000). The representation of objects in the human occipital and temporal cortex, *Journal of Cognitive Neuroscience* **12**: 35–51.

Ito, M. (1976). Mapping unit responses to rewarding stimulation, *in* A. Wauquier and E. T. Rolls (eds), *Brain-Stimulation Reward*, North-Holland, Amsterdam, pp. 89–96.

Ito, M. (1984). *The Cerebellum and Neural Control*, Raven Press, New York.

Ito, M. (1989). Long-term depression, *Annual Review of Neuroscience* **12**: 85–102.

Ito, M. (1993a). Cerebellar mechanisms of long-term depression, *in* M. Baudry, R. F. Thompson and J. L. Davis (eds), *Synaptic Plasticity: Molecular, Cellular and Functional Aspects*, MIT Press, Cambridge, MA, chapter 6, pp. 117–128.

Ito, M. (1993b). Synaptic plasticity in the cerebellar cortex and its role in motor learning, *Canadian Journal of Neurological Science* **Suppl. 3**: S70–74.

Ito, S., Stuphorn, V., Brown, J. W. and Schall, J. D. (2003). Performance monitoring by the anterior cingulate cortex during saccade countermanding, *Science* **320**: 120–122.

Iversen, S. D. (1979). Behaviour after neostriatal lesions in animals, *in* I. Divac (ed.), *The Neostriatum*, Pergamon, Oxford, pp. 195–210.

Iversen, S. D. (1984). Behavioural effects of manipulation of basal ganglia neurotransmitters, *Functions of the Basal Ganglia. CIBA Foundation Symposium*, Vol. 107, Pitman, London, pp. 183–195.

Iversen, S. D. and Mishkin, M. (1970). Perseverative interference in monkey following selective lesions of the inferior prefrontal convexity, *Experimental Brain Research* **11**: 376–

386.

Izard, C. E. (1971). *The Face of Emotion*, Meredity, New York.

Izard, C. E. (1993). Four systems for emotion activation: cognitive and non-cognitive processes, *Psychological Review* **100**: 68–90.

Jacob, S., McClintock, M. K., Zelano, B. and Ober, C. (2002). Paternally inherited HLA alleles are associated with women's choice of male odour, *Nature Genetics* **30**: 175–179.

Jacobsen, C. F. (1936). The functions of the frontal association areas in monkeys, *Comparative Psychology Monographs* **13**: 1–60.

Jahanshahi, M., Jenkins, I. H., Brown, R. G., Marsden, C. D., Passingham, R. E. and Brooks, D. J. (1995). Self-initiated versus externally triggered movements. I: an investigation using measurement of regional cerebral blood flow with pet and movement-related potentials in normal and Parkinson's disease subjects, *Brain* **118**: 913–933.

Jahanshahi, M., Dinberger, G., Fuller, R. and Frith, C. D. (2000). The role of the dorsolateral prefrontal cortex in random number generation: a study with positron emission tomography, *Neuroimage* **12**: 713–725.

Jahr, C. and Stevens, C. (1990). Voltage dependence of NMDA-activated macroscopic conductances predicted by single-channel kinetics, *Journal of Neuroscience* **10**: 3178–3182.

James, W. (1884). What is an emotion?, *Mind* **9**: 188–205.

Jarvis, C. D. and Mishkin, M. (1977). Responses of cells in the inferior temporal cortex of monkeys during visual discrimination reversals, *Society for Neuroscience Abstracts* **3**: 1794.

Jenni, D. A. and Collier, G. (1972). Polyandry in the American jacana, *The Auk* **89**: 743–765.

Johns, T. and Duquette, M. (1991). Detoxification and mineral supplementation as functions of geophagy, *American Journal of Clinical Nutrition* **53**: 448–456.

Johnson-Laird, P. N. (1988). *The Computer and the Mind: An Introduction to Cognitive Science*, Harvard University Press, Cambridge, MA.

Johnson, T. N., Rosvold, H. E. and Mishkin, M. (1968). Projections from behaviorally defined sectors of the prefrontal cortex to the basal ganglia, septum and diencephalon of the monkey, *Experimental Neurology* **21**: 20–34.

Johnston, V. S. and Franklin, M. (1993). Is beauty in the eyes of the beholder?, *Ethology and Sociobiology* **13**: 73–85.

Johnston, V. S., Hagel, R., Franklin, M., Fink, B. and Grammer, K. (2001). Male facial attractiveness: evidence for hormone-mediated adaptive design, *Evolution and Human Behaviour* **22**: 251–267.

Johnstone, S. and Rolls, E. T. (1990). Delay, discriminatory, and modality specific neurons in striatum and pallidum during short-term memory tasks, *Brain Research* **522**: 147–151.

Jones, B. and Mishkin, M. (1972). Limbic lesions and the problem of stimulus–reinforcement associations, *Experimental Neurology* **36**: 362–377.

Jones, E. G. and Peters, A. (eds) (1984). *Cerebral Cortex, Functional Properties of Cortical Cells*, Vol. 2, Plenum, New York.

Jones, E. G. and Powell, T. P. S. (1970). An anatomical study of converging sensory pathways within the cerebral cortex of the monkey, *Brain* **93**: 793–820.

Jones-Gotman, M. and Zatorre, R. J. (1988). Olfactory identification in patients with focal cerebral excision, *Neuropsychologia* **26**: 387–400.

Jouandet, M. and Gazzaniga, M. S. (1979). The frontal lobes, *in* M. S. Gazzaniga (ed.), *Handbook of Behavioural Neurobiology*, Vol. 2, Neuropsychology, Plenum, New York, pp. 25–59.

Julius, D. and Basbaum, A. L. (2001). Molecular mechansims of nociception, *Nature* **413**: 203–210.

Jurgens, U. (2002). Neural pathways underlying vocal control, *Neuroscience and Biobehavioral Reviews* **26**: 235–258.

Kadohisa, M., Rolls, E. T. and Verhagen, J. V. (2004). Orbitofrontal cortex neuronal representation of temperature and capsaicin in the mouth, *Neuroscience* **127**: 207–221.

Kadohisa, M., Rolls, E. T. and Verhagen, J. V. (2005a). Neuronal representations of stimuli in the mouth: the primate insular taste cortex, orbitofrontal cortex, and amygdala, *Chemical Senses* **30**: 401–419.

Kadohisa, M., Rolls, E. T. and Verhagen, J. V. (2005b). The primate amygdala: neuronal representations of the viscosity, fat texture, grittiness and taste of foods, *Neuroscience* **132**: 33–48.

Kagan, J. (1966). Reflection-impulsivity: the generality of dynamics of conceptual tempo, *The Journal of Abnormal Psychology* **1**: 917–924.

Kagel, J. H., Battalio, R. C. and Green, L. (1995). *Economic Choice Theory: An Experimental Analysis of Animal Behaviour*, Cambridge University Press, Cambridge.

Kahneman, D. and Tversky, A. (1984). Choices, values, and frames, *American Psychologist* **4**: 341–350.

Kandel, E. R. (2000). Cellular mechanisms of learning and the biological basis of individuality, *in* E. R. Kandel, J. H. Schwartz and T. H. Jessell (eds), *Principles of Neural Science*, 4th edn, McGraw-Hill, New York, chapter 63, pp. 1247–1279.

Kandel, E. R., Schwartz, J. H. and Jessel, T. H. (2000). *Principles of Neural Science*, 4th edn, McGraw-Hill, New York.

Kanwisher, N., McDermott, J. and Chun, M. M. (1997). The fusiform face area: a module in human extrastriate cortex specialized for face perception, *Journal of Neuroscience* **17**: 4301–4311.

Kapp, B. S., Whalen, P. J., Supple, W. F. and Pascoe, J. P. (1992). Amygdaloid contributions to conditioned arousal and sensory information processing, *in* J. P. Aggleton (ed.), *The Amygdala*, Wiley-Liss, New York, chapter 8, pp. 229–245.

Kappeler, P. M. and van Schaik, C. P. (2004). Sexual selection in primates: review and selective preview, *in* P. M. Kappeler and C. P. van Schaik (eds), *Sexual Selection in Primates*, Cambridge University Press, Cambridge, chapter 1, pp. 3–23.

Karadi, Z., Oomura, Y., Nishino, H., Scott, T. R., Lenard, L. and Aou, S. (1990). Complex attributes of lateral hypothalamic neurons in the regulation of feeding of alert monkeys, *Brain Research Bulletin* **25**: 933–939.

Karadi, Z., Oomura, Y., Nishino, H., Scott, T. R., Lenard, L. and Aou, S. (1992). Responses of lateral hypothalamic glucose-sensitive and glucose-insensitive neurons to chemical stimuli in behaving rhesus monkeys, *Journal of Neurophysiology* **67**: 389–400.

Katz, L. D. (2000). Emotion, representation, and consciousness, *Behavioral and Brain Sciences* **23**: 204–205.

Kawamura, Y. and Kare, M. R. (eds) (1992). *Umami: a Basic Taste*, Dekker, New York.

Keesey, R. E. (1964). Intracranial reward delay and the acquisition rate of a brightness discrimination, *Science* **143**: 702–703.

Kelley, A. E. (1999). Neural integrative activities of nucleus accumbens subregions in relation to learning and motivation, *Psychobiology* **27**: 198–213.

Kelley, A. E. (2004a). Memory and addiction: shared neural circuitry and molecular mechanisms, *Neuron* **44**: 161–179.

Kelley, A. E. (2004b). Ventral striatal control of appetitive motivation: role in ingestive behaviour and reward-related learning, *Neuroscience and Biobehavioral Reviews* **27**: 765–776.

Kelley, A. E. and Berridge, K. C. (2002). The neuroscience of natural rewards: relevance to addictive drugs, *Journal of Neuroscience* **22**: 3306–3311.

Kelly, R. M. and Strick, P. L. (2004). Macro-architecture of basal ganglia loops with the cerebral cortex: use of rabies virus to reveal multisynaptic circuits, *Progress in Brain Research* **143**: 449–459.

Keltikangas-Jarvinen, L., Elovainio, M., Kivimaki, M., Lichtermann, D., Ekelund, J. and Peltonen, L. (2003). Association between the type 4 dopamine receptor gene polymorphism and novelty seeking, *Psychosomatic Medicine* **65**: 471–476.

Kemp, J. M. and Powell, T. P. S. (1970). The cortico-striate projections in the monkey, *Brain* **93**: 525–546.

Kenrick, D. T., DaSadalla, E. K., Groth, G. and Trost, M. R. (1990). Evolution, traits, and the stages of human courtship: qualifying the parental investment model, *Journal of Personality* **58**: 97–116.

Kent, R. and Grossman, S. P. (1969). Evidence for a conflict interpretation of anomalous effects of rewarding brain stimulation, *Journal of Comparative and Physiological Psychology* **69**: 381–390.

Kettlewell, H. B. D. (1955). Selection experiments on industrial melanism in the Lepidoptera, *Heredity* **9**: 323–335.

Keverne, E. B. (1995). Neurochemical changes accompanying the reproductive process; their significance for maternal care in primates and other mammals, *in* C. R. Pryce, R. D. Martin and D. Skuse (eds), *Motherhood in Human and Nonhuman Primates*, Karger, Basel, pp. 69–77.

Keverne, E. B., Nevison, C. M. and Martel, F. L. (1997). Early learning and the social bond, *Annals of the New York Academy of Science* **807**: 329–339.

Kievit, J. and Kuypers, H. G. J. M. (1975). Subcortical afferents to the frontal lobe in the rhesus monkey studied by means of retrograde horseradish peroxidase transport, *Brain Research* **85**: 261–266.

Killcross, S. and Coutureau, E. (2003). Coordination of actions and habits in the medial prefrontal cortex of rats, *Cerebral Cortex* **13**: 400–408.

Killcross, S., Robbins, T. W. and Everitt, B. J. (1997). Different types of fear-conditioned behaviour mediated by separate nuclei within amygdala, *Nature* **388**: 377–380.

Kleinfeld, D. (1986). Sequential state generation by model neural networks, *Proceedings of the National Academy of Sciences of the USA* **83**: 9469–9473.

Kling, A. and Steklis, H. D. (1976). A neural substrate for affiliative behavior in nonhuman primates, *Brain, Behavior, and Evolution* **13**: 216–238.

Kling, A. S. and Brothers, L. A. (1992). The amygdala and social behavior, *in* J. P. Aggleton (ed.), *The Amygdala*, Wiley-Liss, New York, chapter 13, pp. 353–377.

Kluger, A. N., Siegfried, Z. and Ebstein, R. P. (2002). A meta-analysis of the association between DRD4 polymorphism and novelty seeking, *Molecular Psychiatry* **7**: 712–717.

Kluver, H. and Bucy, P. C. (1939). Preliminary analysis of functions of the temporal lobe in monkeys, *Archives of Neurology and Psychiatry* **42**: 979–1000.

Knutson, B., Adams, C. M., Fong, G. W. and Hommer, D. (2001). Anticipation of increasing monetary reward selectively recruits nucleus accumbens, *Journal of Neuroscience* **21**: 1–5.

Koch, C. (1999). *Biophysics of Computation*, Oxford University Press, Oxford.

Koch, C. (2004). *The Quest for Consciousness*, Roberts, Englewood, CO.

Kohonen, T. (1977). *Associative Memory: A System Theoretical Approach*, Springer, New York.

Kohonen, T. (1989). *Self-Organization and Associative Memory*, 3rd (1984, 1st edn; 1988, 2nd edn) edn, Springer-Verlag, Berlin.

Kokko, H., Brooks, R., McNamara, J. M. and Houston, A. I. (2002). The sexual selection continuum, *Proceedings of the Royal Society of London B* **269**: 1331–1340.

Kokko, H., Brooks, R., Jennions, M. D. and Morley, J. (2003). The evolution of mate choice and mating biases, *Proceedings of the Royal Society of London B* **270**: 653–664.

Kolb, B. and Whishaw, I. Q. (2003). *Fundamentals of Human Neuropsychology*, 5th edn, Worth, New York.

Konorski, J. (1967). *Integrative Activity of the Brain: An Interdisciplinary Approach*, University of Chicago Press, Chicago.

Koob, G. F. (1992). Dopamine, addiction and reward, *Seminars in the Neurosciences* **4**: 139–148.

Koob, G. F. and Le Moal, M. (1997). Drug abuse: hedonic homeostatic dysregulation, *Science* **278**: 52–58.

Koob, J. F. (1996). Hedonic valence, dopamine and motivation, *Molecular Psychiatry* **1**: 186–189.

Koski, L. and Paus, T. (2000). Functional connectivity of anterior cingulate cortex within human frontal lobe: a brain mapping meta-analysis, *Experimental Brain Research* **133**: 55–65.

Kowalska, D. M., Bachevalier, J. and Mishkin, M. (1991). The role of the inferior prefrontal convexity in performance of delayed nonmatching-to-sample, *Neuropsychologia* **29**: 583–600.

Kral, T. V. and Rolls, B. J. (2004). Energy density and portion size: their independent and combined effects on energy intake, *Physiology and Behavior* **82**: 131–138.

Kralik, J. D. and Hauser, M. D. (2000). A taste of things to come, *Behavioral and Brain Sciences* **23**: 207–208.

Kraut, R. E. and Johnson, R. E. (1979). Social and emotional messages of smiling: an ethological approach, *Journal of Personality and Social Psychology* **37**: 1539–1553.

Krebs, J. R. and Kacelnik, A. (1991). Decision making, *in* J. R. Krebs and N. B. Davies (eds), *Behavioural Ecology*, 3rd edn, Blackwell, Oxford, chapter 4, pp. 105–136.

Krettek, J. E. and Price, J. L. (1974). A direct input from the amygdala to the thalamus and the cerebral cortex, *Brain Research* **67**: 169–174.

Krettek, J. E. and Price, J. L. (1977). The cortical projections of the mediodorsal nucleus and adjacent thalamic nuclei in the rat, *Journal of Comparative Neurology* **171**: 157–192.

Kringelbach, M. L. and Rolls, E. T. (2003). Neural correlates of rapid reversal learning in a simple model of human social interaction, *Neuroimage* **20**: 1371–1383.

Kringelbach, M. L. and Rolls, E. T. (2004). The functional neuroanatomy of the human orbitofrontal cortex: evidence from neuroimaging and neuropsychology, *Progress in Neurobiology* **72**: 341–372.

Kringelbach, M. L., O'Doherty, J., Rolls, E. T. and Andrews, C. (2003). Activation of the human orbitofrontal cortex to a liquid food stimulus is correlated with its subjective pleasantness, *Cerebral Cortex* **13**: 1064–1071.

Krolak-Salmon, P., Henaff, M. A., Isnard, J., Tallon-Baudry, C., Guenot, M., Vighetto, A., Bertrand, O. and Mauguiere, F. (2003). An attention modulated response to disgust in human ventral anterior insula, *Annals of Neurology* **53**: 446–453.

Krug, R., Plihal, W., Fehm, H. L. and Born, J. (2000). Selective influence of the menstrual cycle on perception of stimuli with reproductive significance: an event-related potential study, *Psychophysiology* **37**: 111–122.

Kruger, T. H., Haake, P., Chereath, D., Knapp, W., Janssen, O. E., Exton, M. S., Schedlowski, M. and Hartmann, U. (2003). Specificity of the neuroendocrine response to orgasm during sexual arousal in men, *Journal of Endocrinology* **177**: 57–64.

Kuhar, M. J., Pert, C. B. and Snyder, S. H. (1973). Regional distribution of opiate receptor binding in monkey and human brain, *Nature* **245**: 447–450.

Kuhn, R. (1990). Statistical mechanics of neural networks near saturation, *in* L. Garrido (ed.), *Statistical Mechanics of Neural Networks*, Springer-Verlag, Berlin.

Kuhn, R., Bos, S. and van Hemmen, J. L. (1991). Statistical mechanics for networks of graded response neurons, *Physical Review A* **243**: 2084–2087.

Kupferman, I. (2000). Reward: Wanted - a better definition, *Behavioral and Brain Sciences* **23**: 208.

Kyl-Heku, L. M. and Buss, D. M. (1996). Tactics as units of analysis in personality psychology: an illustration using tactics of hierarchy negotiation, *Personality and Individual Differences* **21**: 497–517.

LaBar, K. S., Gitelman, D. R., Parrish, T. B., Kim, Y.-H., Nobre, A. C. and Mesulam, M.-M. (1999). Motivational state selectively modulates amygdala activation to appetitive stimuli, *Neuroimage* **9**: S765.

Laibson, D. (1997). Golden eggs and hyperbolic discounting, *Quarterly Journal of Economics* **112**: 443–477.

Laland, K. N. and Brown, G. R. (2002). *Sense and Nonsense. Evolutionary Perspectives on Human Behaviour*, Oxford University Press, Oxford.

Lam, T. K. T., Schwartz, G. J. and Rossetti, L. (2005). Hypothalamic sensing of fatty acids, *Nature Neuroscience* **8**: 579–584.

Lane, R. D., Sechrest, L., Reidel, R., Weldon, V., Kaszniak, A. and Schwartz, G. E. (1996). Impaired verbal and nonverbal emotion recognition in alexithymia, *Psychosomatic Medicine* **58**: 203–210.

Lane, R. D., Fink, G. R., Chau, P. M. L. and Dolan, R. J. (1997a). Neural activation during selective attention to subjective emotional responses, *Neuroreport* **8**: 3969–3972.

Lane, R. D., Reiman, E. M., Ahern, G. L., Schwartz, G. E. and Davidson, R. J. (1997b). Neuroanatomical correlates of happiness, sadness, and disgust, *American Journal of Psychiatry* **154**: 926–933.

Lane, R. D., Reiman, E. M., Bradley, M. M., Lang, P. J., Ahern, G. L., Davidson, R. J. and Schwartz, G. E. (1997c). Neuroanatomical correlates of pleasant and unpleasant emotion, *Neuropsychologia* **35**: 1437–1444.

Lane, R. D., Reiman, E., Axelrod, B., Yun, L.-S., Holmes, A. H. and Schwartz, G. (1998). Neural correlates of levels of emotional awareness. Evidence of an interaction between emotion and attention in the anterior cingulate cortex, *Journal of Cognitive Neuroscience*

10: 525–535.

Lange, C. (1885). The emotions, *in* E. Dunlap (ed.), *The Emotions*, 1922 edn, Williams and Wilkins, Baltimore.

Langlois, J. H., Roggman, L. A., Casey, R. J. and Ritter, J. M. (1987). Infant preferences for attractive faces: Rudiments of a stereotype?, *Developmental Psychology* **23**: 363–369.

Langlois, J. H., Roggman, L. A. and Reiser-Danner, L. A. (1990). Infants' differential social responses to attractive and unattractive faces, *Developmental Psychology* **29**: 153–159.

Langlois, J. H., Ritter, J. M., Roggman, L. A. and Vaughn, L. S. (1991). Facial diversity and infant preferences for attractive faces, *Developmental Psychology* **27**: 79–84.

Langlois, J. H., Kalakanis, L., Rubenstein, A. J., Larson, A., Hallam, M. and Smoot, M. (2000). Maxims or myths of beauty? A meta-analytic and theoretical review, *Psychological Bulletin* **126**: 390–423.

Lanthorn, T., Storn, J. and Andersen, P. (1984). Current-to-frequency transduction in CA1 hippocampal pyramidal cells: slow prepotentials dominate the primary range firing, *Experimental Brain Research* **53**: 431–443.

Lawrence, A. D., Calder, A. J., McGowan, S. W. and Grasby, P. M. (2002). Selective disruption of the recogntion of facial expressions of anger, *NeuroReport* **13**: 881–884.

Lazarus, R. S. (1991). *Emotion and Adaptation*, Oxford University Press, New York.

Leak, G. K. and Christopher, S. B. (1982). Freudian psychoanalysis and sociobiology: a synthesis, *American Psychologist* **37**: 313–322.

LeDoux, J. E. (1987). Emotion, *in* F. Plum and V. B. Mountcastle (eds), *Handbook of Physiology: The Nervous System*, Vol. 5, Higher cortical functions of the brain, American Physiological Society, Bethesda MD, pp. 419–459.

LeDoux, J. E. (1992). Emotion and the amygdala, *in* J. P. Aggleton (ed.), *The Amygdala*, Wiley-Liss, New York, chapter 12, pp. 339–351.

LeDoux, J. E. (1994). Emotion, memory and the brain, *Scientific American* **220 (June)**: 50–57.

LeDoux, J. E. (1995). Emotion: clues from the brain, *Annual Review of Psychology* **46**: 209–235.

LeDoux, J. E. (1996). *The Emotional Brain*, Simon and Schuster, New York.

LeDoux, J. E. (2000). The amygdala and emotion: a view through fear, *in* J. P. Aggleton (ed.), *The Amygdala: a Functional Analysis*, Oxford University Press, Oxford, chapter 7, pp. 289–310.

LeDoux, J. E., Iwata, J., Cicchetti, P. and Reis, D. J. (1988). Different projections of the central amygdaloid nucleus mediate autonomic and behavioral correlates of conditioned fear, *Journal of Neuroscience* **8**: 2517–2529.

Lehrman, D. S. (1965). Reproductive behavior in the ring dove, *Scientific American* **211**: 48–54.

Leibowitz, S. F. and Hoebel, B. G. (1998). Behavioral neuroscience and obesity, *in* G. A. Bray, C. Bouchard and P. T. James (eds), *The Handbook of Obesity*, Dekker, New York, pp. 313–358.

LeMagnen, J. (1956). Hyperphagia produced in the white rat by alteration of the peripheral satiety mechanism, *Comptes Rendues Societé Biologie* **150**: 32–50.

LeMagnen, J. (1971). Advances in studies on the physiological control and regulation of food intake, *in* E. Stellar and J. M. Sprague (eds), *Progress in Physiological Psychology*, Vol. 4, Academic Press, New York, pp. 204–261.

LeMagnen, J. (1992). *Neurobiology of Feeding and Nutrition*, Academic Press, San Diego.

Leonard, C. M., Rolls, E. T., Wilson, F. A. W. and Baylis, G. C. (1985). Neurons in the amygdala of the monkey with responses selective for faces, *Behavioural Brain Research* **15**: 159–176.

Lestang, I., Cardo, B., Roy, M. T. and Velley, L. (1985). Electrical self-stimulation deficits in the anterior and posterior parts of the medial forebrain bundle after ibotenic acid lesion of the middle lateral hypothalamus, *Neuroscience* **15**: 379–388.

Levenson, R. W., Ekman, P. and Friesen, W. V. (1990). Voluntary facial action generates emotion-specific autonomic nervous system activity, *Psychophysiology* **27**: 363–384.

Levin, R. J. (2002). The physiology of sexual arousal in the human female: a recreational and procreational synthesis, *Archives of Sexual Behaviour* **31**: 405–411.

Levine, A. S. and Billington, C. J. (2004). Opioids as agents of reward-related feeding: a consideration of the evidence, *Physiology and Behaviour* **82**: 57–61.

Levy, W. B. (1985). Associative changes in the synapse: LTP in the hippocampus, *in* W. B. Levy, J. A. Anderson and S. Lehmkuhle (eds), *Synaptic Modification, Neuron Selectivity, and Nervous System Organization*, Erlbaum, Hillsdale, NJ, chapter 1, pp. 5–33.

Levy, W. B. and Desmond, N. L. (1985). The rules of elemental synaptic plasticity, *in* W. B. Levy, J. A. Anderson and S. Lehmkuhle (eds), *Synaptic Modification, Neuron Selectivity, and Nervous System Organization*, Erlbaum, Hillsdale, NJ, chapter 6, pp. 105–121.

Liddle, P. F., Barnes, T. R., Morris, D. and Haque, S. (1989). Three syndromes in chronic schizophrenia, *British Journal of Psychiatry* **7**: 119–122.

Lieberman, D. A. (ed.) (2000). *Learning*, Wadsworth, Belmont, CA.

Liebeskind, J. C. and Paul, L. A. (1977). Psychological and physiological mechanisms of pain, *Annual Review of Psychology* **88**: 41–60.

Liebeskind, J. C., Giesler, G. J. and Urca, G. (1985). Evidence pertaining to an endogenous mechanism of pain inhibition in the central nervous system, *in* Y. Zotterman (ed.), *Sensory Functions of the Skin*, Pergamon, Oxford.

Liebman, J. M. and Cooper, S. J. (eds) (1989). *Neuropharmacological Basis of Reward*, Oxford University Press, Oxford.

Lim, M. M., Wang, Z., Olazabal, D. E., Ren, X., Terwilliger, E. F. and Young, L. J. (2004). Enhanced partner preference in a promiscuous species by manipulating the expression of a single gene, *Nature* **429**: 754–757.

Lin, W., Ogura, T. and Kinnamon, S. C. (2003). Responses to di-sodium guanosine 5′-monophosphate and monosodium L-glutamate in taste receptor cells of rat fungiform papillae, *Journal of Neurophysiology* **89**: 1434–1439.

Lisman, J. E., Fellous, J. M. and Wang, X. J. (1998). A role for NMDA-receptor channels in working memory, *Nature Neuroscience* **1**: 273–275.

Liu, Y. and Wang, X.-J. (2001). Spike-frequency adaptation of a generalized leaky integrate-and-fire model neuron, *Journal of Computational Neuroscience* **10**: 25–45.

Logothetis, N. K., Pauls, J., Augath, M., Trinath, T. and Oeltermann, A. (2001). Neurophysiological investigation of the basis of the fMRI signal, *Nature* **412**: 150–157.

Loh, M., Rolls, E. T. and Deco, G. (2007). A dynamical systems hypothesis of schizophrenia.

Lovibond, P. F. (1983). Facilitation of instrumental behaviour by Pavlovian appetitive conditioned stimulus, *Journal of Experimental Psychology* **9**: 225–247.

Lyness, W. H., Friedle, N. M. and Moore, K. E. (1980). Destruction of dopaminergic nerve terminals in nucleus accumbens: effect of D-amphetamine self-administration, *Pharmacology, Biochemistry, and Behavior* **11**: 553–556.

Mackintosh, N. J. (1983). *Conditioning and Associative Learning*, Oxford University Press, Oxford.

Maddison, S., Wood, R. J., Rolls, E. T., Rolls, B. J. and Gibbs, J. (1980). Drinking in the rhesus monkey: peripheral factors, *Journal of Comparative and Physiological Psychology* **94**: 365–374.

Maia, T. V. and McClelland, J. L. (2004). A reexamination of the evidence for the somatic marker hypothesis: what participants really know in the Iowa gambling task, *Proceedings of the National Academy of Sciences* **101**: 16075–16080.

Maia, T. V. and McClelland, J. L. (2005). The somatic marker hypothesis: still many questions but no answers, *Trends in Cognitive Sciences* **9**: 162–164.

Malkova, L., Gaffan, D. and Murray, E. A. (1997). Excitotoxic lesions of the amygdala fail to produce impairment in visual learning for auditory secondary reinforcement but interfere with reinforcer devaluation effects in rhesus monkeys, *Journal of Neuroscience* **17**: 6011–6120.

Malsburg, C. v. d. (1990). A neural architecture for the representation of scenes, *in* J. L. McGaugh, N. M. Weinberger and G. Lynch (eds), *Brain Organization and Memory: Cells, Systems and Circuits*, Oxford University Press, New York, chapter 19, pp. 356–372.

Markram, H. and Siegel, M. (1992). The inositol 1,4,5-triphosphate pathway mediates cholinergic potentiation of rat hippocampal neuronal responses to NMDA, *Journal of Physiology* **447**: 513–533.

Markram, H. and Tsodyks, M. (1996). Redistribution of synaptic efficacy between neocortical pyramidal neurons, *Nature* **382**: 807–810.

Markram, H., Lübke, J., Frotscher, M. and Sakmann, B. (1997). Regulation of synaptic efficacy by coincidence of postsynaptic APs and EPSPs, *Science* **275**: 213–215.

Markram, H., Pikus, D., Gupta, A. and Tsodyks, M. (1998). Information processing with frequency-dependent synaptic connections, *Neuropharmacology* **37**: 489–500.

Marshall, J. (1951). Sensory disturbances in cortical wounds with special reference to pain, *Journal of Neurology, Neurosurgery and Psychiatry* **14**: 187–204.

Marshall, J. F., Richardson, J. S. and Teitelbaum, P. (1974). Nigrostriatal bundle damage and the lateral hypothalamic syndrome, *Journal of Comparative and Physiological Psychology* **87**: 808–830.

Martin, S. J., Grimwood, P. D. and Morris, R. G. (2000). Synaptic plasticity and memory: an evaluation of the hypothesis, *Annual Review of Neuroscience* **23**: 649–711.

Mason, G. J., Cooper, J. and Clareborough, C. (2001). Frustrations of fur-farmed mink, *Nature* **410**: 35–36.

Matsumoto, K., Suzuki, W. and Tanaka, K. (2001). Neuronal correlates of goal-based motor selection in the prefrontal cortex, *Science* **301**: 229–232.

Matthews, G. and Gilliland, K. (1999). The personality theories of H.J.Eysenck and J.A.Gray: a comparative review, *Personality and Individual Differences* **26**: 583–626.

Matthews, G., Zeidner, M. and Roberts, R. D. (2002). *Emotional Intelligence: Science and Myth*, MIT Press, Cambridge, MA.

Mayberg, H. S. (1997). Limbic-cortical dysregulation: a proposed model of depression, *Journal of Neuropsychiatry* **9**: 471–481.

Mayberg, H. S. (2003). Positron emission tomography imaging in depression: a neural systems perspective, *Neuroimaging Clinics of North America* **13**: 805–815.

Mayberg, H. S., Brannan, S. K., Mahurin, R. K., Jerabek, P. A., Brickman, J. S., Tekell, J. L., Silva, J. A., McGinnis, S., Glass, T. G., Martin, C. C. and Fox, P. T. (1997). Cingulate function in depression: a potential predictor of treatment response, *NeuroReport* **8**: 1057–1061.

Mayberg, H. S., Liotti, M., Brannan, S. K., McGinnis, S., Mahurin, R. K., Jerabek, P. A., Silva, J. A., Tekell, J. L., Martin, C. C., Lancaster, J. L. and Fox, P. T. (1999). Reciprocal limbic-cortical function and negative mood: converging PET findings in depression and normal sadness, *American Journal of Psychiatry* **156**: 675–682.

Mayberg, H. S., Lozano, A. M., Voon, V., McNeely, H. E., Seminowicz, D., Hamani, C., Schwalb, J. M. and Kennedy, S. H. (2005). Deep brain stimulation for treatment-resistant depression, *Neuron* **45**: 651–660.

Maynard Smith, J. (1984). Game theory and the evolution of behaviour, *Behavioral and Brain Sciences* **7**: 95–125.

Maynard Smith, J. and Harper, D. (2003). *Animal Signals*, Oxford University Press, Oxford.

McClelland, J. L. and Rumelhart, D. E. (1986). A distributed model of human learning and memory, *in* J. L. McClelland and D. E. Rumelhart (eds), *Parallel Distributed Processing*, Vol. 2, MIT Press, Cambridge, MA, chapter 17, pp. 170–215.

McClure, S. M., Berns, G. S. and Montague, P. R. (2003). Temporal prediction errors in a passive learning task activate human striatum, *Neuron* **38**: 339–346.

McClure, S. M., Laibson, D. I., Loewenstein, G. and Cohen, J. D. (2004). Separate neural systems value immediate and delayed monetary rewards, *Science* **306**: 503–507.

McCormick, D., Connors, B., Lighthall, J. and Prince, D. (1985). Comparative electrophysiology of pyramidal and sparsely spiny stellate neurons in the neocortex, *Journal of Neurophysiology* **54**: 782–806.

McCoy, A. N. and Platt, M. L. (2005). Expectations and outcomes: decision-making in the primate brain, *Journal of Comparative Physiology A* **191**: 201–211.

McDonald, A. J. (1992). Cell types and intrinsic connections to the amygdala, *in* J. P. Aggleton (ed.), *The Amygdala*, Wiley-Liss, New York, chapter 2, pp. 67–96.

McGinty, D. and Szymusiak, R. (1988). Neuronal unit activity patterns in behaving animals: brainstem and limbic system, *Annual Review of Psychology* **39**: 135–168.

McLeod, P., Plunkett, K. and Rolls, E. T. (1998). *Introduction to Connectionist Modelling of Cognitive Processes*, Oxford University Press, Oxford.

Mei, N. (1993). Gastrointestinal chemoreception and its behavioural role, *in* D. A. Booth (ed.), *The Neurophysiology of Ingestion*, Manchester University Press, Manchester, chapter 4, pp. 47–56.

Mei, N. (1994). Role of digestive afferents in food intake regulation, *in* C. R. Legg and D. A. Booth (eds), *Appetite, Neural and Behavioural Bases*, Oxford University Press, Oxford, chapter 4, pp. 86–97.

Melzack, R. and Wall, P. D. (1996). *The Challenge of Pain*, Penguin, Harmondsworth, UK.

Meredith, M. (2001). Human vomeronasal organ function: a critical review of best and worst cases, *Chemical Senses* **26**: 433–445.

Meston, C. M. and Frohlich, P. F. (2000). The neurobiology of sexual function, *Archives of General Psychiatry* **57**: 1012–1030.

Mesulam, M.-M. (1990). Human brain cholinergic pathways, *Progress in Brain Research* **84**: 231–241.

Mesulam, M.-M. and Mufson, E. J. (1982a). Insula of the Old World monkey. I: Architectonics in the insulo-orbito-temporal component of the paralimbic brain, *Journal of Comparative Neurology* **212**: 1–22.

Mesulam, M.-M. and Mufson, E. J. (1982b). Insula of the Old World monkey. III. Efferent cortical output and comments on function, *Journal of Comparative Neurology* **212**: 38–52.

Metcalfe, J. and Mischel, W. (1999). A hot/cool-system analysis of delay of gratification: dynamics of willpower, *Psychological Review* **106**: 3–19.

Meunier, M., Bachevalier, J. and Mishkin, M. (1997). Effects of orbital frontal and anterior cingulate lesions on object and spatial memory in rhesus monkeys, *Neuropsychologia* **35**: 999–1015.

Middleton, F. A. and Strick, P. L. (1994). Anatomical evidence for cerebellar and basal ganglia involvement in higher cognitive function, *Science* **266**: 458–461.

Middleton, F. A. and Strick, P. L. (1996a). New concepts about the organization of the basal ganglia., *in* J. A. Obeso (ed.), *Advances in Neurology: The Basal Ganglia and the Surgical Treatment for Parkinson's Disease*, Raven, New York.

Middleton, F. A. and Strick, P. L. (1996b). The temporal lobe is a target of output from the basal ganglia, *Proceedings of the National Academy of Sciences of the USA* **93**: 8683–8687.

Middleton, F. A. and Strick, P. L. (2000). Basal ganglia output and cognition: evidence from anatomical, behavioral, and clinical studies, *Brain and Cognition* **42**: 183–200.

Millenson, J. R. (1967). *Principles of Behavioral Analysis*, MacMillan, New York.

Miller, E., Gochin, P. and Gross, C. (1993a). Suppression of visual responses of neurons in inferior temporal cortex of the awake macaque by addition of a second stimulus, *Brain Research* **616**: 25–29.

Miller, E. K. and Cohen, J. D. (2001). An integrative theory of prefrontal cortex function, *Annual Review of Neuroscience* **24**: 167–202.

Miller, E. K. and Desimone, R. (1994). Parallel neuronal mechanisms for short-term memory, *Science* **263**: 520–522.

Miller, E. K., Li, L. and Desimone, R. (1993b). Activity of neurons in anterior inferior temporal cortex during a short-term memory task, *Journal of Neuroscience* **13**: 1460–1478.

Miller, E. K., Erickson, C. and Desimone, R. (1996). Neural mechanism of visual working memory in prefrontal cortex of the macaque, *Journal of Neuroscience* **16**: 5154–5167.

Miller, G. A. (1956). The magic number seven, plus or minus two: some limits on our capacity for the processing of information, *Psychological Review* **63**: 81–93.

Miller, G. F. (2000). *The Mating Mind*, Heinemann, London.

Miller, K. D. (1992). Development of orientation columns via competition between ON– and OFF–center inputs, *NeuroReport* **3**: 73–76.

Millhouse, O. E. (1986). The intercalated cells of the amygdala, *Journal of Comparative Neurology* **247**: 246–271.

Millhouse, O. E. and DeOlmos, J. (1983). Neuronal configuration in lateral and basolateral amygdala, *Neuroscience* **10**: 1269–1300.

Milner, A. D. and Goodale, M. A. (1995). *The Visual Brain in Action*, Oxford University Press, Oxford.

Milner, B. (1963). Effects of different brain lesions on card sorting, *Archives of Neurology* **9**: 90–100.

Milner, B. (1982). Some cognitive effects of frontal-lobe lesions in man, *Philosophical Transactions of the Royal Society B* **298**: 211–226.

Minai, A. A. and Levy, W. B. (1993). Sequence learning in a single trial, *International Neural Network Society World Congress of Neural Networks* **2**: 505–508.

Mirenowicz, J. and Schultz, W. (1996). Preferential activation of midbrain dopamine neurons by appetitive rather than aversive stimuli, *Nature* **279**: 449–451.

Miselis, R. R., Shapiro, R. E. and Hand, P. J. (1979). Subfornical organ efferents to neural systems for control of body water, *Science* **205**: 1022–1025.

Mishkin, M. and Aggleton, J. (1981). Multiple functional contributions of the amygdala in the monkey, *in* Y. Ben-Ari (ed.), *The Amygdaloid Complex*, Elsevier, Amsterdam, pp. 409–420.

Mishkin, M. and Manning, F. J. (1978). Non-spatial memory after selective prefrontal lesions in monkeys, *Brain Research* **143**: 313–324.

Miyashita, Y. and Chang, H. S. (1988). Neuronal correlate of pictorial short-term memory in the primate temporal cortex, *Nature* **331**: 68–70.

Miyashita, Y., Rolls, E. T., Cahusac, P. M. B., Niki, H. and Feigenbaum, J. D. (1989). Activity of hippocampal neurons in the monkey related to a conditional spatial response task, *Journal of Neurophysiology* **61**: 669–678.

Mogenson, G., Takigawa, M., Robertson, A. and Wu, M. (1979). Self-stimulation of the nucleus accumbens and ventral tegmental area of Tsai attenuated by microinjections of spiroperidol into the nucleus accumbens, *Brain Research* **171**: 247–259.

Mogenson, G. J., Jones, D. L. and Yim, C. Y. (1980). From motivation to action: functional interface between the limbic system and the motor system, *Progress in Neurobiology* **14**: 69–97.

Moller, A. P. and Thornhill, R. (1998). Male parental care, differential parental investment by females and sexual selection, *Animal Behaviour* **55**: 1507–1515.

Mombaerts, P. (1999). Seven-transmembrane proteins as odorant and chemosensory receptors, *Science* **286**: 707–711.

Moniz, E. (1936). *Tentatives Opératoires dans le Traitment de Certaines Psychoses*, Masson, Paris.

Montague, P. R. and Berns, G. S. (2002). Neural economics and the biological substrates of valuation, *Neuron* **36**: 265–284.

Monti-Bloch, L., Jennings-White, C., Dolberg, D. S. and Berliner, D. L. (1994). The human vomeronasal system, *Psychoneuroendocrinology* **19**: 673–686.

Monti-Bloch, L., Jennings-White, C. and Berliner, D. L. (1998). The human vomeronasal system: a review, *Annals of the New York Academy of Science* **855**: 373–389.

Moore, H. D. M., Martin, M. and Birkhead, T. R. (1999). No evidence for killer sperm or other selective interactions between human spermatozoa in ejaculates of different males in vitro, *Procedings of the Royal Society of London B* **266**: 2343–2350.

Moore, H. D. M., Dvorakova, K., Jenkins, N. and Breed, W. (2002). Exceptional sperm cooperation in the wood mouse, *Nature* **418**: 174–177.

Mora, F. and Myers, R. (1977). Brain self-stimulation: direct evidence for the involvement of dopamine in the prefrontal cortex, *Science* **197**: 1387–1389.

Mora, F., Sanguinetti, A. M., Rolls, E. T. and Shaw, S. G. (1975). Differential effects on self-stimulation and motor behaviour produced by microintracranial injections of a dopamine-receptor blocking agent, *Neuroscience Letters* **1**: 179–184.

Mora, F., Phillips, A. G., Koolhaas, J. M. and Rolls, E. T. (1976a). Prefrontal cortex and neostriatum, *Brain Research Bulletin* **1**: 421–424.

Mora, F., Rolls, E. T. and Burton, M. J. (1976b). Modulation during learning of the responses of neurones in the lateral hypothalamus to the sight of food, *Experimental Neurology* **53**: 508–519.

Mora, F., Rolls, E. T., Burton, M. J. and Shaw, S. G. (1976c). Effects of dopamine-receptor blockade on self-stimulation in the monkey, *Pharmacology, Biochemistry and Behavior* **4**: 211–216.

Mora, F., Sweeney, K. F., Rolls, E. T. and Sanguinetti, M. (1976d). Spontaneous firing rate of neurones in the prefrontal cortex of the rat: evidence for a dopaminergic inhibition, *Brain Research* **116**: 516–522.

Mora, F., Mogenson, G. J. and Rolls, E. T. (1977). Activity of neurones in the region of the substantia nigra during feeding, *Brain Research* **133**: 267–276.

Mora, F., Avrith, D. B., Phillips, A. G. and Rolls, E. T. (1979). Effects of satiety on self-stimulation of the orbitofrontal cortex in the monkey, *Neuroscience Letters* **13**: 141–145.

Mora, F., Avrith, D. B. and Rolls, E. T. (1980). An electrophysiological and behavioural study of self-stimulation in the orbitofrontal cortex of the rhesus monkey, *Brain Research Bulletin* **5**: 111–115.

Moran, J. and Desimone, R. (1985). Selective attention gates visual processing in the extrastriate cortex, *Science* **229**: 782–784.

Morecraft, R. J., Geula, C. and Mesulam, M.-M. (1992). Cytoarchitecture and neural afferents of orbitofrontal cortex in the brain of the monkey, *Journal of Comparative Neurology* **323**: 341–358.

Mori, K., Mataga, N. and Imamura, K. (1992). Differential specificities of single mitral cells in rabbit olfactory bulb for a homologous series of fatty acid odor molecules, *Journal of Neurophysiology* **67**: 786–789.

Mori, K., Nagao, H. and Yoshihara, Y. (1999). The olfactory bulb: coding and processing of odor molecule information, *Science* **286**: 711–715.

Morris, J. A., Jordan, C. L. and Breedlove, M. S. (2004). Sexual differentiation of the vertebrate nervous system, *Nature Neuroscience* **7**: 1034–1039.

Morris, J. S., Frith, C. D., Perrett, D. I., Rowland, D., Young, A. W., Calder, A. J. and Dolan, R. J. (1996). A differential neural response in the human amygdala to fearful and happy facial expressions, *Nature* **383**: 812–815.

Morris, J. S., De Gelder, B., Weiskrantz, L. and Dolan, R. J. (2001). Differential extrageniculostriate and amygdala responses to presentation of emotional faces in a cortically blind field, *Brain* **124**: 1241–1252.

Morris, R. G. M. (1989). Does synaptic plasticity play a role in information storage in the vertebrate brain?, *in* R. G. M. Morris (ed.), *Parallel Distributed Processing: Implications for Psychology and Neurobiology*, Oxford University Press, Oxford, chapter 11, pp. 248–285.

Morrot, G., Brochet, F. and Dubourdieu, D. (2001). The color of odors, *Brain and Language* **79**: 309–320.

Motter, B. C. (1993). Focal attention produces spatially selective processing in visual cortical areas V1, V2, and V4 in the presence of competing stimuli, *Journal of Neurophysiology* **70**: 909–919.

Mufson, E. J. and Mesulam, M.-M. (1982). Insula of the Old World monkey II: Afferent cortical input and comments on the claustrum, *Journal of Comparative Neurology* **212**: 23–37.

Muir, J. L., Everitt, B. J. and Robbins, T. W. (1994). AMPA-induced excitotoxic lesions of the basal forebrain: a significant role for the cortical cholinergic system in attentional function, *Journal of Neuroscience* **14**: 2313–2326.

Munzberg, H. and Myers, M. G. (2005). Molecular and anatomical determinants of central leptin resistance, *Nature Neuroscience* **8**: 566–570.

Murray, E. A., Gaffan, E. A. and Flint, R. W. (1996). Anterior rhinal cortex and amygdala: dissociation of their contributions to memory and food preference in rhesus monkeys, *Behavioral Neuroscience* **110**: 30–42.

Nagai, Y., Critchley, H. D., Featherstone, E., Trimble, M. R. and Dolan, R. J. (2004). Activity in ventromedial prefrontal cortex covaries with sympathetic skin conductance level: a physiological account of a "default mode" of brain function, *Neuroimage* **22**: 243–251.

Nakahara, H., Amari, S. and Hikosaka, O. (2002). Self-organisation in the basal ganglia with modulation of reinforcement signals, *Neural Computation* **14**: 819–844.

Nakamura, K., Kawashima, R., Ito, K., Sugiura, M., Kato, T., Nakamura, A., Hatano, K., Nagumo, S., Kubota, K., Fukuda, H. and Kojima, S. (1999). Activation of the right inferior frontal cortex during assessment of facial emotion, *Journal of Neurophysiology* **82**: 1610–1614.

Nauta, W. J. H. (1961). Fiber degeneration following lesions of the amygdaloid complex in the monkey, *Journal of Anatomy* **95**: 515–531.

Nauta, W. J. H. (1964). Some efferent connections of the prefrontal cortex in the monkey, *in* J. M. Warren and K. Akert (eds), *The Frontal Granular Cortex and Behavior*, McGraw Hill, New York, pp. 397–407.

Nauta, W. J. H. (1972). Neural associations of the frontal cortex, *Acta Neurobiologica Experimentalis* **32**: 125–140.

Nauta, W. J. H. and Domesick, V. B. (1978). Crossroads of limbic and striatal circuitry: hypothalamonigral connections, *in* K. E. Livingston and O. Hornykiewicz (eds), *Limbic Mechanisms*, Plenum, New York, pp. 75–93.

Nemeroff, C. B. (2003). The role of GABA in the pathophysiology and treatment of anxiety disorders, *Psychopharmacology Bulletin* **37**: 133–146.

Nesse, R. M. (2000a). Is depression an adaptation?, *Archives of General Psychiatry* **57**: 14–20.

Nesse, R. M. (2000b). Natural selection, mental modules and intelligence, *Novartis Foundation Symposium: The Nature of Intelligence* **233**: 96–115.

Nesse, R. M. and Lloyd, A. T. (1992). The evolution of psychodynamic mechanisms, *in* J. H. Barkow, L. Cosmides and J. Tooby (eds), *The Adapted Mind*, Oxford University Press, New York, pp. 601–624.

Nicholls, M. E. R., Ellis, B. E., Clement, J. G. and Yoshino, M. (2004). Detecting hemifacial asymmetries in emotional expression with three-dimensional computerised image analysis, *Proceedings of the Royal Society of London B* **271**: 663–668.

Nicolaidis, S. and Rowland, N. (1974). Long-term self-intravenous 'drinking' in the rat, *Journal of Comparative and Physiological Psychology* **87**: 1–15.

Nicolaidis, S. and Rowland, N. (1975). Systemic vs oral and gastro-intestinal metering of fluid intake, *in* G. Peters and J. T. Fitzsimons (eds), *Control Mechanisms of Drinking*, Springer, Berlin, pp. 601–624.

Nicolaidis, S. and Rowland, N. (1976). Metering of intravenous versus oral nutrients and regulation of energy balance, *American Journal of Physiology* **231**: 661–669.

Nicolaidis, S. and Rowland, N. (1977). Intravenous self-feeding: long-term regulation of energy balance in rats, *Science* **195**: 589–591.

Nicoll, R. A. and Malenka, R. C. (1995). Contrasting properties of two forms of long-term potentiation in the hippocampus, *Nature* **377**: 115–118.

Niki, H. and Watanabe, M. (1979). Prefrontal and cingulate unit activity during timing behavior in the monkey, *Brain Research* **171**: 213–224.

Nishijo, H., Ono, T. and Nishino, H. (1988). Single neuron responses in amygdala of alert monkey during complex sensory stimulation with affective significance, *Journal of Neuroscience* **8**: 3570–3583.

Nissen, E., Uvnas-Moberg, K., Svennson, K., Stock, S., Widstrom, A. M. and Winberg, J. (1996). Different patterns of oxytocin, prolactin but not cortisol release during breastfeeding in women delivered by caesarean section or by the vaginal route, *Early Human Development* **45**: 103–118.

Norgren, R. (1984). Central neural mechanisms of taste, *in* I. Darien-Smith (ed.), *Handbook of Physiology - the Nervous System III, Sensory Processes 1*, American Physiological Society, Washington, DC, pp. 1087–1128.

Oatley, K. and Jenkins, J. M. (1996). *Understanding Emotions*, Blackwell, Oxford.

Oatley, K. and Johnson-Laird, P. N. (1987). Towards a cognitive theory of emotions, *Cognition and Emotion* **1**: 29–50.

Oberg, R. G. E. and Divac, I. (1979). "Cognitive" functions of the striatum, *in* I. Divac and R. G. E. Oberg (eds), *The Neostriatum*, Pergamon, New York, pp. 291–314.

O'Brien, C. P., Childress, A. R., Ehrman, R. and Robbins, S. J. (1998). Conditioning factors in drug abuse: can they explain compulsion?, *Journal of Psychopharmacology* **12**: 15–22.

Ochoa, G. and Jaffe, K. (1999). On sex, mate selection and the Red Queen, *Journal of Theoretical Biology* **199**: 1–9.

Odent, M. (1999). *The Scientification of Love*, Free Association Books, London.

O'Doherty, J., Rolls, E. T., Francis, S., Bowtell, R., McGlone, F., Kobal, G., Renner, B. and Ahne, G. (2000). Sensory-specific satiety related olfactory activation of the human orbitofrontal cortex, *NeuroReport* **11**: 893–897.

O'Doherty, J., Kringelbach, M. L., Rolls, E. T., Hornak, J. and Andrews, C. (2001a). Abstract reward and punishment representations in the human orbitofrontal cortex, *Nature Neuroscience* **4**: 95–102.

O'Doherty, J., Rolls, E. T., Francis, S., Bowtell, R. and McGlone, F. (2001b). The representation of pleasant and aversive taste in the human brain, *Journal of Neurophysiology* **85**: 1315–1321.

O'Doherty, J., Deichmann, R., Critchley, H. D. and Dolan, R. J. (2002). Neural response during anticipation of a primary taste reward, *Neuron* **33**: 815–826.

O'Doherty, J., Dayan, P., Friston, K. J., Critchley, H. D. and Dolan, R. J. (2003a). Temporal difference models and reward-related learning in the human brain, *Neuron* **38**: 329–337.

O'Doherty, J., Winston, J., Critchley, H., Perrett, D., Burt, D. M. and Dolan, R. J. (2003b). Beauty in a smile: the role of the medial orbitofrontal cortex in facial attractiveness, *Neuropsychologia* **41**: 147–155.

O'Doherty, J., Dayan, P., Schultz, J., Deichmann, R., Friston, K. and Dolan, R. J. (2004). Dissociable roles of ventral and dorsal striatum in instrumental conditioning, *Science* **304**: 452–454.

O'Donoghue, T. and Rabin, M. (1999). Doing it now or later, *American Economic Review* **89**: 103–124.

O'Kane, D. and Treves, A. (1992). Why the simplest notion of neocortex as an autoassociative memory would not work, *Network* **3**: 379–384.

Olds, J. (1956). Pleasure centers in the brain, *Scientific American* **195**: 105–116.

Olds, J. (1958). Effects of hunger and male sex hormone on self-stimulation of the brain, *Journal of Comparative and Physiological Psychology* **51**: 320–324.

Olds, J. (1961). Differential effects of drive and drugs on self-stimulation at different brain sites, *in* D. E. Sheer (ed.), *Electrical Stimulation of the Brain*, University of Texas Press, Austin, TX.

Olds, J. (1977). *Drives and Reinforcements: Behavioral Studies of Hypothalamic Functions*, Raven Press, New York.

Olds, J. and Milner, P. (1954). Positive reinforcement produced by electrical stimulation of septal area and other regions of the rat brain, *Journal of Comparative and Physiological Psychology* **47**: 419–427.

Olds, J. and Olds, M. (1965). Drives, rewards, and the brain, *in* F. Barron and W. C. Dement (eds), *New Directions in Psychology*, Vol. 2, Holt, Rinehart and Winston, New York.

Olds, J., Allan, W. S. and Briese, A. E. (1971). Differentiation of hypothalamic drive and reward centres, *American Journal of Physiology* **221**: 368–375.

Olds, M. E. and Olds, J. (1969). Effects of lesions in medial forebrain bundle on self-stimulation behaviour, *American Journal of Physiology* **217**: 1253–1264.

Ongur, D. and Price, J. L. (2000). The organisation of networks within the orbital and medial prefrontal cortex of rats, monkeys and humans, *Cerebral Cortex* **10**: 206–219.

Ongur, D., Drevets, W. C. and Price, J. L. (1998). Glial reduction in the subgenual prefrontal cortex in mood disorders, *Proceedings of the National Academy of Sciences USA* **95**: 13290–13295.

Ongur, D., Ferry, A. T. and Price, J. L. (2003). Architectonic subdivision of the human orbital and medial prefrontal cortex, *Journal of Comparative Neurology* **460**: 425–449.

Ono, T. and Nishijo, H. (1992). Neurophysiological basis of the Kluver-Bucy syndrome: responses of monkey amygdaloid neurons to biologically significant objects, *in* J. P. Aggleton (ed.), *The Amygdala*, Wiley-Liss, New York, chapter 6, pp. 167–190.

Ono, T., Nishino, H., Sasaki, K., Fukuda, M. and Muramoto, K. (1980). Role of the lateral hypothalamus and amygdala in feeding behavior, *Brain Research Bulletin* **5, Suppl.**: 143–149.

Ono, T., Tamura, R., Nishijo, H., Nakamura, K. and Tabuchi, E. (1989). Contribution of amygdala and LH neurons to the visual information processing of food and non-food in the monkey, *Physiology and Behavior* **45**: 411–421.

Oomura, Y. and Yoshimatsu, H. (1984). Neural network of glucose monitoring system, *Journal of the Autonomic Nervous System* **10**: 359–372.

Oomura, Y., Nishino, H., Karadi, Z., Aou, S. and Scott, T. R. (1991). Taste and olfactory modulation of feeding related neurons in the behaving monkey, *Physiology and Behavior* **49**: 943–950.

Oring, L. W. (1986). Avian polyandry, **3**: 309–351.

Pager, J. (1974). A selective modulation of the olfactory bulb electrical activity in relation to the learning of palatability in hungry and satiated rats, *Physiology and Behavior* **12**: 189–196.

Pager, J., Giachetti, I., Holley, A. and LeMagnen, J. (1972). A selective control of olfactory bulb electrical activity in relation to food deprivation and satiety in rats, *Physiology and*

Behavior **9**: 573–580.

Pandya, D. N. (1996). Comparison of prefrontal architecture and connections, *Philosophical Transactions of the Royal Society B* **351**: 1423–1432.

Panksepp, J. (1998). *Affective Neuroscience: The Foundations of Human and Animal Emotions*, Oxford University Press, New York.

Panksepp, J. and Trowill, J. A. (1967a). Intraoral self-injection: I, Effects of delay of reinforcement on resistance to extinction and implications for self-stimulation, *Psychonomic Science* **9**: 405–406.

Panksepp, J. and Trowill, J. A. (1967b). Intraoral self-injection: II, The simulation of self-stimulation phenomena with a conventional reward, *Psychonomic Science* **9**: 407–408.

Panksepp, J., Nelson, E. and Bekkedal, M. (1997). Brain systems for the mediation of social separation-distress and social reward, *Annals of the New York Academy of Sciences* **807**: 78–100.

Panzeri, S., Rolls, E. T., Battaglia, F. and Lavis, R. (2001). Speed of feedforward and recurrent processing in multilayer networks of integrate-and-fire neurons, *Network: Computation in Neural Systems* **12**: 423–440.

Pare, D., Quirk, G. J. and LeDoux, J. E. (2004). New vistas on amygala networks in conditioned fear, *Journal of Neurophysiology* **92**: 1–9.

Parker, G. A., Ball, M. A., Stockley, P. and Gage, M. J. (1997). Sperm competition games: a prospective analysis of risk assessment, *Proceedings of the Royal Society of London B* **264**: 1793–1802.

Passingham, R. (1975). Delayed matching after selective prefrontal lesions in monkeys (Macaca mulatta), *Brain Research* **92**: 89–102.

Patton, J. H., Stanford, M. S. and Barratt, E. S. (1995). Factor structure of the Barratt impulsiveness scale, *Journal of Clinical Psychology* **51**: 768–774.

Pearce, J. M. (1997). *Animal Learning and Cognition*, 2nd edn, Psychology Press, Hove, Sussex.

Peck, J. W. and Novin, D. (1971). Evidence that osmoreceptors mediating drinking in rabbits are in the lateral preoptic area, *Journal of Comparative and Physiological Psychology* **74**: 134–147.

Penn, D. and Potts, W. K. (1998). Untrained mice discriminate MHC-determined odors, *Physiology and Behaviour* **64**: 235–243.

Pennartz, C. M., Ameerun, R. F., Groenewegen, H. J. and Lopes da Silva, F. H. (1993). Synaptic plasticity in an in vitro slice preparation of the rat nucleus accumbens, *European Journal of Neuroscience* **5**: 107–117.

Penton-Voak, I. S., Perrett, D. I., Castles, D. L., Kobayashi, T., Burt, D. M., Murray, L. K. and Minamisawa, R. (1999). Menstrual cycle alters faces preference, *Nature* **399**: 741–742.

Percheron, G., Yelnik, J. and François, C. (1984). A Golgi analysis of the primate globus pallidus. III. Spatial organization of the striato-pallidal complex, *Journal of Comparative Neurology* **227**: 214–227.

Percheron, G., Yelnik, J. and François, C. (1984b). The primate striato-pallido-nigral system: an integrative system for cortical information, *in* J. S. McKenzie, R. E. Kemm and L. N. Wilcox (eds), *The Basal Ganglia: Structure and Function*, Plenum, New York, pp. 87–105.

Percheron, G., Yelnik, J., François, C., Fenelon, G. and Talbi, B. (1994). Informational neurology of the basal ganglia related system, *Revue Neurologique (Paris)* **150**: 614–

626.

Perl, E. R. and Kruger, L. (1996). Nociception and pain: evolution of concepts and observations, *in* L. Kruger (ed.), *Pain and Touch*, Academic Press, San Diego, chapter 4, pp. 180–211.

Perrett, D. I. and Rolls, E. T. (1983). Neural mechanisms underlying the visual analysis of faces, *in* J.-P. Ewert, R. R. Capranica and D. J. Ingle (eds), *Advances in Vertebrate Neuroethology*, Plenum Press, New York, pp. 543–566.

Perrett, D. I., Rolls, E. T. and Caan, W. (1982). Visual neurons responsive to faces in the monkey temporal cortex, *Experimental Brain Research* **47**: 329–342.

Perrett, D. I., Smith, P. A. J., Potter, D. D., Mistlin, A. J., Head, A. S., Milner, D. and Jeeves, M. A. (1985). Visual cells in temporal cortex sensitive to face view and gaze direction, *Proceedings of the Royal Society of London, Series B* **223**: 293–317.

Petri, H. L. and Mishkin, M. (1994). Behaviorism, cognitivism, and the neuropsychology of memory, *American Scientist* **82**: 30–37.

Petrides, M. (1996). Specialized systems for the processing of mnemonic information within the primate frontal cortex, *Philosophical Transactions of the Royal Society of London B* **351**: 1455–1462.

Petrides, M. and Pandya, D. N. (1988). Association fiber pathways to the frontal cortex from the superior temporal region in the rhesus monkey, *Journal of Comparative Neurology* **273**: 52–66.

Petrides, M. and Pandya, D. N. (1994). Comparative architectonic analysis of the human and macaque frontal cortex, *in* J. Grafman and F. Boller (eds), *Handbook of Neuropsychology*, Vol. 9, Elsevier, Amsterdam, pp. 17–58.

Petrovich, P., Petersson, K. M., Ghatan, P. H., Ston-Elander, S. and Ingvar, M. (2000). Pain-related cerebral activation is altered by a distracting cognitive task, *Pain* **85**: 19–30.

Pfaff, D. W. (1980). *Estrogens and Brain Function*, Springer, New York.

Pfaff, D. W. (1982). Neurobiological mechanisms of sexual behavior, *in* D. W. Pfaff (ed.), *The Physiological Mechanisms of Motivation*, Springer, New York, pp. 287–317.

Pfaus, J. G., Damsma, G., Nomikos, G. G., Wenkstern, D., Blaha, C. D., Phillips, A. G. and Fibiger, H. C. (1990). Sexual behavior enhances central dopamine transmission in the male rat, *Brain Research* **530**: 345–348.

Phelps, E. (2004). Human emotion and memory: interactions of the amygdala and hippocampal complex, *Current Opinion in Neurobiology* **14**: 198–202.

Phelps, E., O'Connor, K. J., Gatenby, J. C., Gore, J. C., Grillon, C. and Davis, M. (2001). Activation of the left amygdala to a cognitive representation of fear, *Nature Neuroscience* **4**: 437–441.

Phillips, A. G. and Fibiger, H. C. (1976). Long-term deficits in stimulation-induced behaviors and self-stimulation after 6-hydroxydopamine administration in rats, *Behavioral Biology* **16**: 127–143.

Phillips, A. G. and Fibiger, H. C. (1978). The role of dopamine in mediating self-stimulation in the ventral tegmentum, nucleus accumbens and medial prefrontal cortex, *Canadian Journal of Psychology* **32**: 58–66.

Phillips, A. G. and Fibiger, H. C. (1989). Neuroanatomical bases of intracranial self-stimulation: untying the Gordian knot, *in* J. M. Liebman and S. J. Cooper (eds), *The Neuropharmacological Basis of Reward*, Oxford University Press, Oxford, pp. 66–105.

Phillips, A. G. and Fibiger, H. C. (1990). Role of reward and enhancement of conditioned reward in persistence of responding for cocaine, *Behavioral Pharmacology* **1**: 269–282.

Phillips, A. G., Mora, F. and Rolls, E. T. (1979). Intracranial self-stimulation in the orbitofrontal cortex and caudate nucleus of the alert monkey: effects of apomorphine, pimozide and spiroperidol, *Psychopharmacology* **62**: 79–82.

Phillips, A. G., Mora, F. and Rolls, E. T. (1981). Intra-cerebral self-administration of amphetamine by rhesus monkeys, *Neuroscience Letters* **24**: 81–86.

Phillips, A. G., LePiane, F. G. and Fibiger, H. C. (1982). Effects of kainic acid lesions of the striatum on self-stimulation in the substantia nigra and ventral tegmental area, *Behavioural Brain Research* **5**: 297–310.

Phillips, A. G., Blaha, C. D. and Fibiger, H. C. (1989). Neurochemical correlates of brain-stimulation reward measured by ex vivo and in vivo analyses, *Neuroscience and Biobehavioral Reviews* **13**: 99–104.

Phillips, A. G., Pfaus, J. G. and Blaha, C. D. (1991). Dopamine and motivated behavior: insights provided by in vivo analysis, *in* P. Willner and J. Scheel-Kruger (eds), *The Mesolimbic Dopamine System: From Motivation to Action*, Wiley, New York, chapter 8, pp. 199–224.

Phillips, M. I. (1978). Angiotensin in the brain, *Neuroendocrinology* **25**: 354–377.

Phillips, M. I. and Felix, D. (1976). Specific angiotensin II receptive neurones in the cat subfornical organ, *Brain Research* **109**: 531–540.

Phillips, M. L. (2004). Facial processing deficits and social dysfunction: how are they related?, *Brain* **127**: 1691–1692.

Phillips, M. L., Young, A. W., Scott, S. K., Calder, A. J., Andrew, C., Giampetro, V., Williams, S. C. R., Bullmore, E. T., Brammer, M. and Gray, J. A. (1998). Neural responses to facial and vocal expressions of fear and disgust, *Proceedings of the Royal Society of London B* **265**: 1809–1817.

Phillips, M. L., Drevets, W. C., Rauch, S. L. and Lane, R. (2003a). Neurobiology of emotion perception II: Implications for major psychiatric disorders, *Biological Psychiatry* **54**: 515–528.

Phillips, M. L., Williams, L. M., Heining, M., Herba, C. M., Russell, T., Andrew, C., Bullmore, E. T., Brammer, M. J., Williams, S. C., Morgan, M., Young, A. W. and Gray, J. A. (2004). Differential neural responses to overt and covert presentations of facial expressions of fear and disgust, *Neuroimage* **21**: 1484–1496.

Phillips, P. E. M., Stuber, G. D., Heian, M. L. A. V., Wightman, R. M. and Carelli, R. M. (2003b). Subsecond dopamine release promotes cocaine seeking, *Nature* **422**: 614–618.

Phillips, P., Rolls, B. J., Ledingham, J. and Morton, J. (1984). Body fluid changes, thirst and drinking in man during free access to water, *Physiology and Behavior* **33**: 357–363.

Phillips, P., Rolls, B. J., Ledingham, J., Morton, J. and Forsling, M. (1985). Angiotensin-II induced thirst and vasopressin release in man, *Clinical Science* **68**: 669–674.

Phillips, R. R., Malamut, B. L., Bachevalier, J. and Mishkin, M. (1988). Dissociation of the effects of inferior temporal and limbic lesions on object discrimination learning with 24-h intertrial intervals, *Behavioural Brain Research* **27**: 99–107.

Pickens, C. L., Saddoris, M. P., Setlow, B., Gallagher, M., Holland, P. C. and Schoenbaum, G. (2003). Different roles for orbitofrontal cortex and basolateral amygdala in a reinforcer devaluation task, *Journal of Neuroscience* **23**: 11078–11084.

Pinker, S. (1997). *How the Mind Works*, Norton, New York.

Pinker, S. and Bloom, P. (1992). Natural language and natural selection, *in* J. H. Barkow,

L. Cosmides and J. Tooby (eds), *The Adapted Mind*, Oxford University Press, New York, chapter 12, pp. 451–493.

Pinto, S., Roseberry, A. G., Liu, H. Y., Diano, S., Shanabrough, M., Cai, X. L., Friedman, J. M. and Horvath, T. L. (2004). Rapid rewiring of arcuate nucleus feeding circuits by leptin, *Science* **304**: 110–115.

Pitkanen, A. (2000). Connectivitiy of the rat amygdaloid complex, *in* J. P. Aggleton (ed.), *The Amygdala: a Functional Analysis*, Oxford University Press, Oxford, chapter 2, pp. 31–116.

Pitkanen, A., Kelly, J. L. and Amaral, D. G. (2002). Projections from the lateral, basal, and accessory basal nuclei of the amygdala to the entorhinal cortex in the macaque monkey, *Hippocampus* **12**: 186–205.

Pizzari, T., Cornwallis, C. K., Lovlie, H., Jakobsson, S. and Birkhead, T. R. (2003). Sophisticated sperm allocation in male fowl, *Nature* **426**: 70–74.

Platt, M. L. and Glimcher, P. W. (1999). Neural correlates of decision variables in parietal cortex, *Nature* **400**: 233–238.

Potts, W. (2002). Wisdom through immunogenetics, *Nature Genetics* **30**: 130–131.

Potts, W., Manning, J. and Wakeland, E. K. (1991). Mating patterns in seminatural populations of mice influenced by MHC genotype, *Nature* **352**: 619–621.

Preuss, T. M. and Goldman-Rakic, P. S. (1989). Connections of the ventral granular frontal cortex of macaques with perisylvian premotor and somatosensory areas: anatomical evidence for somatic representation in primate frontal association cortex, *Journal of Comparative Neurology* **282**: 293–316.

Price, J. L., Carmichael, S. T., Carnes, K. M., Clugnet, M.-C. and Kuroda, M. (1991). Olfactory input to the prefrontal cortex, *in* J. L. Davis and H. Eichenbaum (eds), *Olfaction: A Model System for Computational Neuroscience*, MIT Press, Cambridge, MA, pp. 101–120.

Priest, C. A. and Pfaff, D. W. (1995). Actions of sex steroids on behaviours beyond reproductive reflexes, *CIBA Foundation Symposium*, Vol. 191, Pitman, London, pp. 74–84.

Pritchard, T. C., Hamilton, R. B., Morse, J. R. and Norgren, R. (1986). Projections of thalamic gustatory and lingual areas in the monkey, *Journal of Comparative Neurology* **244**: 213–228.

Quartermain, D. and Webster, D. (1968). Extinction following intracranial reward: the effect of delay between acquisition and extinction, *Science* **159**: 1259–1260.

Quirk, G. J., Armony, J. L., Repa, J. C., Li, X.-F. and LeDoux, J. E. (1996). Emotional memory: a search for sites of plasticity, *Cold Spring Harbor Symposia on Quantitative Biology* **61**: 247–257.

Rachlin, H. (1989). *Judgement, Decision, and Choice: A Cognitive/Behavioural synthesis*, Freeman, New York.

Rachlin, H. (2000). *The Science of Self-Control*, Harvard Univeristy Press, Cambridge, MA.

Rada, P., Mark, G. P. and Hoebel, B. G. (1998). Dopamine in the nucleus accumbens released by hypothalamic stimulation-escape behavior, *Brain Research* **782**: 228–234.

Rahman, S., Sahakian, B. J., Hodges, J. R., Rogers, R. D. and Robbins, T. W. (1997). Brainstem innervation of prefrontal and anterior cingulate cortex in the rhesus monkey revealed by retrograde transport of HRP, *Brain* **122**: 1469–1493.

Rainville, P., Duncan, G. H., Price, D. D., Carrier, B. and Bushnell, M. C. (1997). Pain affect encoded in human anterior cingulate but not somatosensory cortex, *Science* **277**: 968–971.

Rajkowska, G. (2000). Postmortem studies in mood disorders indicate altered numbers of neurons and glial cells, *Biological Psychiatry* **48**: 766–777.

Ramsay, D. J., Rolls, B. J. and Wood, R. J. (1975). The relationship between elevated water intake and oedema associated with congestive cardiac failure in the dog, *Journal of Physiology (London)* **244**: 303–312.

Rao, S. C., Rainer, G. and Miller, E. K. (1997). Integration of what and where in the primate prefrontal cortex, *Science* **276**: 821–824.

Rauch, A., La Camera, G., Luescher, H.-R., Senn, W. and Fusi, S. (2003). Neocortical pyramidal cells respond as integrate-and-fire neurons to in vivo-like input currents, *Journal of Neurophysiology* **90**: 1598–1612.

Rawlins, J. N., Winocur, G. and Gray, J. A. (1983). The hippocampus, collateral behavior, and timing, *Behavioral Neuroscience* **97**: 857–872.

Reddy, W. M. (2001). *The Navigation of Feeling: A Framework for the History of Emotions*, Cambridge University Press, Cambridge.

Redgrave, P., Prescott, T. J. and Gurney, K. (1999). Is the short-latency dopamine response too short to signal reward error?, *Trends in Neuroscience* **22**: 146–151.

Reid, L. D., Hunsicker, J. P., Kent, E. W., Lindsay, J. L. and Gallistel, C. E. (1973). Incidence and magnitude of the 'priming effect' in self-stimulating rats, *Journal of Comparative and Physiological Psychology* **82**: 286–293.

Reisenzein, R. (1983). The Schachter theory of emotion: two decades later, *Psychological Bulletin* **94**: 239–264.

Renart, A., Parga, N. and Rolls, E. T. (1999a). Associative memory properties of multiple cortical modules, *Network* **10**: 237–255.

Renart, A., Parga, N. and Rolls, E. T. (1999b). Backprojections in the cerebral cortex: implications for memory storage, *Neural Computation* **11**: 1349–1388.

Renart, A., Parga, N. and Rolls, E. T. (2000). A recurrent model of the interaction between the prefrontal cortex and inferior temporal cortex in delay memory tasks, *in* S. Solla, T. Leen and K.-R. Mueller (eds), *Advances in Neural Information Processing Systems*, Vol. 12, MIT Press, Cambridge Mass, pp. 171–177.

Renart, A., Moreno, R., Rocha, J., Parga, N. and Rolls, E. T. (2001). A model of the IT–PF network in object working memory which includes balanced persistent activity and tuned inhibition, *Neurocomputing* **38–40**: 1525–1531.

Rescorla, R. A. (1990a). Evidence for an association between the discriminative stimulus and the response-outcome association in instrumental learning, *Journal of Experimental Psychology* **16**: 326–334.

Rescorla, R. A. (1990b). The role of information about the response-outcome relation in instrumental discrimination learning, *Journal of Experimental Psychology* **16**: 262–270.

Rescorla, R. A. and Solomon, R. L. (1967). Two-process learning theory: relationships between Pavlovian conditioning and instrumental learning, *Psychology Reviews* **74**: 151–182.

Rescorla, R. A. and Wagner, A. R. (1972). A theory of Pavlovian conditioning: the effectiveness of reinforcement and non-reinforcement, *Classical Conditioning II: Current Research and Theory*, Appleton-Century-Crofts, New York, pp. 64–69.

Reynolds, J. and Desimone, R. (1999). The role of neural mechanisms of attention in solving the binding problem, *Neuron* **24**: 19–29.

Reynolds, J. N. and Wickens, J. R. (2002). Dopamine-dependent plasticity of corticostriatal synapses, *Neural Networks* **15**: 507–521.

Ridley, M. (1993a). *Evolution*, Blackwell, Oxford.

Ridley, M. (1993b). *The Red Queen: Sex and the Evolution of Human Nature*, Penguin, London.

Ridley, M. (1996). *The Origins of Virtue*, Viking, London.

Ridley, M. (2003). *Nature via Nurture*, Harper, London.

Ridley, R. M., Hester, N. S. and Ettlinger, G. (1977). Stimulus- and response-dependent units from the occipital and temporal lobes of the unanaesthetized monkey performing learnt visual tasks, *Experimental Brain Research* **27**: 539–552.

Ritter, S. (1986). Glucoprivation and the glucoprivic control of food intake, *in* R. C. Ritter, S. Ritter and C. D. Barnes (eds), *Feeding Behavior: Neural and Humoral Controls*, Academic Press, New York, chapter 9, pp. 271–313.

Robbins, T. W. and Everitt, B. J. (1992). Functions of dopamine in the dorsal and ventral striatum, *Seminars in the Neurosciences* **4**: 119–128.

Robbins, T. W., Cador, M., Taylor, J. R. and Everitt, B. J. (1989). Limbic-striatal interactions in reward-related processes, *Neuroscience and Biobehavioral Reviews* **13**: 155–162.

Roberts, D. C. S., Koob, G. F., Klonoff, P. and Fibiger, H. C. (1980). Extinction and recovery of cocaine self-administration following 6-hydroxydopamine lesions of the nucleus accumbens, *Pharmacology, Biochemistry and Behavior* **12**: 781–787.

Robertson, R. G., Rolls, E. T. and Georges-François, P. (1998). Spatial view cells in the primate hippocampus: Effects of removal of view details, *Journal of Neurophysiology* **79**: 1145–1156.

Robinson, T. E. and Berridge, K. C. (1993). The neural basis of drug craving: an incentive-sensitization theory of addiction, *Brain Research Reviews, Neuroscience and Biobehavioral Reviews* **18**: 247–291.

Robinson, T. E. and Berridge, K. C. (2003). Addiction, *Annual Review of Psychology* **54**: 25–53.

Rodin, J. (1976). The role of perception of internal and external signals in the regulation of feeding in overweight and non-obese individuals, *Dahlem Konferenzen, Life Sciences Research Report* **2**: 265–281.

Rogan, M. T., Staubli, U. V. and LeDoux, J. E. (1997). Fear conditioning induces associative long-term potentiation in the amygdala, *Nature* **390**: 604–607.

Rolls, B. J. and Hetherington, M. (1989). The role of variety in eating and body weight regulation, *in* R. Shepherd (ed.), *Handbook of the Psychophysiology of Human Eating*, Wiley, Chichester, chapter 3, pp. 57–84.

Rolls, B. J. and Rolls, E. T. (1973a). Effects of lesions in the basolateral amygdala on fluid intake in the rat, *Journal of Comparative and Physiological Psychology* **83**: 240–247.

Rolls, B. J. and Rolls, E. T. (1982a). *Thirst*, Cambridge University Press, Cambridge.

Rolls, B. J., Wood, R. J. and Rolls, E. T. (1980a). Thirst: the initiation, maintenance, and termination of drinking, *Progress in Psychobiology and Physiological Psychology* **9**: 263–321.

Rolls, B. J., Wood, R. J., Rolls, E. T., Lind, H., Lind, R. and Ledingham, J. (1980b). Thirst following water deprivation in humans, *American Journal of Physiology* **239**: R476–R482.

Rolls, B. J., Rolls, E. T., Rowe, E. A. and Sweeney, K. (1981a). Sensory specific satiety in man, *Physiology and Behavior* **27**: 137–142.

Rolls, B. J., Rowe, E. A., Rolls, E. T., Kingston, B., Megson, A. and Gunary, R. (1981b).

Variety in a meal enhances food intake in man, *Physiology and Behavior* **26**: 215–221.

Rolls, B. J., Rowe, E. A. and Rolls, E. T. (1982a). How flavour and appearance affect human feeding, *Proceedings of the Nutrition Society* **41**: 109–117.

Rolls, B. J., Rowe, E. A. and Rolls, E. T. (1982b). How sensory properties of foods affect human feeding behavior, *Physiology and Behavior* **29**: 409–417.

Rolls, B. J., Van Duijenvoorde, P. M. and Rowe, E. A. (1983a). Variety in the diet enhances intake in a meal and contributes to the development of obesity in the rat, *Physiology and Behavior* **31**: 21–27.

Rolls, B. J., Van Duijenvoorde, P. M. and Rolls, E. T. (1984a). Pleasantness changes and food intake in a varied four course meal, *Appetite* **5**: 337–348.

Rolls, E. T. (1971a). Absolute refractory period of neurons involved in MFB self-stimulation, *Physiology and Behavior* **7**: 311–315.

Rolls, E. T. (1971b). Contrasting effects of hypothalamic and nucleus accumbens septi self-stimulation on brain stem single unit activity and cortical arousal, *Brain Research* **31**: 275–285.

Rolls, E. T. (1971c). Involvement of brainstem units in medial forebrain bundle self-stimulation, *Physiology and Behavior* **7**: 297–310.

Rolls, E. T. (1974). The neural basis of brain-stimulation reward, *Progress in Neurobiology* **3**: 71–160.

Rolls, E. T. (1975). *The Brain and Reward*, Pergamon Press, Oxford.

Rolls, E. T. (1976a). The neurophysiological basis of brain-stimulation reward, *in* A. Wauquier and E. T. Rolls (eds), *Brain-Stimulation Reward*, North Holland, Amsterdam, pp. 65–87.

Rolls, E. T. (1976b). Neurophysiology of feeding, *Life Sciences Research Report, Dahlem Konferenzen* **2**: 21–42.

Rolls, E. T. (1979). Effects of electrical stimulation of the brain on behaviour, *Psychology Surveys* **2**: 151–169.

Rolls, E. T. (1981a). Central nervous mechanisms related to feeding and appetite, *British Medical Bulletin* **37**: 131–134.

Rolls, E. T. (1981b). Processing beyond the inferior temporal visual cortex related to feeding, learning, and striatal function, *in* Y. Katsuki, R. Norgren and M. Sato (eds), *Brain Mechanisms of Sensation*, Wiley, New York, chapter 16, pp. 241–269.

Rolls, E. T. (1981c). Responses of amygdaloid neurons in the primate, *in* Y. Ben-Ari (ed.), *The Amygdaloid Complex*, Elsevier, Amsterdam, pp. 383–393.

Rolls, E. T. (1982). Neuronal mechanisms underlying the formation and disconnection of associations between visual stimuli and reinforcement in primates, *in* C. Woody (ed.), *Conditioning: Representation of Involved Neural Functions*, Plenum, New York, pp. 363–373.

Rolls, E. T. (1984a). Activity of neurons in different regions of the striatum of the monkey, *in* J. McKenzie, R. Kemm and L. Wilcox (eds), *The Basal Ganglia: Structure and Function*, Plenum, New York, pp. 467–493.

Rolls, E. T. (1984b). Neurons in the cortex of the temporal lobe and in the amygdala of the monkey with responses selective for faces, *Human Neurobiology* **3**: 209–222.

Rolls, E. T. (1986a). Neural systems involved in emotion in primates, *in* R. Plutchik and H. Kellerman (eds), *Emotion: Theory, Research, and Experience*, Vol. 3: Biological Foundations of Emotion, Academic Press, New York, chapter 5, pp. 125–143.

Rolls, E. T. (1986b). Neuronal activity related to the control of feeding, *in* R. Ritter, S. Ritter and C. Barnes (eds), *Feeding Behavior: Neural and Humoral Controls*, Academic Press, New York, chapter 6, pp. 163–190.

Rolls, E. T. (1986c). A theory of emotion, and its application to understanding the neural basis of emotion, *in* Y. Oomura (ed.), *Emotions. Neural and Chemical Control*, Japan Scientific Societies Press; and Karger, Tokyo; and Basel, pp. 325–344.

Rolls, E. T. (1987). Information representation, processing and storage in the brain: analysis at the single neuron level, *in* J.-P. Changeux and M. Konishi (eds), *The Neural and Molecular Bases of Learning*, Wiley, Chichester, pp. 503–540.

Rolls, E. T. (1989a). Functions of neuronal networks in the hippocampus and neocortex in memory, *in* J. Byrne and W. Berry (eds), *Neural Models of Plasticity: Experimental and Theoretical Approaches*, Academic Press, San Diego, chapter 13, pp. 240–265.

Rolls, E. T. (1989b). Information processing and basal ganglia function, *in* C. Kennard and M. Swash (eds), *Hierarchies in Neurology*, Springer-Verlag, London, chapter 15, pp. 123–142.

Rolls, E. T. (1989c). Information processing in the taste system of primates, *Journal of Experimental Biology* **146**: 141–164.

Rolls, E. T. (1989d). The representation and storage of information in neuronal networks in the primate cerebral cortex and hippocampus, *in* R. Durbin, C. Miall and G. Mitchison (eds), *The Computing Neuron*, Addison-Wesley, Wokingham, England, chapter 8, pp. 125–159.

Rolls, E. T. (1990a). Functions of different regions of the basal ganglia, *in* G. Stern (ed.), *Parkinson's Disease*, Chapman and Hall, London, chapter 5, pp. 151–184.

Rolls, E. T. (1990b). Functions of neuronal networks in the hippocampus and of backprojections in the cerebral cortex in memory, *in* J. McGaugh, N. Weinberger and G. Lynch (eds), *Brain Organization and Memory: Cells, Systems and Circuits*, Oxford University Press, New York, chapter 9, pp. 184–210.

Rolls, E. T. (1990c). Theoretical and neurophysiological analysis of the functions of the primate hippocampus in memory, *Cold Spring Harbor Symposia in Quantitative Biology* **55**: 995–1006.

Rolls, E. T. (1990d). A theory of emotion, and its application to understanding the neural basis of emotion, *Cognition and Emotion* **4**: 161–190.

Rolls, E. T. (1992a). Neurophysiological mechanisms underlying face processing within and beyond the temporal cortical visual areas, *Philosophical Transactions of the Royal Society* **335**: 11–21.

Rolls, E. T. (1992b). Neurophysiology and functions of the primate amygdala, *in* J. P. Aggleton (ed.), *The Amygdala*, Wiley-Liss, New York, chapter 5, pp. 143–165.

Rolls, E. T. (1992c). The processing of face information in the primate temporal lobe, *in* V. Bruce and M. Burton (eds), *Processing Images of Faces*, Ablex, Norwood, New Jersey, chapter 3. 41–68.

Rolls, E. T. (1993). The neural control of feeding in primates, *in* D. Booth (ed.), *Neurophysiology of Ingestion*, Pergamon, Oxford, chapter 9, pp. 137–169.

Rolls, E. T. (1994a). Brain mechanisms for invariant visual recognition and learning, *Behavioural Processes* **33**: 113–138.

Rolls, E. T. (1994b). Neurophysiology and cognitive functions of the striatum, *Revue Neurologique (Paris)* **150**: 648–660.

Rolls, E. T. (1995a). Central taste anatomy and neurophysiology, *in* R. Doty (ed.), *Handbook of Olfaction and Gustation*, Dekker, New York, chapter 24, pp. 549–573.

Rolls, E. T. (1995b). A theory of emotion and consciousness, and its application to understanding the neural basis of emotion, *in* M. Gazzaniga (ed.), *The Cognitive Neurosciences*, MIT Press, Cambridge, Mass, chapter 72, pp. 1091–1106.

Rolls, E. T. (1996a). The orbitofrontal cortex, *Philosophical Transactions of the Royal Society B* **351**: 1433–1444.

Rolls, E. T. (1996b). A theory of hippocampal function in memory, *Hippocampus* **6**: 601–620.

Rolls, E. T. (1997a). Consciousness in neural networks?, *Neural Networks* **10**: 1227–1240.

Rolls, E. T. (1997b). Neural processing underlying food selection, *in* H. Macbeth (ed.), *Food Preferences and Intake: Continuity and Change*, Berghahn, Oxford, chapter 4, pp. 39–53.

Rolls, E. T. (1997c). Taste and olfactory processing in the brain and its relation to the control of eating, *Critical Reviews in Neurobiology* **11**: 263–287.

Rolls, E. T. (1999a). *The Brain and Emotion*, Oxford University Press, Oxford.

Rolls, E. T. (1999b). The functions of the orbitofrontal cortex, *Neurocase* **5**: 301–312.

Rolls, E. T. (1999c). Spatial view cells and the representation of place in the primate hippocampus, *Hippocampus* **9**: 467–480.

Rolls, E. T. (2000a). Functions of the primate temporal lobe cortical visual areas in invariant visual object and face recognition, *Neuron* **27**: 205–218.

Rolls, E. T. (2000b). Hippocampo-cortical and cortico-cortical backprojections, *Hippocampus* **10**: 380–388.

Rolls, E. T. (2000c). Memory systems in the brain, *Annual Review of Psychology* **51**: 599–630.

Rolls, E. T. (2000d). Neurophysiology and functions of the primate amygdala, and the neural basis of emotion, *in* J. P. Aggleton (ed.), *The Amygdala: Second Edition. A Functional Analysis*, Oxford University Press, Oxford, chapter 13, pp. 447–478.

Rolls, E. T. (2000e). The orbitofrontal cortex and reward, *Cerebral Cortex* **10**: 284–294.

Rolls, E. T. (2000f). Précis of The Brain and Emotion, *Behavioral and Brain Sciences* **23**: 177–233.

Rolls, E. T. (2001a). The representation of umami taste in the human and macaque cortex, *Sensory Neuron* **3**: 227–242.

Rolls, E. T. (2001b). The rules of formation of the olfactory representations found in the orbitofrontal cortex olfactory areas in primates, *Chemical Senses* **26**: 595–604.

Rolls, E. T. (2002). A theory of emotion, its functions, and its adaptive value, *in* R. Trappl, P. Petta and S. Payr (eds), *Emotions in Humans and Artifacts*, MIT Press, Cambridge, Mass, chapter 2, pp. 11–32.

Rolls, E. T. (2003). Consciousness absent and present: a neurophysiological exploration, *Progress in Brain Research* **144**: 95–106.

Rolls, E. T. (2004a). Convergence of sensory systems in the orbitofrontal cortex in primates and brain design for emotion, *The Anatomical Record Part A* **281**: 1212–1225.

Rolls, E. T. (2004b). The functions of the orbitofrontal cortex, *Brain and Cognition* **55**: 11–29.

Rolls, E. T. (2004c). A higher order syntactic thought (HOST) theory of consciousness, *in* R. J. Gennaro (ed.), *Higher Order Theories of Consciousness*, John Benjamins, Amsterdam, chapter 7, pp. 137–172.

Rolls, E. T. (2004d). Invariant object and face recognition, *in* L. M. Chalupa and J. S. Werner (eds), *The Visual Neurosciences*, MIT Press, Cambridge, Mass, pp. 1165–1178.

Rolls, E. T. (2004e). Multimodal neuronal convergence of taste, somatosensory, visual, olfactory and auditory inputs, *in* G. Calvert, C. Spence and B. Stein (eds), *The Handbook of Multisensory Processes*, MIT Press, Cambridge, MA, chapter 19, pp. 311–331.

Rolls, E. T. (2004f). The operation of memory systems in the brain, *in* J. Feng (ed.), *Computational Neuroscience: A Comprehensive Approach*, CRC Press (UK), London, chapter 16, pp. 491–534.

Rolls, E. T. (2004g). Smell, taste, texture and temperature multimodal representations in the brain, and their relevance to the control of appetite, *Nutrition Reviews* **62**: 193–204.

Rolls, E. T. (2004h). Taste, olfactory, texture and temperature multimodal representations in the brain, and their relevance to the control of appetite, *Primatologie* **6**: 5–32.

Rolls, E. T. (2005). What are emotions, why do we have emotions, and what is their computational basis in the brain?, *in* J.-M. Fellous and M. A. Arbib (eds), *Who Needs Emotions? The Brain Meets the Robot*, Oxford University Press, New York, chapter 5, pp. 117–146.

Rolls, E. T. (2006a). The affective neuroscience of consciousness: higher order linguistic thoughts, dual routes to emotion and action, and consciousness, *in* P. Zelazo, M. Moscovitch and E. Thompson (eds), *Cambridge Handbook of Consciousness*, Cambridge University Press, New York, chapter 29.

Rolls, E. T. (2006b). Brain mechanisms underlying flavour and appetite, *Philosophical Transactions of the Royal Society B* **361**: 1123–1136.

Rolls, E. T. (2006c). Consciousness absent and present: a neurophysiological exploration of masking, *in* H. Ogmen and B. G. Breitmeyer (eds), *The First Half Second*, MIT Press, Cambridge, MA, chapter 6, pp. 89–108.

Rolls, E. T. (2006d). The neurophysiology and functions of the orbitofrontal cortex, *in* D. H. Zald and S. L. Rauch (eds), *The Orbitofrontal Cortex*, Oxford University Press, Oxford, chapter 5, pp. 95–124.

Rolls, E. T. (2007a). The anterior and midcingulate cortices and reward, *in* B. Vogt (ed.), *Cingulate Neurobiology and Disease*, Vol. Volume 1, Infrastructure, Diagnosis and Treatment, Oxford University Press, Oxford, chapter 8.

Rolls, E. T. (2007b). The central representation of flavor, *in* G. Shepherd, S. Firestein and D. V. Smith (eds), *Handbook of the Senses, Vol 2, Olfaction and Taste*, Academic Press, New York.

Rolls, E. T. (2007c). *Memory, Attention and Decision-Making*, Oxford University Press, Oxford.

Rolls, E. T. (2007d). A neuro-biological approach to emotional intelligence, *in* G. Matthews, M. Zeidner and R. Roberts (eds), *The Science of Emotional Intelligence: Knowns and Unknowns*, Oxford University Press, Oxford.

Rolls, E. T. (2007e). The representation of information about faces in the temporal and frontal lobes of primates including humans, *Neuropsychologia* **45**: 124–143.

Rolls, E. T. (2007f). Sensory processing in the brain related to the control of food intake, *Proceedings of the Nutrition Society* **66**: in press.

Rolls, E. T. (2007g). Understanding the mechanisms of food intake and obesity, *Obesity Reviews* **8**: 67–72.

Rolls, E. T. and Baylis, G. C. (1986). Size and contrast have only small effects on the responses to faces of neurons in the cortex of the superior temporal sulcus of the monkey, *Experimental Brain Research* **65**: 38–48.

Rolls, E. T. and Baylis, L. L. (1994). Gustatory, olfactory and visual convergence within the primate orbitofrontal cortex, *Journal of Neuroscience* **14**: 5437–5452.

Rolls, E. T. and Cooper, S. J. (1973). Activation of neurones in the prefrontal cortex by brain-stimulation reward in the rat, *Brain Research* **60**: 351–368.

Rolls, E. T. and Cooper, S. J. (1974). Connection between the prefrontal cortex and pontine brain-stimulation reward sites in the rat, *Experimental Neurology* **42**: 687–699.

Rolls, E. T. and Critchley, H. D. (2007). The representation of olfactory information by populations of neurons in the primate orbitofrontal cortex, *in preparation*.

Rolls, E. T. and de Waal, A. W. L. (1985). Long-term sensory-specific satiety: evidence from an Ethiopian refugee camp, *Physiology and Behavior* **34**: 1017–1020.

Rolls, E. T. and Deco, G. (2002). *Computational Neuroscience of Vision*, Oxford University Press, Oxford.

Rolls, E. T. and Deco, G. (2006). Attention in natural scenes: neurophysiological and computational bases, *Neural Networks* **19**: 1383–1394.

Rolls, E. T. and Johnstone, S. (1992). Neurophysiological analysis of striatal function, *in* G. Vallar, S. Cappa and C. Wallesch (eds), *Neuropsychological Disorders Associated with Subcortical Lesions*, Oxford University Press, Oxford, chapter 3, pp. 61–97.

Rolls, E. T. and Kelly, P. H. (1972). Neural basis of stimulus-bound locomotor activity in the rat, *Journal of Comparative and Physiological Psychology* **81**: 173–182.

Rolls, E. T. and Kesner, R. P. (2006). A theory of hippocampal function, and tests of the theory, *Progress in Neurobiology* **79**: 1–48.

Rolls, E. T. and Milward, T. (2000). A model of invariant object recognition in the visual system: learning rules, activation functions, lateral inhibition, and information-based performance measures, *Neural Computation* **12**: 2547–2572.

Rolls, E. T. and Rolls, B. J. (1973b). Altered food preferences after lesions in the basolateral region of the amygdala in the rat, *Journal of Comparative and Physiological Psychology* **83**: 248–259.

Rolls, E. T. and Rolls, B. J. (1977). Activity of neurones in sensory, hypothalamic and motor areas during feeding in the monkey, *in* Y. Katsuki, M. Sato, S. Takagi and Y. Oomura (eds), *Food Intake and Chemical Senses*, University of Tokyo Press, Tokyo, pp. 525–549.

Rolls, E. T. and Rolls, B. J. (1982b). Brain mechanisms involved in feeding, *in* L. Barker (ed.), *Psychobiology of Human Food Selection*, AVI Publishing Company, Westport, Connecticut, chapter 3, pp. 33–62.

Rolls, E. T. and Rolls, J. H. (1997). Olfactory sensory-specific satiety in humans, *Physiology and Behavior* **61**: 461–473.

Rolls, E. T. and Scott, T. R. (2003). Central taste anatomy and neurophysiology, *in* R. Doty (ed.), *Handbook of Olfaction and Gustation*, 2nd edn, Dekker, New York, chapter 33, pp. 679–705.

Rolls, E. T. and Stringer, S. M. (2000). On the design of neural networks in the brain by genetic evolution, *Progress in Neurobiology* **61**: 557–579.

Rolls, E. T. and Stringer, S. M. (2001a). Invariant object recognition in the visual system with error correction and temporal difference learning, *Network: Computation in Neural Systems* **12**: 111–129.

Rolls, E. T. and Stringer, S. M. (2001b). A model of the interaction between mood and memory, *Network: Computation in Neural Systems* **12**: 89–109.

Rolls, E. T. and Stringer, S. M. (2005). Spatial view cells in the hippocampus, and their idiothetic update based on place and head direction, *Neural Networks* **18**: 1229–1241.

Rolls, E. T. and Stringer, S. M. (2006). Invariant visual object recognition: a model, with lighting invariance, *Journal of Physiology - Paris* **100**: 43–62.

Rolls, E. T. and Tovee, M. J. (1994). Processing speed in the cerebral cortex and the neurophysiology of visual masking, *Proceedings of the Royal Society, B* **257**: 9–15.

Rolls, E. T. and Tovee, M. J. (1995a). The responses of single neurons in the temporal visual cortical areas of the macaque when more than one stimulus is present in the visual field, *Experimental Brain Research* **103**: 409–420.

Rolls, E. T. and Tovee, M. J. (1995b). Sparseness of the neuronal representation of stimuli in the primate temporal visual cortex, *Journal of Neurophysiology* **73**: 713–726.

Rolls, E. T. and Treves, A. (1990). The relative advantages of sparse versus distributed encoding for associative neuronal networks in the brain, *Network* **1**: 407–421.

Rolls, E. T. and Treves, A. (1998). *Neural Networks and Brain Function*, Oxford University Press, Oxford.

Rolls, E. T. and Williams, G. V. (1987a). Neuronal activity in the ventral striatum of the primate, *in* M. B. Carpenter and A. Jayamaran (eds), *The Basal Ganglia II - Structure and Function - Current Concepts*, Plenum, New York, pp. 349–356.

Rolls, E. T. and Williams, G. V. (1987b). Sensory and movement-related neuronal activity in different regions of the primate striatum, *in* J. Schneider and T. Lidsky (eds), *Basal Ganglia and Behavior: Sensory Aspects and Motor Functioning*, Hans Huber, Bern, pp. 37–59.

Rolls, E. T. and Xiang, J.-Z. (2005). Reward–spatial view representations and learning in the primate hippocampus, *Journal of Neuroscience* **25**: 6167–6174.

Rolls, E. T. and Xiang, J.-Z. (2006). Spatial view cells in the primate hippocampus, and memory recall, *Reviews in the Neurosciences* **17**: 175–200.

Rolls, E. T., Kelly, P. H. and Shaw, S. G. (1974a). Noradrenaline, dopamine and brain-stimulation reward, *Pharmacology, Biochemistry and Behavior* **2**: 735–740.

Rolls, E. T., Rolls, B. J., Kelly, P. H., Shaw, S. G. and Dale, R. (1974b). The relative attenuation of self-stimulation, eating and drinking produced by dopamine-receptor blockade, *Psychopharmacologia (Berlin)* **38**: 219–310.

Rolls, E. T., Burton, M. J. and Mora, F. (1976). Hypothalamic neuronal responses associated with the sight of food, *Brain Research* **111**: 53–66.

Rolls, E. T., Judge, S. J. and Sanghera, M. (1977). Activity of neurones in the inferotemporal cortex of the alert monkey, *Brain Research* **130**: 229–238.

Rolls, E. T., Sanghera, M. K. and Roper-Hall, A. (1979a). The latency of activation of neurons in the lateral hypothalamus and substantia innominata during feeding in the monkey, *Brain Research* **164**: 121–135.

Rolls, E. T., Thorpe, S. J., Maddison, S., Roper-Hall, A., Puerto, A. and Perrett, D. (1979b). Activity of neurones in the neostriatum and related structures in the alert animal, *in* I. Divac and R. Oberg (eds), *The Neostriatum*, Pergamon Press, Oxford, pp. 163–182.

Rolls, E. T., Burton, M. J. and Mora, F. (1980c). Neurophysiological analysis of brain-stimulation reward in the monkey, *Brain Research* **194**: 339–357.

Rolls, E. T., Perrett, D. I., Caan, A. W. and Wilson, F. A. W. (1982c). Neuronal responses related to visual recognition, *Brain* **105**: 611–646.

Rolls, E. T., Rolls, B. J. and Rowe, E. A. (1983b). Sensory-specific and motivation-specific satiety for the sight and taste of food and water in man, *Physiology and Behavior* **30**: 185–192.

Rolls, E. T., Thorpe, S. J. and Maddison, S. P. (1983c). Responses of striatal neurons in the behaving monkey. 1. head of the caudate nucleus, *Behavioural Brain Research* **7**: 179–

210.

Rolls, E. T., Thorpe, S. J., Boytim, M., Szabo, I. and Perrett, D. I. (1984b). Responses of striatal neurons in the behaving monkey. 3. Effects of iontophoretically applied dopamine on normal responsiveness, *Neuroscience* **12**: 1201–1212.

Rolls, E. T., Baylis, G. C. and Leonard, C. M. (1985). Role of low and high spatial frequencies in the face-selective responses of neurons in the cortex in the superior temporal sulcus, *Vision Research* **25**: 1021–1035.

Rolls, E. T., Murzi, E., Yaxley, S., Thorpe, S. J. and Simpson, S. J. (1986). Sensory-specific satiety: food-specific reduction in responsiveness of ventral forebrain neurons after feeding in the monkey, *Brain Research* **368**: 79–86.

Rolls, E. T., Scott, T. R., Sienkiewicz, Z. J. and Yaxley, S. (1988). The responsiveness of neurones in the frontal opercular gustatory cortex of the macaque monkey is independent of hunger, *Journal of Physiology* **397**: 1–12.

Rolls, E. T., Miyashita, Y., Cahusac, P. M. B., Kesner, R. P., Niki, H., Feigenbaum, J. and Bach, L. (1989a). Hippocampal neurons in the monkey with activity related to the place in which a stimulus is shown, *Journal of Neuroscience* **9**: 1835–1845.

Rolls, E. T., Sienkiewicz, Z. J. and Yaxley, S. (1989b). Hunger modulates the responses to gustatory stimuli of single neurons in the caudolateral orbitofrontal cortex of the macaque monkey, *European Journal of Neuroscience* **1**: 53–60.

Rolls, E. T., Yaxley, S. and Sienkiewicz, Z. J. (1990). Gustatory responses of single neurons in the orbitofrontal cortex of the macaque monkey, *Journal of Neurophysiology* **64**: 1055–1066.

Rolls, E. T., Hornak, J., Wade, D. and McGrath, J. (1994a). Emotion-related learning in patients with social and emotional changes associated with frontal lobe damage, *Journal of Neurology, Neurosurgery and Psychiatry* **57**: 1518–1524.

Rolls, E. T., Tovee, M. J., Purcell, D. G., Stewart, A. L. and Azzopardi, P. (1994b). The responses of neurons in the temporal cortex of primates, and face identification and detection, *Experimental Brain Research* **101**: 474–484.

Rolls, E. T., Critchley, H. D. and Treves, A. (1996a). The representation of olfactory information in the primate orbitofrontal cortex, *Journal of Neurophysiology* **75**: 1982–1996.

Rolls, E. T., Critchley, H. D., Mason, R. and Wakeman, E. A. (1996b). Orbitofrontal cortex neurons: role in olfactory and visual association learning, *Journal of Neurophysiology* **75**: 1970–1981.

Rolls, E. T., Critchley, H., Wakeman, E. A. and Mason, R. (1996c). Responses of neurons in the primate taste cortex to the glutamate ion and to inosine $5'$-monophosphate, *Physiology and Behavior* **59**: 991–1000.

Rolls, E. T., Robertson, R. G. and Georges-François, P. (1997a). Spatial view cells in the primate hippocampus, *European Journal of Neuroscience* **9**: 1789–1794.

Rolls, E. T., Treves, A. and Tovee, M. J. (1997b). The representational capacity of the distributed encoding of information provided by populations of neurons in the primate temporal visual cortex, *Experimental Brain Research* **114**: 149–162.

Rolls, E. T., Treves, A., Foster, D. and Perez-Vicente, C. (1997c). Simulation studies of the CA3 hippocampal subfield modelled as an attractor neural network, *Neural Networks* **10**: 1559–1569.

Rolls, E. T., Treves, A., Tovee, M. and Panzeri, S. (1997d). Information in the neuronal representation of individual stimuli in the primate temporal visual cortex, *Journal of

Computational Neuroscience **4**: 309–333.

Rolls, E. T., Critchley, H. D., Browning, A. and Hernadi, I. (1998a). The neurophysiology of taste and olfaction in primates, and umami flavor, *Annals of the New York Academy of Sciences* **855**: 426–437.

Rolls, E. T., Treves, A., Robertson, R. G., Georges-François, P. and Panzeri, S. (1998b). Information about spatial view in an ensemble of primate hippocampal cells, *Journal of Neurophysiology* **79**: 1797–1813.

Rolls, E. T., Critchley, H. D., Browning, A. S., Hernadi, A. and Lenard, L. (1999a). Responses to the sensory properties of fat of neurons in the primate orbitofrontal cortex, *Journal of Neuroscience* **19**: 1532–1540.

Rolls, E. T., Tovee, M. J. and Panzeri, S. (1999b). The neurophysiology of backward visual masking: information analysis, *Journal of Cognitive Neuroscience* **11**: 335–346.

Rolls, E. T., Stringer, S. M. and Trappenberg, T. P. (2002). A unified model of spatial and episodic memory, *Proceedings of The Royal Society B* **269**: 1087–1093.

Rolls, E. T., Aggelopoulos, N. C. and Zheng, F. (2003a). The receptive fields of inferior temporal cortex neurons in natural scenes, *Journal of Neuroscience* **23**: 339–348.

Rolls, E. T., Franco, L., Aggelopoulos, N. C. and Reece, S. (2003b). An information theoretic approach to the contributions of the firing rates and the correlations between the firing of neurons, *Journal of Neurophysiology* **89**: 2810–2822.

Rolls, E. T., Kringelbach, M. L. and De Araujo, I. E. T. (2003c). Different representations of pleasant and unpleasant odors in the human brain, *European Journal of Neuroscience* **18**: 695–703.

Rolls, E. T., O'Doherty, J., Kringelbach, M. L., Francis, S., Bowtell, R. and McGlone, F. (2003d). Representations of pleasant and painful touch in the human orbitofrontal and cingulate cortices, *Cerebral Cortex* **13**: 308–317.

Rolls, E. T., Verhagen, J. V. and Kadohisa, M. (2003e). Representations of the texture of food in the primate orbitofrontal cortex: neurons responding to viscosity, grittiness, and capsaicin, *Journal of Neurophysiology* **90**: 3711–3724.

Rolls, E. T., Aggelopoulos, N. C., Franco, L. and Treves, A. (2004). Information encoding in the inferior temporal visual cortex: contributions of the firing rates and the correlations between the firing of neurons, *Biological Cybernetics* **90**: 19–32.

Rolls, E. T., Browning, A. S., Inoue, K. and Hernadi, S. (2005a). Novel visual stimuli activate a population of neurons in the primate orbitofrontal cortex, *Neurobiology of Learning and Memory* **84**: 111–123.

Rolls, E. T., Franco, L. and Stringer, S. M. (2005b). The perirhinal cortex and long-term familiarity memory, *Quarterly Journal of Experimental Psychology B* **58**: 234—-245.

Rolls, E. T., Xiang, J.-Z. and Franco, L. (2005c). Object, space and object-space representations in the primate hippocampus, *Journal of Neurophysiology* **94**: 833–844.

Rolls, E. T., Critchley, H. D., Browning, A. S. and Inoue, K. (2006a). Face-selective and auditory neurons in the primate orbitofrontal cortex, *Experimental Brain Research* **170**: 7487.

Rolls, E. T., Franco, L., Aggelopoulos, N. C. and Jerez, J. M. (2006b). Information in the first spike, the order of spikes, and the number of spikes provided by neurons in the inferior temporal visual cortex, *Vision Research* **46**: 4193–4205.

Rolls, E. T., Critchley, H., Verhagen, J. V. and Kadohisa, M. (2007a). The representation of information about taste in the primate orbitofrontal cortex, *in preparation*.

Rolls, E. T., McCabe, C. and Redoute, J. (2007b). Expected value, reward outcome, and temporal difference error representations in a probabilistic decision task.

Rosenkilde, C. E. (1979). Functional heterogeneity of the prefrontal cortex in the monkey: a review, *Behavioral and Neural Biology* **25**: 301–345.

Rosenkilde, C. E., Bauer, R. H. and Fuster, J. M. (1981). Single unit activity in ventral prefrontal cortex in behaving monkeys, *Brain Research* **209**: 375–394.

Rosenthal, D. (1990). A theory of consciousness, *ZIF Report 40/1990. Zentrum für Interdisziplinaire Forschung, Bielefeld*. Reprinted in Block, N., Flanagan, O. and Guzeldere, G. (eds.) (1997) *The Nature of Consciousness: Philosophical Debates*. MIT Press, Cambridge MA, pp. 729–853.

Rosenthal, D. M. (1986). Two concepts of consciousness, *Philosophical Studies* **49**: 329–359.

Rosenthal, D. M. (1993). Thinking that one thinks, *in* M. Davies and G. W. Humphreys (eds), *Consciousness*, Blackwell, Oxford, chapter 10, pp. 197–223.

Rosenthal, D. M. (2004). Varieties of higher order theory, *in* R. J. Gennaro (ed.), *Higher Order Theories of Consciousness*, John Benjamins, Amsterdam, pp. 17–44.

Routtenberg, A., Gardner, E. I. and Huang, Y. H. (1971). Self-stimulation pathways in the monkey, Macaca mulatta, *Experimental Neurology* **33**: 213–224.

Royet, J. P., Zald, D., Versace, R., Costes, N., Lavenne, F., Koenig, O., Gervais, R., Routtenberg, A., Gardner, E. I. and Huang, Y. H. (2000). Emotional responses to pleasant and unpleasant olfactory, visual, and auditory stimuli: a positron emission tomography study, *Journal of Neuroscience* **20**: 7752–7759.

Rozin, P. and Kalat, J. W. (1971). Specific hungers and poison avoidance as adaptive specializations of learning, *Psychological Review* **78**: 459–486.

Rumelhart, D. E., Hinton, G. E. and Williams, R. J. (1986). Learning internal representations by error propagation, *in* D. E. Rumelhart, J. L. McClelland and the PDP Research Group (eds), *Parallel Distributed Processing: Explorations in the Microstructure of Cognition*, Vol. 1, MIT Press, Cambridge, MA, chapter 8, pp. 318–362.

Rushworth, M. F., Walton, M. E., Kennerley, S. W. and Bannerman, D. M. (2004). Action sets and decisions in the medial frontal cortex, *Trends in Cognitive Sciences* **8**: 410–417.

Rushworth, M. F. S., Hadland, K. A., Paus, T. and Sipila, P. K. (2002). Role of the human medial frontal cortex in task-switching: a combined fMRI and TMS study, *Journal of Neurophysiology* **87**: 2577–2592.

Rushworth, M. F. S., Hadland, K. A., Gaffan, D. and Passingham, R. E. (2003). The effect of cingulate cortex lesions on task switching and working memory, *Journal of Cognitive Neuroscience* **15**: 338–353.

Russchen, F. T., Amaral, D. G. and Price, J. L. (1985). The afferent connections of the substantia innominata in the monkey, Macaca fascicularis, *Journal of Comparative Neurology* **242**: 1–27.

Rusting, C. and Larsen, R. (1998). Personality and cognitive processing of affective information, *Personality and Social Psychology Bulletin* **24**: 200–213.

Rylander, G. (1948). Personality analysis before and after frontal lobotomy, *Association for Research into Nervous and Mental Disorders* **27** (**The Frontal Lobes**): 691–705.

Saint-Cyr, J. A., Ungerleider, L. G. and Desimone, R. (1990a). Organization of visual cortical inputs to the striatum and subsequent outputs to the pallido-nigral complex in the monkey, *Journal of Comparative Neurology* **298**: 129–156.

Saint-Cyr, J. A., Ungerleider, L. G. and Desimone, R. (1990b). Organization of visual cortical inputs to the striatum and subsequent outputs to the pallido-nigral complex in the monkey,

Journal of Comparative Neurology **298**: 129–156.

Salin, P. and Prince, D. (1996). Spontaneous GABA-A receptor mediated inhibitory currents in adult rat somatosensory cortex, *Journal of Neurophysiology* **75**: 1573–1588.

Sanghera, M. K., Rolls, E. T. and Roper-Hall, A. (1979). Visual responses of neurons in the dorsolateral amygdala of the alert monkey, *Experimental Neurology* **63**: 610–626.

Saper, C. B., Loewy, A. D., Swanson, L. W. and Cowan, W. M. (1976). Direct hypothalamo-autonomic connections, *Brain Research* **117**: 305–312.

Saper, C. B., Swanson, L. W. and Cowan, W. M. (1979). An autoradiographic study of the efferent connections of the lateral hypothalamic area in the rat, *Journal of Comparative Neurology* **183**: 689–706.

Sato, T. (1989). Interactions of visual stimuli in the receptive fields of inferior temporal neurons in macaque, *Experimental Brain Research* **77**: 23–30.

Sato, T., Kawamura, T. and Iwai, E. (1980). Responsiveness of inferotemporal single units to visual pattern stimuli in monkeys performing discrimination, *Experimental Brain Research* **38**: 313–319.

Savic, I. (2001). Smelling of odorous sex hormone-like compounds causes sex-differentiated hypothalamic activations in humans, *Neuron* **31**: 661–668.

Savic, I. (2002). Imaging of brain activation by odorants in humans, *Current Opinion in Neurobiology* **12**: 455–461.

Savic, I., Berglund, H., Gulyas, B. and Roland, P. (2001). Smelling of odorous sex hormones-like compounds causes sex-differentiated hypothalamic activations in humans, *Neuron* **31**: 661–668.

Schachter, S. (1971). Importance of cognitive control in obesity, *American Psychologist* **26**: 129–144.

Schachter, S. and Singer, J. (1962). Cognitive, social and physiological determinants of emotional state, *Psychological Review* **69**: 378–399.

Schacter, G. B., Yang, C. R., Innis, N. K. and Mogenson, G. J. (1989). The role of the hippocampal-nucleus accumbens pathway in radial-arm maze performance, *Brain Research* **494**: 339–349.

Schaefer, M. L., Young, D. A. and Restrepo, D. (2001). Olfactory fingerprints for major histocompatibility complex-determined body odors, *Journal of Neuroscience* **21**: 2481–2487.

Schaefer, M. L., Yamazaki, K., Osada, K., Restrepo, D. and Beauchamp, G. K. (2002). Olfactory fingerprints for major histocompatibility complex-determined body odors II: Relationship among odor maps, genetics, odor composition, and behavior, *Journal of Neuroscience* **22**: 9513–9521.

Scherer, K. S. (1999). Appraisal theory, *in* T. Dalgleish and M. J. Power (eds), *Handbook of Cognition and Emotion*, Wiley, New York, pp. 637–663.

Scherer, K. S. (2001). The nature and study of appraisal. A review of the issues, *in* K. S. Scherer, A. Schorr and T. Johnstone (eds), *Appraisal Processes in Emotion*, Oxford University Press, Oxford, pp. 369–391.

Scherer, K. S., Schorr, A. and Johnstone, T. (eds) (2001). *Appraisal Processes in Emotion*, Oxford University Press, Oxford.

Schirmer, A., Zysset, S., Kotz, S. A. and von Cramon, Y. D. (2004). Gender differences in the activation of inferior frontal cortex during emotional speech perception, *Neuroimage* **21**: 1114–1123.

Schmitt, D. P. (2004). The big five related to risky sexual behaviour across 10 world regions: differential personality associations of sexual promiscuity and relationship infidelity, *European Journal of Personality* **18**: 301–319.

Schoenbaum, G. and Eichenbaum, H. (1995). Information encoding in the rodent prefrontal cortex. I. Single-neuron activity in orbitofrontal cortex compared with that in pyriform cortex, *Journal of Neurophysiology* **74**: 733–750.

Schoenbaum, G. and Setlow, B. (2003). Lesions of nucleus accumbens disrupt learning about aversive outcomes, *Journal of Neuroscience* **23**: 9833–9841.

Schoenbaum, G., Chiba, A. A. and Gallagher, M. (1999). Neural encoding in orbitofrontal cortex and basolateral amygdala during olfactory discrimination learning, *Journal of Neuroscience* **19**: 1876–1884.

Schultz, W. (1998). Predictive reward signal of dopamine neurons, *Journal of Neurophysiology* **80**: 1–27.

Schultz, W. (2004). Neural coding of basic reward terms of animal learning theory, game theory, microeconomics and behavioural ecology, *Current Opinion in Neurobiology* **14**: 139–147.

Schultz, W., Apicella, P., Scarnati, E. and Ljungberg, T. (1992). Neuronal activity in the ventral striatum related to the expectation of reward, *Journal of Neuroscience* **12**: 4595–4610.

Schultz, W., Apicella, P., Romo, R. and Scarnati, E. (1995a). Context-dependent activity in primate striatum reflecting past and future behavioral events, *in* J. C. Houk, J. L. Davis and D. G. Beiser (eds), *Models of Information Processing in the Basal Ganglia*, MIT Press, Cambridge, MA, chapter 2, pp. 11–27.

Schultz, W., Romo, R., Ljunberg, T., Mirenowicz, J., Hollerman, J. R. and Dickinson, A. (1995b). Reward-related signals carried by dopamine neurons, *in* J. C. Houk, J. L. Davis and D. G. Beiser (eds), *Models of Information Processing in the Basal Ganglia*, MIT Press, Cambridge, MA, chapter 12, pp. 233–248.

Schultz, W., Dayan, P. and Montague, P. R. (1997). A neural substrate of prediction and reward, *Science* **275**: 1593–1599.

Schultz, W., Tremblay, L. and Hollerman, J. R. (2003). Changes in behavior-related neuronal activity in the striatum during learning, *Trends in Neurosciences* **26**: 312–328.

Schwaber, J. S., Kapp, B. S., Higgins, G. A. and Rapp, P. R. (1982). Amygdaloid and basal forebrain direct connections with the nucleus of the solitary tract and the dorsal motor nucleus, *Journal of Neuroscience* **2**: 1424–1438.

Scott, S. K., Young, A. W., Calder, A. J., Hellawell, D. J., Aggleton, J. P. and Johnson, M. (1997). Impaired auditory recognition of fear and anger following bilateral amygdala lesions, *Nature* **385**: 254–257.

Scott, T. R. and Giza, B. K. (1992). Gustatory control of ingestion, *in* D. A. Booth (ed.), *The Neurophysiology of Ingestion*, Manchester University Press, Manchester.

Scott, T. R., Yaxley, S., Sienkiewicz, Z. J. and Rolls, E. T. (1986a). Gustatory responses in the frontal opercular cortex of the alert cynomolgus monkey, *Journal of Neurophysiology* **56**: 876–890.

Scott, T. R., Yaxley, S., Sienkiewicz, Z. J. and Rolls, E. T. (1986b). Taste responses in the nucleus tractus solitarius of the behaving monkey, *Journal of Neurophysiology* **55**: 182–200.

Scott, T. R., Karadi, Z., Oomura, Y., Nishino, H., Plata-Salaman, C. R., Lenard, L., Giza, B. K. and Aou, S. (1993). Gustatory neural coding in the amygdala of the alert monkey,

Journal of Neurophysiology **69**: 1810–1820.

Scott, T. R., Yan, J. and Rolls, E. T. (1995). Brain mechanisms of satiety and taste in macaques, *Neurobiology* **3**: 281–292.

Seamans, J. K. and Yang, C. R. (2004). The principal features and mechanisms of dopamine modulation in the prefrontal cortex, *Progress in Neurobiology* **74**: 1–58.

Seigel, M. and Auerbach, J. M. (1996). Neuromodulators of synaptic strength, *in* M. S. Fazeli and G. L. Collingridge (eds), *Cortical Plasticity*, Bios, Oxford, chapter 7, pp. 137–148.

Seleman, L. D. and Goldman-Rakic, P. S. (1985). Longitudinal topography and interdigitation of corticostriatal projections in the rhesus monkey, *Journal of Neuroscience* **5**: 776–794.

Seltzer, B. and Pandya, D. N. (1989). Frontal lobe connections of the superior temporal sulcus in the rhesus monkey, *Journal of Comparative Neurology* **281**: 97–113.

Sem-Jacobsen, C. W. (1968). *Depth-Electrographic Stimulation of the Human Brain and Behavior: From Fourteen Years of Studies and Treatment of Parkinson's Disease and Mental Disorders with Implanted Electrodes*, C. C. Thomas, Springfield, Il.

Sem-Jacobsen, C. W. (1976). Electrical stimulation and self-stimulation in man with chronic implanted electrodes. Interpretation and pitfalls of results, *in* A. Wauquier and E. T. Rolls (eds), *Brain-Stimulation Reward*, North-Holland, Amsterdam, pp. 505–520.

Setlow, B., Gallagher, M. and Holland, P. C. (2002). The basolateral complex of the amygdala is necessary for acquisition but not expression of CS motivational value in appetitive Pavlovian second-order conditioning, *European Journal of Neuroscience* **15**: 1841–1853.

Setlow, B., Schoenbaum, G. and Gallagher, M. (2003). Neural encoding in ventral striatum during olfactory discrimination leanring, *Neuron* **38**: 625–636.

Seward, J. P., Uyeda, A. A. and Olds, J. (1959). Resistance to extinction following cranial self-stimulation, *Journal of Comparative and Physiological Psychology* **52**: 294–299.

Seymour, B., O'Doherty, J., Dayan, P., Koltzenburg, M., Jones, A. K., Dolan, R. J., Friston, K. J. and Frackowiak, R. S. (2004). Temporal difference models describe higher-order learning in humans, *Nature* **429**: 664–667.

Shackelford, T. K., Le Blanc, G. L., Weekes-Shackelford, V. A., Bleske-Rechek, A. L., Euler, H. A. and Hoier, S. (2002). Psychological adaptation to human sperm competition, *Evolution and Human Behaviour* **23**: 123–138.

Shallice, T. (1982). Specific impairments of planning, *Philosophical Transactions of the Royal Society of London B* **298**: 199–209.

Shallice, T. and Burgess, P. (1996). The domain of supervisory processes and temporal organization of behaviour, *Philosophical Transactions of the Royal Society B,* **351**: 1405–1411.

Shepherd, G. M. (2004). *The Synaptic Organisation of the Brain*, 5th edn, Oxford University Press, Oxford.

Shidara, M. and Richmond, B. J. (2002). Anterior cingulate: single neuronal signals related to degreee of reward expectancy, *Science* **296**: 1709–1711.

Shiino, M. and Fukai, T. (1990). Replica-symmetric theory of the nonlinear analogue neural networks, *Journal of Physics A: Math. Gen.* **23**: L1009–L1017.

Shima, K. and Tanji, J. (1998). Role for cingulate motor area cells in voluntary movement selection based on reward, *Science* **13**: 1335–1338.

Shimura, T. and Shimokochi, M. (1990). Involvement of the lateral mesencephalic tegmentum in copulatory behavior of male rats: neuron activity in freely moving animals, *Neuroscience Research* **9**: 173–183.

Shizgal, P. and Arvanitogiannis, A. (2003). Gambling on dopamine, *Science* **299**: 1856–1858.

Shizgal, P. and Murray, X. (1989). Neuronal basis of intracranial self-stimulation, *in* J. M. Liebman and S. J. Cooper (eds), *The Neuropharmacological Basis of Reward*, Oxford University Press, Oxford.

Short, R. V. (1998). Review of R. R. Baker and M. A. Bellis, Human Sperm Competition: Copulation, Masturbation and Infidelity, *European Sociobiological Society Newsletter* **47**: 20–23.

Simmen-Tulberg, B. and Moller, A. P. (1993). The relationship between concealed ovulation and mating systems in anthropoid primates: a phylogenetic analysis, *American Naturalist* **141**: 1–25.

Simmons, L. W., Firman, R. C., Rhodes, G. and Peters, M. (2004). Human sperm competition: testis size, sperm production and rate of extra-pair copulations, *Animal Behaviour* **68**: 297–302.

Simpson, J. B., Epstein, A. N. and Camardo, J. S. (1977). The localization of receptors for the dipsogenic action of angiotensin II in the subfornical organ, *Journal of Comparative and Physiological Psychology* **91**: 1220–1231.

Singer, P. (1981). *The Expanding Circle: Ethics and Sociobiology*, Oxford University Press, Oxford.

Singer, T., Seymour, B., O'Doherty, J., Kaube, H., Dolan, R. J. and Frith, C. D. (2004). Empathy for pain involves the affective but not sensory components of pain, *Science* **303**: 1157–1162.

Singer, W. (1987). Activity-dependent self-organization of synaptic connections as a substrate for learning, *in* J.-P. Changeux and M. Konishi (eds), *The Neural and Molecular Bases of Learning*, Wiley, Chichester, pp. 301–335.

Singer, W. (1995). Development and plasticity of cortical processing architectures, *Science* **270**: 758–764.

Singer, W. (1999). Neuronal synchrony: A versatile code for the definition of relations?, *Neuron* **24**: 49–65.

Singh, D. (1993). Adaptive significance of female physical attractiveness: role of waist-to-hip ratio, *Journal of Personality and Social Psychology* **65**: 293–307.

Singh, D. (1995). Female health, attractiveness, and desirability for relationships: role of breast asymmetry and waist-to-hip ratio, *Ethology and Sociobiology* **16**: 465–481.

Singh, D. and Bronstad, M. P. (2001). Female body odour is a potential cue to ovulation, *Proceedings of the Royal Society of London B* **268**: 797–801.

Singh, D. and Luis, S. (1995). Ethnic and gender consensus for the effect of waist-to-hip ratio on judgements of women's attractiveness, *Human Nature* **6**: 51–65.

Singh, D. and Young, R. K. (1995). Body weight, waist-to-hip ratio, breasts and hips: role in judgements of female attractiveness and desirability for relationships, *Ethology and Sociobiology* **16**: 483–507.

Singh, D., Meyer, W., Zambarano, R. J. and Hurlbert, D. F. (1998). Frequency and timing of coital orgasm in women desirous of becoming pregnant, *Archives of Sexual Behaviour* **27**: 15–29.

Sisk, C. L. and Foster, D. L. (2004). The neural basis of puberty and adolescence, *Nature Neuroscience* **7**: 1040–1047.

Small, D. M., Zald, D. H., Jones-Gotman, M., Zatorre, R. J., Petrides, M. and Evans, A. C. (1999). Human cortical gustatory areas: a review of functional neuroimaing data,

NeuroReport **8**: 3913–3917.

Smith, R. L. (1984). Human sperm competiton, *in* R. L. Smith (ed.), *Sperm Competition and the Evolution of Animal Mating Systems*, Academic Press, London, pp. 601–660.

Sobel, N., Prabhakaran, V., Hartley, C. A., Desmond, J. E., Glover, G. H., Sullivan, E. V. and Gabrieli, J. D. (1999). Blind smell: brain activation induced by an undetected air-borne chemical, *Brain* **122**: 209–217.

Sompolinsky, H. and Kanter, I. (1986). Temporal association in asymmetric neural networks, *Physical Review Letters* **57**: 2861–2864.

Spangler, R., Wittkowski, K. M., Goddard, N. L., Avena, N. M., Hoebel, B. G. and Leibowitz, S. F. (2004). Opiate-like effects of sugar on gene expression in reward areas of the rat brain, *Molecular Brain Research* **124**: 134–142.

Spiegler, B. J. and Mishkin, M. (1981). Evidence for the sequential participation of inferior temporal cortex and amygdala in the acquisition of stimulus–reward associations, *Behavioural Brain Research* **3**: 303–317.

Spitzer, H., Desimone, R. and Moran, J. (1988). Increased attention enhances both behavioral and neuronal performance, *Science* **240**: 338–340.

Spruston, N., Jonas, P. and Sakmann, B. (1995). Dendritic glutamate receptor channel in rat hippocampal CA3 and CA1 pyramidal neurons, *Journal of Physiology* **482**: 325–352.

Squire, L. R. (1992). Memory and the hippocampus: A synthesis from findings with rats, monkeys and humans, *Psychological Review* **99**: 195–231.

Squire, L. R., Stark, C. E. L. and Clark, R. E. (2004). The medial temporal lobe, *Annual Review of Neuroscience* **27**: 279–306.

Starkstein, S. E. and Robinson, R. G. (1991). The role of the frontal lobe in affective disorder following stroke, *in* H. M. Eisenberg (ed.), *Frontal Lobe Function and Dysfunction*, Oxford University Press, New York, pp. 288–303.

Stefanacci, L., Suzuki, W. A. and Amaral, D. G. (1996). Organization of connections between the amygdaloid complex and the perirhinal and parahippocampal cortices in macaque monkeys, *Journal of Comparative Neurology* **375**: 552–582.

Stein, L. (1967). Psychopharmacological substrates of mental depression, *in* G. Garattini and M. N. G. Dukes (eds), *Anti-Depressant Drugs*, Excerpta Medica Foundation, Amsterdam.

Stein, L. (1969). Chemistry of purposive behavior, *in* J. Tapp (ed.), *Reinforcement and Behavior*, Academic Press, New York, pp. 328–335.

Stein, N. L., Trabasso, T. and Liwag, M. (1994). The Rashomon phenomenon: personal frames and future-oriented appraisals in memory for emotional events, *in* M. M. Haith, J. B. Benson, R. J. Roberts and B. F. Pennington (eds), *Future Oriented Processes*, University of Chicago Press, Chicago.

Steiner, J. E., Glaser, D., Hawilo, M. E. and Berridge, K. C. (2001). Comparative expression of hedonic impact: affective reactions to taste by human infants and other primates, *Neuroscience and Biobehavioral Reviews* **25**: 53–74.

Stellar, E. (1954). The physiology of motivation, *Psychological Review* **61**: 5–22.

Stellar, J. R. and Rice, M. B. (1989). Pharmacological basis of intracranial self-stimulation, *in* J. M. Liebman and S. J. Cooper (eds), *The Neuropharmacological Basis of Reward*, Oxford University Press, Oxford, pp. 14–65.

Stellar, J. R. and Stellar, E. (1985). *The Neurobiology of Motivation and Reward*, Springer, New York.

Stemmler, D. G. (1989). The autonomic differentiation of emotions revisited: convergent and discriminant validation, *Psychophysiology* **26**: 617–632.

Stent, G. S. (1973). A psychological mechanism for Hebb's postulate of learning, *Proceedings of the National Academy of Sciences USA* **70**: 997–1001.

Stern, C. E. and Passingham, R. E. (1995). The nucleus accumbens in monkeys (Macaca fascicularis): III. Reversal learning, *Experimental Brain Research* **106**: 239–247.

Stern, C. E. and Passingham, R. E. (1996). The nucleus accumbens in monkeys (Macaca fascicularis): II. Emotion and motivation, *Behavioural Brain Research* **75**: 179–193.

Stevens, J. R., Mark, V. H., Ervin, F., Pacheco, P. and Suematsu, K. (1969). Deep temporal stimulation in man, *Archives of Neurology* **21**: 157–169.

Stone, V. E., Baron-Cohen, S., Calder, A., Keane, J. and Young, A. (2003). Acquired theory of mind impairments in individuals with bilateral amygdala lesions, *Neuropsychologia* **41**: 209–220.

Strauss, E. and Moscowitsch, M. (1981). Perception of facial expressions, *Brain and Language* **13**: 308–332.

Strick, P. L., Dum, R. P. and Picard, N. (1995). Macro-organization of the circuits connecting the basal ganglia with the cortical motor areas, *in* J. C. Houk, J. L. Davis and D. G. Beiser (eds), *Models of Information Processing in the Basal Ganglia*, MIT Press, Cambridge, MA, chapter 6, pp. 117–130.

Stricker, E. M. (1984). Brain catecholamines and the central control of food intake, *International Journal of Obesity* **8**: 39–50.

Stricker, E. M. and Zigmond, M. J. (1976). Recovery of function after damage to central catecholamine-containing neurons: a neurochemical model for the lateral hypothalamic syndrome, *Progress in Psychobiology and Physiological Psychology* **6**: 121–188.

Stringer, S. M. and Rolls, E. T. (2000). Position invariant recognition in the visual system with cluttered environments, *Neural Networks* **13**: 305–315.

Stringer, S. M. and Rolls, E. T. (2002). Invariant object recognition in the visual system with novel views of 3D objects, *Neural Computation* **14**: 2585–2596.

Stringer, S. M., Perry, G., Rolls, E. T. and Proske, J. H. (2006). Learning invariant object recognition in the visual system with continuous transformations, *Biological Cybernetics* **94**: 128–142.

Strongman, K. T. (2003). *The Psychology of Emotion*, 5th edn, Wiley, New York.

Suri, R. E. and Schultz, W. (1998). Learning of sequential movements by neural network model with dopamine-like reinforcement signal, *Experimental Brain Research* **121**: 350–354.

Suri, R. E. and Schultz, W. (2001). Temporal difference model reproduces anticipatory neural activity, *Neural Computation* **13**: 841–862.

Sutherland, S. (1997). Emotional displays, *Nature* **390**: 458.

Sutton, R. S. and Barto, A. G. (1981). Towards a modern theory of adaptive networks: expectation and prediction, *Psychological Review* **88**: 135–170.

Sutton, R. S. and Barto, A. G. (1990). Time-derivative models of Pavlovian reinforcement, *in* M. Gabriel and J. Moore (eds), *Learning and Computational Neuroscience*, MIT Press, Cambridge, MA, pp. 497–537.

Sutton, R. S. and Barto, A. G. (1998). *Reinforcement Learning*, MIT Press, Cambridge, Mass.

Suzuki, W. A. and Amaral, D. G. (1994). Perirhinal and parahippocampal cortices of the macaque monkey - cortical afferents, *Journal of Comparative Neurology* **350**: 497–533.

Suzuki, W. A., Miller, E. K. and Desimone, R. (1997). Object and place memory in the macaque entorhinal cortex, *Journal of Neurophysiology* **78**: 1062–1081.

Swaddle, J. P. and Reierson, G. W. (2002). Testosterone increases perceived dominance but not attractiveness in human males, *Proceedings of the Royal Society of London B* **269**: 2285–2289.

Swash, M. (1989). John Hughlings Jackson: a historical introduction, *in* C. Kennard and M. Swash (eds), *Hierarchies in Neurology*, Springer, London, chapter 1, pp. 3–10.

Tabuchi, E., Mulder, A. B. and Wiener, S. I. (2003). Reward value invariant place responses and reward site associated activity in hippocampal neurons of behaving rats, *Hippocampus* **13**: 117–132.

Tagamets, M. and Horwitz, B. (1998). Integrating electrophysical and anatomical experimental data to create a large-scale model that simulates a delayed match-to-sample human brain study, *Cerebral Cortex* **8**: 310–320.

Taira, K. and Rolls, E. T. (1996). Receiving grooming as a reinforcer for the monkey, *Physiology and Behavior* **59**: 1189–1192.

Takagi, S. F. (1991). Olfactory frontal cortex and multiple olfactory processing in primates, *in* A. Peters and E. G. Jones (eds), *Cerebral Cortex*, Vol. 9, Plenum Press, New York, pp. 133–152.

Takeda, K. and Funahashi, S. (2002). Prefrontal task-related activity representing visual cue location or saccade direction in spatial working memory tasks, *Journal of Neurophysiology* **87**: 567–588.

Tanabe, T., Iino, M. and Takagi, S. F. (1975a). Discrimination of odors in olfactory bulb, pyriform-amygdaloid areas, and orbitofrontal cortex of the monkey, *Journal of Neurophysiology* **38**: 1284–1296.

Tanabe, T., Yarita, H., Iino, M., Ooshima, Y. and Takagi, S. F. (1975b). An olfactory projection area in orbitofrontal cortex of the monkey, *Journal of Neurophysiology* **38**: 1269–1283.

Tanaka, D. (1973). Effects of selective prefrontal decortication on escape behavior in the monkey, *Brain Research* **53**: 161–173.

Tanaka, K., Saito, C., Fukada, Y. and Moriya, M. (1990). Integration of form, texture, and color information in the inferotemporal cortex of the macaque, *in* E. Iwai and M. Mishkin (eds), *Vision, Memory and the Temporal Lobe*, Elsevier, New York, chapter 10, pp. 101–109.

Tanaka, S. C., Doya, K., Okada, G., Ueda, K., Okamoto, Y. and Yamawaki, S. (2004). Prediction of immediate and future rewards differentially recruits cortico-basal ganglia loops, *Nature Neuroscience* **7**: 887–893.

Tessman, I. (1995). Human altruism as a courtship display, *Oikos* **74**: 157–158.

Thierry, A. M., Tassin, J. P., Blanc, G. and Glowinski, J. (1976). Selective activation of mesocortical DA system by stress, *Nature* **263**: 242–244.

Thornhill, R. (1983). Cryptic female choice amd its implications in the scorpionfly *Harpobittacus nigriceps*, *American Naturalist* **122**: 765–788.

Thornhill, R. and Gangestad, S. W. (1996). The evolution of human sexuality, *Trends in Ecology and Evolution* **11**: 98–102.

Thornhill, R. and Gangstad, S. W. (1999). The scent of symmetry: a human sex pheromone that signals fitness?, *Evolution and Human Behaviour* **20**: 175–201.

Thornhill, R. and Grammer, K. (1999). The body and face of woman: one ornament that signals quality?, *Evolution and Human Behaviour* **20**: 105–120.

Thornhill, R., Gangestad, S. W. and Comer, R. (1995). Human female orgasm and mate fluctuating asymmetry, *Animal Behaviour* **50**: 1601–1615.

Thorpe, S. J., Rolls, E. T. and Maddison, S. (1983). Neuronal activity in the orbitofrontal cortex of the behaving monkey, *Experimental Brain Research* **49**: 93–115.

Thrasher, T. N., Brown, C. J., Keil, L. C. and Ramsay, D. J. (1980a). Thirst and vasopressin release in the dog: an osmoreceptor or sodium receptor mechanism?, *American Journal of Physiology* **238**: R333–R339.

Thrasher, T. N., Jones, R. G., Keil, L. C., Brown, C. J. and Ramsay, D. J. (1980b). Drinking and vasopressin release during ventricular infusions of hypertonic solutions, *American Journal of Physiology* **238**: R340–R345.

Tiffany, S. T. and Drobes, D. J. (1990). Imagery and smoking urges: the manipulation of affective content, *Addiction and Behaviour* **15**: 531–539.

Tiihonen, J., Kuikka, J., Kupila, J., Partanen, K., Vainio, P., Airaksinen, J., Eronen, M., Hallikainen, T., Paanila, J., Kinnunen, I. and Huttunen, J. (1994). Increase in cerebral blood flow of right prefrontal cortex in man during orgasm, *Neuroscience Letters* **170**: 241–243.

Tinbergen, N. (1951). *The Study of Instinct*, Oxford University Press, Oxford.

Tinbergen, N. (1963). On aims and methods of ethology, *Zeitschrift fur Tierpsychologie* **20**: 410–433.

Tinbergen, N., Broekhuysen, G. J., Feekes, F., Houghton, J. C. W., Kruuk, H. and Szule, E. (1967). Egg shell removal by black-headed gull L*arus ribibundus*, *Behaviour* **19**: 74–117.

Tobler, P. N., Dickinson, A. and Schultz, W. (2003). Coding of predicted reward omission by dopamine neurons in a conditioned inhibition paradigm, *Journal of Neuroscience* **23**: 10402–10410.

Tomkins, S. S. (1995). *Exploring Affect: The Selected Writings of Sylvan S. Tomkins*, Cambridge University Press, New York.

Torrey, E. F., Webster, M., Knable, M., Johnson, N. and Yolken, R. H. (2000). Stanley Foundation Brain Collection and Neuropathology Consortium, *Schizophrenia Research* **44**: 151–155.

Tovee, M. J. and Rolls, E. T. (1992). Oscillatory activity is not evident in the primate temporal visual cortex with static stimuli, *Neuroreport* **3**: 369–372.

Tovee, M. J. and Rolls, E. T. (1995). Information encoding in short firing rate epochs by single neurons in the primate temporal visual cortex, *Visual Cognition* **2**: 35–58.

Tovee, M. J., Rolls, E. T., Treves, A. and Bellis, R. P. (1993). Information encoding and the responses of single neurons in the primate temporal visual cortex, *Journal of Neurophysiology* **70**: 640–654.

Tovee, M. J., Rolls, E. T. and Azzopardi, P. (1994). Translation invariance and the responses of neurons in the temporal visual cortical areas of primates, *Journal of Neurophysiology* **72**: 1049–1060.

Tovee, M. J., Rolls, E. T. and Ramachandran, V. S. (1996). Rapid visual learning in neurones of the primate temporal visual cortex, *NeuroReport* **7**: 2757–2760.

Towbin, E. J. (1949). Gastric distension as a factor in the satiation of thirst in esophagostomized dogs, *American Journal of Physiology* **159**: 533–541.

Tranel, D., Bechara, A. and Denburg, N. L. (2002). Asymmetric functional roles of right and left ventromedial prefrontal cortices in social conduct, decision-making and emotional processing, *Cortex* **38**: 589–612.

Trappenberg, T. P., Rolls, E. T. and Stringer, S. M. (2002). Effective size of receptive fields of inferior temporal visual cortex neurons in natural scenes, *in* T. G. Dietterich, S. Becker and Z. Gharamani (eds), *Advances in Neural Information Processing Systems*, Vol. 14,

MIT Press, Cambridge, MA, pp. 293–300.

Tremblay, L. and Schultz, W. (1998). Modifications of reward expectation-related neuronal activity during learning in primate striatum, *Journal of Neurophysiology* **80**: 964–977.

Tremblay, L. and Schultz, W. (1999). Relative reward preference in primate orbitofrontal cortex, *Nature* **398**: 704–708.

Tremblay, L. and Schultz, W. (2000). Modifications of reward expectation-related neuronal activity during learning in primate orbitofrontal cortex, *Journal of Neurophysiology* **83**: 1877–1885.

Treves, A. (1993). Mean-field analysis of neuronal spike dynamics, *Network* **4**: 259–284.

Treves, A. (1995). Quantitative estimate of the information relayed by the Schaffer collaterals, *Journal of Computational Neuroscience* **2**: 259–272.

Treves, A. and Rolls, E. T. (1991). What determines the capacity of autoassociative memories in the brain?, *Network* **2**: 371–397.

Treves, A. and Rolls, E. T. (1992). Computational constraints suggest the need for two distinct input systems to the hippocampal CA3 network, *Hippocampus* **2**: 189–199.

Treves, A. and Rolls, E. T. (1994). A computational analysis of the role of the hippocampus in memory, *Hippocampus* **4**: 374–391.

Treves, A., Panzeri, S., Rolls, E. T., Booth, M. and Wakeman, E. A. (1999). Firing rate distributions and efficiency of information transmission of inferior temporal cortex neurons to natural visual stimuli, *Neural Computation* **11**: 611–641.

Trivers, R. (1971). The evolution of reciprocal altruism, *Quarterly Review of Biology* **46**: 35–57.

Trivers, R. (1974). Parent-offspring conflict, *American Zoologist* **14**: 249–264.

Trivers, R. L. (1976). Foreword, *The Selfish Gene by R. Dawkins*, Oxford University Press, Oxford.

Trivers, R. L. (1985). *Social Evolution*, Benjamin, Cummings, CA.

Troisi, A. and Carosi, M. (1998). Female orgasm rate increases with male dominance in Japanese macaque, *Animal Behaviour* **56**: 1261–1266.

Tuckwell, H. (1988). *Introduction to Theoretical Neurobiology*, Cambridge University Press, Cambridge.

Udry, J. R. and Eckland, B. K. (1984). Benefits of being attractive: differential pay-offs for men and women, *Psychological Reports* **54**: 47–56.

Ullsperger, M. and von Cramon, D. Y. (2001). Subprocesses of performance monitoring: a dissociation of error processing and response competition revealed by event-related fMRI and ERPs, *Neuroimage* **14**: 1387–1401.

Uma-Pradeep, K., Geervani, P. and Eggum, B. O. (1993). Common Indian spices: nutrient composition, consumption and contribution to dietary value, *Plant Foods and Human Nutrition* **44**: 138–148.

Ungerstedt, U. (1971). Adipsia and aphagia after 6-hydroxydopamine induced degeneration of the nigrostriatal dopamine system, *Acta Physiologia Scandinavica* **81 (Suppl. 367)**: 95–122.

Uvnas-Moberg, K. (1997). Physiological and endocrine effects of social contact, *Annals of the New York Academy of Sciences* **807**: 146–163.

Uvnas-Moberg, K. (1998). Oxytocin may mediate the benefits of positive social interaction and emotions, *Psychneuroendocrinology* **23**: 819–835.

Valenstein, E. S. (1964). Problems of measurement and interpretation with reinforcing brain stimulation, *Psychological Review* **71**: 415–437.

Valenstein, E. S. (1974). *Brain Control. A Critical Examination of Brain Stimulation and Psychosurgery*, Wiley, New York.

Valenstein, E. S., Cox, V. C. and Kakolewski, J. W. (1970). A re-examination of the role of the hypothalamus in motivation, *Psychological Review* **77**: 16–31.

van den Pol, A. N. (2003). Weighing the role of hypothalamic feeding neurotransmitters, *Neuron* **40**: 1059–1061.

van der Berge, P. L. and Frost, P. (1986). Skin colour preferences, sexual dimorphism and sexual selection: a case for gene culture evolution, *Ethnic and Racial Studies* **9**: 87–113.

Van der Kooy, D., Koda, L. Y., McGinty, J. F., Gerfen, C. R. and Bloom, F. E. (1984). The organization of projections from the cortex, amygdala, and hypothalamus to the nucleus of the solitary tract in rat, *Journal of Comparative Neurology* **224**: 1–24.

Van Hoesen, G. W. (1981). The differential distribution, diversity and sprouting of cortical projections to the amygdala in the rhesus monkey, *in* Y. Ben-Ari (ed.), *The Amygdaloid Complex*, Elsevier, Amsterdam, pp. 77–90.

Van Hoesen, G. W., Yeterian, E. H. and Lavizzo-Mourey, R. (1981). Widespread corticostriate projections from temporal cortex of the rhesus monkey, *Journal of Comparative Neurology* **199**: 205–219.

Van Hoesen, G. W., Morecraft, R. J. and Vogt, B. A. (1993). Connections of the monkey cingulate cortex, *in* B. A. Vogt and M. Gabriel (eds), *The Neurobiology of the Cingulate Cortex and Limbic Thalamus: A Comprehensive Handbook*, Birkhauser, Boston, pp. 249–284.

van Veen, V., Cohen, J. D., Botvinick, M. M., Stenger, A. V. and Carter, C. S. (2001). Anterior cingulate cortex, conflict monitoring, and levels of processing, *Neuroimage* **14**: 1302–1308.

Verhagen, J. V., Rolls, E. and Kadohisa, M. (2003). Neurons in the primate orbitofrontal cortex respond to fat texture independently of viscosity, *Journal of Neurophysiology* **90**: 1514–1525.

Verhagen, J. V., Kadohisa, M. and Rolls, E. T. (2004). The primate insular taste cortex: neuronal representations of the viscosity, fat texture, grittiness, and the taste of foods in the mouth, *Journal of Neurophysiology* **92**: 1685–1699.

Voellm, B. A., De Araujo, I. E. T., Cowen, P. J., Rolls, E. T., Kringelbach, M. L., Smith, K. A., Jezzard, P., Heal, R. J. and Matthews, P. M. (2004). Methamphetamine activates reward circuitry in drug naive human subjects, *Neuropsychopharmacology* **29**: 1715–1722.

Vogt, B. A. and Pandya, D. N. (1987). Cingulate cortex of the rhesus monkey: II. Cortical afferents, *Journal of Comparative Neurology* **262**: 271–289.

Vogt, B. A. and Sikes, R. W. (2000). The medial pain system, cingulate cortex, and parallel processing of nociceptive information, *Progress in Brain Research* **122**: 223–235.

Vogt, B. A., Pandya, D. N. and Rosene, D. L. (1987). Cingulate cortex of the rhesus monkey: I. Cytoarchitecture and thalamic afferents, *Journal of Comparative Neurology* **262**: 256–270.

Vogt, B. A., Derbyshire, S. and Jones, A. K. P. (1996). Pain processing in four regions of human cingulate cortex localized with co-registered PET and MR imaging, *European Journal of Neuroscience* **8**: 1461–1473.

Vogt, B. A., Berger, G. R. and Derbyshire, S. W. G. (2003). Structural and functional dichotomy of human midcingulate cortex, *European Journal of Neuroscience* **18**: 3134–

3144.

Waelti, P., Dickinson, A. and Schultz, W. (2001). Dopamine responses comply with basic assumptions of formal learning theory, *Nature* **412**: 43–48.

Wagner, H. (1989). The peripheral physiological differentiation of emotions, *in* H. Wagner and A. Manstead (eds), *Handbook of Social Psychophysiology*, Wiley, Chichester, pp. 77–98.

Wallis, G. and Rolls, E. T. (1997). Invariant face and object recognition in the visual system, *Progress in Neurobiology* **51**: 167–194.

Wallis, J. D. and Miller, E. K. (2003). Neuronal activity in primate dorsolateral and orbital prefrontal cortex during performance of a reward preference task, *European Journal of Neuroscience* **18**: 2069–2081.

Wallis, J., Anderson, K. and Miller, E. (2001). Single neurons in prefrontal cortex encode abstract rules, *Nature* **411**: 953–956.

Walton, M. E., Bannerman, D. M. and Rushworth, M. F. S. (2002). The role of rat medial frontal cortex in effort-based decision making, *Journal of Neuroscience* **22**: 10996–11003.

Walton, M. E., Bannerman, D. M., Alterescu, K. and Rushworth, M. F. S. (2003). Functional specialization within medial frontal cortex of the anterior cingulate for evaluating effort-related decisions, *Journal of Neuroscience* **23**: 6475–6479.

Wang, X. J. (1999). Synaptic basis of cortical persistent activity: the importance of NMDA receptors to working memory, *Journal of Neuroscience* **19**: 9587–9603.

Watanabe, K., Lauwereyns, J. and Hikosaka, O. (2003). Neural correlates of rewarded and unrewarded eye movements in the primate caudate nucleus, *Journal of Neuroscience* **23**: 10052–10057.

Watanabe, M., Hikosaka, K., Sakagami, M. and Shirakawa, S. (2002). Coding and monitoring of motivational context in the primate prefrontal cortex, *Journal of Neuroscience* **22**: 2391–2400.

Watson, J. B. (1929). *Psychology: From the Standpoint of a Behaviorist*, 3rd edn, Lippincott, Philadelphia.

Watson, J. B. (1930). *Behaviorism: Revised Edition*, University of Chicago Press, Chicago.

Wauquier, A. and Niemegeers, C. J. E. (1972). Intra-cranial self-stimulation in rats as a function of various stimulus parameters: II, influence of haloperidol, pimozide and pipamperone on medial forebrain stimulation with monopolar electrodes, *Psychopharmacology* **27**: 191–202.

Wedell, N., Gage, M. J. and Parker, G. (2002). Sperm competition, male prudence and sperm limited females, *Proceedings of the Royal Society of London B* **260**: 245–249.

Weiskrantz, L. (1956). Behavioral changes associated with ablation of the amygdaloid complex in monkeys, *Journal of Comparative and Physiological Psychology* **49**: 381–391.

Weiskrantz, L. (1968). Emotion, *in* L. Weiskrantz (ed.), *Analysis of Behavioural Change*, Harper and Row, New York, pp. 50–90.

Weiskrantz, L. (1998). *Blindsight*, 2nd edn, Oxford University Press, Oxford.

Weiskrantz, L. and Saunders, R. C. (1984). Impairments of visual object transforms in monkeys, *Brain* **107**: 1033–1072.

Weiss, F. and Koob, G. F. (2001). Drug addiction: functional neurotoxicity of the brain reward systems, *Neurotoxicity Research* **3**: 145–156.

West, R. A. and Larson, C. R. (1995). Neurons of the anterior mesial cortex related to faciovocal activity in the awake monkey, *Journal of Neurophysiology* **74**: 1856–1869.

Whitelaw, R. B., Markou, A., Robbins, T. W. and Everitt, B. J. (1996). Excitotoxic lesions of the basolateral amygdala impair the acquisition of cocaine-seeking behaviour under a second-order schedule of reinforcement, *Psychopharmacology* **127**: 213–224.

Whiten, A. and Byrne, R. W. (1997). *Machiavellian Intelligence II: Extensions and Evaluations*, Cambridge University Press, Cambridge.

Wickens, J. and Kotter, R. (1995). Cellular models of reinforcement, *in* J. C. Houk, J. L. Davis and D. G. Beiser (eds), *Models of Information Processing in the Basal Ganglia*, MIT Press, Cambridge, MA, chapter 10, pp. 187–214.

Wickens, J. R., Begg, A. J. and Arbuthnott, G. W. (1996). Dopamine reverses the depression of rat corticostriatal synapses which normally follows high-frequency stimulation of cortex in vitro, *Neuroscience* **70**: 1–5.

Williams, G. V., Rolls, E. T., Leonard, C. M. and Stern, C. (1993). Neuronal responses in the ventral striatum of the behaving macaque, *Behavioural Brain Research* **55**: 243–252.

Wilson, C. J. (1995). The contribution of cortical neurons to the firing pattern of striatal spiny neurons, *in* J. C. Houk, J. L. Davis and D. G. Beiser (eds), *Models of Information Processing in the Basal Ganglia*, MIT Press, Cambridge, MA, chapter 3, pp. 29–50.

Wilson, E. O. (1975). *Sociobiology: The New Synthesis*, Harvard University Press, Cambridge, MA.

Wilson, F. A. W. and Rolls, E. T. (1990a). Learning and memory are reflected in the responses of reinforcement-related neurons in the primate basal forebrain, *Journal of Neuroscience* **10**: 1254–1267.

Wilson, F. A. W. and Rolls, E. T. (1990b). Neuronal responses related to reinforcement in the primate basal forebrain, *Brain Research* **509**: 213–231.

Wilson, F. A. W. and Rolls, E. T. (1990c). Neuronal responses related to the novelty and familiarity of visual stimuli in the substantia innominata, diagonal band of broca and periventricular region of the primate, *Experimental Brain Research* **80**: 104–120.

Wilson, F. A. W. and Rolls, E. T. (1993). The effects of stimulus novelty and familiarity on neuronal activity in the amygdala of monkeys performing recognition memory tasks, *Experimental Brain Research* **93**: 367–382.

Wilson, F. A. W. and Rolls, E. T. (2005). The primate amygdala and reinforcement: a dissociation between rule-based and associatively-mediated memory revealed in amygdala neuronal activity, *Neuroscience* **133**: 1061–1072.

Wilson, F. A. W., O'Sclaidhe, S. P. and Goldman-Rakic, P. S. (1993). Dissociation of object and spatial processing domains in primate prefrontal cortex, *Science* **260**: 1955–1958.

Wilson, F. A. W., O'Scalaidhe, S. P. and Goldman-Rakic, P. (1994). Functional synergism between putative gamma-aminobutyrate-containing neurons and pyramidal neurons in prefrontal cortex, *Proceedings of the National Academy of Science* **91**: 4009–4013.

Wilson, H. R. (1999). *Spikes, Decisions and Actions: Dynamical Foundations of Neuroscience*, Oxford University Press, Oxford.

Wilson, R. I. and Nicoll, R. A. (2002). Endocannabinoid signalling in the brain, *Science* **296**: 678–682.

Winkielman, P. and Berridge, K. C. (2003). What is an unconscious emotion?, *Cognition and Emotion* **17**: 181–211.

Winkielman, P. and Berridge, K. C. (2005). Unconscious affective reactions to masked happy versus angry faces influence consumption behavior and judgments of value, *Personality amd Social Psychology Bulletin* **31**: 111–135.

Winn, P., Tarbuck, A. and Dunnett, S. B. (1984). Ibotenic acid lesions of the lateral hypotha-lamus: comparison with electrolytic lesion syndrome, *Neuroscience* **12**: 225–240.

Winn, P., Clark, A., Hastings, M., Clark, J., Latimer, M., Rugg, E. and Brownlee, B. (1990). Excitotoxic lesions of the lateral hypothalamus made by N-methyl-D-aspartate in the rat: behavioural, histological and biochemical analyses, *Experimental Brain Research* **82**: 628–636.

Winslow, J. T. and Insel, T. R. (2004). Neuroendrocrine basis of social recognition, *Current Opinion in Neurobiology* **14**: 248–253.

Wise, R. A. (1989). Opiate reward: sites and substrates, *Neuroscience and Biobehavioral Reviews* **13**: 129–133.

Wood, R. J., Rolls, B. J. and Ramsay, D. J. (1977). Drinking following intracarotid infusions of hypertonic solutions in dogs, *American Journal of Physiology* **232**: R88–R92.

Wood, R. J., Maddison, S., Rolls, E. T., Rolls, B. J. and Gibbs, J. (1980). Drinking in rhesus monkeys: roles of pre-systemic and systemic factors in control of drinking, *Journal of Comparative and Physiological Psychology* **94**: 1135–1148.

Wood, R. J., Rolls, E. T. and Rolls, B. J. (1982). Physiological mechanisms for thirst in the nonhuman primate, *American Journal of Physiology* **242**: R423–R428.

Woods, S. C., Schwartz, M. W., Baskin, D. G. and Seeley, R. C. (2000). Food intake and the regulation of body weight, *Annual Review of Psychology* **51**: 255–277.

Wrangham, R. W. (1993). The evolution of sexuality in chimpanzees and bonobos, *Human Nature* **4**: 47–49.

Wynne-Edwards, K. E. (2001). Hormonal changes in mammalian fathers, *Hormones and Behaviour* **40**: 139–145.

Xiang, Z., Huguenard, J. and Prince, D. (1998). GABA-A receptor mediated currents in interneurons and pyramidal cells of rat visual cortex, *Journal of Physiology* **506**: 715–730.

Yamaguchi, S. (1967). The synergistic taste effect of monosodium glutamate and disodium 5′-inosinate, *Journal of Food Science* **32**: 473–478.

Yamaguchi, S. and Kimizuka, A. (1979). Psychometric studies on the taste of monosodium glutamate, *in* L. J. Filer, S. Garattini, M. R. Kare, A. R. Reynolds and R. J. Wurtman (eds), *Glutamic Acid: Advances in Biochemistry and Physiology*, Raven Press, New York, pp. 35–54.

Yan, J. and Scott, T. R. (1996). The effect of satiety on responses of gustatory neurons in the amygdala of alert cynomolgus macaques, *Brain Research* **740**: 193–200.

Yaxley, S., Rolls, E. T., Sienkiewicz, Z. J. and Scott, T. R. (1985). Satiety does not affect gustatory activity in the nucleus of the solitary tract of the alert monkey, *Brain Research* **347**: 85–93.

Yaxley, S., Rolls, E. T. and Sienkiewicz, Z. J. (1988). The responsiveness of neurones in the insular gustatory cortex of the macaque monkey is independent of hunger, *Physiology and Behavior* **42**: 223–229.

Yaxley, S., Rolls, E. T. and Sienkiewicz, Z. J. (1990). Gustatory responses of single neurons in the insula of the macaque monkey, *Journal of Neurophysiology* **63**: 689–700.

Yeomans, J. S. (1990). *Principles of Brain Stimulation*, Oxford University Press, New York.

Yokel, R. A. and Wise, R. A. (1975). Increased lever pressing for amphetamine after pimozide in rats: implications for a dopamine theory of reinforcement, *Science* **187**: 547–549.

Young, A. W., Aggleton, J. P., Hellawell, D. J., Johnson, M., Broks, P. and Hanley, J. R.

(1995). Face processing impairments after amygdalotomy, *Brain* **118**: 15–24.

Young, A. W., Hellawell, D. J., Van de Wal, C. and Johnson, M. (1996). Facial expression processing after amygdalotomy, *Neuropsychologia* **34**: 31–39.

Young, L. J. and Wang, Z. (2004). The neurobiology of pairbonding, *Nature Neuroscience* **7**: 1048–1054.

Zahavi, A. (1975). Mate selection: a selection for a handicap, *Journal of Theoretical Biology* **53**: 205–214.

Zahavi, A. and Zahavi, A. (1997). *The Handicap Principle: A Missing Piece of Darwin's Puzzle*, Oxford University Press, Oxford.

Zald, D. H. and Rauch, S. L. (eds) (2006). *The Orbitofrontal Cortex*, Oxford University Press, Oxford.

Zatorre, R. J. and Jones-Gotman, M. (1991). Human olfactory discrimination after unilateral frontal or temporal lobectomy, *Brain* **114**: 71–84.

Zatorre, R. J., Jones-Gotman, M., Evans, A. C. and Meyer, E. (1992). Functional localization of human olfactory cortex, *Nature* **360**: 339–340.

Zatorre, R. J., Jones-Gotman, M. and Rouby, C. (2000). Neural mechanisms involved in odor pleasantness and intensity judgments, *NeuroReport* **11**: 2711–2716.

Zeller, A. C. (1987). Communication by sight and smell, *in* B. S. Smuts, D. L. Cheney, R. M. Seyfarth, R. W. Wrangham and T. T. Stuhsaker (eds), *Primate Societies*, University of Chicago Press, London, pp. 433–439.

Zhang, M., Gosnell, B. A. and Kelley, A. E. (1998). Intake of high-fat food is selectively enhanced by mu opioid receptor stimulation within the nucleus accumbens, *Journal of Pharmacology and Experimental Therapeutics* **285**: 908–914.

Zhang, X. and Firestein, S. (2002). The olfactory receptor gene superfamily of the mouse, *Nature Neuroscience* **5**: 124–133.

Zhao, G. Q., Zhang, Y., Hoon, M. A., Chandrashekar, J., Erlenbach, I., Ryba, N. J. and Zucker, C. S. (2003). The receptors for mammalian sweet and umami taste, *Cell* **115**: 255–266.

Zink, C. F., Pagnoni, G., Martin, M. E., Dhamala, M. and Berns, G. S. (2003). Human striatal responses to salient nonrewarding stimuli, *Journal of Neuroscience* **23**: 8092–8097.

Zink, C. F., Pagnoni, G., Martin-Skurski, M. E., Chappelow, J. C. and Berns, G. S. (2004). Human striatal responses to monetary reward depend on saliency, *Neuron* **42**: 509–517.

Zou, Z., Horowitz, L. F., Montmayeur, J. P., Snapper, S. and Buck, L. (2001). Genetic tracing reveals a stereotyped map in the olfactory cortex, *Nature* **414**: 173–179.

Zuckerman, M. (1994). *Psychobiology of Personality*, Cambridge University Press, New York.

Zuckerman, M. and Kuhlman, D. M. (2000). Personality and risk-taking: common biosocial factors, *Journal of Personality* **68**: 999–1029.

Index